# PROCEDURES *for* NURSE PRACTITIONERS

# PROCEDURES
## *for* NURSE
## PRACTITIONERS

**SPRINGHOUSE CORPORATION** *Springhouse, Pennsylvania*

## STAFF

**Publisher**
Judith A. Schilling McCann, RN, MSN

**Design Director**
John Hubbard

**Editorial Director**
David Moreau

**Clinical Manager**
Joan M. Robinson, RN, MSN, CCRN

**Clinical Editors**
Gwynn Sinkinson, RN,C, MSN, CRNP (project manager); Norma Mann, RN, MSN, NPC; Monica Walter, MSN, NPC; Valerie Winn, RN, NP

**Editors**
Rachel Alexander, Cynthia C. Breuninger, Margaret Eckman, Julie Munden, Laura Poole

**Copy Editors**
Jaime Stockslager (supervisor), Priscilla Dewitt, Amy Furman, Kimberly A.J. Johnson, Judith Orioli, Pamela Wingrod

**Designers**
Arlene Putterman (associate design director), Susan Hopkins Rodzewich (project manager), Joseph John Clark, Donna S. Morris

**Projects Coordinator**
Liz Schaeffer

**Electronic Production Services**
Diane Paluba (manager), Joyce Rossi Biletz

**Manufacturing**
Deborah Meiris (director), Patricia K. Dorshaw (manager), Otto Mezei (book production manager)

**Editorial and Design Assistants**
Tom Hasenmayer, Beverly Lane, Beth Janae Orr, Elfriede Young

**Indexer**
Manjit Sahai

PRONP - D  N

03 02 01 00        10 9 8 7 6 5 4 3 2 1

**Library of Congress Cataloging-in-Publication Data**

Procedures for nurse practitioners.
    p. ; cm.
    Includes index.
    1. Nurse practitioners — Handbooks, manuals, etc. 2. Nursing — Handbooks, manuals, etc.
    [DNLM: 1. Nursing Care—methods — Handbooks. WY 49 P963 2000]
RT82.8 .P755 2000
610.73 — dc21             00-056284
ISBN 1-58255-068-9 (alk. paper)

# CONTENTS

# CONTRIBUTORS AND CONSULTANTS

**Deborah Becker, MSN, CRNP, CS, CCRN**
Lecturer
School of Nursing
University of Pennsylvania
Philadelphia

**Elizabeth Blunt, MSN, CEN, ANP-C**
Assistant Professor
MCP Hahnemann University
Philadelphia

**Alexandria N. Brown, RN, MSN, CRNP**
Nurse Practitioner
Crozer-Chester Medical Center
Upland, Pa.
Temple University Hospital
Philadelphia

**Leanne C. Busby, RN,C, DSN**
Director of Education
Nashville Memorial Hospital
Madison, Tenn.

**Michael A. Carter, RN, DNSc, FAAN, FNP**
Dean and Professor
College of Nursing
University of Tennessee
Memphis

**Maryanne Crowther, RN, MSN, CCRN, CNS, C, NP**
CHF Coordinator
Jersey Shore Medical Center
Neptune, N.J.

**Joseph L. DuFour, RN, MS, CS, FNP**
Lecturer
State University of New York at New Paltz (N.Y.)
Family Nurse Practitioner
Private Practice
Glen Falls, N.Y.

**Leslie Fehan, MS, CNM, WHNP**
Certified Nurse Midwife
Medical College of Virginia
Women's Health at Stony Point
Richmond, Va.

**Anna Fox, MSN, CNP**
Nurse Practitioner
Cardiology Center of Cincinnati

**Susan F. Galiczynski, RN, MSN, ANP, CRNP**
Nurse Practitioner
Temple University Hospital
Philadelphia

**Shelton M. Hisley, RN,C, PhD, ACCE, WHNP**
Assistant Professor
School of Nursing
University of North Carolina at Wilmington

**Michelle Robinson-Jackson, RN, MSN, CRNP, CS**
Independent Consultant
Ambler, Pa.

**Julia Lange Kessler, MS, CM**
Certified Midwife
Private Practice
New Hampton, N.Y.

**Susan J. Kimble, RN, MSN, CS, APN**
Nurse Practitioner
Clinical Instructor
School of Nursing
University of Missouri at Kansas City
Liberty, Mo.

**Norma Mann, RN, NP,C**
Nurse Practitioner
Office of Dr. Neil Levin
Sewell, N.J.

**Kathleen A. Martin, MSN, CRNP**
Nurse Practitioner
Micron Employee Health Clinic —
    Personal Medical
Boise, Idaho

**Patricia McGrath, MSN, CRNP, CCRN, FNP**
Family Nurse Practitioner
Dr. Harman and Associates
Philadelphia

**Geraldine M. Pfeiffer, MSN, CRNP**
Co-Adjutant Faculty Member in Nursing
Delaware County Community College
Media, Pa.

**Jacquelyn Reid, RN, EdD, WHNP,**
Assistant Professor of Nursing
Indiana University Southeast
New Albany, Ind.

**Virginia Richardson, RN, DNS, CPNP**
Assistant Dean for Student Affairs
Indiana University
Indianapolis

**Kristine Bludau Scordo, RN,C, PhD, ACNP**
Assistant Professor
Wright State University
College of Nursing and Health
Dayton, Ohio

**Claire A. Taylor, RN, MSN, NP**
Trauma Nurse Practitioner
Jersey Shore Medical Center
Neptune, N.J.

**Leonora P. Thomas, RN, MS, CS, CCRN**
Acute Care Nurse Practitioner
Department of Cardiology
Hartford (Conn.) Hospital

**Eileen M. Villano, RN, MSN**
Public Health Nurse
La Salle Neighborhood Nursing Center
Philadelphia

**Benita J. Walton-Moss, RN,CS, DNS, FNP**
Assistant Professor
School of Nursing
Johns Hopkins University
Baltimore

**Kathleen M. Woodruff, MS, CRNP**
Instructor
School of Nursing
Johns Hopkins University
Baltimore

**Candace F. Zickler, RN, MSN, CPNP**
Adjunct Faculty
Family Nurse Practitioner Program
College of Nursing and Health
Wright State University
Dayton, Ohio

# FOREWORD

As dramatic changes continue to unfold in our health care system and as the role of the nurse practitioner (NP) continues to evolve, the NP must be well prepared to perform a wider range of procedures, not only in primary care but also in specialty and acute care settings. To meet the myriad of challenges inherent in an ever-changing health care system, the NP must develop the skills and competency to provide more than just health care service to the individual, family, or community; she must also target disease prevention and focus on patient education — a key to promoting health throughout the patient's life.

*Procedures for Nurse Practitioners* delivers what you'll need to gain that edge in your daily practice. Until now, no book has provided NPs with a definitive reference on procedures performed in the major practice areas (adult care and family care) as well as specialty areas (acute care and pediatric, gerontologic, neonatal, and women's health). Now, this comprehensive resource that is brimming with essential facts and guidelines will help you provide safe, competent, cost-effective care. Written by a team of NPs that share their expertise across diverse fields — from trauma NPs to midwives to dermatology specialists, from those who have primary practices in major cities to those who specialize in family practice in rural areas — this book contains a wealth of information that will help you perform procedures more skillfully and allow you to meet patient needs with confidence while enhancing patient comfort. The experienced NP will find it useful in expanding her practice and attaining a broader skill level. The student NP and new NP will also find this an indispensable partner in her evolving profession.

*Procedures for Nurse Practitioners* provides start-to-finish instructions for procedures that NPs perform in various settings. It includes such topics as diagnostic tests and skin care as well as ear, nose, and throat; cardiovascular; GI; and urologic care. In addition to covering adult patients, the book also includes chapters on pediatrics and women's health.

Concise, practical coverage throughout the book's nine chapters includes a full range of procedures that focus on the management of trauma and emergencies as well as special needs and procedural variations for pediatric, maternal-neonatal, and geriatric populations. Procedures such as Doppler evaluation, lumbar puncture, and eyelid eversion as well as DeLee suctioning of the neonate and colposcopy are highlighted in this comprehensive resource.

For your convenience, a consistent format for each procedure presents billing codes, description and purpose, indications, contraindications, equipment, preparation, essential steps, patient teaching, complications, and special considerations. Numerous illustrations and photos provide step-by-step visualization of the procedure and equipment that enhance the text — a valuable adjunct for the new practitioner.

Furthermore, important icons are located throughout the book to highlight cultural tips and alerts for the NP. Cultural differences among patient populations can be managed with the compassion and problem-solving skills that come with comprehension. This information is emphasized at the beginning of specific procedures where it's most useful and offers advice on differences that may affect patient care. Another icon offers advice for the patient.

With the skills and knowledge you gain from *Procedures for Nurse Practitioners*, you can increase community wellness — one patient at a time.

**Michael A. Carter,** RN, DNSc, FAAN, FNP

Dean and Professor
College of Nursing
University of Tennessee
Memphis

# PROCEDURES *for* NURSE PRACTITIONERS

# CARDIOVASCULAR PROCEDURES

Cardiovascular disorders, which affect millions of Americans each year, are the leading cause of death in the United States. Many patients with cardiovascular disorders also have related conditions, such as renal or respiratory disease. This means that you'll find yourself caring for patients with cardiovascular disease in just about every setting. And, with the field of cardiovascular treatment changing rapidly—new diagnostic tests, drugs, and treatments and more sophisticated monitoring equipment—you also face the challenge of keeping up with the latest developments.

As a nurse practitioner, you may perform many cardiac and hemodynamic monitoring procedures that provide critical information about the patient's physical state. Cardiac monitoring allows you to assess cardiac rhythm, gauge a patient's response to drug therapy, and detect and help prevent complications associated with diagnostic and therapeutic procedures. Hemodynamic monitoring allows you to measure pressure, flow, and resistance within the cardiovascular and pulmonary systems to help with diagnosis and guide therapy. Once used only in critical care settings, cardiac monitoring now takes place in high-risk obstetric, urgent care, primary care, and pediatric settings.

You also may perform or assist with cardiopulmonary resuscitation and defibrillation in cardiovascular emergencies. Carrying out these life-saving procedures calls for in-depth knowledge of cardiovascular

anatomy, physiology, and equipment as well as sound assessment and intervention techniques. To perform such procedures safely and effectively, you need to keep up-to-date with information and keep your skills sharp.

Finally, you assume much of the responsibility for preparing patients physically and psychologically for their hospitalization and ongoing care. You play a pivotal role in teaching patients about the disease process and how it affects their bodies, drug therapies and other treatments, test and procedure preparation and follow-up care, disease prevention, and lifestyle modification. By giving a patient the information he needs, you can help him reduce stress, comply with his prescribed therapy, and incorporate disease-preventive measures into his daily life.

 **CULTURAL TIP** Some cultures, such as Native American, view invasive procedures as a last resort and may require additional information and time before consenting. In addition, some cultures, including Native American, Korean, and Russian, frequently prefer to discuss even simple procedures with family members before consenting. You should be aware of this and allow time for this discussion.

People from the Hmong culture generally reject having blood drawn when they feel sick; they believe it will make them weaker because they believe blood is not regenerated. However, others will request blood tests with the belief that they will feel better afterward.

Other cultures, like the Arab American culture, tend to have little tolerance for complications and tend to believe that complications are due to technical error. Thus, it is important to state clearly the potential risks involved in a procedure.

# Diagnostic Testing

## Ambulatory blood pressure and Holter monitoring

CPT CODES
*93784 Ambulatory blood pressure monitoring for 24 hours or longer, including analysis, interpretation, and report*
*93786 Ambulatory blood pressure monitoring for 24 hours or longer, recording only*
*93230 Electrocardiograph (ECG) monitoring for 24 hours by continuous original ECG waveform recording with device producing a full miniaturized printout; includes recording, microprocessor-based analysis with report and physician review and interpretation*
*93231 ECG monitoring for 24 hours by continuous original ECG waveform recording, includes hook-up, recording, and disconnection*
*93232 ECG monitoring for 24 hours by continuous original ECG waveform recording, includes microprocessor-based analysis with report*
*93236 ECG monitoring for 24 hours by continuous computerized monitoring and noncontinuous recording, monitoring, and real-time data analysis with report*

## DESCRIPTION

Ambulatory blood pressure monitoring (ABPM) and Holter monitoring (also called continuous electrocardiograph monitoring) allow measurement of blood pressure and cardiac activity over a period of time without confining a patient to a facility. ABPM records the variations that occur in a patient's blood pressure as well as his average blood pressure during normal activity. Such monitoring more readily allows diagnosis of sustained hypertension and response to treatment than isolated blood pressure measurements taken in your office. Holter monitoring records variations in ECG waveforms during normal activity. A patient can undergo either ABPM or Holter monitoring or both types of monitoring together (as is becoming more common). During monitoring, the patient needs to maintain a log of activities and associated symptoms he may experience.

## INDICATIONS

### ABPM
➤ To identify those who don't require pharmacotherapy
➤ To rule out a diagnosis of sustained hypertension
➤ To determine the range of variability in labile hypertension
➤ To monitor the effectiveness of therapy and evaluate drug-resistant hypertension
➤ To determine diurnal blood pressure variations in patients with diabetes or autonomic insufficiency
➤ To evaluate discrepancies between blood pressure measurements in and out of your office

### Holter monitoring
➤ To determine the status of a patient recuperating from an acute myocardial infarction

➤ To assess pacemaker functioning after implantation

➤ To evaluate cardiac signs and symptoms, such as angina or unexplained fainting

➤ To evaluate the frequency and type of cardiac arrhythmias

➤ To assess the effectiveness of antiarrhythmic drug therapy

➤ To determine the relationship between cardiac events, the patient's activities, and associated symptoms (such as chest pain, light-headedness, syncope or presyncope, and palpitations)

## CONTRAINDICATIONS

### Absolute

➤ Hypertensive crisis that requires immediate intervention

## EQUIPMENT

### ABPM monitoring

Monitor with new battery that contains a cuff, microphone, and microprocessor that pumps the cuff and records measurements ◆ carrying case with strap ◆ 1″ adhesive tape ◆ logbook or diary

### Holter monitoring

Holter unit with new battery ◆ cable wires ◆ disposable pregelled electrodes ◆ carrying case with strap ◆ 4″ × 4″ gauze pad or alcohol wipe ◆ cassette tape ◆ logbook or diary ◆ clippers (optional)

## ESSENTIAL STEPS

➤ Explain the procedure to the patient.

➤ As applicable, ask the patient if he has any allergies to adhesive tape, electrode gel, or alcohol.

➤ Place the equipment into the carrying case, and connect the neck strap.

### PLACING ELECTRODES FOR HOLTER MONITORING

This illustration shows you one method that is used to place electrodes with a 5-leadwire system. Make sure you place the electrodes over bone, not intercostal spaces. The two negative electrodes are placed on the manubrium. Positive electrodes are placed in the $V_1$ and $V_5$ positions. A ground electrode is placed at the lower right rib margin. Refer to your facility's policy or manufacturer instructions for preferred electrode placement.

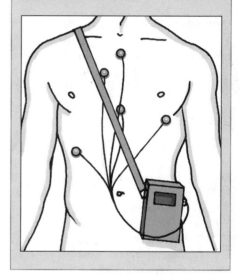

## ABPM

➤ Position the microphone over the brachial artery on the inner aspect of the nondominant arm, just above the elbow. Secure the microphone with tape. Then choose an appropriately sized blood pressure cuff. Manufacturers supply regular adult, obese adult, and pediatric sizes.

➤ Calibrate the monitor while the patient both sits and stands by measuring simultaneous blood pressure readings, using the ABPM unit and a mercury sphygmomanometer attached to the monitor with a T-tube device.

## Holter monitoring

➤ As appropriate, tell the patient that you need to clip the hairs on his chest so that you can place the electrodes properly. After clipping, wash the areas with soap and water to remove body oils.

➤ Connect the wires to the electrodes and to the monitor.

➤ Apply each electrode to the patient's chest by removing the paper backing, securing the edges of the electrode, and then pressing the center to ensure proper contact. (See *Placing electrodes for Holter monitoring,* page 3.)

## Both types of monitoring

➤ Place the strap over the patient's neck and position the unit comfortably. Make sure there isn't too much slack or pull on the cables because artifact may occur.

## PATIENT TEACHING

➤ Explain that the patient will have 24 hours of cardiac activity monitored before the monitor is removed. Tell him that he'll feel no pain from the procedure but that the tape and monitor may cause mild discomfort.

➤ Tell the patient he'll need a follow-up appointment to review results 48 to 72 hours after removal of the monitor.

➤ As appropriate, tell the patient that he'll need to wear a small microprocessor and blood pressure cuff for 24 hours after activation of the monitor. Tell him not to remove the blood pressure cuff, microprocessor, or electrodes unless told to do so. Explain that he'll have a carrying case with strap to carry the 2-lb monitor.

➤ Tell the patient he'll need to maintain an activity log during the 24-hour monitoring period. He should record the time, activities he performs, and any symptoms (such as headache, dizziness, light-headedness, palpitations, or chest pain) that may occur. Explain the importance of maintaining his usual routine, including working, eating, sleeping, using the bathroom, driving, and taking his medication. (See *Using your Holter monitor.*)

➤ Suggest wearing a watch to make it easier to keep an accurate log.

➤ Encourage the patient to wear loose-fitting clothes with tops that open in the front.

➤ Tell the patient that he can sponge bathe but he shouldn't get the equipment wet.

➤ Tell the patient to take the usual steps for medical emergencies (such as taking nitroglycerin and going to the emergency department for chest pain).

## ABPM

➤ Show the patient how to use tape to secure the microphone on the brachial area of his arm in case the microphone becomes loose.

➤ Tell the patient to keep the cuff arm still and free from extraneous noise when he feels the cuff inflating and deflating to ensure that measurements are accurate.

➤ Tell the patient to avoid activities — such as mowing the lawn, golfing, running, and tennis — that call for isometric use of the upper extremities to help avoid erroneous blood pressure measurements during such activities.

## Holter monitoring

➤ Show the patient how to reattach loosened electrodes by depressing the center and tell him to return to the office if an electrode becomes fully dislodged.

➤ Tell the patient to avoid magnets, metal detectors, high-voltage areas, and electric blankets, which may cause artifact or interfere with monitoring.

## COMPLICATIONS

None known

PATIENT-TEACHING AID

## USING YOUR HOLTER MONITOR

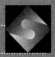

DEAR PATIENT:

Your practitioner has ordered a Holter monitor for you to wear for 24 hours. It works as a continuous electrocardiogram (ECG) by recording any irregular heartbeats you may have. The information from this recording will help your practitioner determine if these abnormal heartbeats are causing your symptoms, such as chest pain or discomfort, dizziness, or weakness. If you are taking heart medication, the Holter monitor can also help your practitioner evaluate how well the medication is working.

The monitor has adhesive patches — called *leads* — that the assistant will attach to your skin. She'll also show you how to wear the monitor on a belt or over your shoulder. If one of the leads becomes loose, secure it with a piece of tape.

While wearing the monitor, you can perform most of your usual activities. You'll even wear it to bed.

Practice these safety measures while you're wearing the Holter monitor.
➤ Don't get the monitor wet — don't shower, bathe, or swim with it.
➤ Avoid high-voltage areas and strong magnetic fields.

While you're wearing the monitor, you'll write down your activities and feelings. You can use the diary below as an example. Your diary will help your practitioner establish a connection between your monitor tracing and your activities and feelings. Jot down the time of day you perform activity, such as taking medication, eating, drinking, having a bowel movement, urinating, engaging in sexual activity, experiencing strong emotions, exercising, and sleeping.

If your monitor has an event button, the assistant will show you how to press it in case you experience anything unusual, such as a sudden, rapid heartbeat.

| DAY | TIME | ACTIVITY | FEELINGS |
|---|---|---|---|
| Tuesday | 10:30 am | Rode from hospital in car | Legs tired, some shortness of breath |
| | 11:30 am | Watched TV in living room | Comfortable |
| | 12:15 pm | Ate lunch, took Inderal | Indigestion |
| | 1:30 pm | Walked next door to see neighbor | Shortness of breath |
| | 2:45 pm | Walked home | Very tired, legs hurt |
| | 3-4:00 pm | urinated, took nap | Comfortable |
| | 5:30 pm | Ate dinner, slowly | Comfortable |
| | 7:20 pm | Had bowel movement | Shortness of breath |
| | 9:00 pm | Watched TV, drank 1 beer | Heart beating fast for about 1 min, no pain |
| | 11:00 pm | Took Inderal, urinated, went to bed | Tired |
| Wednesday | 8:15 am | Awake, urinated, washed face and arms | Very tired, rapid heartbeat for 30 seconds |
| | 10:30 am | Returned to hospital | Felt better |

## SPECIAL CONSIDERATIONS

➤ If the patient's skin is extremely oily, scaly, or diaphoretic, rub the electrode site with a dry 4″ × 4″ gauze pad or alcohol wipe before applying the electrode.

➤ If the patient can't return to the office immediately after the monitoring period, show him how to remove the equipment and store the monitor, blood pressure cuff, and log.

➤ If the patient is wearing a patient-activated Holter monitor, tell him that he can wear the monitor for up to 7 days. Tell him how to initiate the recording manually when symptoms occur.

## DOCUMENTATION

➤ Document the indications for monitoring.

➤ Note the date and time the monitor was applied.

➤ Record the patient's medication regimen and blood pressure before monitoring.

➤ Include the patient's event log in documentation.

➤ Document postprocedure results and actions taken.

## Arterial puncture

CPT CODE
36600   *Arterial puncture and withdrawal of blood for diagnosis*

## DESCRIPTION

Obtaining an arterial blood sample requires percutaneous puncture of the radial, femoral, or brachial artery or withdrawal of a sample from an arterial line. The radial artery is the most commonly used site because it is superficial and generally easily palpated. However, before attempting a radial puncture, Allen's test should be performed (see *Performing Allen's test*).

The femoral artery is the most easily accessible artery during cardiopulmonary resuscitation and in emergencies and may be preferable to radial artery cannulation in a paralyzed or immobile patient. However, it carries a greater risk for such complications as infection. The most difficult to access, the brachial site limits the patient's arm mobility and is generally used only as a last resort.

The arterial blood sample obtained is then sent for arterial blood gas (ABG) analysis, which helps assess alveolar ventilation, oxygenation, and acid-base balance. ABG analysis measures partial pressures of arterial oxygen and carbon dioxide. The blood pH is an indicator of the blood's acid-base balance. ABG samples can also be analyzed for oxygen saturation and bicarbonate levels.

## INDICATIONS

➤ To confirm or diagnose problems with gas exchange or acid-base balance

➤ To monitor physiologic response to treatments or changes in therapy

➤ To provide arterial blood for other laboratory tests, such as ammonia, carbon monoxide, or lactate levels

➤ To provide blood specimens in an emergency situation

## CONTRAINDICATIONS

### Relative

➤ Unpalpable artery

➤ Known or suspected arterial disease at the site, such as aneurysm, atherosclerosis, inflammation, infection, or hematoma

➤ Coagulopathy, anticoagulation therapy, or anticipated thrombolytic therapy

➤ Raynaud's disease

➤ Previous vascular surgery involving the artery

## EQUIPMENT

10-ml glass syringe or plastic luer-lock syringe specifically made for collecting samples for ABG analysis ◆ 1-ml ampule of aqueous heparin (1:1,000) ◆ 20G 1¼″ needle ◆ 25G ⅝″ needle ◆ 22G 1″ needle (for an obese patient or the femoral site) ◆ alcohol pads ◆ povidone-iodine pads ◆ two 2″ × 2″ gauze pads ◆ gloves ◆ rubber cap for syringe hub or rubber stopper for needle ◆ ice-filled plastic bag or cup for sample transport ◆ label ◆ laboratory request form ◆ adhesive bandage ◆ 1% lidocaine solution in 3-ml syringe with 25G ⅝″ needle (optional) ◆ protective eyewear (optional)

*Many facilities use a commercial ABG kit that contains all of the equipment listed (except the adhesive bandage, ice, and lidocaine).*

## PREPARATION OF EQUIPMENT

➤ Prepare the collection equipment before entering the room.
➤ Thoroughly wash your hands.
➤ Open the ABG kit and remove the sample label and plastic bag. On the label, record the patient's name and room number, the date, the collection time, and your name.
➤ Fill the plastic bag with ice and set it aside.
➤ To heparinize the syringe, attach the 20G needle to the syringe and then open the ampule of heparin. Draw all the heparin into the syringe to prevent the sample from clotting. Hold the syringe upright and slowly pull the plunger back to about the 7-ml mark. Rotate the barrel while pulling the plunger back to allow the heparin to coat the inside surface of the syringe. Then slowly force the heparin toward the hub of the syringe and expel all but about 0.1 ml of heparin.

## PERFORMING ALLEN'S TEST

To perform Allen's test, rest the patient's arm on a flat surface and support his wrist with a rolled towel. Have him clench his fist. Then, using your index and middle fingers, press on the radial and ulnar arteries. Hold this position for a few seconds.

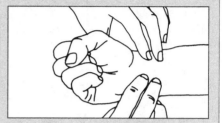

Without removing your fingers from the patient's arteries, ask him to unclench his fist and hold his hand in a relaxed position. The palm will be blanched because pressure from your fingers has impaired the normal blood flow.

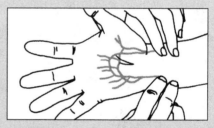

Release pressure on the patient's ulnar artery. If the hand becomes flushed within 15 seconds (an indication that blood is filling the vessels), you can safely proceed with the radial artery puncture. If the hand doesn't flush, this is an abnormal Allen's test and ulnar circulation is impaired. Perform the test on the other arm or choose an alternate site.

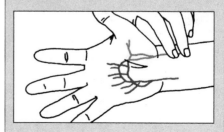

## ARTERIAL PUNCTURE TECHNIQUE

To decrease the patient's discomfort and the number of needlesticks needed to obtain an arterial blood sample, identify the site carefully first. Use both anatomic landmarks and palpation to find a strong pulse, and direct the needle toward the arterial pulsation.

The angle of needle penetration depends on the artery involved. For the radial artery, insert the needle bevel up at a 30- to 45-degree angle, about ½" (1.3 cm) proximal to the wrist crease.

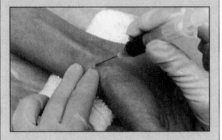

For the right brachial artery, insert the needle bevel up at a 60-degree angle slightly proximal to the elbow crease.

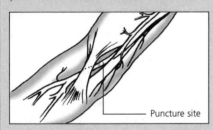

Puncture site

For the femoral artery, insert the needle at a 60- to 90-degree angle, about 1" (2.5 cm) distal to the inguinal ligament, which is marked by the inguinal crease.

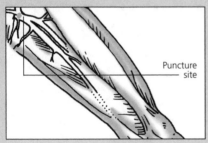

Puncture site

> To heparinize the needle, replace the 20G needle with a 25G or 22G needle and then, holding the syringe upright, tilt it slightly and eject the remaining heparin.

## ESSENTIAL STEPS

> Tell the patient that you need to collect an arterial blood sample, and explain the procedure. Tell him that the needle stick will cause some discomfort but that he must remain still.

> Wash your hands and put on gloves.

> If the patient seems particularly anxious, anesthetize the area with lidocaine before inserting the needle to numb the site.

> If you're using the radial site, place a rolled towel under the patient's wrist for support. Locate the artery and palpate for a strong pulse.

> Using a circular motion, clean the puncture site with an alcohol or povidone-iodine pad. If you're using alcohol, apply it with friction for 30 seconds or until the final pad comes away clean. Allow the skin to dry.

> After cleaning the site with alcohol, you can also apply povidone-iodine to clean the area. Use a circular motion, starting at the center of the site and spiraling outward.

 **ALERT** If you're using povidone-iodine as well as alcohol, use the alcohol first. Using alcohol after povidone-iodine cancels the effect of the povidone-iodine.

> Palpate and immobilize the artery with two or three fingers of one hand while holding the syringe over the puncture site with the other hand.

> Hold the needle bevel up at a 30- to 45-degree angle when puncturing the radial artery. When puncturing the brachial artery, hold the needle at a 60-degree angle. Maintain a 60- to 90-degree angle for the femoral site. (See *Arterial puncture technique*.)

> Puncture the skin and arterial wall in one motion, following the path of the artery.

➤ Watch for blood backflow in the syringe. If possible, don't aspirate blood (although you may have to if the patient is hypotensive) because that increases the chances of obtaining venous blood. Collect a 3- to 5-ml specimen.

➤ If your first attempt isn't successful, withdraw the needle to just below the surface of the skin; then advance it at the same angle but at 1 mm to either side of your previous attempt.

➤ After collecting the sample, press a gauze pad firmly over the puncture site until the bleeding stops (at least 5 minutes). If the patient is receiving anticoagulant therapy or has a blood dyscrasia, apply pressure for 10 to 15 minutes. If necessary, ask a coworker to hold the gauze pad in place while you prepare the sample for transport to the laboratory. Don't ask the patient to hold the pad: If he doesn't apply enough pressure, a large, painful hematoma may form, hindering future arterial punctures at that site.

➤ Check the syringe for air bubbles. If any appear, remove them by holding the syringe upright and slowly ejecting some of the blood onto a 2″ × 2″ gauze pad.

➤ Insert the needle into a rubber stopper or remove the needle and place a rubber cap directly on the needle hub.

➤ Gently rotate the specimen syringe and then put the labeled sample in the ice-filled plastic bag or cup. Attach a properly completed laboratory request form and send the sample to the laboratory immediately.

➤ When the bleeding stops, apply a small adhesive bandage to the site.

➤ Monitor the patient's vital signs, and observe for signs of circulatory impairment, such as swelling, discoloration, pain, numbness, or tingling in the bandaged arm or leg.

➤ Watch for bleeding at the puncture site. Recheck the puncture site in 15 minutes.

## PATIENT TEACHING

➤ Explain the need for and what to expect during the procedure.

➤ Explain the importance of keeping the limb still and the need to apply pressure to the site after the procedure.

➤ Warn the patient that the procedure is painful, but reassure him that the pain should resolve within a few minutes.

## COMPLICATIONS

➤ Using a small-gauge needle and applying prompt, continuous pressure after the procedure can help prevent *hematoma formation and hemorrhage*.

➤ *Thrombosis* occurs more commonly with radial puncture than with femoral or brachial puncture. The patient may need surgical intervention to alleviate ischemia and prevent gangrene.

➤ *Nerve damage from needle trauma or resultant hematoma* may be prevented by immediately responding when the patient complains of considerable pain. Slowly pull back the needle and check for blood return. If there is no return, remove the needle and reattempt insertion at the same site; however, never make more than two attempts at the same site.

➤ Maintaining aseptic technique prevents *infection*.

## SPECIAL CONSIDERATIONS

➤ If arterial spasm occurs, blood won't flow into the syringe and you won't be able to collect the sample. If this happens, replace the needle with a smaller one and attempt to perform arterial puncture again.

➤ Carefully consider the use of lidocaine to anesthetize the site: It delays the procedure, the patient may be allergic to the medication, or the resulting vasoconstriction may prevent successful puncture.

➤ If the patient is receiving oxygen, make sure that he has been receiving oxygen at the same setting for at least 15 minutes before collecting arterial blood.

➤ Unless necessary, don't stop existing oxygen therapy before collecting arterial blood samples. Be sure to indicate on the laboratory request slip the amount and type of oxygen therapy the patient is receiving.

➤ If the patient isn't receiving oxygen, indicate that he's breathing room air.

➤ If the patient has just received a respiratory treatment, performed coughing and deep-breathing exercises, or undergone suctioning, wait 20 minutes before collecting the sample.

➤ When filling out a laboratory request form for ABG analysis, include the patient's temperature, most recent hemoglobin level, respiratory rate and, if the patient is on a ventilator, fraction of inspired oxygen and tidal volume.

➤ To avoid inaccurate results, don't mix venous blood with arterial blood, don't use too much heparin, promptly send the properly chilled sample to the laboratory (delays and improper chilling can allow the blood to metabolize oxygen or allow oxygen to be dissociated from hemoglobin), and make sure the syringe has no air in it. Also, don't use a Vacutainer because it contains a measurable amount of oxygen.

## DOCUMENTATION

➤ Record the results of Allen's test, the time you collected the sample, the patient's temperature, the arterial puncture site, how long you applied pressure to the site to control bleeding, and the type and amount of oxygen therapy in use.

➤ Document the indications for the procedure, the patient's reaction, any medications ordered, the time frame for follow-up evaluation, and patient teaching provided.

## Blood culture

CPT CODES
*87040    Blood culture, bacterial (includes anaerobic screen)*
*87103    Blood culture, fungi, isolation*

## DESCRIPTION

Normally bacteria-free, blood is susceptible to infection from many sources, including contaminated infusion lines, infected shunts, thrombophlebitis, bacterial endocarditis, and local tissue infections. Bacteria can also invade through the lymphatic system and thoracic duct. Blood cultures allow the detection of such bacterial invasion (bacteremia) and the systemic spread of such infection (septicemia) through the bloodstream. Patients at greater risk — including febrile patients with rigors, other seriously ill patients, immunosuppressed patients, and patients suspected of having endocarditis — should have blood samples collected for culturing.

After collection, blood samples are placed in two blood culture bottles. One contains an anaerobic medium and the other, an aerobic medium. An alternative single-tube system, the Isolator system, is also available. (See *Isolator blood-culturing system.*)

The bottles are then incubated, encouraging any organisms in the sample to grow in the medium. These cultures allow identification of about 67% of pathogens within 24 hours and up to 90% within 72 hours. For the most accurate results, some authorities recommend drawing three samples at least 1 hour apart, with the first drawn at the first signs of bacteremia or septicemia (other authorities consider the timing of culture specimens debatable). In cases of suspected bacterial endocarditis, three or four blood samples taken from different sites at 5- to 30-minute intervals before starting antibiotic therapy may produce more positive test results.

## INDICATIONS

➤ To diagnose bacterial invasion
➤ To rule out systemic spread of infection
➤ To detect infection in febrile patients with rigors, seriously ill patients, or immunosuppressed patients
➤ To assess effectiveness of current or recent antibiotic treatment

## CONTRAINDICATIONS

### Relative
➤ Coagulopathies

## EQUIPMENT

Tourniquet ◆ gloves ◆ alcohol pads ◆ povidone-iodine pads ◆ 10-ml syringe (for adult) or 6-ml syringe (for child) ◆ 20G ½″ needles ◆ adhesive bandage ◆ 2″ × 2″ gauze pads ◆ two blood culture bottles (50-ml for adult or 20-ml bottles for infant or child), one aerobic and one anaerobic ◆ labels

## PREPARATION OF EQUIPMENT

➤ Check the dates on the culture bottles to make sure they haven't expired.

## ESSENTIAL STEPS

➤ Tell the patient that you need to collect a series of blood samples to check for infection. Explain the procedure and that you'll need to draw another blood sample later.
➤ Wash your hands and put on gloves.
➤ Tie a tourniquet 1″ (2.5 cm) proximal to the collection site.

### ISOLATOR BLOOD-CULTURING SYSTEM

A single-tube blood-culturing system, the Isolator uses lysis and centrifugation to help detect septicemia and monitor the effectiveness of antibacterial drug therapy. It is indicated for fungus and mycobacterium isolation; however, it is very costly and not readily available.

The Isolator tube used to collect the blood sample contains a substance that lyses red blood cells. Then centrifugation concentrates bacteria and other organisms in the sample onto an inert cushioning pad; the concentrate can then be applied directly onto four agar plates.

The Isolator has several advantages over conventional blood-culturing methods. This system:
➤ eliminates the bottle method's lengthy incubation period, providing faster results
➤ improves bacterial survival
➤ results in more valid positive results through direct application onto agar plates, which dilutes any antibiotic present in the sample to a greater degree and detects more yeast and polymicrobial infections
➤ improves the laboratory's ability to detect organisms that are difficult to grow
➤ is easier to use at the patient's bedside and to transport because blood is drawn directly into the Isolator tube.

➤ Clean the site with just the alcohol pad, or use an alcohol pad followed by povidone-iodine pad. Start at the site and work outward in a circular motion. Allow the site to thoroughly dry.

 **ALERT** If you're using povidone-iodine as well as alcohol, use the alcohol first. Using alcohol after povidone-iodine cancels the effect of the povidone-iodine.
➤ Perform a venipuncture, drawing 10 ml of blood from an adult or 2 to 6 ml from a child.

➤ Apply pressure to the venipuncture site with a 2″ × 2″ gauze pad. When hemostasis is achieved, apply an adhesive bandage.
➤ Wipe the diaphragm tops of the culture bottles with an alcohol sponge.
➤ Replace the needle on the syringe with a new sterile needle. Use a large-gauge needle to prevent hemolysis.
➤ Inject 5 ml of blood into each 50-ml culture bottle or 2 ml into a 20-ml pediatric culture bottle; fill the aerobic bottle first (bottle size may vary, but the sample dilution should never be less than 1:5).
➤ Label the culture bottles with the patient's name and identification number, the site, and the date and time of collection. Indicate the patient's temperature, and note any recent antibiotic therapy.
➤ Immediately send the samples to the laboratory.

## PATIENT TEACHING

➤ Let the patient know that he should feel only minimal pain during the procedure.
➤ Tell the patient that you should have the results in 24 to 72 hours.
➤ Instruct the patient to remove the bandage when bleeding stops.
➤ Describe hematoma formation to the patient, and instruct him to apply a warm compress to the area if a hematoma develops.

## COMPLICATIONS

➤ Place a warm soak over the site and apply pressure to prevent *hematoma formation*.

## SPECIAL CONSIDERATIONS

➤ Obtain each set of cultures from different sites. Ideally, you should take the samples 1 hour apart, but this isn't necessary in emergencies or if the patient is febrile.

➤ Don't take a sample for culturing from an existing line unless you draw the sample when the line is initially inserted. In suspected line sepsis, draw a set of blood cultures from the catheter but also draw a set from a venipuncture site at the same time.
➤ Don't use the femoral vein for blood culture samples because of the difficulty of adequately disinfecting the skin.
➤ Inform the laboratory if you suspect that the patient may have an unusual cause of infection, such as viremia, fungemia, brucellosis, tularemia, or leptospirosis.
➤ If the patient is currently on antibiotic therapy, obtain the blood sample right before administering the next dose so that the sample has a low level of the antibiotic.
➤ Notify the laboratory that the patient is taking antibiotics so that the laboratory can allow for extra dilution or use of an antibiotic removal device. Alternatively, you can use special culture bottles that have resin in the medium that absorbs antibiotics from the blood; however, these bottles are very expensive.
➤ Keep in mind that sample contamination can occur even with careful skin preparation.

## DOCUMENTATION

➤ Document the indications for drawing the cultures.
➤ Record the site, date, and time of blood sample collections; the number of bottles used; the patient's temperature; and any adverse reactions to the procedure.
➤ Record intervening antibiotic or other therapy.
➤ Note the results of the cultures (when available) and any changes or response to therapy.

# Doppler ultrasonography

CPT CODE
*93922  Noninvasive physiologic studies of upper or lower extremity arteries, single-level, bilateral (includes ankle and brachial indices, Doppler waveform analysis, volume plethysmography, and transcutaneous oxygen tension measurement)*

## DESCRIPTION

Doppler ultrasound consists of an audio unit, a volume control, and a transducer that detects the movement of red blood cells. It's useful in critical care settings where vasopressors that constrict peripheral circulation are in use. It's also used when a patient has had trauma to a limb that could impede or divert blood flow.

## INDICATIONS

➤ To determine arterial blood flow when blood flow may be compromised (for instance, in a cool, edematous, pale, cyanotic, or apparently pulseless extremity)
➤ To determine placement for an arterial insertion or puncture

## CONTRAINDICATIONS

### Absolute
➤ Use over an open or draining lesion

## EQUIPMENT

Doppler ultrasound ◆ ultrasound transmission gel (*not* water-soluble lubricant) ◆ marking pen ◆ soft cloth and antiseptic solution or soapy water

## ESSENTIAL STEPS

➤ Explain the procedure to the patient.
➤ Position the patient comfortably with the affected area accessible.
➤ Apply a small amount of coupling or transmission gel to the ultrasound probe.
➤ Position the probe on the skin directly over the selected artery.
➤ Set the volume control to the lowest setting. If your model doesn't have a speaker, plug in the earphones and slowly raise the volume.
➤ To obtain the best signal, tilt the probe at a 45-degree angle from the artery, making sure that you apply gel between the skin and the probe.
➤ Slowly move the probe in a circular motion to locate the center of the artery and the Doppler signal—a hissing noise at the heartbeat. Don't move the probe rapidly because this will distort the signal.
➤ After you've assessed the pulse, clean the probe with a soft cloth soaked in antiseptic solution or soapy water. Don't immerse the probe or bump it against a hard surface.
➤ Wipe the gel from the patient's skin and mark the selected artery with the marking pen.

## PATIENT TEACHING

➤ Tell the patient that he'll feel no pain but that the gel may feel cold. Explain that he may hear loud noises, but that is normal.
➤ Provide further teaching based on the test results, diagnosis, and prognosis.

## COMPLICATIONS

None known

## SPECIAL CONSIDERATIONS

➤ Be aware that failure to position the transducer properly can interfere with results.

➤ If the patient has a threat to vascular integrity, such as recent orthopedic surgery or an indwelling central venous catheter above the affected site, frequently check pulses for any changes in circulation.

➤ If you don't hear any noise when you turn the Doppler ultrasound on, replace the battery.

➤ To avoid a loud static noise, turn the volume all the way down and hold the probe against the skin before turning the Doppler ultrasound on.

## DOCUMENTATION

➤ Document the indication for the procedure, the site of evaluation, whether you found a pulse, a description of the pulse (full and bounding, thready, irregular), and all patient instructions given.

# Electrocardiography

CPT CODES
93000    Electrocardiogram (ECG), routine ECG with at least 12 leads; with interpretation and report
93005    ECG, routine ECG with at least 12 leads; tracing only, without interpretation and report

## DESCRIPTION

The most commonly used test for evaluating cardiac status, the ECG is a graphic recording of the electrical current generated by the heart. This current radiates from the heart in all directions and, on reaching the skin, is measured by electrodes connected to an amplifier and strip chart recorder. The standard resting ECG uses 10 electrodes to measure the electrical potential from 12 different leads: the standard limb leads (I, II, III), the augmented limb leads ($aV_F$, $aV_L$, $aV_R$), and the precordial or chest leads ($V_1$ through $V_6$).

ECG tracings normally consist of three identifiable waveforms: the P wave, the QRS complex, and the T wave. The P wave depicts atrial depolarization, the QRS complex reflects ventricular depolarization, and the T wave indicates ventricular repolarization. The manner in which these waveforms appear, their relationship to one another, and changes in their configuration allow identification of a patient's underlying cardiac status.

## INDICATIONS

➤ To help identify primary conduction abnormalities, cardiac arrhythmias, cardiac hypertrophy, pericarditis, electrolyte imbalances, myocardial ischemia, and the site and extent of myocardial infarction (MI)

➤ To monitor recovery from MI

➤ To evaluate the effectiveness of cardiac medication

➤ To observe pacemaker performance

➤ To determine the effectiveness of thrombolytic therapy and the resolution of ST-segment depression or elevation and T-wave changes

➤ To establish a baseline for a patient who is starting an exercise program, at risk for cardiac problems, or in need of surgery

## EQUIPMENT

Drape ◆ ECG machine ◆ pregelled disposable electrodes or electrodes and paste or gel ◆ alcohol pads ◆ ECG paper ◆ clippers (optional)

## PREPARATION OF EQUIPMENT

➤ Place the ECG machine close to the patient.
➤ Plug the power cord into the wall outlet or confirm that the battery is charged.
➤ Keep the patient away from electrical fixtures and power cords to minimize electrical interference.

## ESSENTIAL STEPS

➤ Explain to the patient that this test evaluates the heart's function by recording its electrical activity and that it doesn't require any special preparation.
➤ Provide privacy and have the patient lie supine in the center of the bed or examination table with his arms relaxed at his sides. You can elevate the head of the bed slightly to make the patient more comfortable.
➤ Drape the patient so that you expose his arms, legs, and chest.
➤ If the bed or examination table is too narrow for the patient to relax or the patient is trembling and is nonresponsive to common measures such as a blanket for warmth, ask him to place his hands under his buttocks to reduce muscle tension, which can interfere with the ECG tracing.
➤ Select flat, fleshy surfaces for placement of the extremity electrodes. Avoid muscular and bony areas. If the patient has an amputated limb, choose a site on the stump.
➤ If you need to place an electrode on a hairy area, clip the patient's hair. Remove the clipped hair; wipe the area with alcohol and allow it to dry.
➤ Apply electrodes to the medial aspects of the wrists and ankles and to the appropriate locations on the chest. Drape the female patient's chest to provide privacy. (See *Positioning chest electrodes.*)

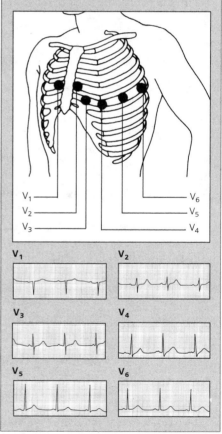

### POSITIONING CHEST ELECTRODES

To ensure accurate test results, position the chest electrodes as follows:
➤ Place $V_1$ at the fourth intercostal space and right sternal border.
➤ Place $V_2$ at the fourth intercostal space and left sternal border.
➤ Place $V_3$ midway between $V_2$ and $V_4$.
➤ Place $V_4$ at the fifth intercostal space and left midclavicular line.
➤ Place $V_5$ at the fifth intercostal space and left anterior axillary line.
➤ Place $V_6$ at the fifth intercostal space and left midaxillary line.

**ALERT** If you're using pregelled disposable electrodes, peel off the contact paper and apply them directly to the prepared sites. If you're using paste or gel, apply it first and then promptly secure the electrodes. Never substitute the recommended paste or gel with another conductive medium because it may impair the quality of the transmission of electrical impulses. Position the electrodes with the lead connection pointing superiorly.

➤ If the patient is a woman, place the electrodes beneath the breast tissue. In a large-breasted woman, displace breast tissue laterally.

➤ Connect the limb leadwires to the electrodes as follows:
– RA to the right arm
– RL to the right leg
– LA to the left arm
– LL to the left leg. Then connect the chest leadwires. Make sure you connect the leadwires properly.

➤ Make sure the paper speed selector is set to the standard 25 mm/second and that the machine is set to full voltage.

➤ Enter requested information into the machine — typically, the patient's name, identification number, and current medications and your name.

➤ Ask the patient to relax, lie still, breathe normally, and not talk while you record the ECG.

➤ Press the AUTO or RECORD button and observe the quality of the tracing. The machine will record all 12 leads automatically, recording 3 consecutive leads simultaneously. Some machines have a display screen so you can preview waveforms before they are recorded on paper.

➤ If the ECG machine display screen reads "check leads" or "lead XX off," make sure the lead connections are secure and attempt to record again.

➤ If the waveform extends beyond the paper during recording, reduce the settings to one-half of the standard and note this on the ECG tracing (it will affect the interpretation).

➤ Make sure all leads are represented on the tracing. If not, determine which lead has become loose, reattach it, and restart the tracing.

➤ When the machine has finished recording, remove the cables from the patient and reposition the patient's gown or clothes. If the patient will have serial ECGs, you may want to leave the electrodes in place to ensure that the next ECG is performed with the same lead placement as the first. If not, remove the electrodes, clean the skin, disconnect the electrodes from the leadwires, and dispose of or clean the electrodes.

## PATIENT TEACHING

➤ Reassure the patient that the test won't hurt and that he won't get an electrical shock. Tell him it will take from 3 to 10 minutes to perform. (See *Learning about an electrocardiogram.*)

➤ Inform the patient that he'll have electrodes attached to his arms, legs, and chest and that the gel or paste may feel cold.

➤ Tell the patient to lie quietly and relax and to breathe normally during the procedure.

➤ Advise the patient not to talk during the test because the movement of his chest and diaphragm may distort the ECG tracing.

➤ Tell the patient that you will interpret the 12-lead ECG for abnormalities or changes and direct the patient's care appropriately.

## COMPLICATIONS

None known

## SPECIAL CONSIDERATIONS

➤ Provide a quiet private area to obtain the ECG.

➤ If the patient has sweaty, oily, or scaly skin, rub the electrode sites with a dry gauze pad or alcohol before applying the electrodes.

PATIENT-TEACHING AID

# LEARNING ABOUT AN ELECTROCARDIOGRAM

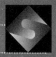

### DEAR PATIENT:

The practitioner has ordered an electrocardiogram for you. (The test is also called an ECG or EKG.) This test tells how well your heart works.

## How your heart beats
Your heart is a pump that has its own built-in pacemaker. This pacemaker is actually a group of special cells in the upper right part of the heart.

About every second, this natural pacemaker releases an electrical impulse that travels down a path of muscle fibers and spreads throughout your heart.

This impulse makes your heart contract and pump blood through its chambers and into the rest of the body through the blood vessels.

## How an ECG works
An ECG records the electrical impulses that travel through your heart. The ECG machine then converts these impulses to pencil-like "tracings" that print on long strips of graph paper. By looking at these tracings, the practitioner can tell whether your heart is healthy or has a problem.

## Before the test
You will be asked to lie on your back, with the skin of your chest, arms, and legs exposed. Lie perfectly still and relax. (Don't even talk.) The test is painless and lasts about 15 minutes.

## During the test
Electrodes will be attached to each wrist and ankle. Six more electrodes are placed on your chest. Thin wires attached to the electrodes lead to the ECG machine.

Don't worry, you can't get a shock because the wires carry a tiny amount of electricity out of your heart. No electricity goes into your heart.

Next, the ECG machine will be turned on to record the heart's electrical impulses, which are picked up by the electrodes on your arms and legs. Then six more electrodes will be attached. The practitioner or another person may perform this test.

## After the test
When the test is over, all equipment will be disconnected. You'll be able to resume your usual activities. The practitioner will probably tell you the results in a day or so.

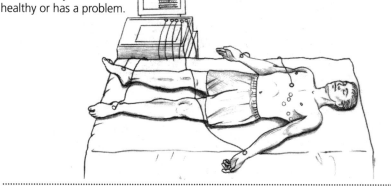

➤ If the patient's respirations interfere with the quality of the recording, ask him to hold his breath briefly while you record the ECG.

➤ If the patient has a pacemaker, you can perform the ECG with or without a magnet. A magnet may be placed over the pacemaker to deactivate it, thereby allowing the underlying heart rhythm to be assessed. If a magnet is not used, the ECG will evaluate the function of the pacemaker as well.

## DOCUMENTATION

➤ Document the indications for performing the ECG.

➤ Note the patient's name, age, and gender and the date on the ECG tracing.

➤ Include a copy of the ECG with any documentation.

➤ Document an interpretation of the ECG, including relevant normal and abnormal results.

➤ List any medications the patient is currently taking, especially those that can affect the heart.

➤ Note any management or treatment initiated or changed based on the results of the ECG.

## Stress echocardiography with dobutamine

CPT CODE
93350   Echocardiography, transthoracic, real-time with image documentation, pharmacologically induced stress test with interpretation and report

## DESCRIPTION

Stress echocardiography with dobutamine is an imaging technique used for patients who can't exercise and for whom adenosine or dipyridamole procedures aren't appropriate. Dobutamine produces hemodynamic changes similar to those produced by exercise. This imaging technique allows assessment of myocardial wall motion abnormalities, ejection fraction, and valvular disease at rest and during exercise.

## INDICATIONS

➤ To assess cardiac function in patients taking drugs (such as beta blockers or calcium channel blockers) that would interfere with adenosine or dipyridamole testing but can't be stopped prior to testing

➤ To assess cardiac function in patients who can't ambulate easily (due to prosthetic limbs, obstructive lung disease, severe peripheral vascular disease, or severe peripheral neuropathy)

➤ To assess the progression of coronary artery disease (CAD)

➤ To assess the significance of known CAD

➤ To evaluate the results of revascularization

➤ To evaluate high-risk patients before surgery

## CONTRAINDICATIONS

### Absolute
➤ Hypersensitivity to dobutamine
➤ Hypertrophic cardiomyopathy
➤ Uncontrolled hypertension
➤ Uncontrolled atrial fibrillation
➤ Malignant ventricular arrhythmia

### Relative
➤ Hypovolemia (correct with volume expanders before initiating infusion)
➤ Poor echogenic window because of funnel chest from emphysema or other conditions (poor visualization of the endocardium prevents accurate identification of myocardial wall motion abnormalities)
➤ Recent myocardial infarction

➤ Hemodynamically significant left ventricle outflow tract obstruction
➤ Large aneurysm

## EQUIPMENT

Echocardiography machine ◆ cardiac stress monitor (such as the Quinton 4000) ◆ electrodes ◆ cable ◆ alcohol pads ◆ clippers ◆ sphygmomanometer and blood pressure cuff ◆ emergency crash cart ◆ emergency medications ◆ infusion pump and tubing ◆ dobutamine ◆ normal saline solution ◆ 20-ml syringe ◆ peripheral I.V. access devices, tape, and gauze

## PREPARATION OF EQUIPMENT

➤ Enter complete patient information on the protocol stress-test sheet, including history, medications, current signs and symptoms, age, predicted stress time to achieve target heart rate, cardiac risk factors, and weight in kilograms.
➤ Enter demographic data into the echocardiography machine and cardiac stress monitor.

## ESSENTIAL STEPS

➤ Explain the procedure to the patient and obtain informed consent.
➤ Wipe the area for electrode placement with alcohol, allow it to dry, and lightly abrade the skin with the electrode pad. If necessary, clip excess hair.
➤ Obtain a baseline electrocardiogram (ECG).
➤ Obtain resting vital signs.
➤ Initiate continuous monitoring with the cardiac stress monitor.
➤ Obtain a resting two-dimensional echocardiograph.
➤ Insert an I.V. catheter or heparin lock.

➤ Prepare the dobutamine solution (4 ml of dobutamine and 16 ml of normal saline solution in a 20-ml syringe).
➤ Enter the patient's weight in kilograms on the volumetric pump.
➤ Enter the starting dobutamine rate (5 mcg/kg/minute).
➤ Using the volumetric pump, begin the infusion at 5 mcg/kg/minute and increase every 3 minutes to 10, then 20, then 30, to a maximum of 40 mcg/kg/minute if the patient doesn't meet the target heart rate. (A high dose of dobutamine helps to achieve a maximal heart rate.)
➤ Monitor vital signs every 3 minutes.
➤ Assess for adverse effects, such as angina and arrhythmias.
➤ Obtain and record a two-dimensional echocardiogram every 3 minutes.
➤ If the patient doesn't reach the target heart rate, inject 0.25 mg of atropine every minute up to a maximum of 1 mg over 4 minutes. Ultrasound is performed after 1 mg of atropine is given or when the maximal heart rate is achieved.

## PATIENT TEACHING

➤ Tell the patient not to eat for 4 hours before the procedure.
➤ Tell the patient that he'll have an I.V. line inserted into an arm vein and that he may feel his heart racing after the dobutamine infusion starts. Explain that these feelings will resolve shortly after the procedure ends (dobutamine has a half-life in plasma of about 2 minutes).
➤ Tell the patient that he should resume normal activities after the procedure.
➤ Advise the patient to schedule an appointment with you a couple of days after the procedure to discuss the results.

## COMPLICATIONS

➤ *Decrease in systolic blood pressure of more than 20 mm Hg, angina, development of or increase in ventricular arrhythmia, excessive tachycardia, or ST-segment depression of 2 mm or more:* Reduce the rate of administration or discontinue the drug. If necessary, administer esmolol, an antagonist to dobutamine, to reverse symptoms.

## SPECIAL CONSIDERATIONS

➤ Coronary steal — uncommon with adenosine or dipyridamole — can occur with dobutamine administration.
➤ Emergency equipment, such as a crash cart and emergency medications, should be readily available.
➤ Depending on results, referral to a cardiologist may be necessary.

## DOCUMENTATION

➤ Before the procedure, document underlying comorbidities, medications, allergies, previous history of and risk factors for CAD, baseline ECG, presenting symptoms, physical examination results, and differential diagnoses.
➤ During the procedure, document the amount of dobutamine infused, the heart rate achieved and blood pressure response, manifestation of symptoms, and any use of atropine or antagonistic medication.
➤ After the procedure, document complications, ECG evaluation, diagnosis, results of the echocardiogram, and the amount of dobutamine administered.

## Stress test

CPT CODES
*93015   Cardiovascular stress testing with continuous electrocardiograph monitoring and interpretation*
*93017   Cardiovascular stress testing with continuous electrocardiograph mon-*

*itoring, tracing only, without interpretation and report*
*93350   Stress echocardiography, real time with image documentation, interpretation, and report*

## DESCRIPTION

Also known as exercise electrocardiography (ECG), stress testing evaluates the heart's action during physical stress, when the demand for oxygen increases. It provides important diagnostic and prognostic information about patients with ischemic heart disease. It is also performed immediately before a stress echocardiogram.

During testing, ECG and blood pressure measurements are recorded while the patient walks on a treadmill or pedals a stationary bicycle. Each type of device has its advantages and disadvantages. (See *Comparing exercise testing devices.*)

The patient's response to a constant or increasing workload is monitored; the test continues until the patient reaches a target heart rate, as determined by an established protocol such as Borg's rate of perceived exertion, or until he experiences chest pain or fatigue. (See *Borg's rate of perceived exertion*, page 22.)

Exercise stress testing allows indirect determination of maximum oxygen uptake ($VO_2$), the greatest amount of oxygen that a person can extract from inspired air. Maximum $VO_2$ is described in terms of metabolic equivalents (METS), with 1 MET equaling 3.5 ml/kg/minute. A moderately active young man walking 2 miles per hour on level ground uses about 2 METS. The patient's maximum $VO_2$ is determined by comparing the number of METS used during exercise stress testing to normal values. Maximum $VO_2$ varies with age, body weight, heredity, gender, and conditioning.

During testing, the patient should have a gradual increase in heart rate to a max-

## COMPARING EXERCISE TESTING DEVICES

The treadmill and stationary bicycle provide information about the heart's action during physical stress. Each device has advantages and disadvantages.

### Treadmill
*Advantages*
➤ Is standardized and provides the most repro-ducible results
➤ Requires the patient to walk, a familiar activity
➤ Maintains a constant pace of activity
➤ Attains the highest maximum oxygen uptake
➤ Involves commonly used muscles, decreasing the chance of fatigue

*Disadvantages*
➤ May result in the patient losing balance and falling off
➤ Results in increased workload with increased weight
➤ Makes obtaining blood pressure readings and electrocardiogram (ECG) readings more difficult be-cause the upper body is in motion
➤ Is more expensive
➤ Is noisy, making communication with the pa-tient more difficult

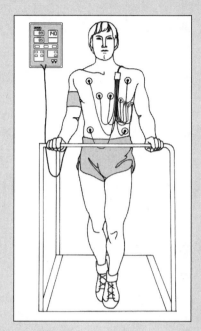

### Stationary bicycle
*Advantages*
➤ Doesn't result in increased workload with in-creased weight
➤ Makes obtaining blood pressure and ECG read-ings easy because the upper body remains relatively still
➤ Is less expensive

*Disadvantages*
➤ Requires a constant rate of pedaling to maintain power
➤ Requires frequent calibration
➤ Induces more stress
➤ Attains a lower maximum oxygen uptake
➤ Involves less commonly used muscles, increasing the chance of fatigue

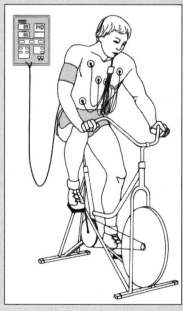

## BORG'S RATE OF PERCEIVED EXERTION

Borg's rate of perceived exertion (RPE), developed by Dr. Gunnar Borg, is a 15-grade scale that assigns a numeric value (ranging from 6 to 20) to subjective feelings of exercise exertion, as shown in the table below. The scale allows the patient to express his perception of fatigue based on all the factors — psychological, musculoskeletal, and environmental — that affect his sense of exertion.

For instance, an RPE of 12 to 13 corresponds to about 60% to 80% of maximal heart rate; an RPE of 16, about 90% of maximal heart rate. A patient typically meets his maximal, or target, heart rate at a level of 12 to 16.

The revised 10-grade scale rates exercise intensity on a scale of 0 to 10. It was developed to simplify terms and make the scale easier to understand.

| ORIGINAL 15-GRADE SCALE | REVISED 10-GRADE SCALE |
|---|---|
| 6 No exertion at all | 0 Nothing at all |
| 7 Extremely light | 0.5 Very, very light |
| 8 | (just noticeable) |
| 9 Very light | 1 Very weak |
| 10 | 2 Weak (light) |
| 11 Light | 3 Moderate |
| 12 | 4 Somewhat |
| 13 Somewhat hard | strong |
| 14 | 5 Strong (heavy) |
| 15 Hard (heavy) | 6 |
| 16 | 7 Very strong |
| 17 Very hard | 8 |
| 18 | 9 |
| 19 Extremely hard | 10 Extremely |
| 20 Maximal exertion | strong (maximal) |

tocols and have advanced cardiac life support (ACLS) certification. The test carries a mortality of approximately 1 in 10,000, and complications from the test — including prolonged chest pain, arrhythmias, and myocardial infarction (MI) — result in about 4 in 10,000 patients, requiring hospital admission.

## INDICATIONS

➤ To aid in the diagnosis of coronary artery disease (CAD)
➤ To determine functional capacity in a patient with known CAD or in a patient who has had an MI, cardiac surgery, or coronary angioplasty
➤ To screen for asymptomatic CAD in a patient who requires a physical examination for his occupation (pilots, air traffic controllers, police officers, and fire fighters) or who is at high risk for developing CAD
➤ To determine a patient's exercise tolerance before he begins an exercise regimen
➤ To evaluate the functional capacity of a patient with congenital or valvular heart disease
➤ To evaluate the functioning of a patient's rate-responsive pacemaker
➤ To determine the presence of exercise-induced arrhythmias in a symptomatic patient
➤ To evaluate the response to medical therapy of a patient with CAD or heart failure
➤ To evaluate blood pressure response in a patient undergoing treatment for hypertension who wishes to begin an exercise program

imum target rate, an increase in systolic pressure, and minimal change in diastolic pressure. After exercise stops, the patient's systolic blood pressure should return to its resting value within about 6 minutes.

To administer such testing, a practitioner should be familiar with exercise pro-

## CONTRAINDICATIONS

### Absolute

➤ Unstable angina
➤ Recent acute MI (generally within previous 6 days)

➤ Symptomatic severe left ventricular dysfunction

➤ Potentially life-threatening cardiac arrhythmias

➤ Acute pericarditis, myocarditis, or endocarditis

➤ Severe aortic stenosis or suspected dissecting aortic aneurysm

➤ Uncontrolled hypertension

➤ Acute pulmonary edema or heart failure

➤ Pulmonary embolism

➤ Acute deep vein thrombosis or thrombophlebitis

➤ Orthopedic, musculoskeletal, neuromuscular, or arthritic conditions that interfere with or impede exercise

➤ Acute systemic illness

➤ Severe hypertrophic obstructive cardiomyopathy

➤ Unavailability of ACLS equipment or an individual certified to perform ACLS

## EQUIPMENT

Treadmill with adjustable speed and grade or bicycle ergometer with adjustable resistance and pedal frequency ◆ cardiac stress monitor with 12-lead ECG recorder and continuous tracing capability (such as the Quinton 4000) ◆ electrodes and cables ◆ sphygmomanometer and stethoscope ◆ emergency equipment (including a defibrillator, oxygen, handheld oxygen resuscitation bag, intubation equipment, suction equipment and catheters, and emergency drug kit with those drugs recommended by ACLS protocols)

## PREPARATION OF EQUIPMENT

➤ Enter complete information on the protocol stress-test sheet, including history, medications, current signs and symptoms, age, predicted time exercising to achieve target heart rate, and cardiac risk factors.

### THE BRUCE PROTOCOL

The Bruce protocol is the most commonly used treadmill protocol for adults. The patient progresses in 3-minute stages from a slow walk at a 10% grade to a slow run at a 16% to 20% grade. The practitioner administering the test takes the patient's heart rate, blood pressure, and electrocardiogram (ECG) readings at the end of each stage and throughout the 4- to 10-minute recovery period.

Before the procedure begins but after monitoring starts, the patient hyperventilates to allow the practitioner to assess the effect of body movement on ECG readings.

| STAGE | SPEED (Km/hour) | GRADE (%) |
|-------|-----------------|-----------|
| 1 | 2.7 | 10 |
| 2 | 4 | 12 |
| 3 | 5.4 | 14 |
| 4 | 6.7 | 16 |
| 5 | 8 | 18 |
| 6 | 8.8 | 20 |
| 7 | 9.6 | 22 |

➤ Enter demographic data into the machine.

## ESSENTIAL STEPS

➤ Explain the procedure to the patient, including using the treadmill (if applicable) and Borg's rate of perceived exertion, and obtain informed consent.

➤ Assess the patient for the appropriate testing protocol (treadmill, bicycle, or arm ergometry).

➤ Determine which protocol to use. If you use the treadmill protocol, make sure it's consistent with the patient's physical capacity and the purpose of the test. Treadmill testing typically uses the Bruce protocol (see *The Bruce protocol*). If the patient would better tolerate it, you can use a modified Bruce protocol with a more gradual workload progression.

## STRESS ECHOCARDIOGRAPHY

This imaging technique allows detection of resting and ischemia-induced wall motion abnormalities, ejection fraction, and valvular disease. It's comparable in sensitivity to stress thallium and sestambi nuclear studies. The patient either exercises or receives a pharmacologic agent to reach the target heart rate and then undergoes imaging. If the patient has severe coronary artery disease, pharmacologic stress echocardiography may be safer because it allows careful titration of the amount of stress.

Stress echocardiography is especially useful in patients with an intermediate or high likelihood of cardiovascular disease; resting ECG abnormalities, such as digitalis effect, severe left ventricular hypertrophy with strain, left bundle-branch block, or Wolff-Parkinson-White syndrome; cardiomyopathy; previous coronary artery bypass surgery or myocardial infarction (MI); or electrolyte abnormalities.

In women, stress echocardiography is preferred because it offers much higher specificity than graded exercise stress testing. It's believed that the similar chemical structures of digoxin and estrogen result in the high false-positive rate in graded stress testing.

### Indications
➤ To determine exercise-induced abnormalities in left ventricular wall motion
➤ To differentiate viable from nonviable myocardial tissue

### Contraindications
*Absolute*
➤ Acute MI
➤ Unstable angina pectoris
➤ Uncontrolled ventricular arrhythmias
➤ Symptomatic severe aortic stenosis
➤ Known or suspected dissecting aneurysm
➤ Active or suspected myocarditis

➤ Thrombophlebitis
➤ Acute systemic or pulmonary embolism
➤ Active infection
➤ Acute pericarditis
➤ Decompensated heart failure
➤ Resting diastolic blood pressure over 120 mm Hg
➤ Severe arthritis or other orthopedic condition that prevents the patient from positioning his arms above his head

*Relative*
➤ Aortic stenosis
➤ Suspected left main coronary artery narrowing
➤ Idiopathic hypertrophic subaortic stenosis
➤ Compensated heart failure
➤ Severe ST-segment depression at rest
➤ Hypertension (systolic blood pressure greater than 200 mm Hg or diastolic blood pressure over 110 mm Hg or both)
➤ Poor echogenic window because of funnel chest from emphysema or other condition (poor visualization of the endocardium prevents accurate identification of myocardial wall motion abnormalities)
➤ Diffuse cardiomyopathy associated with left bundle-branch block

### Essential steps
➤ Have the patient follow the same steps as he would for stress testing, but tell him not to eat for 4 hours before the procedure instead of 2 hours, and tell him not to take any beta blockers unless otherwise directed by the cardiologist.
➤ Before beginning the procedure, show the patient the ECG machine and demonstrate how to dismount from the treadmill and get on the table for the echocardiogram. Emphasize that the patient should move to the table as quickly as possible.

➤ Have the assistant prepare the patient, and connect the exercise 12-lead ECG cables.
➤ If the patient is also having a stress echocardiogram, obtain a resting two-dimensional echocardiogram (see *Stress echocardiography*).
➤ Obtain a baseline blood pressure, heart rate, and 12-lead ECG tracing with the patient in supine and standing positions.

➤ Begin the exercise testing.
➤ Encourage the patient to continue with the testing as long as possible.
➤ Record a 12-lead ECG and blood pressure at the end of each stage of the testing (every 3 minutes), at any indication of a complication, whenever the ECG monitor shows an abnormality, immediately upon ending the testing, and every minute for the first 4 to 10 minutes after exercise stops.
➤ Continuously monitor the patient's ECG, vital signs, signs and symptoms, and heart rate. Tell the patient to report any symptoms and to let you know when he feels he needs to stop the test. If indicated, stop the test early. (See *Indications for stopping stress testing*.) Otherwise, end the test when the patient reaches the target heart rate or completes the protocol. Rather than abruptly stopping the exercise, allow the patient to walk for approximately 1 minute to allow his heart rate to decrease gradually.
➤ If the patient is also undergoing echocardiography, ask him to return immediately to the imaging table for a two-dimensional echocardiogram. These images must be obtained within seconds of stopping the treadmill, so the patient can have no cooling-off period.
➤ Monitor the patient's blood pressure and heart rate, and note any symptoms he may experience during recovery. Continue monitoring until all symptoms disappear, the ECG returns to baseline, or for 4 minutes after ending the testing phase.

## PATIENT TEACHING

➤ Describe the procedure and the reason for it to the patient. Explain that he'll have ECG and blood pressure monitoring during and for a short time after the test. Tell him the entire test usually takes about 20 minutes to complete. (See *Taking an exercise stress test*, page 26.)
➤ Tell the patient not to eat or drink for 2 hours before the test and *not* to take med-

### INDICATIONS FOR STOPPING STRESS TESTING

You would normally end exercise stress testing when the patient reaches the target heart rate or completes the protocol. However, consider ending the test early if the patient develops any of the following:
➤ increasing chest pain
➤ fatigue, shortness of breath, wheezing, leg cramps, or worsening intermittent claudication
➤ a hypertensive response with systolic blood pressure greater than 240 mm Hg or diastolic blood pressure greater than 120 mm Hg
➤ problematic ST-segment changes or increasing QRS changes, QT prolongation, or abnormal beats
➤ bundle-branch block that isn't distinguishable from ventricular tachycardia.
  You must end the test early for any of the following:
➤ systolic blood pressure that drops below resting values during the exercise portion of the test
➤ appearance of or worsening chest pain
➤ light-headedness, dizziness, presyncope, or syncope
➤ signs of poor perfusion, such as pallor and cyanosis
➤ signs of severe intolerance to the workload, such as dyspnea and hyperventilation
➤ serious arrhythmias
➤ electrocardiogram (ECG) readings that show ST-segment depression of more than 3 mm or ST-segment elevation of more than 2 mm
➤ patient's request to stop
➤ technical difficulties in monitoring ECG activity or blood pressure
➤ progressive, reproducible increase in systolic blood pressure.

ications, such as beta blockers and calcium channel blockers.
➤ Instruct the patient to wear comfortable clothes and shoes suitable for walking and jogging.

PATIENT-TEACHING AID

## TAKING AN EXERCISE STRESS TEST

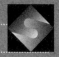

DEAR PATIENT,

If you've never taken an exercise stress test before, you probably have questions. The information below can give you some of the answers you need. Talk to your practitioner if you have additional questions or concerns.

### What is an exercise stress test?
An exercise stress test evaluates the flow of blood through your arteries to your heart. It shows how your heart works under stress and will help your practitioner determine if you are at risk for heart disease.

### What happens during the test?
Usually, you walk on a motorized treadmill or ride a stationary bike. Your heart and blood pressure will be monitored throughout the test. If you're on a treadmill, you'll progress from a walk to a fast pace, probably a slow run, at an increasingly steep grade. (If you can't exercise, you may receive medicine to test your heart. If that is the case, your practitioner can explain the procedure further.) You may also have X-ray-like pictures taken right after the test.

During the test, your practitioner will monitor your electrocardiogram (ECG) and your blood pressure at intervals. The ECG uses electrodes placed on your skin to record your heart's electrical activity. Report any symptoms you experience during the test — such as chest pain, shortness of breath, dizziness, or fatigue. After the test, you will be monitored for a few more minutes. The test typically takes 20 to 45 minutes.

### How do I prepare for the test?
You will be asked to refrain from eating and drinking for several hours before the test. Depending on the type of test, you may be asked to refrain from eating for up to 8 hours before the test. In general, this time will be 2 hours for a graded exercise stress test, 4 hours for dobutamine stress echocardiography, and 8 hours for the first day of the adenosine myoview test. Your practitioner may also tell you not to eat or drink products that contain caffeine — such as coffee, tea, chocolate, and cola drinks — for 24 hours before the test. You may also have to stop taking certain medications for several days before the test. On the day of the test, wear comfortable clothes, including sneakers or other soft, flat-soled shoes for exercise.

Check with your practitioner before taking any of the following drugs for 24 hours before exercise stress testing:
➤ beta blockers, such as acebutolol, atenolol, esmolol, metroprolol, labetalol, pindolol, and propanolol
➤ calcium channel blockers, such as amlodipine, diltiazem, felodipine, nifedipine, and verapamil.

If you are scheduled for an adenosine myoview test, you should also avoid caffeine for 24 hours.

### Is the test safe?
Yes, but because your heart is being tested, you do face some risks. You'll have the risks explained to you before starting, and you'll need to sign a consent form. Experienced personnel are available to handle any emergency.

### When will I learn the results of the test?
Your practitioner or cardiologist will review the results in more detail with you in a few days.

➤ As appropriate, teach the patient how to use the treadmill (see *Using a treadmill*).

➤ Tell the patient to report symptoms — such as chest pain, leg cramping, shortness of breath, dizziness, light-headedness, or fatigue — that he may experience during the test.

➤ Tell the patient that any unusual feelings should resolve within a few minutes after the test ends and that he can resume normal activities.

➤ Advise the patient to schedule an appointment with you a couple of days after the procedure to discuss the results.

## COMPLICATIONS

➤ *Chest pain* or *signs of distress*, such as dizziness, headache, nausea, and dyspnea, require monitoring and possible admission for inpatient monitoring and treatment.

➤ *Arrhythmias* require monitoring. For lethal arrhythmias, initiate ACLS protocols.

## SPECIAL CONSIDERATIONS

➤ Current guidelines for periodic screening (per the U.S. Preventive Services Task Force) don't recommend routine stress testing as a screening tool for the general public.

➤ Performing stress testing on patients with known cardiac disease or cardiac risk factors increases the sensitivity of the test as well as the likelihood of complications during testing.

➤ A patient who feels anxious about the test may have an initial overreaction of heart rate and systolic blood pressure, but this should stabilize after 1 to 2 minutes.

➤ Patients taking digoxin and those with certain conditions, such as left ventricular hypertrophy or left bundle-branch block, are also required to undergo nuclear imaging.

## USING A TREADMILL

If your patient has never been on a treadmill before, she probably won't know the best posture to assume. If she's feeling weak or afraid, she may cling tightly to the handrail, decreasing the workload and possibly leading to a falsely elevated exercise tolerance level.

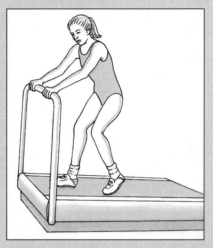

To increase the patient's confidence and obtain more accurate results, show her how to stay erect and close to the front of the treadmill, with her hands resting lightly on the handrail.

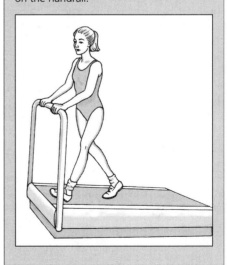

➤ Patients being evaluated for effort–chest pain syndromes may not need to stop their cardiac medications (including drugs such as beta blockers) because the cardiac symptoms (such as breathlessness and epigastric or chest discomfort) are predictably occurring during effort while they're taking their medications. As long as the angina presents, the test can determine if it has ischemic or flow-related etiology.

➤ Stress testing shows changes that occur with increased myocardial vasospasm, ST changes, pulsus alternans, T-wave inversion, early onset of myocardial ischemia (onset in under 3 minutes), prolonged duration of ischemic changes during the recovery phase, and hypotension associated with the ischemic changes.

➤ Imaging tests, such as echocardiography and nuclear imaging, depict ischemia and cardiac defects (such as which vessels are involved). Angiography detects coronary artery changes but doesn't detect ischemia.

➤ A patient with an effort–chest pain syndrome may have a negative angiogram but a positive stress test. This combination of results reveals ischemic effects without large vessel disease and is frequently associated with Syndrome X. Though unresponsive to nitrates, this type of angina may respond favorably to angiotensin-converting enzyme (ACE) inhibitors as well as aggressive reduction of coronary risk factors.

➤ Emergency equipment and medications should be readily available.

➤ Depending on results, referral to a cardiologist may be necessary.

## DOCUMENTATION

➤ Document the indications for exercise stress testing, what medications the patient is presently taking, and medications the patient was told to avoid or take before the test.

➤ Before the test, record baseline vital signs (including blood pressure and heart and respiratory rates), cardiac and pulmonary assessment, and a baseline 12-lead ECG.

➤ Describe the protocol and exercise mode used for testing.

➤ Maintain a log of blood pressures, heart rates, ECG tracings, and symptoms that the patient experienced during the different phases of the exercise stress test.

➤ Note the length of time the patient tolerated the test, stage of the stress test the patient achieved, peak heart rate, and reason for stopping the test.

➤ Document the occurrence of any absolute or relative symptoms or conditions that require the test to be aborted, the time they occurred, the treatment or management of these symptoms, and the patient's response.

➤ List any medications administered during and after the test.

➤ Note the patient's condition at the end of the test.

➤ Record the patient's vital signs and 12-lead ECG tracing at the end of the stress test, results of testing, and recommendations made to the patient.

## Stress test with adenosine

CPT CODES
78460 *Myocardial perfusion imaging; (planar) single study, at rest or stress (exercise or pharmacologic)*
78461 *Myocardial perfusion imaging; multiple studies, at rest or stress (exercise or pharmacologic) and redistribution or rest injection*

# DESCRIPTION

A two-part imaging procedure, adenosine stress testing uses adenosine, radioactive tracers, and a camera connected to a computer to produce pictures of heart muscle perfusion. The adenosine infusion causes vasodilation, decreasing coronary vascular resistance and increasing blood flow to three to four times the normal rate (compared with exercise, which increases blood flow to twice the normal rate). The nuclear imaging reveals areas of hypoperfusion distal to the lesion in stenosed arteries. These regional disparities in blood flow that result from coronary stenosis are called *perfusion defects*.

# INDICATIONS

This test is indicated for patients who have a limited (if any) ability to exercise. Qualifying conditions include disabling arthritis, severe peripheral vascular disease, severe peripheral neuropathy, a prosthetic limb, systemic muscular disease, aortic aneurysm, aortic stenosis, severe hypertension, or left bundle-branch block. It's used to evaluate:
➤ atypical cardiac symptoms
➤ the significance of known coronary artery disease (CAD)
➤ the progression of CAD
➤ the likely outcome for symptomatic patients
➤ the results of surgical revascularization
➤ high-risk patients before major surgery.

# CONTRAINDICATIONS

## Absolute
➤ Second-degree or third-degree heart block, except in patients with a functioning atrial pacemaker (adenosine can induce first-degree and second-degree atrioventricular block)

➤ Sinus node disease, except in patients with a functioning atrioventricular pacemaker
➤ Known or suspected bronchoconstrictive or bronchospastic lung disease (adenosine may induce bronchospasm)
➤ Hypersensitivity to adenosine
➤ Systolic blood pressure lower than 90 mm Hg

## Relative
➤ Recent myocardial infarction (caution required)

# EQUIPMENT

Cardiac stress monitor (such as the Quinton 4000) ◆ gamma camera ◆ sphygmomanometer and blood pressure cuff ◆ cable and electrodes ◆ alcohol pads ◆ clippers (if needed) ◆ emergency crash cart with defibrillator, emergency medications, airway, handheld resuscitation bag, oxygen, and suction equipment ◆ aminophylline (direct antagonist to adenosine) ◆ peripheral I.V. access supplies ◆ volumetric infusion pump and tubing ◆ adenosine and dose calibrator ◆ radioisotope

# PREPARATION OF EQUIPMENT

➤ Enter complete information on the stress-test sheet, including history, medications, current signs and symptoms, age, predicted test time to achieve target heart rate, stress time, and cardiac risk factors.
➤ Enter demographic data into the machine.

# ESSENTIAL STEPS

➤ Explain the procedure to the patient and obtain informed consent.
➤ Before the procedure, verify that the patient has had nothing by mouth for the past 4 hours and has refrained from medications as directed.

## INDICATIONS FOR DECREASING OR STOPPING ADENOSINE INFUSION

Certain signs and symptoms call for you to decrease or stop the adenosine infusion.
➤ *Chest pain:* Decrease the infusion from 140 mcg/kg/minute to 100 mcg/kg/minute.
➤ *ST-segment depression of 2 mm or more with angina:* Stop the infusion and administer sublingual nitroglycerin.
➤ *Atrioventricular heart block, dizziness, or headache accompanied by hypotension or worsening nausea or dyspnea:* Decrease the infusion rate. If the adverse effect worsens, stop the infusion but complete the imaging.

➤ Wipe the skin with alcohol, abrade it lightly by scraping skin with the electrode, and apply the electrodes. If necessary, clip excess hair.
➤ Obtain a baseline electrocardiogram (ECG) and resting vital signs.
➤ Initiate continuous cardiac monitoring.
➤ Insert an I.V. line into the patient's arm.
➤ Instruct the nuclear technologist to start the infusion (the nuclear technologist calculates the dose of adenosine per kilogram of body weight and prepares the volumetric pump for infusion).
➤ Once the infusion has started, record vital signs every minute.
➤ Monitor the patient's ECG rhythm, blood pressure, heart rate, and symptoms. If necessary, stop the test early. (See *Indications for decreasing or stopping adenosine infusion.*)
➤ After waiting 3 minutes to ensure the patient doesn't receive a bolus dose, the nuclear technologist slowly injects the radioisotope (such as thallium) without stopping the adenosine infusion.
➤ The patient undergoes nuclear imaging 30 to 45 minutes after injection of the radioisotope.

➤ The next day, the patient undergoes the second part of the procedure. The nuclear technologist injects the radioisotope into a peripheral vein, and the patient undergoes nuclear imaging about 45 minutes later.

## PATIENT TEACHING

➤ Before the day of testing, tell the patient to take nothing by mouth for 4 hours before testing, to discontinue nitrates 12 hours before testing, to avoid caffeine for at least 48 hours before testing (caffeine has properties similar to aminophylline), and to discontinue dipyridamole 48 hours before testing.
➤ Before the procedure, inform the patient that he'll have an I.V. line inserted in his arm and undergo continuous cardiac monitoring during the infusion of adenosine. Tell him the effects of the medication will last only a few seconds. After the adenosine has been infusing for 3 minutes, the radioisotope will be injected. After the infusion, he'll need to wait for 35 to 40 minutes and then undergo the first scan. For the second part of the procedure (which may take place on the following day, depending on the facility), the patient will have a radioisotope injected and wait about 45 minutes for the tracer to circulate. Then he'll undergo a scan of the tracer.
➤ Inform the patient that the radioactive exposure received from the procedure is about the same as the average background radiation exposure received in 8 years, or less than half the annual radiation exposure allowed for X-ray and nuclear medicine technologists.

## COMPLICATIONS

➤ *Chest pain, ST-segment depression, atrioventricular heart block, dizziness, headache, nausea, flushing, dyspnea,* and *hy-*

*potension* are adverse effects of medication and require monitoring.
➤ *Arrhythmias* require monitoring and treatment as indicated by the rhythm.

## SPECIAL CONSIDERATIONS

➤ Preliminary results may be available within 2 hours after completion of the test.
➤ Severe ischemia may cause a persistent defect up to 4 hours after the test is completed.
➤ Delayed images at 6 to 24 hours may reveal the reversible pattern of ischemia.
➤ Thallium imaging can't differentiate scarring from acute infarction, so it can't reveal the age of a persistent defect.
➤ Emergency equipment and medications should be readily available.
➤ Referral to a cardiologist may be necessary if the test is abnormal.

## DOCUMENTATION

➤ Before the procedure, document underlying comorbidities, medications, allergies, risk factors for CAD, baseline ECG, presenting symptoms, physical examination results, and differential diagnoses.
➤ During the procedure, document the amount of adenosine infused, heart rate achieved and blood pressure response, manifestation of symptoms, any use of antagonistic medication, and ECG changes.
➤ After the procedure, document blood pressure and heart rate response, ECG interpretation, arrhythmias, heart block, tolerance to the procedure, complications, dissipation of symptoms, diagnosis, and results of the nuclear scan. Normal findings are homogenous distribution of isotope throughout all segments of the left ventricle, with no transient or fixed regional perfusion defects.

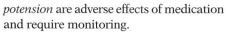

# Stress test with thallium

CPT CODES
*78464   Myocardial perfusion imaging tomographic (SPECT), single study*
*78465   Myocardial perfusion imaging tomographic (SPECT), multiple studies*

## DESCRIPTION
This procedure uses nuclear scanning to assess ischemic heart disease and myocardial perfusion. It differentiates areas of infarction from areas of ischemia in the ventricle and is useful in evaluating the health and function of the myocardium. The procedure works by distributing the nuclear agent thallium or radioactive technetium 99m to the myocardial cells in proportion to the blood supply they receive. Nuclear scanning then reveals myocardial perfusion by displaying the radioisotopes attached to cell proteins.

## INDICATIONS
➤ To help diagnose ischemic heart disease in asymptomatic or symptomatic patients
➤ To assess the efficacy of various medical and surgical procedures and therapies
➤ To further evaluate cardiac perfusion in a patient whose resting electrocardiogram (ECG) exhibits paced rhythm or who has left bundle-branch block, digoxin effect, severe left hypertrophy with strain, or baseline ST-T wave abnormalities
➤ To determine risk in a patient with known coronary artery disease

## CONTRAINDICATIONS
### Absolute
➤ Pregnancy
➤ Acute myocardial infarction (MI)
➤ Unstable angina pectoris

➤ Uncontrolled ventricular arrhythmia
➤ Symptomatic severe aortic stenosis
➤ Suspected or known dissecting aneurysm
➤ Active or suspected myocarditis
➤ Thrombophlebitis
➤ Active infection
➤ Acute pericarditis
➤ Decompensated heart failure
➤ Resting diastolic blood pressure higher than 120 mm Hg
➤ Weight of more than 325 lb (147.4 kg) (weight limit depends on the camera or table being used and should be checked before scheduling the procedure)
➤ Severe arthritis or other orthopedic condition that prevents the patient from positioning his arms above his head
➤ Extreme claustrophobia

**Relative**
➤ Left main coronary stenosis
➤ Moderate to severe stenotic valvular heart disease
➤ Electrolyte abnormalities
➤ Severe arterial hypertension (systolic blood pressure above 200 mm Hg or diastolic blood pressure above 110 mm Hg or both)
➤ Tachyarrhythmias or bradyarrhythmias
➤ Hypertrophic cardiomyopathy and other forms of outflow obstruction
➤ Mental or physical impairment that leads to inability to exercise adequately
➤ High-degree atrioventricular block

## EQUIPMENT

Cardiac stress monitor (such as the Quinton 4000) ◆ treadmill ◆ sphygmomanometer and blood pressure cuff ◆ electrodes ◆ alcohol pads ◆ clippers (optional) ◆ peripheral I.V. supplies ◆ thallium supplies ◆ emergency cart

## PREPARATION OF EQUIPMENT

➤ Enter complete information on the stress-test sheet, including history, medications, current signs and symptoms, age, predicted time to achieve the target heart rate, and cardiac risk factors.
➤ Enter demographic data into the machine.

## ESSENTIAL STEPS

➤ Explain the procedure to the patient, including Borg's rate of perceived exertion, and obtain informed consent. (See the entry "Stress test," page 20, for more information on Borg's rate of perceived exertion.) If the patient is a woman under age 50, also have her sign the pregnancy release form.
➤ Wipe the chest area with alcohol and abrade the skin lightly with the electrode. Clip excess hair if necessary.
➤ Apply the electrodes, and obtain a baseline ECG and blood pressure.
➤ With the patient lying down, ask him to hyperventilate for 30 seconds and record a second ECG.
➤ Set the cardiac monitor to leads II, $V_1$, and $V_5$.
➤ Program the standard Bruce protocol (you can use an accelerated or modified protocol, depending on the patient's needs).
➤ Demonstrate how to use the treadmill.
➤ The nuclear technologist will insert an I.V. line into a peripheral vein.
➤ Instruct the patient to tell you about dizziness, leg cramping, chest pain, dyspnea, or other symptoms that occur during the test, and instruct the patient to begin walking on the treadmill.
➤ Record the patient's blood pressure every 2 minutes or if symptoms occur.
➤ Instruct the nuclear technologist to inject the isotope when the patient reaches the target heart rate.

➤ Instruct the patient to ambulate for 1 minute after the injection.

➤ After the procedure, monitor the patient's blood pressure, rhythm, and heart rate for 4 minutes or until the ECG readings return to baseline.

➤ Have the patient wait 20 minutes and then lie under the nuclear camera so that the technologist can take the perfusion images.

➤ The following day, the patient will receive an injection of the radioisotope while he is at rest, wait about 45 minutes, and then undergo nuclear imaging again.

## PATIENT TEACHING

➤ Tell the patient that the whole procedure takes 2 days. On the first day, he'll undergo the stress portion of the procedure, in which he'll ambulate on the treadmill before injection of the radioisotope. After the injection, he'll wait 20 minutes and undergo nuclear imaging. On the second day, he'll receive the injection while resting, wait 45 minutes for the isotope to circulate, and then undergo imaging.

➤ Instruct the patient to discontinue beta blocking and calcium channel blocking agents 48 hours before the procedure so that they don't interfere with reaching the target heart rate. Tell him to take nothing by mouth after midnight the night before the test (with the exception of patients with diabetes, who may need to fast for only 4 hours before the test and may have juice if needed).

➤ Tell the patient to wear comfortable, loose-fitting clothing, along with sneakers or rubber-soled walking shoes.

➤ Tell the patient you'll need to weigh him before scheduling the procedure.

➤ Explain to the patient that he'll have to ambulate for at least 1 minute after injection of the radioisotope; this means that 1 minute before he reaches peak exercise or fatigue, he'll need to inform the test supervisor or nuclear technologist so that he can receive the injection. Indications include angina; feeling dizzy, fatigued, or short of breath; or leg cramps.

➤ Instruct the patient to resume normal activities after the procedure.

➤ Advise the patient to schedule a follow-up appointment with you to discuss results.

## COMPLICATIONS

➤ *Mild headache* and *chest discomfort* may be experienced but can be relieved with aminophylline.

➤ *MI* or signs of cardiac distress may require inpatient evaluation and treatment.

➤ *Arrhythmias* are treated as indicated by the rhythm.

## SPECIAL CONSIDERATIONS

➤ If necessary, modify the stress portion of the test by adjusting the Bruce protocol to meet the patient's needs.

➤ Keep in mind that, if necessary, the injection of the radioisotope can be made within 10% of the target heart rate.

➤ Remember the following as absolute indications for terminating the exercise portion of the test:
– patient request to stop
– failure of monitoring system
– moderate to severe angina
– increasing nervous symptoms (ataxia, dizziness, or near syncope)
– drop in systolic blood pressure of more than 10 mm Hg from baseline despite an increase in workload, when accompanied by other evidence of ischemia
– sustained ventricular tachycardia
– indications of poor perfusion, including pallor, dyspnea, and dizziness
– ST elevation (greater than 1 mm) in leads without diagnostic Q waves (other than $aV_R$ or $V_1$).

➤ Use the following relative indications for terminating the exercise portion of the test:

– ST or QRS changes, such as excessive ST depression (greater than 2 mm of horizontal or downsloping ST-segment depression) or marked axis shift
– fatigue, shortness of breath, wheezing, or leg cramps
– development of bundle-branch block that can't be distinguished from ventricular tachycardia
– arrhythmias other than sustained ventricular tachycardia, including multifocal premature ventricular contractions (PVCs), triplets of PVCs, supraventricular tachycardia, and onset of second-degree or third-degree heart block
– drop in systolic blood pressure of more than 10 mm Hg from baseline in the absence of ischemia
– hypertensive response (systolic blood pressure greater than 250 mm Hg or diastolic blood pressure greater than 115 mm Hg or both)
➤ Emergency equipment and medications should be readily available.
➤ Referral to a cardiologist may be necessary depending on results.

## DOCUMENTATION

➤ Before the procedure, document underlying comorbidities, medications, risk factors, previous history of coronary artery disease, baseline ECG and blood pressure, presenting symptoms, physical examination results, differential diagnoses, predicted heart rate, stage, and average time to achieve target heart rate correlated with gender and age.
➤ During the procedure, document Borg's rate of perceived exertion, test duration, heart rate achieved at completion of the procedure, blood pressure response (blunted, paradoxical, or hypertensive), indications for terminating the procedure, and arrhythmias.
➤ After the procedure, document any arrhythmias or symptoms that occurred and the length of time for symptoms to resolve,

referral to a cardiologist for an equivocal or positive test, results of the nuclear scan, and diagnosis.

# EMERGENCY PROCEDURES

## Defibrillation

CPT CODE
*92950    Cardiopulmonary resuscitation*

## DESCRIPTION

Always an emergency procedure, defibrillation delivers a controlled, untimed transcutaneous electrical charge to the myocardium, depolarizing the heart muscle and often allowing the sinoatrial node to resume its inherent rhythm. Its effectiveness depends on the amount of elapsed time from cardiac arrest to defibrillation. Because the patient requiring defibrillation is in a pulseless state, the rescuers should continue to perform cardiac compressions between attempts at defibrillation and should also maintain an airway.

Conditions that may contribute to lethal arrhythmias include hypoxia, severe acidosis, and electrolyte imbalance. If possible, the patient should receive treatment for the underlying cause while the resuscitation effort continues.

 **ALERT** Defibrillation is the most important intervention for a patient in ventricular fibrillation or pulseless ventricular tachycardia; the patient's chances of survival decrease with any delay in defibrillation.

## INDICATIONS

➤ To terminate ventricular fibrillation and pulseless ventricular tachycardia

## CONTRAINDICATIONS

None known

## EQUIPMENT

Defibrillator with anterior-posterior or transverse paddles (manual or external automatic defibrillator) ◆ conductive medium pads or gel ◆ electrocardiogram (ECG) monitor with recorder ◆ I.V. line and solution ◆ oxygen administration and suction equipment ◆ oral or nasal airway or intubation equipment ◆ handheld resuscitation bag with 100% oxygen adapter and face mask ◆ emergency drugs, such as epinephrine, atropine, lidocaine, and vasopressors

## ESSENTIAL STEPS

➤ Check that the patient is unresponsive.
➤ Open the airway, and assess for absence of spontaneous breathing.
➤ Provide two full ventilations.
➤ Assess the patient for the absence of a carotid pulse (adult or child) or brachial pulse (infant). .
➤ Call for help and initiate cardiopulmonary resuscitation (CPR) until a monitor and defibrillator are available.
➤ Expose the chest wall.
➤ Apply the ECG monitor leads to the chest wall (avoiding paddle placement sites) or use "quick-look" paddles to determine cardiac rhythm. Quick-look paddles allow for single-lead interpretation of the cardiac rhythm.
➤ Apply conductive pads to the chest wall, using transverse or anterior-posterior placement. If conductive pads aren't available, apply conductive gel to the paddles and place them in the transverse or anterior-

posterior position. For anterolateral placement, place one paddle to the right of the upper sternum, just below the right clavicle, and the other over the fifth or sixth intercostal space at the left anterior axillary line. For anteroposterior placement, place the anterior paddle directly over the heart at the precordium, to the left of the lower sternal border. Place the posterior paddle under the patient's body beneath the heart and immediately below the scapulae (but not under the vertebral column).
➤ Turn on the defibrillator.
➤ Select the appropriate energy level for defibrillation.
➤ Charge the defibrillator for manual defibrillation.
➤ Warn everyone to step back from the patient. Then quickly scan the area to make sure that everyone and all unnecessary equipment are clear of the patient and bed.
➤ Make sure the rhythm is still ventricular fibrillation or pulseless ventricular tachycardia.
➤ Activate the discharge buttons on the paddles of the manual defibrillator, and keep the paddles on the chest wall until the paddles discharge.
➤ Assess the rhythm on the monitor and check the patient for a pulse.
➤ If defibrillation doesn't succeed, repeat three countershocks at increasing energy levels in rapid succession, after making sure everyone and all nonessential equipment are clear of the patient and bed.
➤ If the three rapid countershocks don't succeed, reinitiate CPR, provide manual ventilation, administer emergency drugs, and continue to defibrillate according to advanced cardiac life support (ACLS) protocol while transporting the patient to an acute care facility.
➤ If defibrillation succeeds, assess the patient's vital signs, peripheral pulses, level of consciousness, and respiratory effort. Administer emergency cardiac medications, oxygen or ventilation, and I.V. fluids and

continue cardiac monitoring while transporting the patient to an acute care facility.
➤ Obtain a postdefibrillation ECG rhythm strip or 12-lead ECG.

## PATIENT TEACHING

➤ After successful defibrillation, explain to the patient or family that the patient will be admitted to an acute care facility or a critical care unit.
➤ Explain that the patient may feel muscle soreness for a few days after defibrillation.
➤ Address the patient's and family's other educational needs after the initial crisis has passed.

## COMPLICATIONS

➤ *Chest wall injury or burns:* The patient may require pain management, surgical intervention, rib stabilization, or treatment (such as the application of silver sulfadiazine [Silvadene] to burns) to prevent infection.

## SPECIAL CONSIDERATIONS

➤ Make sure you're familiar with the defibrillator before using it.
➤ As needed, treat hypoxia, hypothermia, and acidosis because these may inhibit the success of defibrillation.
➤ Select correct energy levels sequentially from 200 to 360 joules according to ACLS protocol for external defibrillation in adults. Use 2 joules/kg for children.

 **ALERT** If you've successfully defibrillated a patient at 300 (or 360) joules and now need to defibrillate him again, start at the higher energy level; don't go back to 200 joules.
➤ Maintain about 25 p.s.i. on each paddle during defibrillation.
➤ Try to avoid a pacemaker or implanted cardioverter-defibrillator generator because defibrillating over the device may interfere with its functioning. However, the need for defibrillation takes precedence.

## DOCUMENTATION

➤ Document the patient's ECG, rhythm, and absence of pulse both before and after defibrillation, the time of each defibrillation, the energy levels used, the results of each defibrillation, and all other resuscitation measures used.
➤ Document the final outcome of the resuscitative effort.

# Stabilization of a cardiovascular penetrating injury

CPT CODES
*20101    Exploration of penetrating wound, chest (separate procedure)*
*20103    Exploration of penetrating wound, extremity (separate procedure)*

## DESCRIPTION

Injuries are the most common cause of death for people ages 1 to 44. A large portion of these deaths result from penetrating trauma—gunshot wounds, punctures, lacerations, and amputations. Even if at first assessment a cardiovascular penetrating injury appears insignificant, it's important not to underestimate such an injury, which could rapidly lead to death. However, most penetrating chest injuries aren't fatal, with 75% to 85% of such patients requiring only a chest tube for stabilization. When death does result, it's usually from hemorrhage, making hemostasis the primary treatment goal, followed by immediate surgical intervention if indicated.

 **ALERT** Any patient who presents to an ambulatory setting with a penetrating cardiovascular injury requires immediate assessment and stabilization. Activate the emergency medical services (EMS) system and transport the patient to the nearest hospital for further evaluation.

## INDICATIONS

➤ To stabilize a patient until he can be transported to the appropriate emergency department

## CONTRAINDICATIONS

### Absolute
➤ A patient for whom any delay to stabilize injury would lead to irreparable harm or death

## EQUIPMENT

2 L lactated Ringer's solution ◆ large-bore I.V. catheters (16G to 18G for adults, 18G to 21G for children) and I.V. tubing ◆ 500 to 1,000 ml normal saline solution for irrigation ◆ oxygen with nasal cannula, mask, or rebreather mask ◆ pulse oximeter (if available) ◆ cardiac monitor (if available) ◆ intubation tray and handheld resuscitation bag with mask (if available) ◆ catheter-tip syringe ◆ sterile gloves ◆ mask ◆ gown ◆ goggles ◆ 4″ × 4″ sterile gauze sponges ◆ adhesive tape ◆ sterile drapes ◆ nasogastric (NG) tube (if available) ◆ urinary catheter (if available)

## PREPARATION OF EQUIPMENT

➤ Assemble emergency resuscitation kit and the equipment.
➤ Put on protective equipment, including eyewear, gown, mask, and gloves.

## ESSENTIAL STEPS

➤ Evaluate the patient's ABCs (airway, breathing, and circulation).

➤ Establish an airway, intubate if necessary, and provide ventilation via handheld resuscitation bag and oxygen.
➤ Assess the patient's vital signs and initiate cardiopulmonary resuscitation (CPR), if necessary.
➤ Activate the EMS system, if indicated.
➤ Apply oxygen at high concentration. Use a handheld resuscitation bag and provide oxygenated breaths if needed.
➤ Monitor cardiac rhythm and rate, blood pressure, respiration rate, mental status, and oxygen saturation.
➤ Establish two large-bore I.V. catheters. If possible, use the antecubital fossa, which is the preferred site because of the size of the veins. Perform a venous cutdown if you can't obtain I.V. access using the venipuncture method.
➤ Begin I.V. fluid resuscitation with lactated Ringer's solution, if indicated.
➤ Remove any constricting clothing from the site of the injury.
➤ If you can, provide direct pressure over the wound to control hemorrhage and attempt hemostasis.
➤ If time allows and you suspect major organ trauma, insert an NG tube and urinary catheter.
➤ Transport the patient as soon as possible.
➤ If the patient has an open pneumothorax or sucking chest wound, tape a nonporous dressing around three sides of the wound to allow air to escape during exhalation. This will help prevent a tension pneumothorax.
➤ If the patient has a wound on an extremity, stabilize the extremity in an anatomically correct position. If able, gently irrigate the wound with normal saline solution using a catheter-tip syringe to remove dirt or other debris. Cover the wound with a sterile dressing and apply direct pressure to control bleeding.
➤ Assess for a bruit or thrill, suggesting an arteriovenous fistula; active or pulsatile hemorrhage; pulsatile or expanding hematoma; signs of limb ischemia; and dimin-

ished or absent pulses. Any of these indicates that the patient needs further vascular intervention.

## Patient Teaching

➤ Provide patient teaching after the crisis period, except as the patient's needs and status dictate.
➤ Provide reassurance and emotional support to the patient and family. Give a brief assessment of the situation, severity, potential problems, and need for emergency care.

## Complications

➤ *Arteriovenous fistula or pseudoaneurysm:* Apply pressure and consult a vascular surgeon.
➤ *Intimal tear:* Maintain pressure; the patient may require surgery.
➤ *Hypovolemia or shock:* Replace lost blood and fluids as rapidly as possible and keep the patient warm.
➤ Decompress *tension pneumothorax* with a needle and insert a chest tube.
➤ *Hemothorax:* Insert a chest tube.
➤ *Cardiovascular collapse and shock:* Perform CPR as needed and follow advanced cardiac life support protocols regarding vasopressors and treatments.
➤ *Neurologic impairment or paralysis:* Immobilize the patient and consult a neurologist. The patient requires rehabilitation.

## Special Considerations

➤ Elicit a history of recent alcohol or drug use, past medical history, allergies, mechanism of injury, use of seat belts (if relevant), and use of anticoagulant therapy in your assessment.
➤ Leave any impaled object in place and stabilize it with a dressing. Carefully protect the object during transport.
➤ Keep in mind that few prehospital interventions exist for suspected hemothorax,

tension pneumothorax, and cardiac tamponade except support and careful assessment.
➤ Delayed diagnosis and treatment of severe peripheral vascular injury may result in thrombosis, embolization, or hemorrhage.
➤ Consider penetrating peripheral vascular injuries to the following areas high risk for developing complications if not treated early:
–*lower extremity:* inguinal region, medial thigh, and popliteal fossa
–*upper extremity:* axilla, medial or anterior upper arm region, and antecubital fossa. As a general rule, extremity tissues can tolerate up to 6 hours of ischemia.

## Documentation

➤ Document the initial presentation of the patient, the mechanism of injury, the initial assessment (vital signs, mental status, and location of injury), a secondary assessment (vital signs, mental status, pulse oximetry, breath sounds, and presence of pulses), past medical history, alcohol or drug use, treatments performed, and patient response.
➤ Note the disposition of the patient and his condition on transport.

# INVASIVE PROCEDURES

## Arterial line placement

CPT CODE
*36620   Arterial catheterization or cannulation for sampling, monitoring, or transfusion (separate procedure); percutaneous*

# DESCRIPTION

Direct arterial pressure monitoring permits continuous measurement of systolic, diastolic, and mean pressures and allows arterial blood sampling. Because direct measurement reflects systemic vascular resistance as well as blood flow, it's generally more accurate than indirect methods (such as palpation and auscultation of Korotkoff's, or audible pulse, sounds), which are based on blood flow.

An arterial line may be inserted to perform arterial dye studies, monitor vital signs, or provide access for obtaining blood samples. Radial arteries are preferred because they're relatively easy to access, lack excessive organisms, and allow the patient more freedom of motion. However, the femoral and dorsalis pedis arteries can also be used.

## INDICATIONS

➤ To allow constant blood pressure monitoring
➤ To provide continuous access for blood samples, especially for tests that require arterial samples, such as arterial blood gas analysis
➤ To provide accurate blood pressure readings in patients receiving potent dilators or pressors

## CONTRAINDICATIONS

### Absolute
➤ Severe injury to the extremity
➤ Positive Allen's test
➤ Injury proximal to the vessel
➤ Local skin compromise

### Relative
➤ Atherosclerotic or vasospastic arterial disease
➤ Hypercoagulable state

# EQUIPMENT

Arterial line catheter ◆ 4″ × 4″ gauze pads ◆ alcohol swab ◆ povidone-iodine solution ◆ sterile gloves ◆ rolled towel ◆ tape ◆ site care kit (containing sterile dressing, antimicrobial ointment, and hypoallergenic tape) ◆ 1% lidocaine ◆ 5-ml syringe ◆ 25G ⅝″ needle ◆ gown and mask ◆ protective eyewear ◆ sterile drapes ◆ prepared pressure transducer system ◆ linen saver pad

# PREPARATION OF EQUIPMENT

➤ Before setting up and priming the monitoring system, wash your hands thoroughly. Wear personal protective equipment throughout the procedure.
➤ Set the alarms on the bedside monitor according to your facility's policy.

# ESSENTIAL STEPS

➤ Explain the procedure to the patient, including its benefits and risks. Obtain informed consent.
➤ Maintain aseptic technique throughout the procedure.
➤ For a radial artery insertion, position the patient on his back, with his nondominant arm extended, palm up. Perform Allen's test; choose a different site if vascular compromise is detected. Place a linen-saver pad under the site. Put a rolled towel beneath the dorsum of the wrist, and gently tape across the fingers to secure the hand.
➤ Clean the area with an alcohol swab; use a circular motion, moving outward from the site.
➤ Anesthetize the skin over the site of planned insertion with lidocaine using the 5-ml syringe and 25G ⅝″ needle.
➤ Put on sterile gloves.
➤ Use povidone-iodine solution and gauze to clean the area over the radial artery.

➤ Cover the area surrounding the insertion site with sterile drapes or towels.

➤ Palpate and immobilize the artery with two to three fingers of one hand while holding the needle over the puncture site with the other.

➤ Puncture the skin at a 45- to 60-degree angle and access the artery with the needle. A bright red flashback indicates arterial puncture. If your first attempt isn't successful, withdraw the needle to just below the surface of the skin and advance the needle at the same angle but at 1 mm to either side of the previous attempt.

➤ Grasp the cannula hub to hold it in the artery, and withdraw the needle as you advance the cannula up to the hub.

➤ Attach the pressure transducer system and flush the catheter. Visually assess the waveform on the monitor.

➤ Suture the catheter in place, or secure it with tape.

➤ Using the site care kit, apply antimicrobial ointment and cover the insertion site with a dressing.

➤ Immobilize the insertion site. With a radial or brachial site, use an arm board and a soft wrist restraint (if the patient's condition requires). With a femoral site, assess the need for an ankle restraint; maintain the patient on bed rest, with the head of the bed raised no more than 30 degrees to prevent the catheter from kinking.

➤ Level the zeroing stopcock of the transducer with phlebostatis axis. Then zero the system to atmospheric pressure.

➤ Activate the monitor alarms, as appropriate.

## PATIENT TEACHING

➤ Tell the patient that pain associated with this procedure typically resolves quickly but that the site may remain sore or the vessel may have spasms for up to 2 days later.

➤ Tell the patient that he'll initially feel a sting but that it should resolve quickly. Assure him that you'll anesthetize the area before beginning the procedure.

➤ If the patient is alert, tell him to remain still to maintain the integrity of the dressing and the position of the wrist.

## COMPLICATIONS

➤ *Local infection or sepsis* may require antibiotic ointment or a systemic antibiotic.

➤ *Nerve damage:* The patient may require physical therapy or rehabilitation.

➤ *Hematoma:* Apply pressure; warm compresses can help relieve discomfort.

➤ *Tissue necrosis with ischemia distal to the insertion:* The patient may require surgical intervention.

➤ *Embolism or arterial thrombosis:* The patient may need surgical intervention or systemic anticoagulation therapy.

➤ *Aneurysm:* The patient may require ultrasonic compression or surgical intervention.

## SPECIAL CONSIDERATIONS

➤ If the patient is noncompliant or can't hold still, have another person maintain the arm's position.

➤ Observing the pressure waveform on the monitor can enhance assessment of arterial pressure. An abnormal waveform may reflect an arrhythmia (such as atrial fibrillation) or other cardiac problems, such as aortic stenosis, aortic insufficiency, pulsus alternans, or pulsus paradoxus.

➤ Be aware that erroneous pressure readings may result from a catheter that is clotted or from positional, loose connections; addition of extra stopcocks or extension tubing; inadvertent entry of air into the system; or improper calibration, leveling, or zeroing of the monitoring system. If the catheter lumen clots, the flush system may be improperly pressurized.

## DOCUMENTATION

➤ Document the need for the procedure and the patient's status, including Allen's test results if cannulating the radial artery.
➤ Document the waveform, site of insertion, and needle size.
➤ Record the patient's condition after the procedure, including systolic, diastolic, and mean pressures as well as circulation in the extremity distal to the site, which is determined by assessing color, pulses, and sensation.

## Femoral sheath removal

**CPT CODE**
No specific code has been assigned.

## DESCRIPTION

Sometimes after cardiac catheterization, a sheath (a large-bore device for venous access similar to a central venous catheter introducer) is left in the femoral vessel until the activated clotting time (ACT) is below 150 to 180 seconds, depending on your protocol. Femoral sheaths vary in size from #5 or #6 French (small) to #8 or #9 French (large). Generally speaking, the bigger the sheath, the longer the procedure, and the more catheter changes there were, the longer the compression time should be after removal of a femoral device.

## INDICATIONS

➤ To terminate the sheath when coagulation times return to acceptable range: ACT greater than 150 to 180 seconds (depending on protocol) after cardiac catheterization

## CONTRAINDICATIONS

**Relative**
➤ Coagulopathy

## EQUIPMENT

Drape ◆ Gauze pads ◆ povidone-iodine solution ◆ two to four packages of 4″ × 4″ cotton gauze ◆ #11 scalpel or suture removal kit ◆ linen-saver pad ◆ clean and sterile gloves ◆ gown and mask ◆ protective eyewear ◆ bacitracin ointment ◆ adhesive bandage ◆ compression clamp with compression disk (optional) ◆ 10-lb sandbag covered with a pillowcase (optional)

## ESSENTIAL STEPS

➤ Check laboratory results for prothrombin, partial thromboplastin, or actual clotting time and platelet count before removing any femoral device to avoid unnecessary bleeding. Remove the device when the international normalized ratio is less than 1.8 seconds, the ACT is less than 150 to 180 seconds, or the platelet count is greater than 100 to 200 × 10³/µl (per protocol).
➤ Explain the procedure to the patient. Administer an analgesic and an anxiolytic (such as oxycodone or midazolam) 20 to 30 minutes before the procedure.
➤ Wash your hands and put on gown, mask, and protective eyewear. Maintain aseptic technique throughout the procedure.
➤ Close the curtain or door and drape the area to provide privacy.
➤ Place the linen-saver pad on the patient below the level of the sheath. Place your equipment on the pad.
➤ Wearing clean gloves, remove and discard the dressing.
➤ If you're using a compression clamp, position it under the mattress at the level of the patient's hip so that the arm of the compression clamp reaches over the arterial puncture site. The patient may need

to be moved closer to the bed's edge to better accommodate the length of the compression clamp's arm.

➤ Put on sterile gloves and use the scalpel blade or scissors from the suture removal kit to cut and remove the retention suture.

➤ Use povidone-iodine solution to clean the femoral area over and around the sheath, moving outward in concentric circles. Allow the skin to dry.

➤ Apply firm pressure inferior to and just superior to the puncture site with several folded 4″ × 4″ cotton gauze pads, and pull the sheath out with one steady motion.

➤ Hold firm pressure at the site, occluding the vessel for several minutes. If you're applying manual pressure only, maintain pressure for another 15 to 40 minutes, depending on the size of the sheath removed and the duration of femoral artery cannulation.

➤ If you're using a compression clamp, apply it to the femoral site after several minutes of manual pressure, when bleeding is controlled. Apply the clamp arm loaded with a compression disk just above the puncture site, leaving the folded 4″ × 4″ gauze pad over the site and under the disk. Tighten the compression clamp, obliterating distal pulses for 1 or 2 minutes. Then gradually release pressure until distal pulses are palpable, keeping pressure firm enough to prevent arterial bleeding or oozing at the site.

➤ Leave the clamp in place for 15 to 60 minutes. Generally, the larger the diameter of the device and the longer the cannulation time, the longer pressure needs to be held over the site.

➤ Order frequent vital signs and leg checks for color, temperature, and pulses. The compression clamp may be loosened slightly if needed to ensure palpable arterial pulses at all times.

 **ALERT** Move the compression device laterally if distal venous congestion occurs. This measurement will release pressure on the femoral vein.

➤ If the patient complains of neurogenic pain, position the clamp more medially to release pressure on the femoral nerve.

➤ Release the compression clamp slowly and steadily. Reapply pressure as needed if bleeding starts again.

➤ Once you've released the clamp or manual pressure, apply bacitracin ointment and an adhesive bandage over the site.

➤ To help promote hemostasis after compression and serve as a reminder to the patient to keep his leg straight and still, you can place the covered 10-lb sandbag over the site.

➤ Wash your hands.

➤ Order vital sign assessment of the affected limb, including pulse, color, and temperature, every 15 minutes for the first hour, with a note to report abnormal findings at once. Routine follow-up orders then include vital sign, groin, and leg checks every 30 minutes for the next 2 hours, then every hour for 4 hours, and then every 4 hours for 16 hours.

➤ Remove the sandbag, and inspect the groin site for local complications, including hematoma, bleeding, arteriovenous fistula, and pseudoaneurysm, as part of the groin and leg checks.

## PATIENT TEACHING

➤ Tell the patient that he'll receive pain medication so that he should feel minimal discomfort during the procedure.

➤ Explain the procedure before removing the femoral sheath. Let the patient know that he'll feel some discomfort and tenderness at the site and that the pressure (necessary to achieve hemostasis) can also feel uncomfortable.

➤ Tell the patient he must keep his head flat on the bed; raising his head would increase pressure in the groin area and possibly lead to bleeding. Explain that after removal of the sheath, the head of the bed must remain at less than 45 degrees until the patient is allowed out of bed.

➤ Direct the patient to report any warmth or wetness at the site while he's on bed rest, an indication of bleeding that calls for the reapplication of pressure.

➤ Tell the patient to immediately report any progressively enlarging mass at the site that occurs over the next 2 weeks; a flat bruise may be expected.

## COMPLICATIONS

 **ALERT** Removing the femoral sheath may induce a *vasovagal response* in some patients, causing hypotension or bradycardia or both. Be prepared to administer atropine for sustained bradycardia or an I.V. fluid bolus for persistent hypotension.

➤ Indicated by a pulsatile mass over the artery, *pseudoaneurysm* causes local tenderness, ecchymosis of surrounding tissue, and systolic bruit. Ultrasound confirms the diagnosis, and ultrasound-guided sonography can successfully compress the pseudoaneurysm about 85% of the time. The remaining 15% require surgical repair.

➤ An *arteriovenous fistula* causes systolic or diastolic bruit or both, but it doesn't cause a pulsatile mass and usually doesn't cause ecchymosis. It requires monitoring and possibly surgical repair.

➤ *Uncontrolled bleeding:* Reapply pressure over the site for another 10 to 20 minutes. Significant blood loss requires transfusion, so the patient may need typing and crossmatching.

➤ *Hematoma:* Mark the edges with a pen and have the size monitored at each vital sign and site check. If the hematoma doesn't enlarge, it's probably benign, unless the patient develops blood loss (signs of hypovolemia include low blood pressure, shock, light-headedness, dizziness, decreased pulse oximetry readings, tachycardia, pallor, and diaphoresis) or such symp-

toms as sharp pain or a palpable mass (which might indicate arterial thrombosis). Serial examinations should ideally reveal slow and steady resolution of the hematoma.

➤ If *arterial laceration with retroperitoneal bleeding* is significant, a potentially life-threatening problem occurs: Notify your collaborative physician and consult a vascular surgeon at once. Order typing and crossmatching for transfusion of packed cells, assess the patient's vital signs frequently, and replace volume as necessary.

➤ *Arterial thrombosis or peripheral embolization and limb ischemia:* The affected extremity looks pale and mottled and is pulseless, cold, and painful. This complication requires anticoagulation therapy until the patient's body can reabsorb the thrombus. Order frequent pulse checks and a vascular consultation.

➤ Proper clamp placement should prevent *femoral neuropathy.* If the patient does complain of pain or numbness over the compression site, reposition the clamp as necessary. Femoral neuropathy may be temporary or permanent. Physical therapy may be helpful for some patients.

➤ To help prevent *infection,* use aseptic technique when removing devices and changing dressings. If the patient develops erythema, purulent drainage, or fever, obtain a culture specimen from the wound bed and begin broad-spectrum antibiotic therapy while you wait for culture and sensitivity results.

## SPECIAL CONSIDERATIONS

 **ALERT** You may find erythema difficult to assess in a dark-skinned patient; make sure you palpate the area for warmth. Pallor in a dark-skinned patient produces an ashen-gray color.

➤ Because most patients find the compression clamp very uncomfortable, provide analgesics, such as oxycodone, and anxiolytics, such as midazolam, as needed during this time.

➤ Although the duration of bed rest may vary, it usually isn't less than 6 hours. Consider longer bed rest for longer procedures, for procedures performed with a large-French sheath catheter, or for instances when many catheter changes have been performed.

➤ Keep in mind that a flat bruise that spreads gradually isn't necessarily clinically significant if the patient has no other signs and symptoms of vascular compromise, such as sharp pain or a palpable mass, and vital signs remains stable.

➤ Remember that the risk of complications increases with age, female gender, thrombolytic therapy, postprocedural anticoagulation, decreased platelet count, a faulty low cannulation site, and multiple procedures.

## DOCUMENTATION

➤ Document the procedure, the patient's vital signs before and after the procedure, the initial groin site, the leg appearance and presence of distal pulses, and the patient's response to the procedure.

➤ Include the method and duration of manual or mechanical compression, and indicate whether you used a sandbag.

➤ Record type and amount of analgesia or sedation given to the patient.

➤ Indicate any complications and actions taken.

## Intra-aortic balloon removal

CPT CODE
No specific code has been assigned.

## DESCRIPTION

The intra-aortic balloon pump (IABP) provides mechanical circulatory support for the failing myocardium. The counterpulsation action of the IABP improves cardiac output by decreasing afterload and increasing coronary artery perfusion during diastole and by displacing blood toward the periphery. The patient should have a stable heart rate and rhythm, mean pulmonary artery and wedge pressures, stable mixed venous oxygen saturation, and a urine output of least 30 ml/hour. The balloon must be kept in motion at all times before removal to prevent the development of clots on and around the catheter.

## INDICATIONS

➤ To terminate therapy when cardiac output is stable, the IABP counterpulsation ratio is 1:3, and hemodynamics are stable (see *Optimal hemodynamic parameters for intra-aortic balloon removal*)

➤ To replace a malfunctioning intra-aortic balloon

## CONTRAINDICATIONS

### Absolute

➤ Electrolyte, hemoglobin, and hematocrit values abnormal

➤ Arrhythmia present

➤ Deterioration during weaning to preinsertion clinical and hemodynamic parameters

➤ Abnormal blood pressure, heart rate, cardiac output, and cardiac index

➤ Chest X-ray revealing congestion

## EQUIPMENT

#11 scalpel or suture removal kit ◆ povidone-iodine solution ◆ two to four packages of 4″ × 4″ gauze pads ◆ clean and sterile gloves ◆ gown and mask ◆ protective eyewear ◆ absorbent pad to set supplies on and to collect drainage ◆ bacitracin ointment ◆ adhesive bandage ◆ compression clamp with compression disk (optional) ◆ 10-lb sandbag with a pillowcase (optional)

## ESSENTIAL STEPS

➤ Make sure that the international normalized ratio is less than 1.8 seconds, the activated clotting time is less than 150 to 180 seconds (depending on protocol), and the platelet count is greater than 100 to 200 × 10³/µl (per protocol) before removing the device.
➤ Discontinue I.V. anticoagulation 4 to 6 hours before removal or until all of the above values are reached.
➤ Explain the procedure to the patient.
➤ Administer an analgesic and an anxiolytic (such as oxycodone or midazolam) before the procedure.
➤ Close the curtain or door, and drape the patient to provide privacy.
➤ Wash your hands and put on the gown, mask, and protective eyewear. Maintain aseptic technique.
➤ Place an absorbent pad on the bed, over the patient, and below the balloon insertion site. Arrange your supplies on the pad.
➤ If you're using a mechanical compression clamp, place it under the mattress at the level of the patient's hip. If necessary, move the patient closer to the edge of the bed to accommodate the length of the clamp arm.
➤ Wearing clean gloves, remove and dispose of the dressing.
➤ Open your supplies, and put on sterile gloves. Clean the area over and around the femoral cannulation site with gauze soaked in povidone-iodine, moving outward in concentric circles. Allow the area to dry.
➤ Use the scalpel blade or scissors from the suture removal kit to cut the suture holding the balloon and sheath in place.
➤ Turn off the balloon pump and disconnect the tubing from the balloon to allow any remaining air to escape passively from

### OPTIMAL HEMODYNAMIC PARAMETERS FOR INTRA-AORTIC BALLOON REMOVAL

After vasoactive drugs have been discontinued, these hemodynamic values must be achieved before removal of the intra-aortic balloon.

| PARAMETER | VALUE |
|---|---|
| Systolic arterial pressure | > 90 mm Hg |
| Cardiac index | > 2 L/min/m² |
| Systemic vascular resistance | < 2,100 dynes/sec/cm⁻⁵ |
| Heart rate | < baseline, no arrhythmias |
| Pulmonary capillary wedge pressure | < 18 mm Hg |

the balloon. Alternatively, use a syringe to withdraw any remaining air from the balloon.

 **ALERT** Once you've turned off the balloon pump, you must remove the balloon promptly to prevent the development of clots on the inactive balloon.
➤ Remove the balloon and sheath with one slow, steady motion.
➤ If you're applying manual pressure only, maintain pressure for 1 to 2 minutes to ensure hemostasis and control of the artery. Release pressure gradually until the distal foot pulses become palpable.
➤ If you're using a compression clamp, release it slowly and steadily.
➤ Nonocclusive manual pressure or the compression clamp is used for another 50 minutes or longer.
➤ Occlusive pressure is reapplied for 1 to 2 minutes if bleeding reoccurs.

➤ Once you've released the clamp or manual pressure, apply bacitracin ointment and an adhesive bandage over the site.

➤ To help promote hemostasis and serve as a reminder to the patient to keep his limb straight and still, you can place the 10-lb sandbag over the site.

➤ Wash your hands.

➤ Order vital sign checks, including the patient's distal pulse, color, and temperature, and assessment of the insertion site for hematoma or bleeding every 15 minutes for the first hour, every 30 minutes for 2 hours, and then every 4 hours for 16 hours.

## PATIENT TEACHING

➤ Tell the patient he will feel some discomfort during the procedure.

➤ Tell the patient he must lie flat for the duration of compression and for at least 24 hours after that. He must keep his head flat to avoid any increase in pressure in the groin, which could lead to bleeding.

➤ Direct the patient to report any warmth or wetness at the groin, which could indicate further bleeding.

## COMPLICATIONS

 **ALERT** Removing a femoral device may induce a **vasovagal response** in some patients, causing hypotension or bradycardia. Be prepared to administer atropine for sustained bradycardia or an I.V. fluid bolus for persistent hypotension.

➤ *Ischemic limb:* Slowly release compression on the limb. If ischemia remains, consult with a vascular surgeon. The patient may need to receive anticoagulation and may require a thrombectomy.

➤ Keep the area clean and dry after decannulation to avoid *infection.* Use aseptic technique to remove the device and for dressing changes. If you note erythema, purulent drainage, or fever, suspect infection. Collect a culture specimen from the wound bed, and begin broad-spectrum antibiotic therapy while awaiting culture and sensitivity results.

➤ Indications for *pseudoaneurysm* include an enlarged pulsatile mass over the arterial site, with ecchymosis and a systolic bruit. Ultrasound confirms the diagnosis, and ultrasound-guided sonography can successfully compress the pseudoaneurysm about 85% of the time. The remaining 15% require surgical arterial repair.

➤ Second in frequency only to pseudoaneurysm, *arteriovenous fistula* causes systolic or diastolic bruits or both but without a pulsatile mass and usually without significant ecchymosis. The condition may require surgical repair.

➤ *Uncontrolled bleeding:* Reapply pressure over the site for another 10 to 20 minutes until bleeding completely stops. Significant blood loss may require transfusion of packed cells.

➤ *Arterial laceration and retroperitoneal bleeding* requires immediate consultation with a vascular surgeon. Order typing and crossmatching for transfusion of packed cells, replace volume as necessary, and provide symptomatic support.

➤ Symptoms of *arterial thrombus and peripheral embolism* include a lack of pulse, pallor, paresthesia, and pain in the extremity. Begin anticoagulation according to the physician's specifications, and consult a vascular surgeon. Order frequent assessments of the affected area and vital signs, and provide pain relief.

➤ Careful clamp positioning during compression should prevent *femoral neuropathy.* Reposition the clamp medially to relieve pressure on the nerve. Femoral neuropathy may be temporary or permanent. Some patients may benefit from physical therapy.

➤ *Ischemic bowel* requires surgical consultation and probable surgery. Early recognition is essential; assess for abdominal pain perceived as more painful than elicited on examination, guarding of the abdomen, and lack of bowel sounds.

## SPECIAL CONSIDERATIONS

 **ALERT** If the balloon was inserted by direct cutdown method, don't attempt to remove the balloon. The balloon must be removed in conjunction with operative repair of the femoral artery.

➤ Note any resistance during removal of the balloon. If you feel resistance, try twisting the catheter slightly and attempting to withdraw it again. If resistance persists, stop your attempts and ask for immediate assistance from the collaborative physician or consulted vascular surgeon. The patient must have the device removed promptly to avoid complications. If this occurs, continue to assess for leg pulses, color, temperature, and sensation in the affected extremity as well as for hemostasis.

➤ After withdrawing the tip of the balloon, some practitioners hold pressure distally to the insertion site only, allowing the free flow of blood out of the leg for several seconds, followed by constant proximal pressure on the vessel. The purpose is to divert potential clots out of the body instead of into the leg, but this practice and its usefulness remain controversial.

➤ If you're using a sandbag on the groin after removal of the balloon, remember to look under the bag when assessing the groin because the sandbag may prevent the patient from noticing active bleeding at the site.

➤ Assess for complications such as pseudoaneurysm or arteriovenous fistula for up to 1 week after removal of the device.

## DOCUMENTATION

➤ Document the procedure, vital signs, distal pulses, and leg color before and after the procedure and how the patient tolerated the procedure.

➤ Describe the method of femoral compression and millimeters of pressure used to maintain compression (if indicated on the compression device). Note whether you used a sandbag.

➤ Indicate any complications and treatment provided if indicated.

## Peripherally inserted central catheter insertion

**CPT CODE**
*36489   Placement of central venous catheter (subclavian, jugular, or other vein) percutaneous, age 2 or older*

## DESCRIPTION

For a patient who requires I.V. therapy for 5 days to 3 months or who requires repeated venous access, a peripherally inserted central catheter (PICC) line may be a good option. A PICC line also may be ideal for a patient who has suffered trauma or burns resulting in chest injury, has a coagulopathy, or is at increased risk for developing complications from central venous access. With any of these conditions, a PICC line helps avoid complications that may occur with a central venous catheter (CVC). The device is also easier to insert than a CVC and provides safe, reliable access for medications and blood sampling. A single catheter may be used for the entire course of therapy (less than 3 months), with greater convenience and at a lower cost than CVCs.

Made of silicone or polyurethane, PICCs range from 16G to 23G in diameter and from 16″ to 24″ (41 to 61 cm) in length. They're radiopaque and nonpyrogenic and come in single- and double-lumen versions, with and without a guide wire. A guide wire stiffens the catheter, easing its advancement through the vein, but it can damage the vessel if improperly used. A PICC line allows infusion of medications, total parenteral nutrition, chemotherapy, antibiotics, narcotics, analgesics, blood products, and inotropic agents.

A PICC offers the most advantage when introduced early in treatment. It shouldn't be considered a last resort for a patient with sclerotic or repeatedly punctured veins. A patient considered for PICC therapy must have a peripheral vein large enough to accept a 14G or 16G introducer needle and a 3.8G to 4.8G catheter. The PICC is inserted via the basilic, median antecubital, cubital, or cephalic vein. It's then threaded to the superior vena cava or subclavian vein, although it can also be advanced to a non-central site, such as the axillary vein.

## INDICATIONS

➤ To provide continuous or intermittent I.V. therapy for 3 months or less
➤ To infuse medications or solutions that can lead to peripheral vein sclerosis, inflammation, and irritation

## CONTRAINDICATIONS

### Absolute
➤ Conditions that impede venous return from the arms, such as paralysis, dialysis, grafts, or lymphedema after mastectomy
➤ Venous thrombosis or infection in the intended vein
➤ Orthopedic or neurologic conditions that affect the intended arm
➤ Lack of surface anatomy secondary to obesity or edema
➤ Extremity that may receive graft placement

### Relative
➤ Indefinite duration infusion needs
➤ Need for blood pressure monitoring

## EQUIPMENT

PICC insertion kit ◆ three alcohol and povidone-iodine swabs ◆ povidone-iodine ointment ◆ vial of heparin (100 units/ml) ◆ latex injection port with short extension tubing for each lumen ◆ sterile and nonsterile measuring tape ◆ vial of normal saline solution for injection ◆ syringes (5 ml) and needles ◆ sterile gauze pads (2 containers) ◆ tape ◆ linen-saver pad ◆ sterile drapes ◆ tourniquet or blood pressure cuff ◆ sterile transparent semipermeable dressing ◆ two pairs of sterile gloves ◆ sterile gown ◆ mask ◆ goggles ◆ local anesthetic (such as 1% lidocaine) ◆ 3-ml syringe ◆ 25G 1" needle (optional)

## ESSENTIAL STEPS

➤ Explain the procedure to the patient, answer all questions, and obtain informed consent.
➤ Check the expiration dates on all sterile packages and solutions.
➤ Wash your hands and maintain aseptic technique.
➤ Position the patient supine, with the head of the bed raised to about 30 degrees. Position the patient's nondominant arm (use the dominant arm if necessary) at a 45- to 90-degree angle from his body, and place a linen-saver pad under his arm.
➤ Assess each antecubital fossa for an appropriate vein. Tie a tourniquet around the upper arm to enhance venous dilation and improve visualization and palpation of the vessels. Locate the brachial artery to avoid puncturing it inadvertently.
➤ Once you've located a vein, remove the tourniquet.
➤ Determine the length of catheter to insert. Take the nonsterile measuring tape and measure the distance from the insertion site to the shoulder and then from the shoulder to the sternal notch. (See *Determining PICC length*.)

➤ Open the PICC insertion kit. Open and drop the other sterile supplies onto a sterile field. Draw up several normal saline flushes, using sterile technique. Put on the mask, goggles, and sterile gown and gloves.

➤ Cut the distal end of the catheter to the appropriate length (determine length by using the sterile measuring tape).

 **ALERT** Don't cut the tip at an angle. Doing so may cause the catheter to lie against the vessel wall and possibly obstruct the infusion flow. Inspect the tip to ensure that there are no loose fragments.

➤ Using sterile technique, withdraw 5 ml of the normal saline solution and flush the extension tubing and the cap.

➤ Remove the needle from the syringe. Attach the syringe to the hub of the catheter and prime each lumen of the PICC.

➤ Set the PICC, cap, and tubing aside on the sterile field.

➤ Prepare the insertion site by cleaning the area with three alcohol swabs. Using a circular motion, scrub outward from the intended site about 6″ (15.2 cm). Repeat the process with three povidone-iodine swabs for a total of 2 minutes. Pat the area dry with sterile gauze pads.

 **ALERT** Make sure you use the alcohol first, followed by the povidone-iodine. Using alcohol after povidone-iodine cancels the effect of the povidone-iodine.

➤ Remove the sterile gloves. Tie a tourniquet around the arm about 4″ (10 cm) above the antecubital fossa.

➤ Put on a new pair of sterile gloves. Place a sterile drape under the patient's arm and on top of the arm distal to the insertion site. Drop a sterile 4″ × 4″ gauze pad over the tourniquet.

➤ Administer a local anesthetic (such as lidocaine), if needed. Inject 0.5 ml of 1% lidocaine intradermally, slightly distal to the site, forming a small intradermal bleb.

➤ Stabilize the vein with two fingers and insert the catheter introducer into the bleb,

## DETERMINING PICC LENGTH

To determine the length of a peripherally inserted central catheter (PICC), first determine where the catheter tip will rest after insertion. For subclavian vein placement, use the nonsterile measuring tape to measure the distance from the insertion site to the shoulder and from the shoulder to the sternal notch. For placement in the superior vena cava, add 3″ (7.6 cm) to this number.

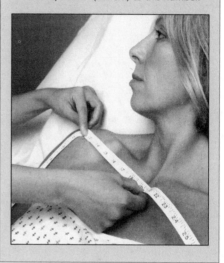

tunneling upward toward the vein at a 10-degree angle.

➤ You will see blood return in the flashback chamber once you've accessed the vein. At this point, gently advance the introducer until the tip is well within the vein.

➤ Carefully withdraw the needle, holding the introducer firmly in place. Apply pressure on the vein just beyond the distal end of the introducer sheath to minimize bleeding.

➤ Using sterile forceps, insert the PICC into the introducer sheath and advance the catheter into the vein. Loosen the tourniquet using the sterile gauze pad.

➤ Continue advancing the catheter. Once you've reached the shoulder, have the patient turn his head toward the insertion

## PLACING A PICC

When you place a peripherally inserted central catheter (PICC), you'll typically insert it into the basilic or cephalic vein and then thread it up toward the heart, as shown.

The tip of the PICC should rest in central circulation, typically the superior vena cava, as shown, or the subclavian vein.

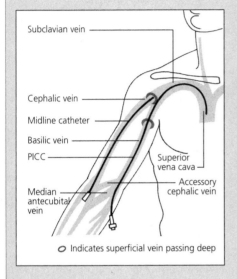

Subclavian vein

Cephalic vein

Midline catheter

Basilic vein

PICC

Superior vena cava

Accessory cephalic vein

Median antecubital vein

○ Indicates superficial vein passing deep

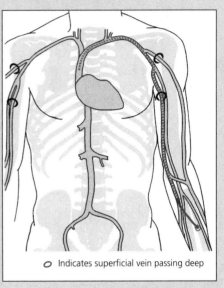

○ Indicates superficial vein passing deep

arm and place his chin on his chest. This will occlude the jugular vein and promote catheter advancement into the subclavian vein. (See *Placing a PICC.*)

 **ALERT** Don't advance the catheter if you meet resistance. Applying excessive force could perforate the vein or myocardium. If you're unsure about placement, send the patient to an interventional radiology department for fluoroscopic insertion of the catheter or remove the catheter.

➤ Advance the catheter until 4″ (10 cm) remain outside the skin. Pull the introducer sheath completely out of the vein and away from the insertion site.

➤ Grasp the tabs of the introducer sheath and flex them toward its distal end to split the sheath. Discard the sheath.

➤ Continue to advance the catheter until about 2″ (5 cm) remain exposed. Flush the

catheter with normal saline solution and instill 2 ml of the heparin.

➤ Attach the latex cap and extension tubing to the catheter. Position the patient's arm below heart level and clamp the lumen to prevent air from entering the catheter.

➤ Place a dab of povidone-iodine ointment at the insertion site. Place a sterile, occlusive dressing on the insertion site using sterile gauze and transparent dressing. Leave the first dressing in place for 24 hours as appropriate. Order dressing changes every 7 days thereafter for a hospitalized patient (or as per hospital policy) and every 5 to 7 days for an outpatient.

➤ If desired, you may suture the distal end of the PICC with one suture. Tie one loose loop through the skin using nylon suture material. Then tie the suture around the catheter, taking care not to occlude the lumen of the line.

➤ Secure the extension tubing to allow for adequate arm movement.
➤ If you advanced the catheter to a central vein, obtain a chest X-ray to confirm catheter tip position before using. If you didn't advance the catheter to a central vein, the patient doesn't need an X-ray.

## PATIENT TEACHING

➤ Reinforce to the patient that the PICC will remain in place for the duration of the I.V. medication therapy.
➤ Reassure the patient that the catheter won't restrict arm movement.
➤ Direct the patient to avoid strenuous activities that use the arm, such as tennis, golf, or weight lifting. (See *Caring for your catheter,* page 52.)

## COMPLICATIONS

➤ *Phlebitis:* Apply warm compresses.
➤ *Air embolism:* Immediately turn the patient to the left lateral Trendelenburg position and aspirate the air.
➤ *Malposition or migration of the catheter:* Adjust or remove the catheter.
➤ *Catheter occlusion:* First try to flush the catheter with heparin or saline solution. If the catheter is still occluded, try to clear the obstruction by instilling 2.5 mg tissue plasminogen activator (tPA) in the catheter and allowing it to dwell there for 1 to 2 hours. Then withdraw the solution and try to access the catheter again. If this doesn't work, the patient may need the catheter removed.
➤ *Localized pain:* Apply warm compresses to the site and give the patient acetaminophen.
➤ *Hematoma:* Apply pressure to the site.
➤ *Infection, bacteremia, or sepsis:* For a local infection, apply an antibiotic ointment. For a suspected infection, draw blood from the line for culturing and administer a broad-spectrum antibiotic until you get the results. If the line is infect-

ed, remove it and administer systemic antibiotics.
➤ *Vein thrombosis:* Begin anticoagulant therapy.

## SPECIAL CONSIDERATIONS

➤ How much fluid you need to prime the catheter depends on the diameter of the lumen and the length of the catheter. Check the manufacturer's guidelines for the exact volume you'll need to prime the catheter.
➤ For a hospitalized patient receiving intermittent PICC therapy, flush the catheter with 6 ml of normal saline solution before and after each use and 2 ml of heparin (100 units/ml) after each use. For a catheter not being used, a weekly flush of 2 ml of heparin (1,000 units/ml) will maintain patency. Refer to hospital or home health agency policies regarding frequency of flushing.

 **ALERT** When accessing a port not currently in use, withdraw any dwelling solution to avoid inadvertent administration of heparin.
➤ Add an extension tubing set to all PICC lines so that an infusion can be started and stopped distal to the infusion site. An extension set will also make using the PICC easier for the patient who'll be administering infusions or medications himself.
➤ Assess the insertion site through the transparent semipermeable dressing every 24 hours. Check the site for bleeding, redness, drainage, and swelling. Ask your patient if he's having any pain associated with infusions.

## DOCUMENTATION

➤ Document the indications for the procedure.
➤ Document the entire procedure, including any problems encountered during catheter placement. Include the size and type of catheter, lumen size, and length of catheter inserted as well as the length from

## CARING FOR YOUR CATHETER

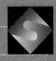

DEAR PATIENT:

You have a special catheter inserted into one of the major blood vessels of your body. Now that it's in place, you need to know how to spot potential problems and care for your catheter.

### Potential problems

Occasionally, a problem can develop with the catheter. Below are potential complications to watch for.

➤ *Bleeding*: If you notice bleeding from the insertion site, place light pressure over it. It's normal to see a little blood under the dressing, but you shouldn't see active bleeding. If you do, call your practitioner.

➤ *Swelling in your arm, shoulder, or neck on the side of your body where you have the catheter:* If you notice swelling, call your practitioner at once.

➤ *Signs and symptoms of infection:* Fever, chills, and sweating indicate infection and warrant an immediate call to the practitioner. Also call if you develop tenderness, redness, or drainage at the insertion site.

➤ *Pain:* Report pain at the insertion site or along your arm. If the pain occurs while fluids are running through the catheter, stop the fluids.

➤ *Inability to flush or run fluids or medications through catheter:* If this happens, call your practitioner. Don't try to force any solution into the catheter or the catheter may break.

➤ *Torn or leaking catheter:* Fold the catheter above the break and tape it to prevent air from entering your bloodstream; then call your practitioner.

➤ *Catheter that slipped out of place:* If your catheter has slipped out of place—

even by a small amount—don't try to push it back in. Instead, stop any fluids running into the catheter, secure it, and call your practitioner.

➤ *Development of severe shortness of breath, chest pain, or pain with breathing:* Call 911.

### Safeguarding your catheter

Following some basic guidelines can help you keep your catheter in place and free from infection. If you have any questions or concerns about catheter care, call your practitioner.

*Activity*

The catheter won't restrict your arm movements. However, don't take part in activities that involve vigorous arm movement—such as tennis, golf, and weight lifting—or you may accidentally reposition the catheter or lodge the catheter against a blood vessel wall.

*Showering and bathing*

When you take a shower or bath, take steps to keep the catheter area dry to discourage bacteria growth. Wrap the catheter in a plastic bag and tape the bag securely closed; then cover the insertion site with plastic wrap and tape the ends. If the area does get wet, carefully blot it dry and notify your practitioner.

*Hand washing*

To help prevent infection, make sure you thoroughly wash your hands before handling your catheter.

exit to hub, insertion location, and patient instructions.

➤ Document any dwelling solution in the catheter line. Follow up on chest X-ray findings, and chart PICC tip position.

## Central venous catheter insertion

**CPT CODES**
*36010    Introduction of catheter, superior or inferior vena cava*
*36011    Catheter placement, venous branch (renal, jugular)*
*36489    Central venous catheter placement; over age 2*

## DESCRIPTION

A central venous catheter (CVC) is a sterile catheter made of polyurethane, polyvinyl chloride, or silicone rubber (silastic). It's inserted through a large vein to enable central venous access, which serves several purposes. It allows the delivery of fluids and drugs to the central circulation through large vessels, makes collecting blood samples easier, and allows for sophisticated monitoring of critical care patients. Sites for CVC insertion include the subclavian, jugular, and femoral veins.

The right subclavian site is most frequently used because the right lung is usually lower than the left and the thoracic duct isn't exposed. For patients with coagulopathies, the jugular site is preferred because it's easily compressible. It's also preferred during cardiopulmonary resuscitation (CPR) because it's accessible and doesn't require that the rescuer stop compressions. In an awake and alert patient, however, the jugular site limits neck motion. Plus, a hematoma at this site is more likely to interfere with airway management. Also easily compressible and accessible during CPR,

the femoral site can be used but it carries an increased risk of infection and limits the range of motion of the affected limb, making this site less desirable.

## INDICATIONS

➤ To provide high-volume fluid resuscitation (for instance, in a severely burned patient)
➤ To allow for central venous pressure monitoring
➤ To place a pulmonary artery catheter
➤ To provide emergency venous access
➤ To infuse hyperosmolar or irritating solutions (such as total parenteral nutrition or chemotherapy)
➤ To provide plasmapheresis or hemodialysis
➤ To place a transvenous pacemaker
➤ To prevent the need for frequent venipuncture for I.V. access or laboratory samples

## CONTRAINDICATIONS

### Absolute
➤ Trauma at the access area
➤ Trauma to adjacent structures
➤ Full-thickness burn, infection, or cellulitis over the insertion site
➤ Uncooperative or agitated patients (increases the incidence of serious complications)
➤ Distorted local anatomy or landmarks at insertion site (as a result of surgery, irradiation, trauma, or congenital malformation)
➤ Previous use of the vessel for a sclerosing agent (such as some chemotherapeutic agents)
➤ Suspected or actual injury to the superior vena cava (requires central access below the diaphragm)
➤ Significant carotid artery disease in the internal jugular vein
➤ Recent unsuccessful contralateral cannulation (because of the possibility of bi-

lateral hematomas and the threat to airway patency) in the internal jugular vein

### Relative

➤ Coagulopathy or anticoagulant therapy

➤ Hemothorax or pneumothorax on contralateral side (ipsilateral side would be preferred). *Note:* If you have a pneumothorax already on right side, you have no added risk of causing one by trying a central line on the right.
➤ Suspected or known prior injury to the vein
➤ Anticipated mastectomy on the side of central access
➤ Vasculitis
➤ Previous recent long-term cannulation of the vessel

## EQUIPMENT

Rolled towel or sheet ◆ sterile drapes ◆ povidone-iodine ◆ sterile 4" × 4" gauze pads ◆ 1% lidocaine ◆ gown, mask, and sterile gloves ◆ CVC insertion kit (typically containing a 7.5 or 8.5 French catheter) ◆ single-lumen or triple-lumen CVC catheter ◆ 5-ml syringes, needles, and normal saline solution ◆ central line dressing kit ◆ linen-saver pad ◆ hair clippers
*For a CVC kit that doesn't contain a syringe with lidocaine:* alcohol pads ◆ 3-ml syringe with 25G 1" needle ◆ 1% or 2% injectable lidocaine

## PREPARATION OF EQUIPMENT

➤ Before inserting a central venous line, confirm the catheter type and size, and then choose the site (see *Choosing a central venous catheter site*).
➤ Notify the radiology department that a portable X-ray will be needed (for a subclavian or jugular insertion).

## ESSENTIAL STEPS

➤ Explain the procedure and risks to the patient, and obtain informed consent. Verify allergies, particularly to latex, iodine, or local anesthetic.
➤ Thoroughly wash your hands.

## USING CLAVICULAR LANDMARKS

Clavicular landmarks, such as the triangle formed by the clavicle with the trapezius and stern-ocleidomastoid muscles, can help you locate the subclavian venous access site.

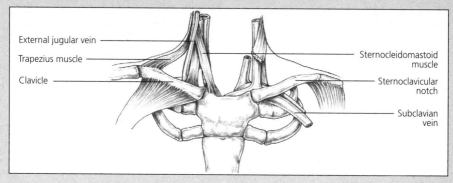

> ➤ Establish a sterile field on a table, using a sterile towel or the wrapping from the instrument tray.
> ➤ Place a linen-saver pad under the area to be cannulated.

### Subclavian site
> ➤ To dilate the patient's neck veins and reduce the risk of air embolism, place the patient in a 10- to 20-degree Trendelenburg position or raise the patient's lower extremities. If the patient can't tolerate the Trendelenburg position, lay the head of the bed flat.
> ➤ Place a rolled sheet or towel vertically beneath the patient's shoulder blades to promote posterior shoulder retraction and provide improved access to the neck veins.
> ➤ Turn the patient's head to the opposite side to prevent contamination and make the site more accessible.
> ➤ Prepare the insertion site. As needed, clip the hairs close to the skin and wash the skin with soap and water.
> ➤ Put on the mask and sterile gloves and gown; then clean the area around the insertion sites with alcohol pads followed by povidone-iodine solution. Clean in a circular motion outward from the site.

> ➤ Maintaining sterile technique, drape the patient so that you can readily see and palpate the suprasternal notch.
> ➤ If you're using a CVC insertion kit that doesn't contain a syringe with lidocaine, you may need an assistant. Maintaining sterile technique, place a 3-ml syringe and a 25G needle in the field. Have the assistant wipe the lidocaine vial with an alcohol sponge and invert it. Then fill the 3-ml syringe with lidocaine to anesthetize the site.
> ➤ Use one of the following landmarks to determine the entry site (see *Using clavicular landmarks*):
> – the point just lateral to the midclavicular line along the inferior surface of the clavicle
> – the point 1 cm below the junction of the middle and medial thirds of the clavicle
> – the point just inferior to the tubercle of the clavicle (palpate along the inferior surface of the clavicle, starting at the sternoclavicular notch one-third to one-half way laterally).
> ➤ Anesthetize the skin at the insertion site, advance the needle, and anesthetize the subcutaneous tissue and the periosteum of the clavicle. Align the markings of your

## ACCESSING THE INTERNAL JUGULAR SITE

When you access the internal jugular vein, make sure you maintain a straight insertion at a shallow needle angle, as shown here. The internal jugular vein rests under the apex of the triangle formed by the two heads of the sternocleidomastoid muscle. You can use the ipsilateral nipple as a reference for the needle direction.

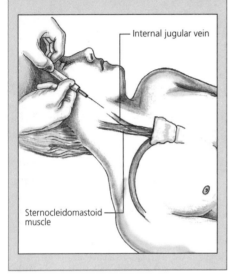

Internal jugular vein

Sternocleidomastoid muscle

syringe with the bevel of your needle so that you can infer the angle of the needle once you've punctured the skin (the angle is the same as for an I.V. line, usually 45 degrees above the skin).

➤ Once the area is numbed, insert the introducing needle with the syringe attached and advance it along the inferior surface of the clavicle, using the contralateral ear as reference.

➤ Advance the needle under the clavicle, applying negative pressure on the syringe until a flashback of blood indicates entry into the subclavian vein.

 **ALERT** Bright red pulsatile blood indicates inadvertent puncture an artery. If this happens, withdraw the

needle and apply direct pressure for 10 minutes.

➤ Stabilize the needle and remove the syringe, capping the hub of the needle with your gloved finger to prevent the entry of air or particulate matter.

➤ Slowly insert the guide wire through the needle (also known as the Seldinger technique). If the wire doesn't pass smoothly, the bevel of the needle may be against the wall of the vessel or angled upward. If so, reposition the bevel and try to advance the wire again.

➤ When you've successfully advanced the wire so 10 cm of wire lies within the central vein, remove the needle, maintaining contact with the wire at all times to prevent wire movement.

➤ Make a small incision with the scalpel at the wire insertion site, taking care not to damage the guide wire.

➤ Advance the dilator over the wire to enlarge the skin opening.

➤ Remove the dilator, again maintaining contact with the wire.

➤ Pass the introducer or catheter over the wire using a slight twisting motion, 5″ to 6″ (12.7 to 15.2 cm) for the right subclavian vein or 6″ to 7″ (15.2 to 17.8 cm) for the left subclavian vein.

➤ Slowly remove the wire, holding the CVC in place.

➤ Aspirate blood from each of the ports and then flush with 5 ml of normal saline solution to confirm that the catheter is in a vein.

➤ Set the flow rate at a keep-vein-open rate, or cap the catheter and flush it with heparin.

➤ Suture the line in place, using the holes provided on the hub of the CVC.

➤ Dress the site using a central line dressing kit.

➤ Obtain a chest X-ray to confirm line placement. Don't infuse fluids through the line beyond a keep-vein-open rate until the X-ray confirms placement.

## Internal jugular site

➤ Except for locating the insertion site and the depth of insertion, you'll follow the same steps as for the subclavian site. Begin by positioning the patient as you would for subclavian insertion. However, you don't need to elevate his shoulders with a towel.

➤ To find the appropriate site for insertion, palpate the triangle formed by the clavicle and the two heads of the sternocleidomastoid muscle with your left index finger. The internal jugular vein rests under the apex of this triangle and travels inferomedially.

 **ALERT** Keep in mind that on the patient's left side, the thoracic duct is more prominent, the pleural cupula is higher, and the internal jugular vein enters the subclavian vein at a more perpendicular angle. The subclavian vein generally follows a straighter course on the patient's right side, making the right side easier to cannulate and less prone to complications.

➤ Use the ipsilateral nipple as reference and maintain a shallow angle of insertion (20 to 30 degrees above the skin; see *Accessing the internal jugular site*).

➤ Aspirate with the syringe for a venous flashback, usually ⅜″ to 1⅛″ (1 to 2.9 cm) deep.

## Femoral site

➤ Follow the same guidelines as for a subclavian insertion except for positioning the patient and locating the insertion site. You also don't need to check the insertion site with an X-ray.

➤ Position the patient flat in bed and locate the femoral vein by palpating for the inguinal ligament and the femoral artery. The femoral vein runs just medial to the femoral artery at the level of the inguinal ligament. (See *Locating the femoral vein*.)

**LOCATING THE FEMORAL VEIN**

Palpation of the inguinal ligament and femoral artery can help you locate the femoral vein. Use care in locating these landmarks so that you don't traumatize any adjacent structures.

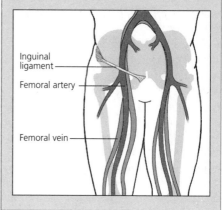

## PATIENT TEACHING

➤ Reassure the patient that the local anesthetic will keep him as comfortable as possible during the procedure.

➤ Instruct the patient to report pain not related to the needle stick, dyspnea, or excessive pain or burning at the insertion site.

➤ If the patient or a family member will care for the catheter, provide hands-on practice with site care or fluid or medication administration as needed.

## COMPLICATIONS

➤ *Pneumothorax* may require chest tube insertion.

➤ If *tension pneumothorax in a patient on positive-pressure ventilation* develops, the patient would require needle decompression and a chest tube.

➤ *Air embolism:* Immediately turn the patient to the left lateral Trendelenburg position and aspirate the air through the catheter.

➤ *Local or systemic infection:* The patient may require treatment with antibiotics.

➤ *Hemorrhage or hematoma:* Apply pressure to the site.

➤ *Venous thrombosis:* The patient may require anticoagulation therapy.

➤ *Arterial puncture:* Apply direct pressure to the site.

➤ *Laceration of the subclavian, carotid, or internal mammary artery:* Apply direct pressure; the patient may also need surgical repair.

➤ *Puncture an endotracheal tube cuff:* Maintain the patient's airway and reintubate him.

➤ *Perforation of the trachea* requires surgical intervention.

➤ *Cannulation (retrograde) of the internal jugular vein* can be used for I.V. fluids but can't be used to monitor central venous pressure, so it is usually removed.

➤ *Injury to the phrenic nerve or brachial plexus:* The patient may require physical therapy or rehabilitation.

➤ *Cardiac arrhythmias:* Withdraw the catheter.

➤ *Catheter kinking or knotting:* Withdraw the catheter and attempt to advance it again.

## SPECIAL CONSIDERATIONS

➤ Consider sedating the patient to reduce the anxiety and pain associated with any invasive procedure.

➤ In an emergency, you may not be able to maintain sterility. If you suspect contamination, consider changing the site once the patient has been stabilized.

➤ If you suspect infection, consider prophylactic antibiotic use.

## DOCUMENTATION

➤ Document the patient's status before the procedure and the need for the procedure. Include a note detailing the entire insertion in the progress notes, including

vital signs before and after the procedure, the status of the insertion site, the gauge of catheter inserted, and the number and type of sutures.

➤ Document the patient's response to the procedure and any complications.

## Central venous catheter blood collection

### CPT CODES
*Use laboratory code for specific diagnostic test.*
80051   *Electrolyte panel (4 tests)*
80053   *Comprehensive metabolic panel (12 tests)*
85025   *Complete blood count (including white blood cell differential and platelet count)*
85610   *Prothrombin time (PT) test*
85730   *Partial thromboplastin time (PTT) test*

## DESCRIPTION

A central venous catheter (CVC) provides easy access for blood specimens and spares the patient the pain and anxiety associated with frequent venipunctures. However, a direct relationship exists between the frequency of system interruptions and the increased risk of infection. Because of this, practitioners must maintain sterile technique when collecting blood and use the CVC only when necessary.

## INDICATIONS

➤ To obtain blood samples for analysis to assess the patient's medical condition and response to therapy

➤ To determine if the line is a source of infection

## CONTRAINDICATIONS

### Absolute

➤ Indications of catheter infection or phlebitis

## EQUIPMENT

Gloves ◆ ethyl alcohol swabs ◆ povidone-iodine swabs ◆ 10-ml vial of normal saline solution for injection ◆ vial of heparin flush solution (100 units/ml) ◆ 10-ml syringes with needles or needleless system hub (if available) ◆ hemostat with rubber on clamps (optional) ◆ blood collection tubes or blood culture vials

## PREPARATION OF EQUIPMENT

➤ Note the volume of blood needed to perform all indicated tests.
➤ Assemble all equipment, and check expiration dates on all sterile supplies, solutions, and tubes.

## ESSENTIAL STEPS

➤ Tell the patient that you're going to collect a blood sample, and explain the procedure.
➤ Place the patient in a supine position, with the head of the bed slightly elevated.
➤ Wash your hands and put on gloves.
➤ Aspirate normal saline solution into a 10-ml syringe.
➤ Clamp the catheter lumens.
➤ Clean the catheter hubs or tubing connection with povidone-iodine swabs. *Note:* Use alcohol pads first if drawing blood cultures.
➤ Attach an empty 10-ml syringe to the hub of the CVC, release the clamp, and aspirate 5 ml of blood.
➤ Clamp the catheter. Remove the syringe and discard it.

➤ Connect an empty syringe to the catheter, release the clamp, and withdraw the blood sample.
➤ Clamp the catheter and remove the syringe. Set the sample aside.
➤ Connect the syringe containing normal saline solution and release the clamp.
➤ Flush the catheter with 5 ml of normal saline solution, connect the clamp, and remove the syringe. If the patient doesn't have a continuous infusion, flush the catheter with 2 ml of heparin flushing solution unless otherwise indicated and replace the cap on the hub. If the patient does have a continuous infusion, reconnect and restart it.
➤ Attach a needle to the syringe with the blood sample and inject the blood into the appropriate blood collection tubes or blood culture mediums.
➤ Label all collection tubes with the patient's name and room number and the date and time of collection.

## PATIENT TEACHING

➤ Explain the procedure, what blood tests will be performed, and how the results will contribute to the medical treatment plan.

## COMPLICATIONS

➤ *Occlusion of the line* may require the placement of a new line. You can sometimes clear a line by flushing it with normal saline solution or heparin flush. If that is ineffective, instill 2.5 mg of tissue plasminogen activator (tPA) into the catheter. Allow the tPA to stay in the line for 1 to 2 hours; then withdraw the solution and reattempt to draw blood. Don't push too hard to clear the line or you may dislodge a clot.
➤ *Air embolism:* Immediately turn the patient to the left lateral Trendelenburg position and aspirate the air.
➤ *Extravasation of fluid into surrounding subcutaneous tissue:* Apply warm compresses. Keep in mind that extravasation

may indicate that the line is poorly positioned; make sure you can aspirate blood from the catheter, or have the placement checked with a chest X-ray, if indicated. The line may need to be removed.

## SPECIAL CONSIDERATIONS

➤ If you're having difficulty aspirating blood from the catheter, it may be poorly positioned with the catheter tip lodged against the vessel wall. If you suspect this problem, there are three options for trying to dislodge a catheter from a vessel wall. You can ask the patient to cough or bear down; you can reposition him on his side, turn his head, raise his arms above his head, or have him assume a sitting position; or you can place the bed in Trendelenburg's position.

➤ Flush the catheter with normal saline solution before drawing a waste specimen. If you need a sample for a prothrombin or partial thromboplastin time, draw that sample last to allow any heparin in the line to clear.

➤ Never reinject withdrawn blood back into catheter.

➤ When drawing blood from a multilumen catheter, temporarily stop any other infusions.

➤ If there isn't a clamp on the catheter, use a hemostat with rubber on the clamps to occlude the catheter.

## DOCUMENTATION

➤ Record the indications for the procedure and any complications that occur.

➤ Document the presence or absence of a blood return, the ease of blood withdrawal, and any special maneuvers required to obtain a sample.

➤ Record the date and time of blood sample collection.

## Central venous catheter change

CPT CODES
36010   Introduction of catheter, superior or inferior vena cava
36011   Catheter placement, venous branch (renal, jugular)
36489   Central venous catheter placement; over age 2

## DESCRIPTION

A patient who has limited alternative sites for cannulation or who requires a change in type of catheter (from a single to a triple-lumen catheter, for instance) may need this procedure.

## INDICATIONS

➤ To enlarge the lumen size of the existing catheter to allow entrance of a pulmonary artery catheter or transvenous pacemaker

➤ To provide a multilumen catheter instead of a single-lumen catheter

## CONTRAINDICATIONS

### Absolute
➤ Line sepsis
➤ Infection at the insertion site
➤ Suspected or actual injury to the superior vena cava (requires access from below the diaphragm, in the femoral vein)

### Relative
➤ A catheter that has been in place longer than the institution's recommended time (most facilities have protocols requiring that central lines routinely be changed at a specified time, although this isn't always possible)

➤ Mastectomy anticipated on the same side

## EQUIPMENT

Povidone-iodine solution ◆ sterile 4″ × 4″ gauze pads ◆ 1% lidocaine ◆ prepared kit (Cordis 8.5 French kit, single-lumen catheter kit, or triple-lumen catheter kit) ◆ 5-ml syringes ◆ needles and normal saline solution ◆ sterile drape ◆ central-line dressing kit ◆ gown ◆ mask ◆ sterile gloves

## PREPARATION OF EQUIPMENT

➤ Notify the radiology department that a portable X-ray will be needed.

## ESSENTIAL STEPS

➤ Explain the procedure to the patient and obtain informed consent.
➤ Place the patient flat in bed.
➤ Place a rolled sheet or towel beneath the shoulder blades of the patient. This allows the shoulders to retract posteriorly and provides improved access.
➤ If possible, turn the patient's head to the opposite side.
➤ Put on mask, gown, and sterile gloves.
➤ Prepare the area by cleaning around the insertion site with gauze pads soaked with povidone-iodine solution; work in a circular motion outward from the site. Drape the area with the sterile drape.
➤ Remove the stitches holding the present line in place.
➤ Aspirate blood from the present line to confirm placement.
➤ Pass the guide wire through the port of the existing line.
➤ Observe the cardiac rhythm on a monitor for any ectopia, which could indicate that the wire is in too far.
➤ Maintaining contact with the wire, remove the existing catheter. You may have

to use the scalpel to enlarge the skin opening if you need to insert a larger catheter.
➤ Pass the new catheter over the wire maintaining contact with the wire. Insert the catheter 5″ to 6″ (12.7 to 15.2 cm) if you're using the right subclavian vein, 6″ to 7″ (15.2 to 17.8 cm) if you're using the left subclavian vein.
➤ Slowly remove the wire.
➤ Anesthetize the skin before suturing.
➤ Flush the ports of the catheter with 5 ml of normal saline solution, aspirating blood to ensure that the catheter is in the vein.
➤ Suture the catheter in place.
➤ Dress the site with a central-line dressing kit.
➤ Obtain a chest X-ray to confirm placement.

 **ALERT** Don't infuse through the line until an X-ray of the new central venous catheter has confirmed placement.

## PATIENT TEACHING

➤ Tell the patient you'll make him as comfortable as possible by using a local anesthetic before suturing the line in place.
➤ Instruct the patient to remain as still as possible with his head turned to avoid contaminating the site and to provide better access.

## COMPLICATIONS

➤ *Pneumothorax:* The patient may require chest tube insertion.
➤ *Tension pneumothorax in a patient on positive-pressure ventilation:* The patient requires needle decompression and a chest tube.
➤ *Air embolism:* Immediately place the patient in the left lateral Trendelenburg position and aspirate through the catheter.
➤ *Local or systemic infection:* Provide treatment with antibiotics.

➤ *Hemorrhage or hematoma:* Apply pressure.
➤ *Venous thrombosis:* The patient may require anticoagulation therapy.
➤ *Subclavian artery puncture:* Apply direct pressure.
➤ *Laceration of the thoracic duct (on the left) or lymphatic duct (on the right):* The patient requires surgical intervention.
➤ *Laceration of the subclavian, carotid, or internal mammary artery:* Apply direct pressure; the patient may need surgical repair.
➤ *Puncture of the cuff of an endotracheal tube:* Maintain the patient's airway and reintubate.
➤ *Perforation of the trachea:* The patient requires surgical intervention.
➤ *Cannulation (retrograde) of the internal jugular vein:* This can't be used to monitor central venous pressure and should be removed as soon as possible.
➤ *Injury to phrenic nerve, brachial plexus:* The patient may require physical therapy or rehabilitation.
➤ *Cardiac arrhythmias:* Withdraw the catheter.
➤ *Catheter kinking or knotting:* Withdraw and attempt to advance again.

## SPECIAL CONSIDERATIONS

➤ To prevent venous air embolism when changing connections in a central venous line, create a temporary positive pressure by having the patient hum.

## DOCUMENTATION

➤ Document the patient's status that indicated the need for the procedure.
➤ Document the entire insertion in the progress notes, including the chest X-ray reading.
➤ Detail the status of the insertion site, noting color, temperature, any drainage, and the presence or absence of a hematoma.

➤ Document a reading of the chest X-ray and the patient's status following the procedure.
➤ Note any complications.

# Central venous or peripherally inserted central catheter removal

**CPT CODE**
No specific code has been assigned.

## DESCRIPTION

Removal of a central venous catheter (CVC) or a peripherally inserted central catheter (PICC), a sterile procedure, takes place at the end of therapy or at the onset of a complication. The patient's most recent chest X-ray should be checked before removal to trace the catheter's path as it exits the body. Also, assistance should be available in case a complication such as uncontrolled bleeding occurs during catheter removal because some vessels (such as the subclavian vein) can be difficult to compress.

## INDICATIONS

➤ To replace a malfunctioning, occluded, or malpositioned catheter
➤ To treat local or systemic infection, lymphatic fistula, or unexplained fever
➤ To decrease the risk of infection from a CVC that was placed under nonsterile conditions during an emergency (should be removed within 24 hours)
➤ To terminate therapy

## CONTRAINDICATIONS

**Relative**
➤ Severe coagulopathy

## EQUIPMENT

### CVC

Gloves (clean and sterile) ◆ suture removal kit (includes sterile scissors and forceps) ◆ sterile 4″ × 4″ gauze pads ◆ adhesive tape ◆ mask ◆ sterile drape ◆ antiseptic solution (ethyl alcohol or povidone-iodine) ◆ povidone-iodine ointment ◆ sterile specimen cup (optional)

### PICC

Gloves ◆ sterile 4″ × 4″ gauze pads ◆ adhesive tape ◆ povidone-iodine ointment ◆ sterile specimen cup (optional)

## ESSENTIAL STEPS

➤ Tell the patient that you're going to remove the catheter, and explain the procedure.
➤ Make sure you have patent alternative I.V. access, if needed.

### CVC

➤ Place the patient in the supine position. Keep the bed flat or put it in the Trendelenburg position to increase intrathoracic pressure.
➤ Wash your hands and put on gloves and a mask. Maintain aseptic technique.
➤ Turn off all infusions and prepare a sterile field, using a sterile drape.
➤ Remove and discard the old dressing and change to sterile gloves.
➤ Clean the site with an alcohol sponge or a gauze pad soaked in povidone-iodine solution. Inspect the site for signs of drainage or inflammation.
➤ Clip the anchor sutures close to the skin on one side, using forceps to pull the short side through the skin to minimize the amount of contaminated suture material pulled beneath the skin.

**ALERT** If you meet resistance, stop the procedure. The catheter may be knotted. Obtain a chest X-ray to confirm catheter integrity.

➤ Have the patient perform Valsalva's maneuver and remove the catheter using a slow, even motion. If the patient is on mechanical ventilation, time the catheter removal to coincide with exhalation.
➤ Apply firm pressure to the insertion site until bleeding stops (for at least 5 minutes). You may raise the head of the bed at this point.
➤ If a culture is needed, cut the tip of the catheter using sterile scissors and let the tip drop into the sterile specimen cup. Label the cup with the patient's name, room number, hospital identification number, your name, the date and time, and what the specimen is and send it to the microbiology laboratory for analysis.
➤ When bleeding stops, cover the insertion site with an occlusive dressing. Label the dressing with the date and time of the removal and your initials.
➤ Keep the site covered for 24 to 48 hours. (The longer the catheter was in place, the greater the risk of subcutaneous tract formation, and the longer the dressing should stay in place.)
➤ Inspect the catheter to ensure that no portion broke off during removal. Monitor the patient closely for signs of respiratory distress and, if any occurs, obtain a chest X-ray.
➤ Dispose of equipment and supplies in the appropriate receptacles.

### PICC

➤ Wash your hands. Place a linen-saver pad under the patient's arm.
➤ Remove the tape holding the extension tubing. Open two sterile gauze pads on a clean, flat surface; then put on gloves. Stabilize the catheter at the hub with one hand. Without dislodging the catheter, use your other hand to gently remove the dressing by pulling it toward the insertion site. Next, withdraw the catheter using smooth, gentle pressure in small increments. It should come out easily. If you feel resistance, stop. Apply slight tension to the line by taping it

down. Then try to remove it again in a few minutes. If you still feel resistance, consult with your collaborating physician.

➤ Once you successfully remove the catheter, apply manual pressure to the site for 1 minute using a sterile gauze pad.

➤ Measure and inspect the catheter after you remove it to ensure that the line has been removed intact. If any part has broken off during removal, notify your collaborating physician or initiate a surgical consult immediately and monitor the patient for signs of distress.

➤ Cover the site with povidone-iodine ointment, and tape a new folded gauze pad in place. Dispose of used items properly, and wash your hands.

## PATIENT TEACHING

➤ Briefly go over the steps involved in the procedure, and teach the patient how to perform Valsalva's maneuver. You may want to have him practice it once or twice to make sure he understands. Explain that he'll need to perform the maneuver as you remove the catheter.

➤ Tell the patient that the procedure won't cause much pain but that he'll have the sensation of something being drawn out of his skin. Tell him the site may feel sore for a few days.

➤ Tell the patient to report signs of infection, including redness, swelling, drainage, odor at the site, opening of the wound, or a fever greater than 101° F (38.3° C).

## COMPLICATIONS

➤ *Air embolism:* Immediately lay the patient in the left lateral Trendelenburg position. Observe him for signs and symptoms of cardiac arrest, and initiate advanced cardiac life support as indicated. Notify the attending or collaborating physician. This potentially fatal complication can be avoided by following the protocol.

➤ *Pulmonary embolism:* Administer oxygen; the patient may require intubation or anticoagulation therapy.

➤ *Local infection:* Apply warm compresses. The patient may require antibiotic ointment or systemic antibiotics.

## SPECIAL CONSIDERATIONS

➤ Don't keep a CVC in place for a prolonged period. Fibrous tracts may form, leading to subcutaneous tract formation and increasing the risk of pulmonary or air embolism when the dressing is removed.

➤ Watch for signs of an air embolism, including sudden onset of pallor, cyanosis, hypoxia, dyspnea, coughing, and tachycardia; this complication can quickly progress to cardiovascular collapse.

## DOCUMENTATION

➤ After removing the CVC or PICC, record the time and date of removal and the type of dressing applied.

➤ Document the patient's response to the procedure and any complications.

➤ Note the condition of the catheter and insertion site and whether you collected a culture specimen.

## Venous cutdown

CPT CODE
36425   *Venipuncture, cutdown; age 1 or older*

## DESCRIPTION

Venous cutdown allows infusion of blood products or colloids when venipuncture at a peripheral site or central venous access are unavailable. It's typically used in emergency situations to infuse large volumes rapidly, which isn't possible with standard venipuncture. The greater saphenous vein at the ankle is the first choice, especially when speed is essential. Alternative sites include the basilic vein in the antecubital space and the greater saphenous vein in the groin.

## INDICATIONS

➤ To provide emergency venous access or multiple I.V. access for hypotensive patients whose veins can't be visualized, palpated, or cannulated percutaneously

## CONTRAINDICATIONS

### Relative
➤ The possibility of less invasive alternatives
➤ A patient for whom the time needed to perform standard venipuncture would cause irreversible harm

## EQUIPMENT

Sterile catheter (#2, #3, or #4 French, depending on the size of vein to be cannulated) ◆ needle holder ◆ curved hemostat ◆ tissue dissection and suture scissors ◆ mosquito hemostat ◆ absorbable skin sutures (4-0) ◆ silk ligatures (4-0) ◆ #11 or #15 scalpel with handle ◆ 1% lidocaine without epinephrine ◆ 3-ml syringe with 25G ⅝" needle ◆ I.V. fluids and tubing ◆ tourniquet ◆ antiseptic solution, such as povidone-iodine ◆ sterile gloves and drapes ◆ sterile 4" × 4" gauze pads ◆ antibiotic ointment ◆ adhesive tape ◆ goggles ◆ soft restraints (optional)

## PREPARATION OF EQUIPMENT

➤ Assemble all supplies and equipment, and check the expiration dates on all sterile packages and medication containers.

## ESSENTIAL STEPS

➤ Explain the need for I.V. access and the procedure. Obtain informed consent.
➤ Place the patient in the supine position.
➤ Position the appropriate extremity flat on the bed or stretcher and ensure adequate stabilization. To ensure immobility of patient's limb during the procedure, use soft restraints only if absolutely necessary.
➤ If accessing the antecubital or distal saphenous vein, apply a tourniquet proximal to the intended incision site to allow better visualization and palpation. Release the tourniquet once you've punctured the vein to minimize bleeding. (See *Locating veins for cutdown,* page 66.)
➤ Clean the area around the vein and intended incision site with povidone-iodine, moving outward in concentric circles. Allow the area to dry.
➤ Position the sterile drapes distally and proximally to provide a wide sterile field.
➤ Put on goggles and sterile gloves; then administer a local anesthetic to the area.

 **ALERT** Veins used in venous cutdown are in superficial fat layers. If the incision exposes muscle fascia, it's too deep. The vein will appear pulseless and thin-walled and should blanch when you apply distal traction. If necessary, have an assistant tighten the proximal tourniquet to make the vein more apparent. In all cutdowns, you should dissect the vein free and isolate it for at least ¾" (2 cm) along its axis.

### To locate the vein

DISTAL SAPHENOUS VEIN
➤ The distal saphenous vein is located above the medial malleolus. To find it, make a full-thickness, 1⅛" (3 cm) transverse skin incision approximately ¾" anterior and superior to the medial malleolus between the anterior and posterior border of the tibia.
➤ Using a curved, closed hemostat, insert anterolaterally to the vein.

## LOCATING VEINS FOR CUTDOWN

To access the distal saphenous vein, make an incision above the medial malleoulus, beginning at the anterior tibial border and extending toward the posterior tibial border.

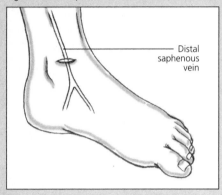

Distal saphenous vein

To access the basilic vein, make a horizontal, superficial incision across the groove of the medial arm between the triceps and biceps muscles.

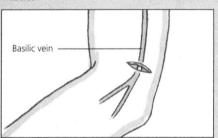

Basilic vein

To access the proximal greater saphenous vein, make a transverse incision in the groin, as shown above right. Again, note the proximity of the surrounding structures, in this case the femoral artery, vein, and nerve.

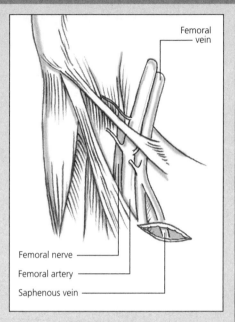

Femoral vein

Femoral nerve

Femoral artery

Saphenous vein

The vein is exposed and separated from surrounding structures. This allows for ligation and also minimizes the risk of trauma. For example, note the position of the saphenous nerve in relation to the saphenous vein.

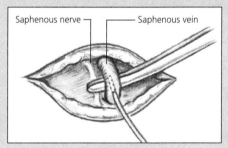

Saphenous nerve

Saphenous vein

➤ Rotate the point of the hemostat upward and spread open. This will reveal the distal saphenous vein, nerve, and tissue.
➤ Bluntly dissect to identify the vein by sliding the hemostat posteromedially.
➤ Dissect the vein free from the surrounding tissue. Take care not to involve the saphenous nerve, using sterile 4″ × 4″ gauze pads to remove blood and maintain visibility.

BASILIC VEIN
➤ The basilic vein lies in the groove of the medial area between the triceps and the

biceps muscles. It follows a course slightly anterior and superficial to the brachial artery. To find it, divide the distance between the tip of the olecranon and the acromion into thirds and find the biceps or triceps groove in the middle of the distal third segment.

➤ Make a full-thickness, 1⅛" (3 cm) transverse skin incision at this level from the biceps muscle across the groove to the triceps muscle.

➤ Dissect the superficial fat layer until you see the basilic vein. If you see muscle fascia and the radial artery, the incision is too deep.

### PROXIMAL OR GREATER SAPHENOUS VEIN

➤ The saphenous vein lies anteromedially to the saphenofemoral junction. To find it, make a full-thickness, 3-cm transverse skin incision centered just medial to a palpable femoral pulse. If you can't palpate the femoral pulse, you can approximate the location of the femoral artery at a position halfway between the anterior iliac spine and the pubic tubercle.

➤ Insert the closed hemostat under the vein to expose it, and free it from the surrounding tissue.

➤ Insert the catheter.

### To insert the catheter

➤ Dissect aside any loose adipose or adventitial tissue and isolate the intended vein to the length of ¾" (2 cm).

➤ Pass the silk ties under the exposed vein at the proximal and distal points of the incision.

➤ Place light traction on the proximal ligature to minimize bleeding and provisionally ligate the distal vein.

➤ Release the tourniquet (if applicable).

➤ At a 45-degree angle, incise approximately one-third of the diameter of the vessel with a scalpel or fine scissors in a distal-to-proximal direction. Gently dilate the venotomy with the closed tips of the

## VENOUS CUTDOWN CANNULATION

Once you've exposed the vein, you must isolate it, occlude it briefly during cannulation, and then evaluate it before securing it.

1. Isolate and ligate the intended vein. Then make a venotomy in the anterior wall of the vein while maintaining traction with the ligatures.

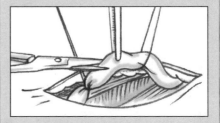

2. Introduce catheter through the wedge cut.

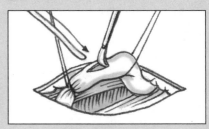

3. Advance the catheter into the vein and loosen traction on the proximal ligature.

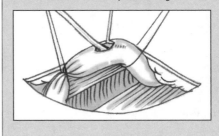

mosquito hemostat while maintaining proximal traction on the ligature. (See *Venous cutdown cannulation*.)

## DRESSING AND ANCHORING THE LINE

After venous cutdown, you must anchor the line to minimize the risk for traumatic dislocation, infection, and vascular compromise.

1. Here the incision is closed and the catheter to the distal greater saphenous vein is sutured.

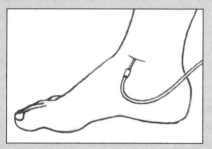

2. This shows how to dress the area to prevent inadvertent removal of the catheter.

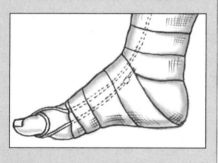

 **ALERT** When cannulating the proximal greater saphenous vein, don't block the lumen of the femoral vein, which would impede venous return from the lower extremities. Also, position the catheter so that it isn't advanced into the femoral vein.

➤ Insert the catheter into the vein at a 45-degree angle, making sure you have the right size catheter for the vein. Loosen the traction on the proximal ligature as needed to advance the catheter (typically the most difficult portion of the procedure). If you can't advance the catheter smoothly, you may have chosen a catheter too large for the lumen, punctured the posterior wall, or created a false lumen.

➤ After you've adequately advanced the catheter, aspirate air from the catheter by withdrawing blood.

➤ Anchor both the vein and the catheter by sliding the proximal ligature down and forming a suboccluding ligature. Cut the long ends of the proximal ligature and remove the distal ligature. Suture the incision.

➤ Infuse I.V. solution into the catheter and watch for leakage.

➤ Secure the catheter to the skin with another stitch, and apply antibacterial ointment and a sterile dressing (see *Dressing and anchoring the line*).

## PATIENT TEACHING

➤ Tell the patient to keep the affected limb as immobile as possible to avoid tension on the incision and tubing.

➤ Explain that the area will look red and may feel itchy or painful, especially if the surrounding tissue is edematous.

## COMPLICATIONS

➤ *Hematoma:* Apply pressure.

➤ *Local infection:* Apply antibiotic ointment.

➤ *Thrombophlebitis:* Apply a warm compress and elevate the limb.

➤ *Bacteremia and sepsis:* Administer broad-spectrum antibiotics until culture results become available.

➤ *Embolism:* The patient requires systemic anticoagulation.

## SPECIAL CONSIDERATIONS

➤ Keep in mind that accessing the distal saphenous vein allows uninterrupted resuscitation while performing the procedure, involves minimal risk of complications compared with a central venous access procedure, and doesn't threaten any vital structures. However, accessing the basilic vein poses less risk of infection than accessing the saphenous vein.

➤ When attempting to access the proximal saphenous vein, take care not to dissect too deeply to avoid damaging the femoral nerve, artery, or vein.

➤ If the patient had previous surgery involving the saphenous vein, such as coronary artery bypass grafting, peripheral bypass grafting, or saphenous vein stripping, choose an alternate site.

## DOCUMENTATION

➤ Describe the indications for the procedure.

➤ Outline the steps of the procedure, including the site selected, the size of the catheter, and any complications.

# PREVENTION

## Bacterial endocarditis prophylaxis

CPT CODE
No specific code has been assigned.

## DESCRIPTION

Bacterial endocarditis prophylaxis is prescribing or administering antibiotics be-

### CONDITIONS THAT INCREASE THE RISK OF ENDOCARDITIS

Certain cardiac conditions increase the risk of endocarditis and increase the likelihood of a poor outcome from the disease. Patients at high risk include those with:
➤ a prosthetic cardiac valve (bioprosthetic or homograft)
➤ previous bacterial endocarditis
➤ complex cyanotic congenital heart disease (single ventricle malfunction states, such as tricuspid atresia, transposition of the great vessels, or tetralogy of Fallot)
➤ a surgically constructed systemic-pulmonary shunt or conduit.
    Patients at moderate risk include those with:
➤ many congenital cardiac malformations not included in the high-risk categories
➤ acquired valvular dysfunction
➤ hypertrophic cardiomyopathy
➤ mitral valve prolapse with insufficiency or thickened redundant leaflets.

fore certain procedures to minimize a patient's risk of contracting bacterial endocarditis, an infection that results in vegetative growths on the heart valves or the wall of the endocardium. Prophylaxis may be necessary before surgery or dental work that increases the chance of bacterial entering the bloodstream. Patients who are at high risk for the disease should also receive prophylactic treatment (see *Conditions that increase the risk of endocarditis*). The recommendations listed here are from the American Heart Association as revised in 1997.

The disease can occur in acute or subacute forms. *Acute endocarditis* typically affects functional valves and results from infection with staphylococci; *subacute endocarditis* tends to occur in a previously damaged endothelium and typically results from infection with *Streptococcus*

## WHEN TO ADMINISTER ENDOCARDITIS PROPHYLAXIS

Endocarditis prophylaxis is recommended for many—but not all—dental, genitourinary, GI, and respiratory procedures. Listed below are procedures that call for prophylaxis and those that don't call for it.

**Prophylaxis recommended**
*Dental**
➤ Dental extractions
➤ Periodontal procedures
➤ Dental implant placement and reimplantation of avulsed teeth
➤ Endodontic instrumentation or surgery beyond the apex
➤ Subgingival placement of antibiotic fibers or strips
➤ Initial placement of orthodontic bands (but not brackets)
➤ Intraligamentary local anesthetic injections
➤ Prophylactic teeth cleaning or implants in which bleeding is expected

*Genitourinary*
➤ Prostatic surgery
➤ Cystoscopy
➤ Urethral dilatation

*GI***
➤ Sclerotherapy for esophageal varices
➤ Esophageal stricture dilation
➤ Endoscopic retrograde cholangiography with biliary obstruction
➤ Biliary tract surgery
➤ Surgery that involves the intestinal mucosa

*Respiratory*
➤ Tonsillectomy or adenoidectomy
➤ Surgery that involves respiratory mucosa
➤ Rigid bronchoscopy

**Prophylaxis not recommended**
*Dental*
➤ Restorative dentistry
➤ Local anesthetic injections (nonintraligamentary)
➤ Intracanal endodontic treatment
➤ Placement of rubber dams
➤ Postoperative suture removal
➤ Placement of removable prosthodontic or orthodontic appliances
➤ Oral impressions
➤ Oral radiographs
➤ Orthodontic appliance adjustment

*Cardiovascular*
➤ Implanted cardiac pacemakers, defibrillators, and coronary stents
➤ Cardiac catheterization and angioplasty

*Genitourinary*
➤ Vaginal hysterectomy†
➤ Vaginal delivery† or cesarean section
➤ Urethral catheterization, uterine dilatation and curettage, therapeutic abortion, sterilization procedures, and insertion or removal of intrauterine devices (in uninfected tissue)

*GI*
➤ Transesophageal echocardiogram
➤ Endoscopy†

*Respiratory*
➤ Endotracheal intubation
➤ Flexible bronchoscopy†
➤ Tympanostomy tube insertion

**KEY**
* Prophylaxis is recommended for high- and moderate-risk cardiac conditions.
** Prophylaxis is recommended for high-risk patients; is optional for moderate-risk patients.
† Prophylaxis is optional for high-risk patients.

Source: *Prevention of Bacterial Endocarditis* (1997). American Heart Association.

*viridans*. Appropriate therapy usually reduces such signs and symptoms as fever and results in a return to negative blood cultures.

Bacterial endocarditis can also be classified as native or prosthetic valve. (A form of the disease can also develop in I.V. drug abusers, but the infecting organism in these cases isn't clear, and such patients generally don't receive endocarditis prophylaxis.) *Native valve endocarditis* affects the mitral valve more often than the aortic valve. It almost always results from infection with streptococci, although staphylococci, enterococci, and (rarely) fungi can also cause this form of the disease. Only 60% to 80% of patients with native valve endocarditis have identified cardiac lesions. *Prosthetic valve endocarditis* can develop in any patient who has an intravascular prosthesis, such as a prosthetic valve. The incidence is highest during the first 6 to 12 months after valve replacement. Regardless of whether the patient has a mechanical or bioprosthetic valve or has the prosthesis in the mitral or aortic position, the infection rate doesn't vary much. However, the prosthesis makes curing the disease more difficult, increasing the importance of prevention.

## INDICATIONS

➤ To prevent infection during traumatic procedures, particularly those involving epithelial surfaces colonized by flora (such as the oropharynx, the GI and genitourinary tracts, and the skin)
➤ To prevent infection during procedures that involve the prostate or female reproductive tract (such as cystoscopy, urethral dilatation, and catheterization)
➤ To prevent infection during procedures that can cause transient bacteremia, such as certain dental, diagnostic, and therapeutic procedures (see *When to administer endocarditis prophylaxis*)

## CONTRAINDICATIONS

### Absolute

➤ Allergy or hypersensitivity to any component of the antibiotic (an alternative drug should be used)

## ESSENTIAL STEPS

➤ Obtain a complete history from the patient, including any past or present heart disease, previous cardiac surgery, and drug allergies.
➤ Perform a comprehensive cardiovascular examination, including special maneuvers to elicit heart murmurs.
➤ Review available records for results of echocardiograms, electrocardiograms, and operations.
➤ Determine the patient's risk for developing endocarditis by evaluating the risk of the procedure coupled with the nature of the existing heart disease.
➤ Discuss the risk of developing endocarditis and the benefits of antibiotic prophylaxis with the patient. (See *Preventing infection with antibiotics*, page 72.)
➤ Prescribe the appropriate antibiotic regimen based on the type of procedure the patient will undergo. (See *Endocarditis prophylaxis regimens,* pages 73 and 74.)

## PATIENT TEACHING

➤ Explain to the patient his specific risks for endocarditis, the seriousness of the disease, and the usefulness of prophylactic treatment.
➤ Tell the patient to take the complete prescribed dosage of medication within the prescribed time before the procedure.
➤ Discuss the signs and symptoms of an allergic reaction to the antibiotic the patient will take, and instruct him to notify you if any occur.

*(Text continues on page 74.)*

## PREVENTING INFECTION WITH ANTIBIOTICS

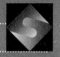

**DEAR PATIENT:**

Your practitioner is giving you this because you are at risk for getting an infection, which could harm your heart valves. By taking an antibiotic drug, you can protect yourself from infection.

### When to take an antibiotic
Take your antibiotic drug exactly as your practitioner directs. This lets the drug do its job of fighting infection. If you've been exposed to an infection, an antibiotic helps your body defend itself by killing bacteria before they multiply and make you sick.

Your practitioner may also tell you that you need to take antibiotics before you have dental work or any kind of surgery. Dental work, for instance, may allow germs to enter your bloodstream through your gums. Make sure you let your dentist or other practitioner know you have a heart-valve disorder *before* any treatments.

### If you forget your antibiotic
If you forget to finish or renew your prescription, let your practitioner know right away. She can decide whether you need to continue your medicine.

### When to call your practitioner
Let your practitioner know if you have any break in your skin or if you feel sick. That is

because a cut, a puncture, a rash, or an abscess can introduce germs. A sore throat, fever, cold, or flu means that germs are already at work.

Be alert for signs and symptoms that your heart valves may be infected again. These include:
➤ shortness of breath
➤ fatigue
➤ weakness
➤ swollen ankles
➤ sudden weight gain, such as 5 pounds in a week or 1 pound overnight.

If you have any of these signs or symptoms, let your practitioner know right away or go to the nearest emergency room.

### An important reminder
Get a card from your local American Heart Association that tells dentists (and other health care providers) which antibiotics you need to prevent heart valve infection. Always carry the card with you. Each year, have the card checked to make sure you're carrying the latest advice.

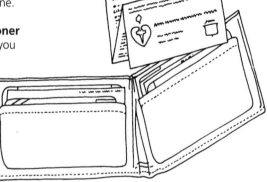

## ENDOCARDITIS PROPHYLAXIS REGIMENS

This table details the type of medication and regimen for various types of patients requiring endocarditis prophylaxis. Note that the total children's dose should not exceed the adult dose, and cephalosporins shouldn't be used in patients with immediate-type hypersensitivity reaction (such as urticaria, angioedema, or anaphylaxis) to penicillins.

| PATIENT TYPE | MEDICATION | REGIMEN |
| --- | --- | --- |
| FOR DENTAL, ORAL, RESPIRATORY TRACT, AND ESOPHAGEAL PROCEDURES (NO FOLLOW-UP DOSE RECOMMENDED) | | |
| Requires standard prophylaxis | amoxicillin | *Adults:* 2 g; *children:* 50 mg/kg P.O. 1 hour before procedure |
| Can't take medications by mouth | ampicillin | *Adults:* 2 g I.M. or I.V.; *children:* 50 mg/kg I.M. or I.V. within 30 minutes before procedure |
| Allergic to penicillin | clindamycin OR cephalexin or cefadroxil OR azithromycin or clarithromycin | *Adults:* 600 mg; *children:* 20 mg/kg P.O. 1 hour before procedure *Adults:* 2 g; *children:* 50 mg/kg P.O. 1 hour before procedure *Adults:* 500 mg; *children:* 50 mg/kg P.O. 1 hour before procedure |
| Allergic to penicillin and can't take medications by mouth | clindamycin OR cefazolin | *Adults:* 600 mg; *children:* 20 mg/kg I.V. within 30 minutes before procedure *Adults:* 1 g; *children:* 25 mg/kg I.M. or I.V. within 30 minutes before procedure |
| FOR GENITOURINARY AND GI (EXCLUDING ESOPHAGEAL) PROCEDURES | | |
| High risk | ampicillin plus gentamicin | *Adults:* ampicillin 2 g I.M. or I.V. plus gentamicin 1.5 mg/kg (not to exceed 120 mg) within 30 minutes of starting procedure. 6 hours later, ampicillin 1 g I.M. or I.V. or amoxicillin 1 g P.O. *Children:* ampicillin 50 mg/kg I.M. or I.V. (not to exceed 2 g) plus gentamicin 1.5 mg/kg within 30 minutes of starting procedure. 6 hours later, ampicillin 25 mg/kg I.M. or I.V. or amoxicillin 25 mg/kg P.O. |
| High risk and allergic to ampicillin or amoxicillin | vancomycin plus gentamicin | *Adults:* vancomycin 1 g I.V. over 1 to 2 hours and gentamicin 1.5 mg/kg I.M. or I.V. (not to exceed 120 mg) completed within 30 minutes of starting procedure *Children:* vancomycin 20 mg/kg I.V. over 1 to 2 hours plus gentamicin 1.5 mg/kg I.M. or I.V. completed within 30 minutes of starting procedure |

*(continued)*

| PATIENT TYPE | MEDICATION | REGIMEN |
|---|---|---|

**ENDOCARDITIS PROPHYLAXIS REGIMENS** *(continued)*

FOR GENITOURINARY AND GI (EXCLUDING ESOPHAGEAL) PROCEDURES *(continued)*

| PATIENT TYPE | MEDICATION | REGIMEN |
|---|---|---|
| Moderate risk | amoxicillin<br>**OR**<br>ampicillin | *Adults:* amoxicillin 2 g P.O. 1 hour before procedure<br>*Children:* amoxicillin 50 mg/kg P.O. 1 hour before procedure<br>*Adults:* ampicillin 2 g I.M. or I.V. within 30 minutes of starting procedure<br>*Children:* ampicillin 50 mg/kg I.M. or I.V. within 30 minutes of starting procedure |
| Moderate risk and allergic to ampicillin or amoxicillin | vancomycin | *Adults:* vancomycin 1 g I.V. over 1 to 2 hours completed within 30 minutes of starting procedure<br>*Children:* vancomycin 20 mg/kg I.V. over 1 to 2 hours completed within 30 minutes of starting procedure |

## COMPLICATIONS

➤ If the patient develops an *allergic reaction* to the prescribed antibiotic, he should contact you at once.

## SPECIAL CONSIDERATIONS

➤ For genitourinary procedures, consider the most likely pathogen and prescribe an antibiotic specific to that pathogen as well.
➤ Consider prescribing antibiotics prophylactically for low-risk procedures involving the lower respiratory, GI, or genitourinary tract for patients with prosthetic heart valves, surgically constructed cardiac shunts, or a history of endocarditis.
➤ The 1997 revision of the guidelines of the American Heart Association states that patients with certain conditions are no longer considered to be at increased risk and don't need prophylactic measures beyond those for the general population. These patients include those with isolated atrial defect; surgical repair of atrial septal defect, ventricular septal defect, or patent ductus arteriosus (without residual effects beyond 6 months); previous coronary artery bypass graft surgery; mitral valve prolapse without valvar regurgitation; benign heart murmurs; previous Kawasaki disease or rheumatic fever without valvar dysfunction; or cardiac pacemakers or implanted defibrillators.

## DOCUMENTATION

➤ Document the type of procedure and the patient's risk factors for endocarditis.
➤ Thoroughly document the cardiac examination, including a description of heart murmurs.
➤ List the type and amount of antibiotic prescribed.
➤ Note the patient's response to teaching.
➤ Document the procedure and follow-up assessment, noting the presence or lack of infection.

# Respiratory Procedures

## 2

No matter where you work, you're sure to encounter patients with respiratory conditions. Such conditions may be acute or chronic and may have developed as a primary disorder or resulted from a cardiac or other body system malfunction.

Caring for the patient with a respiratory condition will challenge your assessment and disease management skills. Not only is his oxygenation compromised, but he may develop other problems as well. For instance, the patient with chronic obstructive pulmonary disease may develop bronchitis and then heart failure. He may cut back on fluids to decrease nocturia and become dehydrated. Shortness of breath may cause him to decrease his activities and eat less, leading to progressive generalized weakness and compromised nutrition. He may also feel anxious, cope ineffectively, and have an impaired ability to communicate. For such a patient, you'll need to develop a management plan that ensures optimal gas exchange and physical independence.

To meet patient needs, you need to have a working knowledge of the many therapies available to respiratory patients. Then you'll understand the rationale behind a patient's treatment and be able to order or perform procedures, recognize complications, and quickly implement corrective actions. You'll also work with other members of the health care team to teach the patient and his family about equipment and procedures necessary for his care.

## DIAGNOSTIC TESTING

### Peak flow meter use

CPT CODE
*94150    Vital capacity, total*

## DESCRIPTION

Peak expiratory flow rate (PEFR) is the maximum force and speed that a patient can exhale air from his lungs. It's a valuable measurement because it can demonstrate a decrease in lung function 1 to 3 days before other respiratory signs become apparent. It's measured with a spirometer or a peak flow meter (PFM). Although not as accurate as a spirometer, a PFM is a simple, portable, and inexpensive device (see *Peak flow meter,* page 76).

The practitioner can use a PFM to determine the patient's individual range of PEFR values and customize it to define a patient's "personal best." Individualized guidelines can be developed in conjunction with his practitioner to allow the patient to adjust the dose according to his PEFR. Using a system that divides PEFRs into three ranges, the practitioner defines the treatment according to the patient's

## PEAK FLOW METER

Once your patient uses a particular brand of flow meter, make sure she sticks with that brand. If she must switch to a new brand, she'll need to establish a new "personal best" because different brands assign different values to the results. This illustration shows a typical peak flow meter, with a bar graph on the top where the sliding indicator stops after the patient reaches her peak expiratory flow rate.

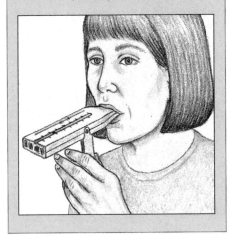

current PEFR. Using a PFM can reduce the frequency, duration, and severity of asthma attacks as well as the number of visits to the emergency department. (See *Obtaining your peak expiratory flow rate.*)

## INDICATIONS

➤ To determine the severity of asthma
➤ To check response to treatment during an acute episode
➤ To detect unrecognized decrease in lung function
➤ To diagnose asthma triggers such as exercise

## CONTRAINDICATIONS

### Absolute

➤ Respiratory distress
➤ Asthma attack

## EQUIPMENT

PFM

## ESSENTIAL STEPS

➤ Explain the procedure to the patient and answer any questions.
➤ Make sure the patient remains inactive for 5 minutes before testing.
➤ Check that the PFM indicator is set to the zero mark.
➤ Have the patient stand up, if possible. If he can't, have him assume a position that allows maximal chest expansion and stay in that position for all maneuvers.
➤ Tell the patient to inhale as deeply as possible.
➤ Have the patient bring the PFM to his mouth, hold it in the proper direction (according to the manufacturer's instructions), and form a tight seal around the mouthpiece with his lips; remind the patient not to cough or let his tongue block the mouthpiece.
➤ Tell the patient to exhale as hard and fast as possible for 1 to 2 seconds.
➤ Note the PEFR.
➤ Have the patient repeat the procedure two more times.
➤ Record the highest of the three values obtained, and note it in the patient's medical records. If the patient keeps his own diary to chart progress, record results there as well.
➤ Determine the zone of lung function, and instruct the patient on which medications to take based on PEFR values obtained. (See *Lung function zones*, page 78.)
➤ Clean the PFM according to the manufacturer's instructions to prevent bacter-

## OBTAINING YOUR PEAK EXPIRATORY FLOW RATE

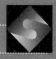

DEAR PATIENT:

The practitioner needs to obtain your peak expiratory flow (PEFR) rate to determine your level of lung functioning.

### How PEFR works

PEFR combines deep breathing and normal breathing with forced expiration. This demonstrates your ability to cough effectively and evaluates the volume of air you can move out of your lungs at a given time. The procedure isn't hard to learn. Just remember to concentrate so that you get an accurate measurement.

### When to perform PEFR

*Never* perform PEFR during an asthma attack; it could trigger coughing or worsen your symptoms. Generally, you'll perform PEFR daily for 2 to 3 weeks to perfect your technique and develop guidelines with your practitioner based on your personal values. During those weeks, record your peak expiratory flow measurements at least twice daily. Your "personal best" is the highest reading (usually reached in the afternoon or evening).

After that, continue to perform PEFR daily during times when you're normally prone to respiratory problems, during respiratory infections, and when you notice a change in your respiratory status.

Your personal best measurement needs periodic reevaluation to see if it has changed. If your personal best measurement decreases, you may need your medications changed or your dose increased to prevent your asthma from getting worse. If it improves significantly, you may need less anti-inflammatory medication.

A child needs his personal best measurement checked about every 6 months to account for growth.

### How to perform PEFR

Follow these steps to perform PEFR.
➤ Set the flow meter to zero.
➤ Stand up.
➤ Inhale as deeply as possible.
➤ Bring the flow meter to your mouth, hold it in the proper direction, and form a tight seal around the mouthpiece with your lips.
➤ Don't cough or let your tongue block the mouthpiece.
➤ Exhale as hard and fast as possible for 1 to 2 seconds.
➤ Note the PEFR.
➤ Repeat two more times.
➤ Record the highest of the three values in your diary.
➤ Determine your zone of lung function and follow the practitioner's guidelines.
➤ Clean the flow meter according to the manufacturer's instructions to prevent the growth of bacteria and fungi and ensure accuracy. Typical instructions call for you to wash the meter in soapy water every 2 weeks.

**ADDITIONAL INSTRUCTIONS:**

......................................................................

......................................................................

......................................................................

......................................................................

......................................................................

......................................................................

## LUNG FUNCTION ZONES

The following three charts can help you determine appropriate lung function zones for your patient. The first two charts list expected "normal" peak expiratory flow rates (PEFRs) that you can use to evaluate your patient's PEFR. The first chart includes values for both sexes under age 20 based on height.

### NORMAL PEFR FOR THOSE UNDER AGE 20

| HEIGHT (IN.) | PEFR (L/MINUTE) | HEIGHT | PEFR | HEIGHT | PEFR |
|---|---|---|---|---|---|
| 43 | 147 | 51 | 254 | 59 | 360 |
| 44 | 160 | 52 | 267 | 60 | 373 |
| 45 | 173 | 53 | 280 | 61 | 387 |
| 46 | 187 | 54 | 293 | 62 | 400 |
| 47 | 200 | 55 | 307 | 63 | 413 |
| 48 | 214 | 56 | 320 | 64 | 427 |
| 49 | 227 | 57 | 334 | 65 | 440 |
| 50 | 240 | 58 | 347 | 66 | 454 |

The second chart lists the different values for men and women at age 20. After age 20, the normal predicted PEFR decreases from 5 to 15 L/minute every 5 years. Keep in mind that a "normal" PEFR can vary widely among individuals.

### NORMAL PEFR AT AGE 20

| HEIGHT (IN.) | PEFR (L/MINUTE) |
|---|---|
| Males 60 | 554 |
| 65 | 602 |
| 70 | 649 |
| 75 | 693 |
| 80 | 740 |
| Females 55 | 390 |
| 60 | 423 |
| 65 | 460 |
| 70 | 496 |
| 75 | 529 |

ial and fungal growth and to ensure accuracy.

## PATIENT TEACHING

➤ Teach the patient proper technique for obtaining his PEFR, and have him demonstrate his ability use the PFM.

➤ If the patient is a child, tell his parents or caregivers to obtain three roughly similar readings to ensure that the child made a good effort each time.

➤ Tell the patient he'll need to determine his PEFR twice daily for 2 to 3 weeks to perfect his technique and develop guidelines with his practitioner based on those values.

## LUNG FUNCTION ZONES (continued)

This last chart uses the patient's "personal best" to determine his lung function zones. A patient's personal best is the highest value he can reach in the middle of a good day after inhaling a bronchodilator (if prescribed). Once you and your patient have established his personal best, this chart can help him maintain 80% or more of that value or intervene as needed if he falls below that. The chart uses a familiar color-coded system — green for go, yellow for caution, and red for danger — to help keep the patient on track, even when he's under stress.

| ZONE | RANGE OF PEFR VALUES | TREATMENT GUIDELINES |
|------|----------------------|----------------------|
| *Green:* All systems GO | 80% to 100% of personal best | ➤ Continue current management plan.<br>➤ If on chronic medications and constantly in the green zone with minimal variation, consider gradually decreasing daily medication. |
| *Yellow:* Lung function decreasing, CAUTION | 50% to 80% of personal best | ➤ Temporarily increase asthma medication; refer to individualized guidelines for patient (for instance, use bronchodilator, inhaled steroid, or oral steroid burst).<br>➤ Have patient notify practitioner.<br>➤ If constantly in the yellow zone using chronic medications, increase maintenance therapy. |
| *Red:* Asthma control is failing, DANGER | Below 50% of personal best | ➤ Instruct patient to use inhaled bronchodilator. If PEFR doesn't return to yellow or green zone, patient requires medically supervised aggressive therapy. If unable to contact practitioner, patient to go to an urgent care center or walk-in clinic.<br>➤ Adjust maintenance therapy. |

➤ Explain what individualized treatment steps the patient should follow for each of the three ranges of PEFR.

➤ Explain to the patient that he can expect a significant decline in acute exacerbations within 1 month of using PEFR-guided treatment. He'll know his asthma is controlled when he has no more asthma symptoms (including nocturnal symptoms) and can maintain a normal activity level.

➤ Tell the patient to follow up with you within 2 days of an emergency department visit for a physical examination and to assess his technique, diary, and treatment protocol.

➤ Tell the patient to call you for persistent, changing, worsening, or anxiety-producing signs and symptoms. Explain that he should follow the guidelines listed in the yellow and red zones.

➤ Tell the patient to measure his PEFR twice daily (upon awakening and between noon and 2 p.m.) after exposure to asthma triggers, when he has a respiratory infection, and when his asthma management plan changes.

➤ To identify asthma triggers, tell the patient to write down his PEFR before and

## BREATHING EASILY—AND SAFELY—AT WORK

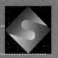

DEAR PATIENT:

Breathing dirty air on the job can damage your lungs. To protect yourself, try to reduce or eliminate your exposure to breathing hazards. Here are some tips.

### Identify breathing hazards
Keep alert for air pollution signs at work, including:
➤ *Dust clouds.* Inhaling dust particles can irritate your lungs. Repeated exposure over months or years can cause serious disease.
➤ *Unusual fumes.* The first warning of a breathing hazard may be a strange odor as you enter your work area.
➤ *Burning eyes, throat, and lungs.* If your eyes start to smart and your throat and chest feel tight as soon as you enter the workplace, suspect a breathing hazard.
➤ *Chronic cough or shortness of breath.* See your practitioner if you have these symptoms. They may be job-related if they occur or get worse when you're at work or if your co-workers have the same symptoms.

### Safeguard your lungs
Follow these tips to avoid inhaling dust, smoke, and noxious gases:
➤ Stay away from unnecessary dust, fumes, and vapors, if possible.
➤ Wash your skin thoroughly after working with hazardous materials — especially before you eat or drink. Also change into clean clothing. Wash contaminated clothing separately from other laundry.
➤ Insist on good ventilation at work. An open window or cooling fan may not be enough to remove air pollutants. If your work area has an exhaust system to re-

move contaminated air, make sure the system works. If you're given a respirator, wear it properly. Also insist on and use other protective equipment for the job.
➤ Don't smoke. Cigarette smoke injures lungs and contains carbon monoxide. By smoking, you also breathe in other airborne pollutants.

### Work safely with chemicals
Your employer is responsible for providing training and equipment to do your job safely. But you can help too.
➤ Read label warnings on chemical containers before you open them. Then heed them.
➤ Ask for and follow your employer's instructions on how to use chemicals safely to avoid illness and injury.
➤ Make sure you read the Material Safety Data Sheet that the law says your employer must keep on file (or post) for all hazardous chemicals. This sheet identifies the chemical's physical properties and health effects. It tells how to use, store, and handle the chemical safely on the job and in emergencies.
➤ Ask your employer to set up a workplace safety and health training program for employees if you don't have one yet.

### ADDITIONAL INSTRUCTIONS:

...........................................................................

...........................................................................

...........................................................................

...........................................................................

...........................................................................

after exposure to allergens, irritants, exercise, and other suspected triggers. Once identified, triggers should be avoided at all times. (See *Breathing easily — and safely — at work*.)

➤ Tell the patient to wash the PFM in soapy water every 2 weeks or according to the manufacturer's instructions.

## COMPLICATIONS

➤ If left untreated, *acute respiratory distress* can cause hypoxia, brain damage, or death. If signs of respiratory distress occur, stop the procedure and institute emergency medical procedures as needed.

 **ALERT** This procedure can exacerbate *respiratory distress* in a patient already short of breath.

## SPECIAL CONSIDERATIONS

➤ The patient doesn't need to wear noseclips during the procedure.

➤ If patient can't achieve 80% of PEFR during the initial 2 to 3 weeks, he'll need a course of oral corticosteroids to help determine his personal best measurement.

➤ The patient doesn't have to wake up at night to determine if nocturnal asthma occurred. If the morning reading is 15% or more below the reading from the night before, he experienced nocturnal asthma.

➤ Evaluating the PEFR during different seasons can help identify such seasonal triggers as pollen, cold, and dry air.

 **CULTURAL TIP** Before seeking outside medical help, some patients from different cultures may try folk medicine, which may affect PEFR measurements. For instance, massage therapy has been shown to increase PEFR, whereas Lobelia (also known as asthma weed and touted as a spasmolytic and antiasthmatic agent) can cause respiratory depression.

➤ A child's PEFR shouldn't decrease; he should undergo reevaluation every 6 months to assess changes that occur with growth.

➤ To simplify reading the PFM for a child or visually impaired patient, colored tape or lines can indicate the green, yellow, and red zones on the PFM.

## DOCUMENTATION

➤ Record the patient's current PEFR.

➤ Record whether the patient demonstrated proper technique and described appropriate actions for each range of PEFR.

➤ Document the management plan for each zone of lung function.

# Pulmonary function testing

CPT CODES
*94010    Spirometry (includes graphic record, total and timed vital capacity, expiratory flow rate measurements [including calculation of forced vital capacity and forced expiratory volume] and interpretation)*
*94060    Spirometry before and after bronchodilator (or before and after exercise)*
*94150    Vital capacity screening test*
*94375    Respiratory flow volume loop*

## DESCRIPTION

Pulmonary function testing (PFT) uses standardized measures to evaluate lung function. Complete PFT includes static and dynamic lung volumes, diffusing capacity, flow volume loop, maximal voluntary ventilation, and maximal inspiratory and expiratory pressures.

PFT uses spirometry to obtain measurements. Spirometry can classify processes as normal, restricted, or obstructive, but it can't yield specific diagnoses. Airflow measurements reflect airway patency, elasticity of the respiratory muscles, and the conscious muscular effort exerted by the patient. These measurements don't, however, indicate the adequacy of gas exchange (diffusing capacity and arterial blood gas measurements indicate gas exchange). Electronic spirometers produce flow volume loops by generating continuous recordings of flow and volume during forced inspiration and expiration. (See *Understanding pulmonary function test results.*)

To obtain accurate, reproducible results (based on the standards set by the American Thoracic Society [ATS]), the patient must exert his maximal inspiratory effort. Because the results depend on the patient's effort, active coaching increases the likelihood of obtaining valid results.

## INDICATIONS

➤ To evaluate lung function
➤ To detect obstructive or restrictive lung disease
➤ To assess the presence and extent of reversibility of airway obstruction
➤ To evaluate and monitor therapeutic interventions (for instance, to evaluate the success of bronchodilators)
➤ To determine the presence and extent of drug-induced toxicity (for instance, from chemotherapy)
➤ To assess patients at risk for respiratory complications before surgery
➤ To screen for occupational lung disease
➤ To motivate a patient to stop smoking
➤ To screen for disability

## CONTRAINDICATIONS

### Relative
➤ Severe shortness of breath or bronchoconstriction related to effort
➤ Severe fatigue

➤ Recent myocardial infarction and acute illness, including viral infection in the past 2 to 3 weeks
➤ Large pulmonary blebs or bullae
➤ History of marked vasovagal responsiveness
➤ History of spontaneous pneumothorax
➤ Uncontrolled hypertension

## EQUIPMENT

Volume-based spirometer (spirometer meets ATS accuracy standards and fulfills National Institute of Occupational Safety and Health requirements; it must have at least a 7-L and 15-second strip capacity and be regularly checked for leaks) or flow-based pneumotachygraph ◆ noseclip

## ESSENTIAL STEPS

➤ At least 6 hours before the test, withhold bronchodilators (if possible), unless the purpose of the test is to evaluate the bronchodilator's effectiveness.
➤ Make sure the patient understands that he shouldn't smoke, drink beverages, or eat a heavy meal for at least 1 hour before the test or he won't be able to produce his maximal breathing effort.
➤ Explain the purpose of the specific test to the patient and what he'll need to do.
➤ Make sure the patient isn't so tired that he can't follow directions.
➤ Record the patient's age, gender, height, and race. If the patient can't stand or has a spinal deformity, you can approximate his height from his arm span.
➤ Have the patient sit or stand. If he sits, make sure that his legs aren't crossed and that he has both feet solidly on the floor.
➤ Have the patient remove poorly fitting dentures and loosen or remove any constricting clothing, such as a belt or necktie.
➤ Tell the patient to slightly elevate his chin, with his neck slightly extended; he

# UNDERSTANDING PULMONARY FUNCTION TEST RESULTS

These graphs show the results of pulmonary function testing (PFT). However, to understand the results, you first need to understand the terminology.

➤ *Total lung capacity (TLC):* The total volume of air remaining in the lungs after maximum inspiration.

➤ *Vital capacity (VC):* The maximum volume of air an individual can completely (and slowly) exhale after a maximum inspiration; normal is 3.88 to 5 L.

➤ *Forced vital capacity (FVC):* The same as VC but using maximum forceful expiration. The FVC may be less than the VC because of premature closure of the terminal airways, reflecting obstructive disease. A reduced FVC may also indicate the presence of restrictive disease.

➤ *Tidal volume (TV):* Airflow in a resting individual; normal is 500 ml.

➤ *Forced expiratory volume in 1 second (FEV₁):* The FVC volume exhaled in 1 second; normal is 3.12 to 3.96 L; it primarily reflects the condition of the large airway.s

➤ *Percentage of FEV₁ (FEV₁/FVC):* $FEV_1$ compared to FVC; normal is at least 75%; less than 75% suggests obstruction.

➤ *Mean forced expiratory flow (FEF₂₅%-₇₅%):* Formally called midexpiratory flow; a sensitive indicator of the condition of the small airways. Decreased values are an indication of obstruction disease, especially in asthma and bronchitis.

When interpreting PFT results, keep in mind the criteria for acceptable results and reproducibility.

## Acceptable results

➤ The tracing doesn't reflect coughing, early glottic closure (see figure 7), a hesitant start, or problems with equipment.

➤ Forceful expiration occurs with 6 seconds of smooth, continuous exhalation or a plateau of at least 2 seconds or both.

## Reproducibility

➤ The largest FVC is within 0.2 L of the next largest FVC.

➤ The largest $FEV_1$ is within 0.2 L of the next largest FEV₁.

**FIGURE 1: NORMAL SPIROMETRY (VOLUME-BASED)**

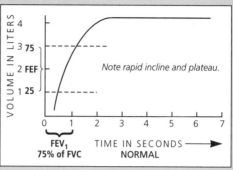

**FIGURE 2: NORMAL SPIROMETRY (FLOW-BASED)**

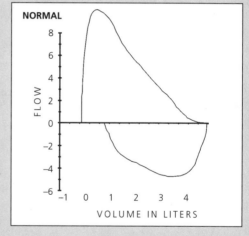

**FIGURE 3: SPIROMETRY REFLECTING OBSTRUCTIVE DISEASE**

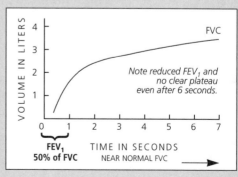

*(continued)*

## UNDERSTANDING PULMONARY FUNCTION TEST RESULTS (continued)

**FIGURE 4: SPIROMETRY REFLECTING RESTRICTIVE DISEASE**

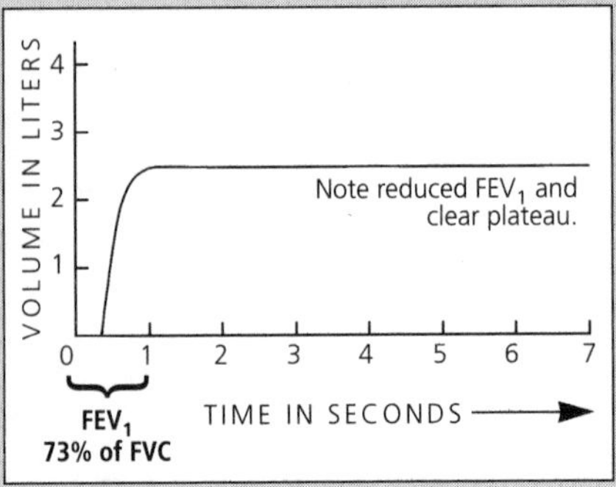

Note reduced FEV₁ and clear plateau.

FEV₁ 73% of FVC

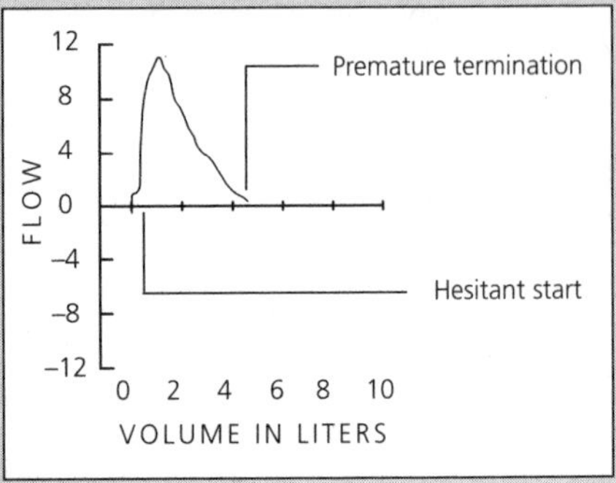

**FIGURE 5: ABRUPT DECREASES IN TRACING BECAUSE OF COUGHING**

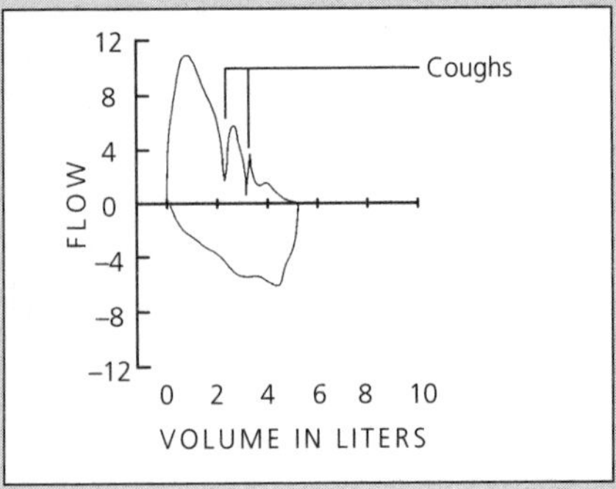

Coughs

**FIGURE 6: HESITANT START**

Premature termination

Hesitant start

**FIGURE 7: EARLY GLOTTIC CLOSURE**

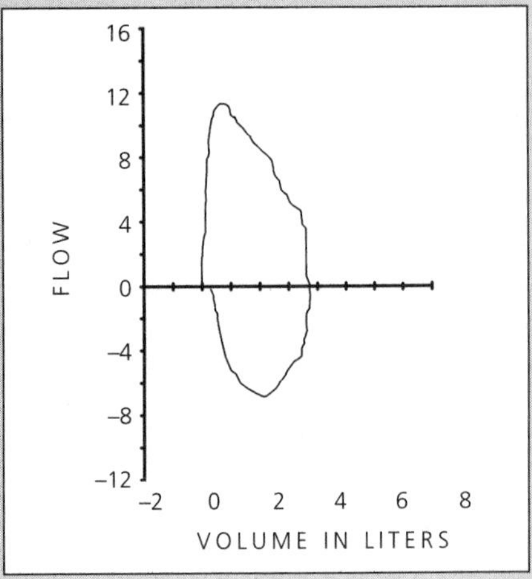

shouldn't have his chin down toward the chest.

➤ Calibrate the machine based on instructions from the manufacturer.

➤ Put the noseclip on the patient and have him make sure that he can't pass any air through his nose.

➤ Tell the patient to seal his lips tightly around the mouthpiece with his teeth around the outside. For a cardboard mouthpiece, tell the patient not to bite

down so that he doesn't obstruct the hole in the tubing. Tell him not to protrude his tongue into the mouthpiece.

➤ Tell the patient to exhale forcibly into the tube. If necessary, demonstrate how to do this.

➤ Actively coach the patient to blow out all his air as hard and as fast as possible.

➤ Make sure the patient exhales for at least 6 seconds, up to 20 seconds.

➤ Repeat the procedure until you achieve three acceptable trials, but don't do more than eight trials or the patient may become fatigued.

➤ Record the measurements on the spirometer. Note the measurement on the spirometer recording at 1 second as forced expiratory volume in 1 second ($FEV_1$).

➤ Evaluate the strips. The tracing needs to last at least 6 seconds with at least 2 seconds of plateau.

➤ Make sure the two best tracings don't vary by more than 100 ml, or 5%; this suggests consistent best effort. Note whether the patient coughed, which could interfere with some tests.

➤ If you didn't obtain any acceptable tracings after eight trials, select the best one, noting its limitations.

➤ Compare the patient's results (and previous test results if available) with standardized norms. Norms vary according to race, height, age, and gender.

### Bronchodilator evaluation

➤ If you're evaluating the patient's response to bronchodilators, administer the medication after selecting the initial two tracings.

➤ Wait 15 minutes and then repeat the procedure until you've obtained three acceptable trials.

➤ Interpret the two best tracings. A positive response to bronchodilators is generally considered to be an increase in forced vital capacity (FVC) of at least 15% and an increase in $FEV_1$ of at least 12%.

 **ALERT** Keep in mind that exceptionally fit lungs might have to deteriorate by as much as 40% of their capacity to fall out of normal range.

## PATIENT TEACHING

➤ Tell the patient he may experience some fatigue but no other adverse effects. (See *Preparing for pulmonary function tests*, page 86.)

➤ Demonstrate how to blow out hard right at the start of the test and repeat the trial, coaching the patient. (See Figure 6 in *Understanding pulmonary function test results*.)

➤ Tell the patient he should try to keep the flow as fast and as consistent as possible and repeat trials as necessary.

➤ Tell the patient to follow up based on his indication for PFT.

➤ Make sure the patient contacts you if he experiences persistent fatigue or any breathing difficulties. Explain that this may stem from the pulmonary disorder rather than the testing.

## COMPLICATIONS

➤ Prevent *fainting* by allowing the patent to decrease expiration after the initial 3 seconds and continue exhaling without forcing it. If the patient faints, ease him to the floor and elevate his legs until consciousness returns. Defer testing, if possible, for another day.

➤ *Test-induced bronchospasm (each subsequent effort demonstrates declining airflow):* Select the best effort and note the problem. The patient is usually scheduled for further testing after administration of a bronchodilator.

➤ *Machine malfunction:* Check for air leaks and recalibrate the machine.

## SPECIAL CONSIDERATIONS

➤ Children younger than age 5 typically can't cooperate well enough to ensure valid results.

➤ Blacks and Asians have spirometry and lung volumes 15% lower than Whites.

➤ A cough peak expiratory flow rate (PEFR) approximates the peak flow you should observe during testing. For this measurement, the patient should take a deep

## PREPARING FOR PULMONARY FUNCTION TESTS

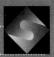

DEAR PATIENT:

The practitioner has ordered pulmonary (or lung) function tests for you. These tests measure how well your lungs work. Here is what to expect.

### How the tests work

You will be asked to breathe as deeply as possible into a mouthpiece that is connected to a machine called a spirometer. This measures and records the rate and amount of air inhaled and exhaled.

Or you may sit in a small, telephone booth–like enclosure for a test called body plethysmography. Again, you'll be asked to breathe in and out, and the measurements will be recorded.

### Before the tests

Avoid smoking for at least 4 hours before the tests. Eat lightly, and don't drink a lot of fluid. Wear loose, comfortable clothing. Remember to use the bathroom.

To make the tests go quickly, give your full cooperation. Tell the technician if you don't understand the instructions. If you wear dentures, keep them in — they'll help you keep a tight seal around the spirometer's mouthpiece.

### During the tests

During spirometry, you'll sit upright, and you'll wear a noseclip to make sure you breathe only though your mouth. During body plethysmography, you won't need a noseclip.

If you feel too confined in the small chamber, keep in mind that you can't suffocate. You can talk to the technician through a window.

The tests have several parts. For each test, you'll be asked to breathe a certain way — for example, to inhale deeply and exhale completely or to exhale quickly. You may need to repeat some tests after inhaling a bronchodilator medicine to expand the airways in your lungs. Also, the practitioner may take a sample of blood from an artery in your arm. This sample will be used to measure how well your body uses the air you breathe.

### How will you feel?

During the tests, you may feel tired or short of breath. However, you'll be able to take rest breaks between measurements.

Tell the practitioner right away if you feel dizzy, begin wheezing, or have chest pain, a racing or pounding heart, an upset stomach, or severe shortness of breath.

Also tell her if your arm swells or you're bleeding at the spot where a blood sample was taken or if you experience weakness or pain in that arm.

### After the tests

When the tests are over, rest if you feel like it. Then plan to resume your usual activities when you regain your energy.

### ADDITIONAL INSTRUCTIONS:

...........................................................................

...........................................................................

...........................................................................

...........................................................................

breath and then cough into the mouthpiece. If the observed **PEFR** isn't more than 1 L/second more than cough PEFR, the patient may not be exerting his best effort.

➤ Normal FEVs peak for women at age 20 and for men at age 22. Such values then decrease approximately 20 to 30 ml per year and shouldn't demonstrate more than a 15% change per year.

➤ FVC and $FEV_1$ values greater than 80% of the predicted values are considered normal. The highest FVC and $FEV_1$ should be reported, even if they're from two separate trials. Forced expiratory flow$_{25\%-75\%}$, however, must be reported from the most acceptable test curve with the largest sum of FVC and $FEV_1$.

➤ If the patient coughs during testing, repeat the trial if possible, especially if the coughing occurs during the 1st second of testing. If the patient can't control coughing, note that in the comments. (See Figure 5 in *Understanding pulmonary function test results*, page 84.)

➤ If the patient puts forth a poor effort, explain once again the importance and purpose of the test and repeat trial as necessary.

➤ If the patient stops exhaling too early, explain the problem and its significance and increase your coaching as you repeat the trial.

➤ If the results show variable peak flow rates, repeat the trial as necessary and increase your coaching during each trial (for instance, say, "Keep blowing, don't stop!").

## DOCUMENTATION

➤ Document the patient's age, gender, height, and race.
➤ Note the patient's position during trials and the number of trials.
➤ Record the patient's effort.
➤ Note whether you administered any bronchodilator, including the dose and timing.

➤ Record the spirometry results.
➤ Note the patient's appearance after testing.

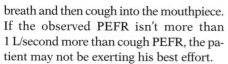

# Chest X-ray interpretation

CPT CODES
*71010    Radiologic exam, chest, frontal*
*71020    Radiologic exam, chest, frontal and lateral*

## DESCRIPTION

Used in conjunction with patient history and physical examination, chest X-rays can help a practitioner arrive at a more accurate diagnosis. For a chest X-ray to provide the most useful information, the practitioner needs a basic knowledge of how X-rays work and how to read films to detect the pathologies that chest X-rays can reveal. (See *X-ray terminology*, page 88.)

To produce a chest X-ray film, the X-ray machine sends a stream of X-rays (or photons) through the chest. Structures in the chest then absorb these X-rays to a greater or lesser degree. Denser structures such as bone absorb more X-rays; less dense structures, such as soft tissue and fat, allow more X-rays to pass through; and the least dense structures such as air allow the most X-rays to pass through. X-rays that pass through the chest strike a film, turning it darker. The areas of film behind the densest structures (such as bone) appear the lightest because the dense structure absorbed most of the X-rays before they could reach the film. As a result, a typical chest X-ray film shows ribs and other bones as white against a darker background.

The patient typically stands or lies in a supine position for a chest X-ray and re-

## X-RAY TERMINOLOGY

To evaluate a chest X-ray, you need to understand the terminology involved:
➤ *Density:* Brightness or any area of whiteness on an image.
➤ *Lucency:* Blackness or any area of blackness on an image.
➤ *Shadow:* Anything visible on an image; any specific density or lucency.
➤ *Edge:* Any visible demarcation between a density on one side and a lucency on the other.
➤ *Line:* A thin density with lucency on both sides, or a thin lucency with density on both sides.
➤ *Stripe:* Any edge or line.
➤ *Silhouette:* Another term for edge; the ability to see an edge is the silhouette sign.

quires no special preparation. Basic chest views include the posterior-anterior and lateral views (for a standing patient) and the anterior-posterior view (for a supine patient). During the procedure, the patient is exposed to approximately 20 milliroentgens of radiation. (See *Chest X-ray case studies,* pages 89 to 93.)

## INDICATIONS

➤ To assess chest trauma
➤ To detect and assess lung disease
➤ To verify the placement of devices

## CONTRAINDICATIONS

### Absolute
➤ Pregnancy

## EQUIPMENT

X-ray films ◆ photographic light box

## ESSENTIAL STEPS

➤ Before reading the film, verify patient information and the position of left and right markers on the film.
➤ Place the films on the illuminated photographic light box.
➤ Judge the technical quality of the film, especially the adequacy of penetration (vertebral bodies should appear clear).
➤ Look briefly at films for obvious abnormalities.

### Scanning the frontal view
➤ Study the lungs, looking both up and down and side to side. Include lung volume and symmetry of markings.
➤ Check the periphery of the lungs for pneumothorax and effusions.
➤ Evaluate the edges and shape of the mediastinal contour; note the diaphragm.
➤ Evaluate heart size and location.
➤ Follow the trachea to the carina and main stem bronchus.
➤ Look at both hili for enlargement and abnormal bulges.
➤ Begin at the neck and review the periphery of chest, include the shoulders, ribs, and clavicle.
➤ Check the upper abdomen for free air and abnormal air collection.

### Scanning the lateral view
➤ Follow the airway from the neck to the hilum. Note lung markings and look for fissures.
➤ Look down to the heart and up the anterior mediastinum to the neck.
➤ Follow the spine and posterior ribs to the costophrenic angle.
➤ Judge the shape of the diaphragm and the upper abdomen.
➤ Check the anterior chest wall and sternum.

## CHEST X-RAY CASE STUDIES

These eight chest X-rays can help you recognize what various pathologies look like on film. The first shows the structures you'll see in a normal chest X-ray, and the next seven show pathology ranging from lobar pneumonia to lung cancer.

### Normal posteroanterior chest X-ray

This X-ray shows certain normal, soft, and bony structures in the chest and upper abdomen.

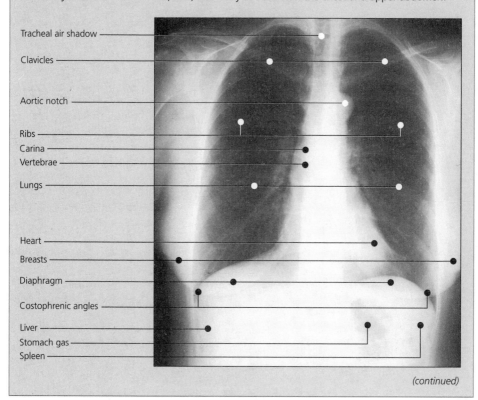

Tracheal air shadow

Clavicles

Aortic notch

Ribs
Carina
Vertebrae

Lungs

Heart

Breasts

Diaphragm

Costophrenic angles

Liver
Stomach gas
Spleen

*(continued)*

### Evaluating the frontal view

➤ Evaluate lung markings (vessels) and minor fissures. Specifically, evaluate the:
– mediastinum
– airways (trachea, carina, and main bronchi)
– hili (left and right pulmonary arteries)
– soft tissues (in the neck and chest walls, breast shadows, diaphragms, and intestinal gas)
– bones (ribs, clavicles, scapula, humerus, spine, vertebral bodies, and disk spaces).

### Evaluating the lateral view

➤ Evaluate the airways, including the trachea and main and left bronchi. Also evaluate:
– hili (left and right pulmonary arteries)
– lung (major and minor markings and fissures)
– left ventricle of the heart.
➤ On the posterior chest view, evaluate the spine, ribs, diaphragms, and intestinal gas.
➤ Evaluate the anterior chest.

### Lobar pneumonia
This chest X-ray of a 79-year-old woman shows classic findings of lobar pneumonia involving the left lower lobe. These signs include the silhouette sign, in which the left hemidiaphragm and heart shadow borders can't be seen, mild atelectasis (note the smaller left lung), and depressed left hilum with mediastinal shift to the left ➡.

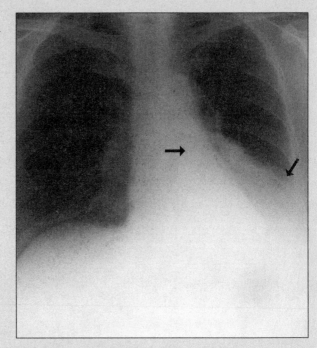

### Pulmonary changes with asthma
In this posteroanterior chest X-ray of a young woman with asthma, note the hyperinflated lungs ➤, small heart ➡, and depressed diaphragm ➡➤.

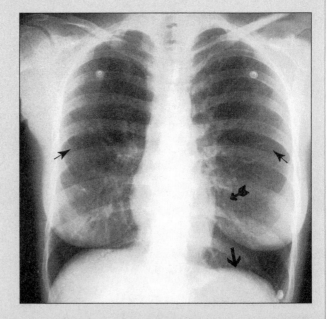

### Pneumothorax with subcutaneous emphysema

In this posteroanterior chest X-ray of a patient with a pneumothorax, the chest tube ⇨ has migrated outside of the pleural space. As a result, the patient has a larger pneumothorax ➡ than he originally had. He has also developed subcutaneous and mediastinal emphysema ➜.

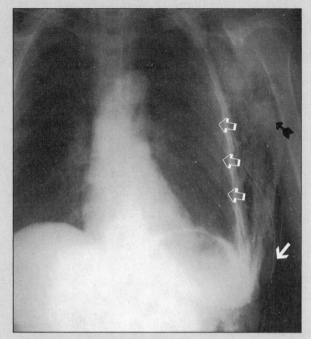

### Pleural effusion

This is a posteroanterior chest X-ray of a 58-year-old man with a history of heart failure. The patient has right-side pleural fluid blunting the right costophrenic angle due to the pleural fluid. Note the concavity of the upper border of the pleural fluid ➜.

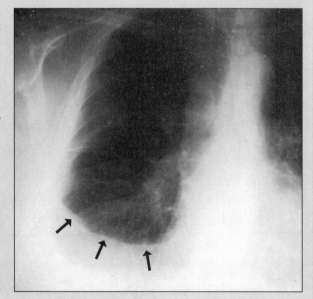

(continued)

### Rib fractures

This anteroposterior chest X-ray of a trauma patient after a motor vehicle accident shows left fifth ➤➤ and sixth ⇨ lateral rib fractures. Note the separation at fracture sites from displacement and associated left clavicle ➜ and left scapula fractures ➤.

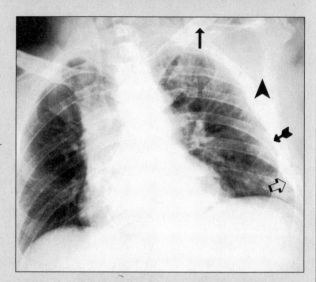

### Lung cancer

This is a chest X-ray of a 67-year-old woman with bronchogenic lung cancer. Note the large mass ➜ with cavitation at the center ➤➤ in the right hilum area. The right lower lobe is opaque, which indicates atelectasis caused by the tumor.

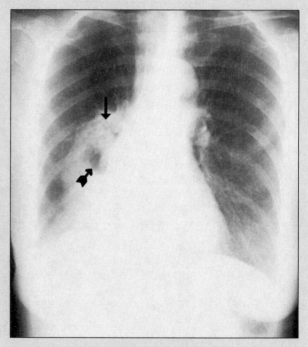

**Foreign body**
This is a classic inspiratory and expiratory anteroposterior chest X-ray of a 17-month-old child with a ball-valve-type foreign body in the left bronchus. Inspiratory film is essentially normal, but expiratory film shows the left lung hyperinflated ➤ by the foreign body because air is being trapped. You can also see a shift of the mediastinum to the right ➤➤ and relative increased lucency, or dark air-filled area, on the left.

**INSPIRATION**

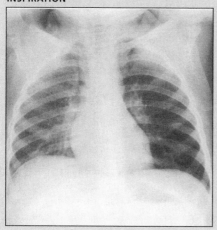

**EXPIRATION**

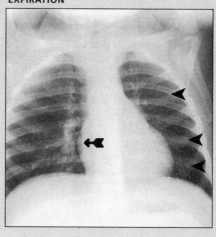

➤ Evaluate the chest wall and sternum.

## PATIENT TEACHING

➤ Tell the patient he'll feel only minimal discomfort from the position he must maintain and the cold metal of the X-ray table touching his body.
➤ Discuss the results of the X-ray study with patient.

## COMPLICATIONS

None known

## SPECIAL CONSIDERATIONS

➤ Always interpret a patient's chest X-rays in light of his history and physical examination.
➤ Compare any X-ray film with previous films, particularly when assessing the progression of a disorder, such as pneumonia or a pneumothorax. Keep in mind the position the film was taken in; a structure on an anterior-posterior view may appear to be a different size than on a posterior-anterior view because of the distance from the X-ray source. For instance, the heart may appear enlarged in an anterior-posterior projection because it was closer to the X-ray tube (and farther from the film) when exposed.

➤ Establish a pattern for evaluating chest films to make it less likely to miss a pathology.

➤ Include both frontal and lateral views in most evaluations.

➤ Remember that plain films have limitations; they aren't extremely sensitive so they may miss many pathologies. Know when to move to further studies such as a computed tomography scan.

➤ Four general patterns of pulmonary disease can be seen on a chest X-ray: a distinct mass, consolidative (alveolar) pattern, interstitial pattern, and vascular pattern.

## DOCUMENTATION

➤ Document the details of your X-ray analysis, comparisons with previous films, and the correlation with clinical findings.

# TREATMENTS

## Oropharyngeal airway insertion and removal

CPT CODE
No specific code has been assigned.

## DESCRIPTION

An oropharyngeal airway, a curved rubber or plastic device, is inserted into the mouth to the posterior pharynx to establish or maintain a patent airway. In an unconscious patient, the tongue usually obstructs the posterior pharynx. The oropharyngeal airway conforms to the curvature of the palate, removing the obstruction and allowing air to pass around and through the tube. It also facilitates oropharyngeal suctioning.

## INDICATIONS

➤ To establish or maintain a patent airway in an unconscious patient, such as after anesthesia, a seizure, or a stroke

➤ To allow oropharyngeal suctioning

➤ To help prevent the orally intubated patient from biting the endotracheal tube

## CONTRAINDICATIONS

### Relative

➤ Loose or avulsed teeth

➤ Recent oral surgery

➤ A conscious or semiconscious state

## EQUIPMENT

Oral airway of appropriate size ◆ regular and padded tongue blades ◆ gloves ◆ suction equipment ◆ handheld resuscitation bag or oxygen-powered breathing device ◆ cotton-tipped applicator

## PREPARATION OF EQUIPMENT

➤ Select an appropriately sized airway for your patient. Usually, you'll select a small size (size 1 or 2) for an infant or child, a medium size (size 4 or 5) for the average adult, and a large size (size 6) for the large adult.

➤ Confirm the correct size of the airway by placing the airway flange beside the patient's cheek, parallel to his front teeth. If the airway is the right size, the airway curve should reach to the angle of the jaw.

## ESSENTIAL STEPS

➤ Explain the procedure to the patient even though he may not appear to be alert.

➤ Maintain privacy and standard precautions.

➤ Put on gloves.

➤ If the patient is wearing dentures, remove them so they don't cause further airway obstruction.

➤ Suction the patient if necessary.

➤ Place the patient in the supine position with his neck hyperextended if this isn't contraindicated.

➤ Insert the airway using the cross-finger or tongue blade techniques. (See *Inserting an oral airway.*)

 **ALERT** Immediately after inserting the airway, auscultate the lungs to ensure adequate ventilation. If the patient has no respirations or they're inadequate, initiate artificial positive-pressure ventilation using mouth-to-mask technique, a handheld resuscitation bag, or an oxygen-powered breathing device.

➤ If the patient has adequate ventilation, position him on his side to decrease the risk of aspiration of vomitus.

➤ Monitor the patient constantly while the airway is in place.

➤ When the patient regains consciousness and can swallow, remove the airway by pulling it outward and downward, following the mouth's natural curvature.

➤ After removing the airway, test the patient's cough and gag reflexes to ensure that removal of the airway wasn't premature and that the patient can maintain his own airway. To test the gag reflex, use a cotton-tipped applicator to touch both sides of the posterior pharynx. To test the cough reflex, gently touch the posterior oropharynx with the cotton-tipped applicator.

## PATIENT TEACHING

➤ Patient teaching will have to wait until the patient regains consciousness; specifics will depend on the precipitating event.

➤ Advise the patient that his throat may be sore for a few days.

## INSERTING AN ORAL AIRWAY

Unless this position is contraindicated, hyperextend the patient's head (as shown) before using either the cross-finger or tongue blade insertion method.

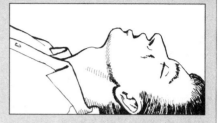

To insert an oral airway using the cross-finger method, place your thumb on the patient's lower teeth and your index finger on his upper teeth. Gently open his mouth by pushing his teeth apart (as shown).

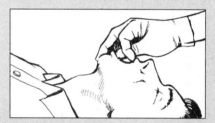

Insert the airway upside down to avoid pushing the tongue toward the pharynx, and slide it over the tongue toward the back of the mouth. Rotate the airway as it approaches the posterior wall of the pharynx so that it points downward (as shown).

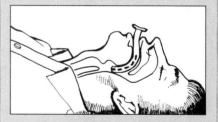

To use the tongue blade technique, open the patient's mouth and depress his tongue with the blade. Guide the airway over the back of the tongue as you did for the cross-finger technique.

## COMPLICATIONS

➤ *Tooth damage or loss, tissue damage, or bleeding* may result from insertion of the airway. Remove and save the tooth, suction as needed, and monitor respirations until the patient is stable.

➤ *Complete airway obstruction* may result if the airway is too long and presses the epiglottis against the entrance of the larynx. If this happens, remove the airway and insert another airway of the correct size. Improper insertion may block the airway by pushing the tongue posteriorly. Remove and reinsert the airway if this happens.

➤ To prevent *traumatic injury to the lips and tongue,* make sure that the patient's lips and tongue aren't between his teeth and the airway. Surgical repair may be needed to repair lacerations.

## SPECIAL CONSIDERATIONS

 **ALERT** An oversized airway can obstruct breathing by depressing the epiglottis into the laryngeal opening.

➤ Auscultate for the patient's breath sounds; clear breath sounds indicate that the patient's airway is the proper size and in the correct position.

➤ Don't tape the airway in place. The time it takes to remove the tape (as the patient regains consciousness) could delay airway removal, increasing the risk of aspiration.

➤ Monitor the patient constantly while the airway is in place, and use the patient's behavior to let you know when to remove the airway. When the patient gags or coughs, he is becoming more alert, indicating that he no longer needs the airway.

## DOCUMENTATION

➤ Record the indications for procedure, the date and time of insertion, and the size of airway used.

➤ Document the date and time of airway's removal, the presence of positive gag and cough reflexes, the condition of the patient's mucous membranes, any suctioning performed, any adverse reactions and actions taken, and the patient's tolerance of the procedure. Also document the patient's general condition.

# Cricothyrotomy

**CPT CODE**
*31605    Tracheostomy, emergency procedure; cricothyroid membrane*

## DESCRIPTION

When endotracheal intubation or a tracheotomy can't be performed quickly to establish an airway, an emergency cricothyrotomy may be necessary. Performed rarely, this procedure involves puncturing the trachea through the cricothyroid membrane. Ideally, cricothyrotomy is performed using sterile technique but, in an emergency, this may not be possible.

## INDICATIONS

➤ To correct airway obstruction

## CONTRAINDICATIONS

### Relative

➤ Children under age 12 (scalpel cricothyrotomy could damage the cricoid cartilage, which is the only circumferential support to the upper trachea; needle cricothyrotomy should be used instead)

## EQUIPMENT

### Scalpel and needle cricothyrotomy

Sterile gloves ◆ povidone-iodine solution ◆ sterile 4" × 4" gauze pads ◆ tracheal dilator ◆ tape ◆ oxygen source with tubing and handheld resuscitation bag ◆ cardiac monitor (if available) ◆ pulse oximeter (if available) ◆ oral-tip suction apparatus ◆ mask ◆ goggles

### Scalpel cricothyrotomy

Scalpel ◆ #6 or smaller tracheostomy tube or endotracheal tube (if available) ◆ syringe ◆ handheld resuscitation bag or T tube and wide-bore oxygen tubing

### Needle cricothyrotomy

14G (or larger) through-the-needle or over-the-needle catheter ◆ 10-ml syringe ◆ I.V. extension tubing ◆ hand-operated release valve or pressure-regulating adjustment valve

## ESSENTIAL STEPS

➤ Place the patient on a cardiac monitor and pulse oximeter (if available).
➤ Explain the procedure in a few short, simple sentences while offering emotional support.
➤ Help the patient into the supine position, and hyperextend his neck to expose the incision site.
➤ Identify the cricothyroid membrane, located between the thyroid and cricoid cartilages (the first indentation inferior to the hard thyroid cartilage).
➤ Put on sterile gloves, mask, and goggles.
➤ Clean the skin overlying the cricothyroid membrane using povidone-iodine solution and sterile gauze. To reduce the risk of contamination, use a circular motion, working outward from the incision site.
➤ Have someone hold the patient's head in the correct position while you perform the procedure.

**LOCATING THE INCISION SITE FOR CRICOTHYROTOMY**

This illustration shows the incision site (through the cricothyroid membrane) for scalpel cricothyrotomy.

Thyroid cartilage — Cricothyroid membrane — Cricoid ring — Incision site — First tracheal ring

➤ Locate the precise insertion site by sliding your thumb and fingers down to the thyroid gland. (See *Locating the incision site for cricothyrotomy.*) You'll know you've located its outer borders when the space between your fingers and thumb widens. Move your finger across the center of the gland, over the anterior edge of the cricoid ring.

### Scalpel cricothyrotomy

➤ Make a horizontal incision, less than ½" (1.3 cm) long, in the cricothyroid membrane just above the cricoid ring.
➤ Insert a dilator to prevent tissue from closing around the incision. If a dilator isn't available, hemostats with the points facing into the incision may be used, or insert the handle of the scalpel and rotate it 90 degrees. A rush of air indicates a patent airway has been established.
➤ Insert the tracheostomy tube or endotracheal tube into the opening until the cuff just disappears. Inflate the cuff with a syringe while securing the tube to help maintain a patent airway. If a tube isn't available, tape the dilator or scalpel han-

dle in place until a tracheostomy or endotracheal tube is available.

➤ If the patient can't breathe spontaneously, attach a handheld resuscitation bag. The cuff of the tube must be inflated to provide positive-pressure ventilation. Inflate the cuff with air until you don't hear any audible leaks.

➤ If the patient can breathe spontaneously, attach a humidified oxygen source to the tracheostomy tube with the T tube. If you use an endotracheal tube, remove the adapter, shorten the tube, replace the cap, and then attach the oxygen.

➤ Suction the trachea.

➤ Auscultate bilaterally for breath sounds, and take the patient's vital signs. If you don't hear breath sounds, reposition the tube so that it isn't obstructing the airway.

➤ Obtain arterial blood gas levels and a chest X-ray as soon as possible. Dispose of the gloves and wash your hands.

### Needle cricothyrotomy

➤ Attach a 10-ml syringe to a 14G (or larger) through-the-needle or over-the-needle catheter. Then insert the catheter into the cricothyroid membrane just above the cricoid ring.

➤ Direct the catheter downward at a 45-degree angle to the trachea to avoid damaging the vocal cords. Maintain negative pressure by pulling back the syringe plunger as you advance the catheter. You'll know the catheter has entered the trachea when air enters the syringe.

➤ When the catheter reaches the trachea, advance it and remove the needle and syringe. Tape the catheter in place.

➤ Attach the catheter hub to one end of the I.V. extension tubing. At the other end, attach a hand-operated release valve or a pressure-regulating adjustment valve. Connect the entire assembly to an oxygen source.

➤ Press the release valve to introduce oxygen into the trachea and inflate the lungs.

When you can see that they're inflated, release the valve to allow passive exhalation. Adjust the pressure-regulating valve to the minimum pressure needed for adequate lung inflation.

➤ Auscultate bilaterally for breath sounds, and take the patient's vital signs. If you can't hear breath sounds, reposition the tube so that it isn't obstructing the airway.

➤ Dispose of waste and wash your hands.

## PATIENT TEACHING

➤ Tell the patient (or family members) that the procedure should immediately allow the patient to breathe spontaneously.

➤ Provide further patient teaching after the crisis resolves.

## COMPLICATIONS

➤ *Hemorrhage:* Apply direct pressure.

➤ *Obstructed airway from an incorrectly positioned tube:* Auscultation reveals this complication; immediately reposition the tube to prevent asphyxiation.

➤ *Perforation of the thyroid or esophagus:* Consult with a physician.

➤ *Subcutaneous or mediastinal emphysema:* Monitor the patient for respiratory distress.

➤ *Infection* may develop up to several days after the procedure. Obtain a culture from the site and administer a broad-spectrum antibiotic; refine treatment when culture and sensitivity reports are available.

## SPECIAL CONSIDERATIONS

➤ Immediately after the procedure, check for bleeding at the insertion site, subcutaneous emphysema or inadequate ventilation, and tracheal or vocal cord damage.

## DOCUMENTATION

➤ Note the date, time, and reason for the procedure.
➤ Document whether you had time to explain the procedure to the patient.
➤ Record physical findings, including vital signs, breath sounds, and bleeding.
➤ Note whether the patient initiated spontaneous respirations after the procedure.
➤ Record how much and by what method oxygen was delivered.
➤ Note any procedures performed after the airway was established, such as endotracheal intubation.

# Metered-dose inhaler use

**CPT CODE**
*94640   Nonpressurized inhalation treatment for acute airway obstruction*

## DESCRIPTION

A metered-dose inhaler (MDI) is a device that consists of a metal canister that is placed in a plastic container with a mouthpiece. It's used to administer medication to the lungs for conditions such as asthma. Children younger than age 9 and some adults may need to use a spacer device with the MDI. The spacer device (which may have a small mask attached to it) attaches to the MDI to increase the amount of medicine that reaches the lungs. The MDI propels the medicine into the spacer; the patient then inhales the medicine into his lungs.

## INDICATIONS

➤ To improve delivery of asthma, bronchitis, and allergy medication

## CONTRAINDICATIONS

### Absolute
➤ Inability to follow directions for MDI use

### Relative
➤ Difficulty using proper technique

## EQUIPMENT

MDI canister ◆ canister holder ◆ spacer (optional)

## ESSENTIAL STEPS

➤ Explain the procedure to the patient and answer any questions. If necessary, demonstrate the procedure.
➤ Make sure the metal canister is placed securely in the plastic holder.
➤ Shake the MDI well.
➤ Remove the cap.
➤ Have the patient exhale completely.
➤ Have the patient hyperextend his head slightly and place the mouthpiece about two fingerwidths in front of his mouth.
➤ Have the patient start taking long, slow, deep breaths with his mouth open. About one-third of the way into a breath, have him compress the canister and holder to release a puff of medication while he continues to inhale fully. Then have him hold his breath for up to 10 seconds.
➤ If the patient needs more than one puff, tell him to wait 30 seconds and repeat the procedure.
➤ After the last puff, tell the patient to gargle and rinse his mouth with water — particularly important after steroid administration to decrease the risk of thrush.

## PATIENT TEACHING

➤ Teach the patient how to clean his MDI. Explain that he should remove the canister from the plastic holder every 1 to 2 days and set it aside. He should then rinse the plastic holder and cap with warm water, allow it to dry, and replace the canister. Explain that cleaning the MDI helps prevent clogging.

➤ Teach the patient how to determine the approximate amount of medication remaining in the MDI. He should remove the canister, place a finger on top, and shake it gently to feel the liquid moving inside. If he feels little movement, the MDI is almost empty. Alternatively, he can remove the canister and place it in clean water. The more buoyant it is, the emptier it is; if it floats on its side, it's almost empty.

## COMPLICATIONS

➤ *Thrush* usually results from steroid inhalation. Prevent this by having the patient gargle and rinse his mouth after using the MDI. If thrush occurs, treat it with an antifungal such as nystatin liquid.

## SPECIAL CONSIDERATIONS

➤ Each patient's response varies with the medication in the MDI.
➤ A patient who can't master proper MDI technique may benefit from using a spacer device. A spacer may also decrease the risk of thrush for a patient taking steroids with the MDI. Some experts recommend that all patients using an MDI use a spacer device.
➤ If a patient has difficulty taking long, slow, deep breaths and holding his breath, it may help to have him take five breaths before removing the spacer from his mouth.
➤ If mist escapes from the patient's mouth during inhalation, medication is escaping and he isn't receiving the full dose.
➤ The patient must aim the MDI properly or the medication won't reach his lungs. If the patient reports a strong medicine taste in his mouth after using the MDI, the medicine has only reached his mouth, not

his lungs, and he needs to improve his technique.

## DOCUMENTATION

➤ Document the patient's baseline knowledge, specific instructions he received, his response to the drug, and his ability to use the MDI independently (usually through reverse demonstration).
➤ Note whether the patient needed to use a spacer device.

# Nebulizer therapy

CPT CODES
*94664   Aerosol inhalation, initial*
*94665   Aerosol inhalation, subsequent*

## DESCRIPTION

An established component of respiratory care, nebulizer therapy aids bronchial hygiene by restoring and maintaining mucus blanket continuity; hydrating dried, retained secretions; promoting expectoration of secretions; humidifying inspired oxygen; and delivering medications. The therapy may be administered through nebulizers that have a large or small volume, are ultrasonic, or are placed inside ventilator tubing.

An *ultrasonic nebulizer* is electrically driven and uses high-frequency vibrations to break up surface water into particles. The resultant dense mist can penetrate the smaller airways and is useful for hydrating secretions and inducing a cough. A *large-volume nebulizer* can provide humidity for an artificial airway, such as a tracheostomy; a *small-volume nebulizer* allows delivery of medications such as bronchodilators. (See *Comparing nebulizers.*)

## COMPARING NEBULIZERS

Each type of nebulizer has different pluses and minuses, as seen in this chart.

| TYPE | DESCRIPTION AND USES | ADVANTAGES AND DISADVANTAGES |
|---|---|---|
| Ultrasonic 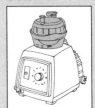 | Uses high-frequency sound waves to create an aerosol mist | **Advantages**<br>➤ Provides 100% humidity<br>➤ About 20% of its particles reach the lower airways.<br>➤ Loosens secretions<br>**Disadvantages**<br>➤ May precipitate bronchospasms in the asthmatic patient<br>➤ Increased risk of overhydration in infants |
| Large volume (Venturi jet) 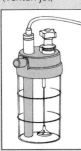 | Supplies cool or heated moisture to a patient whose upper airway has been by-passed by endotracheal in-tubation or a tracheostomy, or who has recently been extubated | **Advantages**<br>➤ Provides 100% humidity with cool or heated devices<br>➤ Provides oxygen and aerosol therapy<br>➤ Can be used for long-term therapy<br>**Disadvantages**<br>➤ Nondisposable units increase risk of bacterial growth.<br>➤ Condensate can collect in large-bore tubing.<br>➤ If correct water level isn't maintained in reservoir, mucosal irritation may result from breathing hot, dry air.<br>➤ Infants have an increased risk of overhydration from mist. |
| Small volume (mini-nebulizer, Maxi-mist) 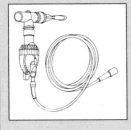 | Delivers aerosolized medication and is handheld | **Advantages**<br>➤ Conforms to patient's physiology, allowing him to inhale and exhale on his own<br>➤ Can cause less air trapping than medication administered by intermittent positive-pressure breathing<br>➤ May be used with compressed air, oxygen, or compressor pump<br>➤ Is compact and disposable<br>**Disadvantages**<br>➤ Takes a long time if patient needs assistance<br>➤ Medication is distributed unevenly if patient doesn't breathe properly. |

Many questions still exist regarding aerosol therapy, including what type of fluid to use, the type of medications that can be delivered, and the effectiveness of therapy.

## INDICATIONS

➤ To relieve bronchospasm
➤ To provide relief to a symptomatic patient with a hyperresponsive airway
➤ Liquefaction and clearance of tenacious secretions

## CONTRAINDICATIONS

### Relative
➤ Tachycardia

## EQUIPMENT

Air compressor ◆ mask or mouthpiece ◆ medication (typically beta agonists such as albuterol, corticosteroids such as methylprednisolone, or cromoglycates such as cromolyn sodium) ◆ normal saline solution ◆ peak flow meter ◆ pulse oximeter

### For an ultrasonic nebulizer
Ultrasonic gas-delivery device ◆ large-bore oxygen tubing ◆ nebulizer couplet compartment

### For a large-volume nebulizer (such as Venturi jet)
Pressurized gas source ◆ flowmeter ◆ large-bore oxygen tubing ◆ nebulizer bottle ◆ sterile distilled water ◆ heater (if indicated) ◆ in-line thermometer (if using heater)

### For a small-volume nebulizer (such as a mini-nebulizer)
Pressurized gas source ◆ flowmeter ◆ oxygen tubing ◆ nebulizer cup ◆ mouthpiece or mask ◆ normal saline solution or sterile distilled water

## PREPARATION OF EQUIPMENT

### For an ultrasonic nebulizer
➤ Fill the couplet compartment on the nebulizer to the level indicated.

### For a large-volume nebulizer
➤ Fill the water chamber to the indicated level with sterile distilled water. Avoid using saline solution to prevent corrosion.
➤ Add a heating device, if ordered, and place a thermometer in-line between the outlet port and the patient, as close to the patient as possible, to monitor the actual temperature of the inhaled gas and to avoid burning the patient.
➤ If the unit will supply oxygen, analyze the flow at the patient's end of the tubing to ensure delivery of the prescribed oxygen percentage.

### For a small-volume nebulizer
➤ Draw up the prescribed medication and inject it into the nebulizer cup.
➤ Add the prescribed amount of normal saline solution or water.
➤ Attach the mouthpiece or mask.

## ESSENTIAL STEPS

➤ Explain the procedure to the patient and wash your hands.
➤ Determine whether to use a mask or mouthpiece. If possible, place the patient in a sitting or high Fowler's position to encourage full lung expansion and promote aerosol dispersion. Obtain baseline data including vital signs, pulse oximetry, and peak expiratory flow rate (PEFR). Perform screening history and physical, including percussion and auscultation of lung fields.
➤ Before beginning, administer an inhaled bronchodilator as indicated, using a metered-dose inhaler or small-volume nebulizer to prevent bronchospasm.
➤ Turn on the machine and check the outflow port to ensure fine misting.

➤ Attach the pulse oximeter and monitor throughout treatment.
➤ Attach the delivery device to the patient.
➤ Encourage the patient to cough and expectorate, or suction as needed.
➤ Encourage the patient to take slow, deep breaths.
➤ After treatment, auscultate the patient's lungs and repeat the PEFR to evaluate the effectiveness of therapy.

### For an ultrasonic nebulizer

➤ Instruct the patient to inhale until the mist disappears and then slowly exhale. Repeat until the medication and the mist disappears.
➤ Check the patient frequently during the procedure to observe for adverse reactions. Watch for labored respirations because ultrasonic nebulizer therapy may hydrate retained secretions and obstruct airways.

### For a large-volume nebulizer

➤ Attach the delivery device to the patient.
➤ Encourage the patient to cough and expectorate, or suction as needed.
➤ Check the water level in the nebulizer at frequent intervals and refill or replace as indicated. When refilling a reusable container, discard the old water to prevent infection from bacterial or fungal growth and refill the container to the indicator line with sterile distilled water.
➤ Change the nebulizer unit and tubing according to policy to facility prevent bacterial contamination.
➤ If the nebulizer is heated, tell the patient to report any warmth, discomfort, or hot tubing because these may indicate a heater malfunction. Use the in-line thermometer to monitor the temperature of the gas the patient is inhaling. If you turn off the flow for more than 5 minutes, unplug the heater to avoid overheating the water and burning the patient when the aerosol is resumed.

### For a small-volume nebulizer

➤ After attaching the flowmeter to the gas source, attach the nebulizer to the flowmeter and then adjust the flow to at least 10 L/minute to ensure adequate functioning but not more than 14 L/minute to prevent excess venting.
➤ Check the outflow port to ensure fine misting.
➤ Attach the delivery device to the patient and remain with him during the treatment, which lasts 15 to 20 minutes. Monitor his vital signs (including pulse and respirations within 5 minutes of treatment initiation) to detect any adverse reaction to the medication.
➤ Encourage the patient to cough and expectorate, or suction as necessary. Change the nebulizer cup and tubing according to facility policy to prevent bacterial contamination.

## PATIENT TEACHING

➤ Tell the patient that difficulty breathing, chest tightness, and shortness of breath should ease within 15 minutes of treatment. If he doesn't feel significant relief, the PEFR remains unacceptable, or improvement doesn't last for 4 hours, he may need another treatment or more aggressive action.
➤ Tell the patient treated at an emergency department or urgent care center to follow up with you within 1 to 2 days to evaluate the treatment regimen.
➤ Explain that slow, deep breaths enhance medication administration and reduce adverse effects.
➤ Explain that the treatment is complete when the medication and mist disappear.
➤ Tell the patient to perform nebulizer treatments at home using medications as prescribed. Tell him to notify you of any changes in his condition or if he experiences such adverse effects as nervousness, edginess, rapid heart rate, or palpitations.

PATIENT-TEACHING AID

# HELPING A CHILD USE A COMPRESSOR-DRIVEN NEBULIZER

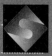

**DEAR PATIENT:**

A very young child may have a hard time using a metered-dose inhaler. He may have trouble timing his breathing so that he breathes in when the device dispenses the medicated mist, and the bad taste of the medication may make it hard for him to take the necessary long, slow, deep breaths. To avoid these problems, your child may instead use a device called a compressor-driven nebulizer. This special nebulizer produces a fine mist that your child can inhale while breathing normally and can even be used when your child is asleep.

## Recognizing respiratory distress

Because of your child's condition, you need to recognize the signs of respiratory distress:
➤ wheezing while breathing in and breathing out
➤ intercostal retractions; when this happens, the skin between the ribs is sucked in as your child breathes (you can pull up your child's shirt to check for this sign)
➤ exhalations that take longer than inhalations
➤ rapid breathing.

If nebulizer treatment doesn't result in a significant improvement in these signs within 15 minutes or if the improvement doesn't last for 4 hours, contact your child's primary care provider.

## Giving a nebulizer treatment

Give your child a nebulizer treatment every __ hours. To do so, follow these steps:
➤ Use the dropper that comes with the medication to draw up __ ml of the medication and put it into the nebulizer cup.
➤ Next, measure out __ ml of normal saline solution and add that to the cup.

➤ Replace the nebulizer cap and tighten it.
➤ Attach the connector (it looks like the letter "T") and the mouthpiece or mask to the nebulizer cup.
➤ Attach the ends of the tubing to the machine and the bottom of the nebulizer cup.
➤ Start the treatment; if it takes longer than 20 minutes, you may need to replace the nebulizer cup.

## Maintaining the equipment

To keep the nebulizer working its best, follow these steps:
➤ After each use, take the nebulizer cup apart and clean it with hot water.
➤ Each day, clean the cup and mouthpiece with diluted dishwashing detergent. Let it soak for a few minutes and then rinse the nebulizer cup with water and set aside to air-dry.
➤ Once a week, clean the nebulizer cup and tubing with a solution made up of 1 cup vinegar and 3 cups water. To do this, submerge the nebulizer cup and tubing in a tub or pan of the solution, let them soak for 10 minutes, and then rinse them under warm running water.
➤ Keep extra nebulizer cups on hand in case one breaks. This also makes it easy to set up several doses for a caregiver who isn't familiar with giving nebulizer treatments.

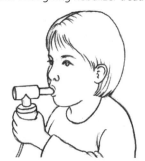

➤ Tell the patient to seek emergency treatment for nasal flaring, intercostal retractions (the skin between the ribs sinks in during inhalation), or blue nail beds or lips. He should call you for wheezing during inspiration and expiration, breathing out that takes longer than breathing in, and rapid breathing.

➤ If the patient is a child who needs to use a compressor-driven nebulizer, a special type of nebulizer, review its use with his parents. (See *Helping a child use a compressor-driven nebulizer.*)

## COMPLICATIONS

➤ *Airway burns (when heating elements are used)* require further evaluation and treatment depending on the severity of the burn.

➤ Adverse reactions from medications require you to stop the medication, decrease the dosage, or wean as soon as possible.

## SPECIAL CONSIDERATIONS

➤ When using a high-output nebulizer (such as an ultrasonic nebulizer) for a child or a patient with a delicate fluid balance, watch for signs of overhydration. These include unexplained weight gain that occurs over several days after the beginning of therapy, pulmonary edema, crackles, and electrolyte imbalance.

➤ If the patient is receiving oxygen concomitantly, he may need a higher oxygen flow to maintain his fraction of inspired oxygen ($FIO_2$); increase the oxygen flow if the mist disappears when the patient inhales.

## DOCUMENTATION

➤ Record the time of the treatment, the type and amount of medication given, and the patient's response to treatment.

➤ Document baseline and subsequent vital signs and breath sounds.

➤ Note the $FIO_2$ or oxygen flow, if administered.

➤ Record baseline and posttreatment vital signs, PEFR, pulse oximetry, and breath sounds.

## Thoracentesis

CPT CODES
*32000    Thoracentesis, puncture of pleural cavity for aspiration, initial or subsequent*
*32002    Thoracentesis with insertion of tube*

## DESCRIPTION

In thoracentesis, a needle is inserted into the pleural space to remove abnormal fluid or air. It's done therapeutically to relieve pulmonary restriction and respiratory distress and diagnostically to help determine the etiology of pleural effusion.

## INDICATIONS

➤ To assess a pleural fluid of unknown etiology

➤ To provide relief from and assess a large symptomatic effusion

➤ To treat a stable spontaneous pneumothorax

## CONTRAINDICATIONS

### Absolute
➤ Bleeding dyscrasias
➤ Lack of patient cooperation

### Relative
➤ Anticoagulant use

## POSITIONING THE PATIENT FOR THORACENTESIS

Before you can perform thoracentesis, you need to help the patient find a position he can maintain in reasonable comfort. Typically, he'll sit on the bed and lean forward on the overbed table.

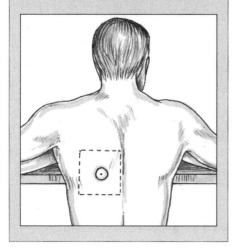

## EQUIPMENT

Most hospitals use a prepackaged thoracentesis tray, which typically includes the following: povidone-iodine and isopropyl alcohol solution ◆ 1% or 2% lidocaine ◆ 5-ml syringe with 21G and 25G needles for anesthetic injection ◆ 15G (for fluid) or 18G (for air) thoracentesis needles for aspiration 50-ml syringe ◆ 3-way stopcock ◆ tubing ◆ sterile specimen containers ◆ sterile hemostat ◆ 4″ × 4″ pads. Additional supplies include: adhesive tape ◆ shaving supplies ◆ fenestrated drape or sterile towels ◆ sphygmomanometer ◆ stethoscope ◆ sterile gloves, gown, and mask ◆ 500- to 1,000-ml vacuum collection bottles ◆ Teflon catheter (18G for air, 15G for fluid) if not included in the kit ◆ specimen tubes, including one red-top tube, one lavender-top tube, culture tubes (aerobic and anaerobic), one green-top

tube, and a 10-ml tube ◆ povidone-iodine ointment ◆ 4″ × 4″ sterile gauze pads ◆ analgesia such as fentanyl and sedative such as lorazepam (optional)

## PREPARATION OF EQUIPMENT

➤ Assemble all equipment at the patient's bedside or in the treatment area.
➤ Check the expiration date on each sterile package, and inspect for tears.
➤ Prepare the necessary laboratory request forms. Be sure to list current antibiotic therapy on the forms because this will be considered in analyzing the specimens.
➤ Have the patient's chest X-rays available.

## ESSENTIAL STEPS

➤ Explain the procedure to the patient and obtain informed consent (check your state regulations regarding the appropriate practitioner to obtain consent). Verify allergies such as latex, iodine, and lidocaine.
➤ Inform the patient that he'll feel some pressure and discomfort during needle insertion.
➤ Assess the patient's vital signs and respiratory status before the procedure. If appropriate, administer analgesia and a sedative.
➤ Confirm the location and extent of effusion or air by percussion, auscultation, and assessment of chest X-rays (posterior-anterior and lateral films). Use a lateral decubitus film to differentiate fluid effusion from consolidation. Review the film with a collaborative physician or radiologist if needed and document clinical findings.
➤ Position the patient upright if possible. Typically, the patient sits leaning forward on the bed, with his feet down and his head and folded arms supported on a pillow on the overbed table. (See *Positioning the patient for thoracentesis*.)

➤ If the patient can't sit, turn him onto his unaffected side, with the arm of the affected side raised over his head and his palm against the back of his head. Then elevate the head of the bed to at least 30 degrees but as close as possible to 90 degrees. (Proper positioning stretches the chest or back, allowing easier access to the intercostal spaces.) For air removal air, position the patient supine at a 30- to 45-degree angle.

➤ Apply oxygen for supplemental support because it's common for arterial saturation to drop transiently during and after the procedure.

➤ Wash your hands and maintain aseptic technique.

➤ Select the insertion site. To remove air, choose a site at the second or third intercostal space at the midclavicular line or more laterally. To remove fluid, choose a site one to two intercostal spaces below the level of the fluid (but not below the eighth intercostal space) and 5 to 10 cm lateral to the spine.

➤ Clip hair close to the site if necessary.

➤ Put on sterile gloves, gown, and mask; open the thoracentesis tray; and set up the equipment. Keep the specimen containers nearby. Set up the three-way stopcock with the 50-ml syringe on one end and tubing for vacuum collection bottles on the other end. Turn the stopcock off to the vacuum collection bottle tubing.

➤ Clean the skin with povidone-iodine solution, working outward in concentric circles. Allow the area to dry.

➤ Drape the area with the fenestrated drape or sterile towels.

➤ Draw up the 1% to 2% lidocaine into a 5-ml syringe with a large-gauge needle. Switch to the 1½" 23G or 25G skin needle, and inject a wheal of solution under the skin and deeper into the tissue, and over the rib.

 **ALERT** Never insert a needle under the rib because the intercostal nerve bundles and blood vessels that

## INJECTING LOCAL ANESTHESIA

When you're injecting anesthesia for thoracentesis, alternate injecting and aspirating anesthetic as you advance the needle. This allows the anesthetic to infiltrate the area, prevents injecting anesthesia into a vessel, and confirms correct placement when you observe fluid during aspiration. At this point, you should mark the proper depth for thoracentesis needle insertion by clamping the needle with hemostats.

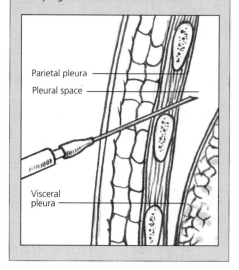

run on the inferior rib borders could be damaged.

➤ Infiltrate the area through the wheal with a downward angle. The needle should rub against the superior edge of the rib. Alternate aspiration and injection to prevent inadvertently administering lidocaine into the circulation. Continue infiltrating the anesthetic into the intercostal space and intercostal muscle. When you enter the parietal pleura, you may feel a pop, and air or fluid may rush into the syringe. The patient may feel an uncomfortable sensation at this point; encourage him to remain still. (See *Injecting local anesthesia*.)

➤ Place a clamp on the needle at the level of the skin to mark the depth of needle

## THE NEEDLE METHOD

As you advance the needle, it slides over the superior end of the rib and then into the pleural space, as shown, while the patient exhales.

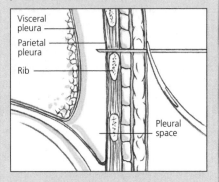

Fluid can then travel from the pleural space and through the needle to the three-way stopcock. From there, you can draw it into a syringe or allow it to drain into the collection bottle, as shown.

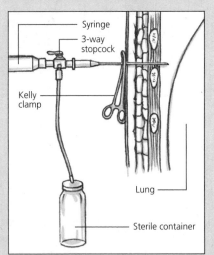

You can also draw fluid up into a syringe, reposition the stopcock, and then inject the fluid into the collection bottle.

penetration. Withdraw the needle and observe the depth of penetration necessary to enter the pleural space.

➤ Use one of several methods to drain the thoracic cavity.

### Needle method

➤ Attach the clamp to the 15G or 18G needle and mark it at the depth of the first needle. This prevents you from penetrating too deeply into the thoracic cavity, which can lead to pneumothorax. (See *The needle method.*)

➤ Attach the three-way stopcock to the needle, a 50-ml syringe, and tubing for connection to vacuum collection bottles.

➤ With the stopcock off to the tubing, insert the procedure needle through the anesthetized zone, advancing the needle over the rib to the level of the clamp.

➤ Withdraw fluid with the syringe, and then turn the stopcock off to the patient. Push fluid into the specimen tubes and vacuum collection bottles from the syringe. Set aside the first specimen to send to the laboratory, if appropriate. Continue the process until you can't remove much more fluid or until you've withdrawn 1,000 to 1,500 ml (the amount depends on the patient's size). Alternatively, allow fluid to drain from the needle directly into the vacuum collection bottles, and use the syringe once to withdraw a fluid sample for specimens. With the stopcock turned off to the patient, withdraw the needle.

### Catheter-within-a-needle method

➤ Place a 10-ml syringe onto an introducer needle. Mark the depth of insertion with a clamp, and insert the needle to the level of the clamp, bevel down, over the anesthetized site. Use the syringe to withdraw fluid and confirm proper placement of the needle.

➤ Remove the syringe. Use your gloved finger to cover the needle hub when chang-

ing equipment to prevent air from entering the pleural space.
➤ While the patient exhales, insert the catheter through the needle; then remove the needle.
➤ Attach the end of the catheter to a three-way stopcock turned off to the patient, and attach a syringe and collection bottle tubing to the other end.
➤ Drain fluid from the hemothorax.

## Needle-within-catheter method
➤ Attach the 10-ml syringe to the needle and insert it throughout the anesthetized zone (as previously described) until you withdraw fluid.
➤ Advance the catheter into the pleural space and remove the needle during exhalation. Place a gloved finger over the catheter hub until you can attach the three-way stopcock, 50-ml syringe, and vacuum collection bottle tubing.
➤ Drain fluid into the vacuum collection bottles.

## All methods
➤ No matter which method you use, support the patient verbally through the procedure.
➤ Watch for signs of distress during the procedure, including pallor, vertigo, weak or rapid pulse, hypotension, dyspnea, tachypnea, diaphoresis, chest pain, blood-tinged mucus, and excessive coughing. If any of these signs or symptoms occur and are sustained, suspend the procedure and provide symptomatic treatment.
➤ After the procedure, dress the site with povidone-iodine ointment, 4″ X 4″ sterile gauze pads, and adhesive tape. Order a chest X-ray to assess the degree of removal and to check for such complications as pneumothorax or hemothorax.
➤ Place the patient into a comfortable position. Order vital signs and respiratory assessment every 15 minutes for 1 hour af-

ter the procedure, with instructions to call you at once with any change in condition.
➤ Send sterile fluid specimens for analysis. Diagnostic studies include cell count, Gram stain, tuberculin and fungal smears, aerobic and anaerobic cultures, cytology, cell block for immunochemical staining, and protein, glucose, pH, lactate dehydrogenase, and amylase levels.

## PATIENT TEACHING
➤ Explain the procedure to the patient. (See *Learning about thoracentesis*, pages 110 and 111.)
➤ Encourage the use of analgesia and sedatives to promote comfort during the procedure and full chest expansion.
➤ Explain the importance of holding still during the procedure.
➤ Tell the patient to expect feelings of pressure and a need to cough. Tell him to let you know if he feels the need to cough or shortness of breath during the procedure so that you can stop the procedure momentarily to allow him to recover and to avoid inadvertently puncturing lung tissue.
➤ Tell him he should feel relief from respiratory distress after the procedure. Explain that he may cough briefly during and after the procedure but should recover shortly after the procedure. Tell him that chest X-rays after the procedure should demonstrate less effusion or pneumothorax.
➤ Have him report shortness of breath or chest discomfort after the procedure; this requires reassessment and another chest X-ray.
➤ Continue to provide supplemental oxygen, if needed, after the procedure.

## COMPLICATIONS
➤ *Pleuritic or shoulder pain* indicates that the needle's point is causing pleural irritation. The pain isn't clinically significant and resolves spontaneously.

*(Text continues on page 112.)*

## LEARNING ABOUT THORACENTESIS

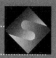

DEAR PATIENT:

Your practitioner wants you to have thoracentesis. In this procedure, the practitioner uses a needle to remove extra fluid from the area around your lung called the pleural space. She'll send a sample of this fluid to the laboratory where it will be studied to find out what is causing your disorder.

    The procedure is usually done in your hospital room, and it takes about 10 to 15 minutes.

**Getting ready**

The assistant will ask you to put on a hospital gown that opens down the back so the practitioner can easily reach the right location for the procedure.

    Then the assistant will take your vital signs. She'll take your temperature and pulse rate. She'll also check your breathing rate and your blood pressure.

    Next, the practitioner will examine your back and chest and choose an area for inserting the needle. Then that area will be shaved and cleaned.

    Just before the procedure, the assistant will help you to assume a special position. If the practitioner decides to perform thoracentesis from your back, you may sit on the edge of the bed and lean forward on your overbed table. The assistant will help you rest your arms on a pillow and your feet on a stool (as shown above right, or she may ask you to straddle a chair (as shown bottom right).

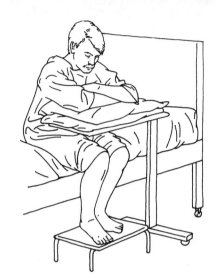

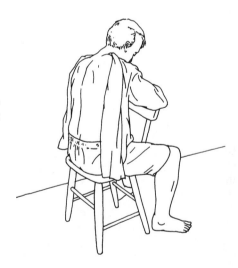

## LEARNING ABOUT THORACENTESIS *(continued)*

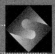

If the practitioner decides to perform thoracentesis by obtaining a fluid sample from your chest, the assistant will help you sit up in bed with the head of your bed raised. This is called the semi-Fowler's position.

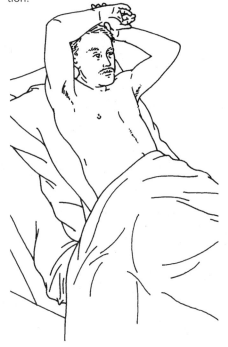

### During the procedure

Immediately before thoracentesis, the practitioner will clean your chest or back with a cold antiseptic solution. She'll numb the area by injecting a local anesthetic. This may cause a slight stinging or burning sensation.

Then she'll perform thoracentesis by inserting a special needle between your ribs and into your chest cavity where the fluid lies. You shouldn't feel much discomfort, but you may feel some pressure when the needle is inserted.

Don't move and don't breathe deeply or cough when the needle is in place because this could damage your lung.

Be sure to let the practitioner or assistant know if you feel short of breath, dizzy, weak, or sweaty or if your heart is racing.

Now, the practitioner will use the needle and a syringe to withdraw excess pleural fluid. If you have lots of fluid, she may also use a suction device. Usually, she'll take out 1 to 2 quarts of fluid. If your lung holds more, you may need thoracentesis again later.

### After the procedure

When the practitioner removes the needle, you may feel the urge to cough. (Go ahead. It's safe to do so.) Then she'll apply pressure and a snug bandage to the wound.

Immediately after thoracentesis, you'll have an X-ray to monitor your progress and check for complications. The assistant will check your vital signs frequently for the next few hours.

If the practitioner withdrew a lot of fluid, you may notice that you're breathing more easily.

### What to watch for

If you feel faint, tell the practitioner. She may give you some oxygen. And be sure to report any other discomfort, such as difficult breathing, chest pain, or uncontrollable coughing — these can signal complications.

➤ *Pneumothorax* occurs in 5% to 20% of patients undergoing thoracentesis and can result from the needle puncturing the lung. About 20% of patients with this complication will need a chest tube inserted. Observe for tachypnea, shortness of breath, decreased arterial saturation, tracheal shift from the midline, or clinical deterioration. Order a portable chest X-ray and evaluate it.

➤ *Hemothorax* can result from laceration of thoracic vasculature and requires that a chest tube be inserted. Evaluate and provide the same treatment that you would for a pneumothorax.

➤ Faulty low-needle entry into the thorax can result in *laceration of the liver, spleen, or diaphragm,* which requires immediate surgical consultation. Prevent this complication by inserting needles only above the level of the eighth rib.

➤ *Reexpansion pulmonary edema and hypotension* results from excessive fluid removal. Prevent this by removing no more than 1,000 to 1,500 ml of fluid depending on the size of the patient. Provide supportive therapy including oxygen therapy, I.V. fluid replacement, pressors if needed, and diuretics if persistent.

➤ Avoid *infection* by using aseptic technique during the procedure.

➤ *Hypoxia* results from a ventilation-perfusion mismatch in the reexpanded lung. Administer oxygen temporarily during and after the procedure until pulse oximetry levels stabilize.

## SPECIAL CONSIDERATIONS

 **CULTURAL TIP** Because this procedure requires ongoing instruction and reassurance, a patient who doesn't speak English needs an interpreter during the procedure. A patient who speaks English as a second language may also benefit from an interpreter during this stressful procedure.

➤ If the patient coughs, briefly halt the procedure and withdraw the needle slightly to prevent puncture.

➤ The diagnostic pleural fluid tests needed for each patient vary with the clinical situation. Some practitioners recommend sending fluid for basic testing (such as white blood cell and cell counts) and storing remaining fluid for further testing as indicated by those results.

➤ To minimize the risk of hypoxia, the patient should have his oxygenation monitored after the procedure with pulse oximetry and arterial blood gas levels. He may benefit from prophylactic oxygen administration for several hours after the procedure.

## DOCUMENTATION

➤ Document informed consent.

➤ Note the date, time, and the location of the insertion site.

➤ Document the indication for the procedure, describe the fluid withdrawn, indicate the amount withdrawn, and note specimens you sent to the laboratory.

➤ Record the patient's vital signs and respiratory status before and after the procedure, chest X-ray results, the patient's reaction to the procedure, and any complications, including actions taken to remedy the situation.

## Chest tube insertion

CPT CODE
*32020 Tube thoracostomy with or without water seal (for example, for abscess, hemothorax, empyema) (separate procedure)*

# DESCRIPTION

Normally, the pleural space contains a thin layer of lubricating fluid that allows the lungs to move without friction during breathing. However, if air, fluid, or both enter this space, they increase pressure, causing the lungs to collapse either partially or completely. Inserting a chest tube helps correct the collapsed lung by allowing the air or fluid to drain from the pleural space and permitting the lungs to reinflate. Performed therapeutically for pathology or to prevent complications, chest tube insertion requires technical skill and a calm, reassuring manner.

# INDICATIONS

➤ To relieve or prevent buildup of pressure from:
– tension pneumothorax
– hemothorax
– simple pneumothorax occupying more than 20% of the lung
– hemopneumothorax
– empyema
– pleural effusion
– chylothorax
– penetrating thoracic trauma
– postthoracotomy.

# CONTRAINDICATIONS

## Relative

➤ Systemic anticoagulation or coagulopathy
➤ Small (less than 20%), stable pneumothorax

# EQUIPMENT

Closed thoracotomy tray ◆ povidone-iodine ◆ #10 or #11 scalpel with mounted blade ◆ curved clamp ◆ 1% lidocaine (1 vial) ◆ 1-0 or 2-0 silk on a straight or curved cutting needle ◆ closed-drainage system ◆ suction setup and tubing ◆ white petroleum-impregnated gauze ◆ sterile

## CHEST TUBE INCISION SITE

Make the incision for chest tube insertion at the rib below the pleural insertion site to allow for angulation of the chest tube. This is the pathway for anesthesia infiltration.

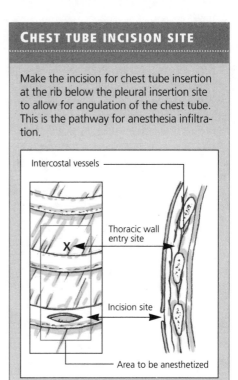

drain dressings (4" × 4" gauze pads with slit) ◆ 3" or 4" sturdy elastic tape ◆ adhesive tape for connections ◆ appropriate size chest tube ◆ sterile gloves and gown ◆ surgical mask and goggles

## Pneumothorax
Adult, #24 to #28 French chest tube ◆ child, #20 to #24 French chest tube ◆ infant, #8 to #10 French chest tube

## Hemothorax
Adult, #32 to #36 French chest tube ◆ child, #10 to #34 French chest tube per height and weight ◆ infant, #10 to #14 French chest tube

# PREPARATION OF EQUIPMENT

➤ Check the expiration dates on sterile packages and inspect for tears.

## GUIDING THE CLAMP INTO THE PLEURAL CAVITY

Use your fingertip to guide the clamp and catheter tip into the pleural cavity (as shown here).

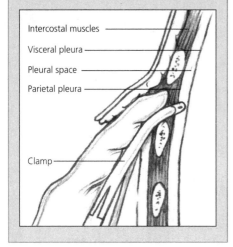

Intercostal muscles

Visceral pleura

Pleural space

Parietal pleura

Clamp

➤ Assemble all equipment and set up the throacic drainage system. Place it next to the patient's bed, below chest level.

## ESSENTIAL STEPS

➤ If the procedure is elective and not an emergency, explain the procedure to the patient, answer any questions, and obtain written informed consent before beginning. Then wash your hands.

➤ If the patient appears anxious, consider administering an anxiolytic (such as midazolam) or analgesic either by mouth or I.V. line 30 minutes before the procedure.

➤ Obtain baseline vital signs and assess respiratory function.

➤ Position the patient sitting up, leaning over a bedside table or lying in a lateral position (if possible) with the affected side uppermost and the arm flexed with the palm of the ipsilateral hand behind the ear. Mark the insertion site. (See *Chest tube incision site*, page 113.)

➤ Put on goggles, gown, mask, and gloves, and maintain aseptic technique throughout.

➤ Thoroughly clean a wide area of the chest with an antiseptic solution such as povidone-iodine.

➤ Infiltrate lidocaine at the insertion site by inserting the needle and slowly injecting anesthesia as you withdraw the needle. Make sure you infuse the intercostal musculature and periosteum.

➤ Estimate the length of tube to insert by measuring the tube against the chest.

➤ Make a small transverse incision through the skin and subcutaneous tissue of the fifth or sixth rib in the middle or anterior axillary line, keeping it as small as possible to ensure a tight fit for the chest tube to prevent leakage around the insertion site.

➤ Introduce a curved clamp into the incision and open it, advancing it to form an oblique subcutaneous tunnel to the periosteum over the selected rib.

➤ Puncture the parietal pleura with the curved clamp; this usually allows air or fluid to escape from the pleural space.

➤ Introduce a finger into the tunnel and sweep it to lyse any adhesions, separate any adherent lung tissue, and ensure entry into the pleural spaces. (See *Guiding the clamp into the pleural cavity*.)

➤ Using your nondominant hand and a curved clamp, grasp the clamped chest tube far enough back to allow the tube to advance adequately (the distance from the skin to the rib plus ¾" [2 cm]) and advance it through the skin and into the pleural cavity. Using your dominant hand, take the medial end of the tube and use firm, steady pressure and a back-and-forth, twisting motion to gain controlled entry. Make sure all drainage holes on the tube are within the cavity. Confirm positioning inside the pleural space by noting an efflux of air or "fogging" of the tube.

➤ For dependent effusion or fluid, direct the tube posteriorly; for pneumothorax, direct the tube apically. Apply a clamp to the free end of the chest tube to prevent an uncontrolled efflux until the tube can be connected to the closed-suction or water-seal system.

➤ Attach the tube to the assembled drainage system. Set the suction at 15 to 20 cm $H_2O$. You'll note gentle bubbling of the water chamber, which indicates adequate suction for air and fluid. (See *Disposable drainage system*.)

➤ Using 1-0 or 2-0 silk suture on a straight or curved cutting needle, place the first suture next to the chest tube and tie it firmly.

➤ Leave both suture ends long and wind the ends around the tube several times. Tie the ends of the suture tightly around the tube and cut the ends.

➤ With a second suture, place a purse-string stitch around the tube at the skin incision site that can be used later to close the skin when the tube is removed. Pull both ends of this suture together, and close the skin around the tube with a knot. Wind this suture around the chest tube and tie it. (See *Suturing the chest tube,* page 116.)

➤ Wrap the petroleum-impregnated gauze around the chest tube, creating a seal at the skin, and apply sterile drain dressings. Cover with gauze pads and tape securely to the lateral chest wall.

➤ Securely tape the connection site between the chest tube and the suction tubing. Then tape the chest tube to the patient's side.

➤ Have the patient take several deep breaths to inflate the lungs.

➤ Order a chest X-ray (with the patient erect if possible) to confirm placement of the tube.

## PATIENT TEACHING

➤ If the patient had an effusion, tell him the chest tube will most likely be removed after 24 to 48 hours without drainage. If the patient had a pneumothorax, tell him

### DISPOSABLE DRAINAGE SYSTEM

Commercially prepared disposable systems combine a drainage collection, water seal, and suction control in one unit, as shown here. These systems ensure patient safety with positive- and negative-pressure relief valves and have a prominent air-leak indicator. Some systems produce no bubbling sound.

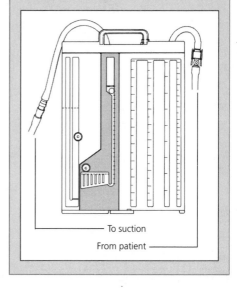

To suction

From patient

the tube can be switched from suction to water seal for 24 hours when his lung has fully expanded; if the follow-up X-ray shows that his lung remains fully expanded, he can have the tube removed.

➤ Tell the patient to schedule a follow-up visit with you and have a chest X-ray 7 to 10 days after removal of tube.

➤ Tell the patient that the occlusive dressing should remain in place for 24 to 48 hours after tube removal.

➤ Explain to the patient that he'll receive pain medication so that pain doesn't interfere with pulmonary hygiene (including respiratory treatments, use of incen-

## SUTURING THE CHEST TUBE

Securing the chest tube in place minimizes the risk of dislocation, infection, hemothorax, and pneumothorax. To secure it, place the first suture adjacent to the tube, leave the ends long, and then wind them around the tube and tie the tube snug to the suture.

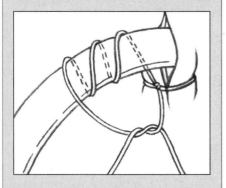

Then place a purse-string stitch around the incision site. You can use this later when you withdraw the chest tube to maintain a seal.

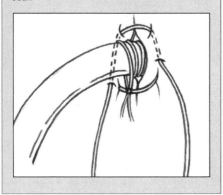

tive spirometry, coughing, and deep breathing) while he has a chest tube in place. (See *How to do controlled coughing exercises*.)

➤ Warn the patient not to fly on an airplane or scuba dive for 6 months after removal of the tube.

➤ Teach the patient the rationale for and how to perform incentive spirometry; explain that, while the chest tube is in place, he'll need to perform incentive spirometry at least 10 times per hour when awake.

➤ Tell the patient to report the sudden onset of shortness of breath or chest pain as well as such signs of infection as excessive drainage or warmth and redness at the insertion site.

## COMPLICATIONS

➤ If *injury to heart and great vessels or lung* occurs, the patient needs an immediate open thoracotomy.

➤ *Bleeding from the chest wall* can result from laceration of an internal mammary vessel or an intercostal artery. If this occurs, apply direct pressure to control bleeding; if this doesn't work, the patient may require surgical exploration and repair.

➤ *Continuing air leak:* Check and secure all connections.

➤ *Occlusion of the chest tube* may result from large clots or kinking of the tubing. Gently apply direct suction, but don't milk the chest tube.

➤ *Subcutaneous air pocketing* may result from a distal hole in the subcutaneous tissue or from inadequate decompression of a pneumothorax, which allows air to continue to leak into the subcutaneous space. It may require placement of a second tube.

➤ *Persistent pneumothorax* indicates a failure of the lung to expand. It may require placement of a second tube and investigation into possibly more serious pathology, such as a defect in a large bronchus, that requires surgical repair.

➤ *Local or systemic infection:* As needed, obtain a culture specimen from the wound site, and administer a broad-spectrum antibiotic until the pathogen and sensitivities are identified.

➤ *Injury to the liver, spleen, or diaphragm,* result of a low or caudal insertion site, may require surgical intervention.

➤ *Contralateral tension pneumothorax* requires needle decompression and insertion of another chest tube.

PATIENT-TEACHING AID

# HOW TO DO CONTROLLED COUGHING EXERCISES

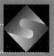

DEAR PATIENT:

Learning how to do coughing exercises will help you save energy and remove mucus from your airways. Here is what to do.

**1** Sit on the edge of your chair or bed. Rest your feet flat on the floor or use a stool if your feet don't touch the floor. Lean slightly forward.

**2** To help stimulate your cough reflex, slowly take a deep breath. Place your hands on your stomach. Breathe in through your nose, letting your stomach expand as far as it can.

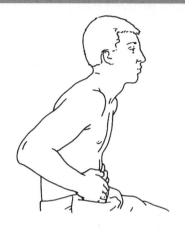

**4** Cough twice with your mouth slightly open. Once isn't enough: The first cough loosens mucus; the second cough helps remove it.

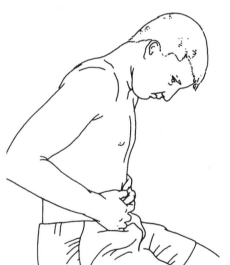

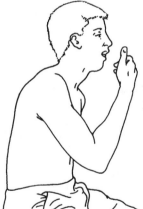

**3** Next, purse your lips and slowly breathe out through your mouth, as shown above right. Concentrate on pulling your stomach inward. Try to exhale twice as long as you inhaled.

**5** Pause for a moment. Then breathe in through your nose by sniffing gently. Don't breathe deeply. If you do, the mucus you brought up may slide back into your lungs.

## SPECIAL CONSIDERATIONS

➤ The patient should receive daily chest X-rays to monitor the resolution of pathology.
➤ These factors can affect how long the chest tube remains in place:
– air leaks that result from a fault in the suction system
– a shift in the chest tube so that one of the chest tube's holes is in subcutaneous tissue rather than the chest cavity
– air leaking through a bronchiole; this may indicate a more serious injury, such as a tear in the main stem bronchus or a ruptured esophagus.
➤ If available, a quick way to determine the correct chest tube size for a child is to measure with the Broselow Pediatric Emergency Tape. It's based on the principle that a child's length is related to lean body weight. The practitioner measures the child head to toe and then turns the tape over. The reverse side lists the correct size equipment and precalculated resuscitation drugs and infusion rates, along with cardiopulmonary resuscitation standards.

 **ALERT** For a large patient in whom the tube must penetrate a lot of subcutaneous tissue before reaching the pleura, use a trocar to insert a chest tube. Trocars come with #32 French or larger chest tubes, but keep in mind that trocar use can lead to further complications, such as vascular injuries.

## DOCUMENTATION

➤ Document the patient's status before the procedure and specify the indications for the procedure. Include vital signs, chest X-ray results, and breath sounds. Note whether you obtained informed consent.
➤ Write a procedural note that details the insertion in the progress notes. Include the type and amount of anesthesia given; the size and location of the chest tube; the amount, color, and consistency of initial drainage; the number of sutures; and the type of drainage system used.
➤ Document the patient's condition following the procedure. Include vital signs, breath sounds, chest tube patency, pain medications, whether or not incentive spirometry was ordered, and instructions given.
➤ Document the results of postprocedure chest X-rays.

## Chest tube removal

CPT CODE
No specific code has been assigned.

## DESCRIPTION

When a patient's lung has reexpanded and chest tube drainage has dropped below 100 ml in 24 hours, the chest tube can be removed. Clinical indications that document improvement in the patient's status include resolving arterial blood gas levels; stable vital signs; regular, nonlabored breathing; symmetrical chest expansion; and the absence of air leaks in the chest tube container. Before removal, the patient should have a posterior-anterior and lateral chest X-ray to document reexpansion or clearing of the affected lung (if the patient can't go to the X-ray department, undergoing an upright portable X-ray at his bedside may be acceptable). If there is any doubt about the interpretation of the X-ray, the film should be reviewed with the radiologist or collaborating physician. Unless you have had a lot of practice, you may have difficulty finding a pneumothorax, which can be easily mistaken for a reexpanded or clear lung.

# INDICATIONS

➤ To terminate therapy because of reexpanded lung with minimal chest tube drainage and stable vital signs

# CONTRAINDICATIONS

## Absolute
➤ Air leak

# EQUIPMENT

#11 scalpel blade or suture removal set ◆ package of petroleum gauze ◆ package of 4″ × 4″ sterile gauze pads ◆ several 2″ or 3″ wide strips of silk tape ◆ linen-saver pads ◆ clean and sterile gloves ◆ povidone-iodine solution ◆ tube clamp (such as a Hoffman gate clamp) ◆ trash bag ◆ analgesic (such as fentanyl) ◆ antianxiety drug (such as lorazepam)

# ESSENTIAL STEPS

➤ Explain the procedure to the patient.
➤ Administer an analgesic and antianxiety drug (such as 1 mg lorazepam and 25 to 50 mg fentanyl I.V.) 15 minutes before the procedure.
➤ Monitor vital signs, electrocardiogram, and pulse oximetry throughout the procedure.
➤ Place the patient in semi-Fowler's position, lying on his unaffected side, or in the same position as when the tube was inserted.

 **ALERT** Before removing the tube, assess the drainage system's water-seal chamber for air leaks. With a water seal and no suction, ask the patient to cough, and look for bubbles in the water-seal chamber. Bubbles or fluctuations in the water-seal chamber indicate an air leak. If you find a leak, determine whether it's in the system (tubing leak) or in the patient (pleural cavity leak). If the leak is in the

patient, the chest tube MUST stay in place for another 24 to 48 hours while a fibrin layer forms around the tube site. If you don't detect an air leak, you can safely remove the tube.

➤ Wash your hands and maintain aseptic technique.
➤ Cover the patient's bed and lower body with linen-saver pads to protect them from drainage and to provide a place to put the chest tube after removal.
➤ With clean gloves, remove the dressing covering the chest tube insertion site. Discard the soiled dressing.
➤ Put on sterile gloves and clean the area around the chest tube with povidone-iodine solution using 4″ × 4″ sterile gauze pads. If you see a purse-string suture, use the scalpel blade to cut both sides of the knot holding the tube in place.
➤ If the patient has more than one tube connected with a Y-connector, use a chest tube clamp to clamp the remaining tubes closed to the air. Remove one chest tube at a time.
➤ If you're removing mediastinal tubes connected with a Y-connector to one or more pleural tubes, clamp tube connections distally to prevent air from entering the pleural tube at the connection with the mediastinal tubes. You can pull out the mediastinal tubes together or separately. With either technique, remove the tubes carefully to avoid disturbing operative structures.
➤ Clamp the tube securely with the tube clamp. Before pulling the tube, tell the patient either to exhale fully or inhale fully. Then have him hold his breath and bear down while you completely remove the tube. (Valsalva's maneuver increases intrathoracic pressure and prevents sudden involuntary inhalation from pain or anxiety during the procedure.) Make sure the patient understands that inhaling could result in another pneumothorax.

**CULTURAL TIP** Because of the importance of the patient not inhaling during removal of the tube, you may want to have someone translate for a patient who doesn't speak English so that the patient can cooperate fully with the procedure.

➤ For the patient on a positive-pressure ventilator, negative pressure is less during inspiration and greater during expiration, so you should pull the chest tube during inspiration. Alternatively, have someone momentarily pause the ventilator during the procedure to prevent entry of air into the thorax during removal.

 **ALERT** Don't allow air to enter the pleural cavity during chest tube removal. For the patient on a positive-pressure ventilator, pull the tube at the end of inspiration, when negative pressure is the least. For all others, emphasize that they can't inhale during the removal.

➤ Unwrap the suture from the tube and tighten it to mold the skin around the tube. This prepares the suture for retying.

➤ With a single and steady motion, quickly pull out the tube. If the tube was sutured, gently and immediately close the skin by pulling the purse-string suture closed as the tube exits the body. Tie the suture and clip the ends so that they're short but long enough to grasp with forceps for later removal.

➤ When no purse-string suture is present, immediately place petroleum gauze over the exit site to prevent air from entering the pleural space. Remember to tell the patient when it's safe to breathe again.

➤ Complete the occlusive dressing with a 4″ × 4″ gauze pad and tape.

➤ Order and review a postprocedure chest X-ray to assess for a new pneumothorax or hemothorax that may have resulted from the procedure.

➤ Have the patient's vital signs monitored, and compare the results to previous data. Assess the patient's postprocedure respi-

ratory status and arterial oxygen saturation ($SaO_2$) levels. Identify abnormalities.

## PATIENT TEACHING

➤ Explain the procedure to the patient before performing it. Tell him that chest tube removal causes discomfort, which usually lasts less than 15 minutes. Emphasize that he probably will feel discomfort but that it won't last; it's generally better to overestimate the pain to the patient rather than underestimate it so patient won't accidentally inhale from pain during removal. It's better to have the patient say "it wasn't so bad" rather than "you didn't tell me it would be like that."

➤ Encourage analgesia or sedation before the procedure to minimize procedural pain.

➤ Explain and demonstrate breath holding and Valsalva's maneuver, and ask for a return demonstration. Have the patient practice if necessary.

➤ Explain to the patient that he'll undergo chest X-rays after the procedure to check for fully reexpanded lungs.

➤ Order the petroleum dressing to remain in place for 48 hours; then soap and water can be used for daily wound care. You don't need to give any special wound care instructions.

➤ Remove the sutures 5 to 7 days after chest tube removal.

➤ Tell the staff nurse or patient to call you if signs or symptoms of a complication develop — particularly fever, erythema, or new drainage from the wound site, which could indicate infection.

## COMPLICATIONS

Because complications from chest tube removal can be serious or life-threatening, contact the collaborating physician if any of the following occur.

➤ *Recurrent pneumothorax:* If it's small (under 10% to 15%), it may resolve with no treatment. If it's large or causes respiratory distress, the patient may need another chest tube inserted. He should undergo daily X-rays to assess the progress of resorption and to rule out progression of the pneumothorax. A large pneumothorax may cause a change in vital signs, tachypnea, decreased oxygen saturation, or decompensation. Intubation may be needed.

➤ Although *subcutaneous emphysema* may not be significant by itself, you should continue to assess the patient for expansion of subcutaneous emphysema up to the neck and face or throughout the thorax. It this occurs, the asymptomatic patient may require serial chest X-rays. Development of rapid, symptomatic, or persistent subcutaneous emphysema may indicate an air leak from the thoracic cavity and, if serious, may require endotracheal intubation and placement of a new chest tube.

➤ *Sudden respiratory distress* requires immediate evaluation and stabilization. Consider endotracheal intubation while you assess the cause of the respiratory distress, and assess the need for insertion of another chest tube.

➤ Fever, purulent or foul-smelling drainage, and erythema at the removal site indicate *infection*. Obtain a culture specimen from the wound, and place the patient on a broad-spectrum antibiotic until the laboratory can identify the pathogen and sensitivities.

➤ *Hemorrhage:* Consult a surgeon immediately to help identify and correct the cause of bleeding, and assess the patient's vital signs, hemoglobin, and hematocrit. When appropriate, order typing and crossmatching for transfusion of packed red blood cells. Infuse blood and I.V. fluids to replace lost volume. Obtain a chest X-ray to assess for hemothorax; if the patient has a hemothorax, he'll need a new chest tube inserted to collect related drainage from the thorax.

➤ *Lung damage:* Consult a thoracic surgeon to further assess the lung.

➤ *Injury of the heart or mediastinal structures:* Immediately consult the cardiothoracic surgeon to further assess the damage. Assess the patient's vital signs, and look for signs of arrhythmia, bleeding, and ischemia.

## SPECIAL CONSIDERATIONS

➤ Analgesic effects will resolve within 1 hour of start of procedure.

➤ A chest tube left in place for more than 7 days increases the risk of infection along the chest tube tract.

➤ In mediastinal chest tube removal, air can leak through the mediastinum into the pleural space. Therefore, after heart surgery, mediastinal tubes can be removed like regular chest tubes, but pull the tubes more slowly to avoid interruption of surgical sutures in the chest cavity.

## DOCUMENTATION

➤ Document the procedure in the patient's record, including vital signs and respiratory status before and after the procedure. Document the rate and quality of the patient's respirations after tube removal, including $SaO_2$.

➤ Also document the patient's tolerance for the procedure and analgesia given. Include the results of the chest X-rays taken before and after the procedure.

## Flail chest stabilization

### CPT CODE
*21810  Treatment of rib fracture requiring external fixation (flail chest)*

## LIFE-THREATENING INJURIES FROM CHEST TRAUMA

When caring for a patient with flail chest, be alert for other life-threatening injuries that may have resulted from the same chest trauma that caused the multiple rib fractures. Injuries to watch for include:
➤ sternal fracture
➤ aortic rupture
➤ pulmonary contusion
➤ cardiac rupture
➤ myocardial contusion
➤ tamponade
➤ pneumothorax
➤ hemothorax
➤ interruption of the great vessels
➤ bleeding
➤ tracheal injuries
➤ esophageal injury
➤ rupture of diaphragm
➤ chest wall contusions.

## DESCRIPTION

In flail chest, multiple rib or sternal fractures result in a segment of the chest wall becoming unstable. Flail chest may occur in the front, back, or side of the chest and results from direct trauma to the chest.

The hallmark of flail chest is paradoxical movement of the chest wall; a portion of the chest wall moves in toward the injury when the patient inhales and out when the patient exhales. This happens because changes in the structural integrity of the chest wall and changes in intrathoracic pressure cause that area to move in the opposite direction from the rest of the chest wall. The patient with flail chest typically complains of severe pain on inspiration or from palpation of the ribs. X-rays confirm fractures or pneumothorax.

 **ALERT** Because it typically takes a great deal of force to fracture multiple ribs, the practitioner should look for other life-threatening injuries that may have resulted from the chest trauma.

Mortality rates range from 5% to 50% and stem from underlying lung injury or other related injuries. Pulmonary contusion, for instance, occurs in 90% of all flail chest injuries, and a patient with a sternal fracture may have cardiac injuries. (See *Life-threatening injuries from chest trauma.*)

## INDICATIONS

➤ To treat rib and associated chest wall injuries from blunt trauma
➤ To prevent respiratory compromise
➤ To prevent life-threatening complications from chest trauma

## CONTRAINDICATIONS

None known

## EQUIPMENT

Pulse oximeter ◆ oxygen with nasal cannula, mask, or nonrebreather mask ◆ cardiac monitor (if available) ◆ two large-bore I.V. catheters (14G to 18G for adults, 20G to 18G for children) ◆ I.V. infusion tubing ◆ 500 ml of normal saline or lactated Ringer's solution for fluid resuscitation ◆ abdominal dressings (3" × 12" or larger) ◆ 2" tape ◆ small pillow ◆ morphine, injectable (optional)

### Intubation equipment (optional)

Endotracheal tubes (sizes 6 to 8) ◆ laryngoscope with blade ◆ end-tidal carbon dioxide monitor (if available) ◆ chest tube (#32 French chest tube for adults, #10 to #34 French chest tube for children, depending on height and weight of child)

## ESSENTIAL STEPS

➤ Monitor the patient's airway, breathing, and circulation to ensure appropriate treatment.

➤ Activate the emergency medical services system.

➤ If the patient is awake, talk to him and tell him what you're doing to help him.

➤ Remove clothing from the patient to completely assess his injuries.

➤ Note the patient's effort of breathing, look for paradoxical chest movement, and assess for changes in breath sounds.

➤ Look for any penetrating wounds and treat accordingly

➤ Administer high-flow oxygen (10 ml/ minute).

➤ If necessary, prepare to intubate and assist the patient with ventilation.

➤ Establish two large-bore I.V. access lines. Start I.V. fluids according to the patient's needs.

➤ Draw blood from the I.V. line for a complete blood count (CBC), electrolyte levels, and typing and crossmatching.

➤ Continuously monitor pulse oximetry; when available, monitor serial electrocardiogram (ECG) readings and arterial blood gas (ABG) levels.

➤ Assess the patient's pain level and provide injectable morphine for adequate pain relief without suppressing respiratory effort.

➤ Look for signs of cardiogenic shock and provide treatment as indicated.

➤ If possible, treat any cardiac arrhythmias.

➤ Use gentle palpation to locate the edges of the flail segment.

➤ Apply a 3″ to 12″ (7.6 to 30.5 cm) or larger abdominal dressing over the site. Use a small pillow to support the patient.

➤ Tape the dressing in place with a 5″ to 6″ (12.5 to 15 cm) long piece of 2″ tape. Don't bind the chest wall with a constricting dressing, don't place sandbags, tape, straps, or belts around the chest and back. Although they may provide temporary relief, they prevent adequate expansion of the rib cage and lead to atelectasis.

➤ Continue to reevaluate the patient frequently for changes.

➤ Transport the patient to the nearest emergency department as soon as possible.

➤ Once the patient arrives at the emergency department, he may need a chest tube inserted for crepitus or pneumothorax. He'll also need chest X-rays, serial ABG levels, ECG readings, echocardiography (if he may have a cardiac injury), creatine kinase and troponin levels, a CBC, and possibly an arteriogram and transesophageal echocardiogram.

➤ If possible, provide conservative management in the hospital to prevent respiratory compromise; provide adequate ventilation, ensure airway patency, treat underlying injuries, and continuously monitor the patient's respiratory status.

➤ Administer morphine to control pain; increase effective coughing, vital capacity, and forceful inspiration; help alleviate respiratory compromise and paradoxical motion by decreasing the work of breathing; and sedate the patient. As appropriate, administer the morphine I.V., as an intercostal nerve block, through an epidural catheter, or as patient-controlled analgesia.

➤ Provide oxygen therapy in conjunction with pain management; don't resort to mechanical ventilation if possible. However, if decompensation, severe head injury, inability to maintain a patent airway, the need for general anesthesia, or obvious respiratory failure occur, the patient may need intubation or positive-pressure ventilation.

➤ Provide aggressive pulmonary hygiene to help move secretions and prevent atelectasis. To do this, turn the patient frequently and provide incentive spirometry, postural drainage, and nasotracheal suctioning. Also, provide chest physiotherapy by having the patient inhale deeply and then exhale in four short "huff coughs" to increase forceful expirations.

➤ Use fluid resuscitation cautiously because it increases the potential for pulmonary edema and adult respiratory distress syndrome in patients with pulmonary contusion. Restrict fluids when the patient is hemodynamically stable, with a urine output of 30 ml/hour.

## PATIENT TEACHING

➤ If the patient's condition allows it, explain the procedure. Address other patient-teaching needs after the crisis, including instructions to contact you if he experiences shortness of breath, signs of respiratory compromise, increasing pain, or any other change in condition that makes him anxious.

➤ After the flail chest is stabilized, tell the patient his chest wall should be stable in 2 to 3 weeks. Instruct the patient to schedule a follow-up visit in less than 1 week (the time frame varies depending on clinical presentation).

➤ At the follow-up visit, teach the patient about safety measures, including using seatbelts at all times, following posted speed limits, wearing protective gear for contact sports, and avoiding any situation that could lead to violence

## COMPLICATIONS

➤ *Increased work to breathe:* Emphasize need for analgesia and pulmonary exercises.

➤ *Restricted chest wall motion* usually results from pain, so the analgesia should be adjusted.

➤ *Pulmonary contusion:* Use I.V. fluid judiciously to avoid further decrease in respiratory function. Mechanical ventilation, analgesia, pulmonary exercise, and treatments may be required. Steroids are occasionally used.

## SPECIAL CONSIDERATIONS

➤ The primary indication for intubation and ventilation is respiratory decompen-

sation, which leads to atelectasis and hypoxia.

➤ Surgical stabilization with internal fixation of the fractured bones is used only in patients with grossly displaced fractures or floating segments that have the potential to cause life-threatening injuries.

➤ For pediatric patients, determine appropriate equipment sizes and doses quickly using the Broselow Pediatric Emergency Tape. It was developed on the principle that a child's length is related to lean body weight. The practitioner measures the child head to toe and then turns the tape over. The reverse side lists the correct size equipment and precalculated resuscitation drugs and infusion rates, along with cardiopulmonary resuscitation standards.

## DOCUMENTATION

➤ Document signs and symptoms and physical findings before and after treatment, including vital signs, breath sounds, mechanism of injury, and actions taken.

# GASTROINTESTINAL PROCEDURES

# 3

GI conditions affect just about everyone at one time or another. These conditions, so intimately tied to psychological health and stability, range from simple changes in bowel habits to life-threatening disorders that require major surgery and radical lifestyle changes.

Patient care for GI conditions also varies widely. For example, the patient with simple constipation may need only brief teaching about diet and exercise. The patient with irritable bowel syndrome may need extensive history taking, frequent followup to establish a trusting relationship between you and your patient, encouragement with lifestyle changes, and reassurance about the benign nature of the disease. However, the patient with colorectal cancer may need expeditious referral, encouragement and support during the diagnostic workup, collaboration with multiple specialists, and coordination of services to minimize visits and needlesticks while covering his special and routine preventive health needs.

## Your role in GI procedures

Therapeutic GI procedures reflect the wide spectrum of clinical settings in which nurse practitioners practice. These procedures may include inserting a feeding tube in a nursing home, performing a scheduled anoscopy or an abdominal paracentesis in an office, or performing gastric lavage in an emergency department.

To successfully carry out responsibilities such as these, you need to address the emotional and physical needs of the patient. When you notice patient discomfort or reluctance to undergo needed procedures, your knowledge of anatomy and physiology as well as your familiarity with the patient's individual risk factors, diagnostic prognosis, and viable options will allow you to communicate his needs and options effectively.

A patient who is undergoing certain GI procedures, especially uncomfortable or embarrassing ones, requires a considerable amount of emotional support. Helping such a patient maintain his sense of dignity while eliciting his cooperation requires a skillful blend of compassion and judgment. Your sensitivity to the patient's emotional and cultural issues as well as to his physical needs may be crucial in determining how he ultimately responds and may also assist him in providing informed consent.

 **CULTURAL TIP** Many cultural groups have a high degree of modesty regarding emesis, constipation, diarrhea, and other bowel-related topics. Some cultural groups, such as Cambodians and Iranians, may interpret nausea and vomiting as a balance problem within the GI system and are likely to restrict particular foods. You should ask if the patient feels in balance to elicit this information. Members of other cultural groups, such as Central Americans, may use laxatives to purge when experiencing nausea or vomiting.

## DIAGNOSTIC TESTING

## Anoscopy

CPT CODE
*46600   Anoscopy*

## DESCRIPTION

Anoscopy is the direct visualization of the anus with the use of a speculum. This procedure is performed to diagnose and evaluate diseases of the perianal and distal anal canal. Anoscopes are tubular metal or plastic instruments about 2 ¾″ (7 cm) long and ¾″ (2 cm) in diameter. Some have built-in fiber-optic light sources; others require an external light source.

## INDICATIONS

➤ To evaluate perianal or anal pain, hemorrhoids, rectal prolapse, rectal bleeding, or abnormality in the anal canal on digital examination
➤ To identify perianal abscess or condyloma

## CONTRAINDICATIONS

**Absolute**
➤ Acute cardiovascular problems (anoscopy may stimulate a vasovagal response)
➤ Anal canal stenosis
➤ Severe rectal pain

## EQUIPMENT

Anoscope with obturator ◆ gloves ◆ drape ◆ water-soluble lubricant or anesthetic ointment (such as 2% lidocaine) ◆ large cotton-tipped applicators

## ESSENTIAL STEPS

➤ Explain the procedure to the patient. Inform him that he may feel fullness in the rectal area during the examination. Answer any questions he has about the procedure. Obtain informed consent.
➤ Position the patient in the left lateral decubitus position with knees bent up toward the chest.
➤ Drape him so that only the perianal area is exposed to promote privacy.
➤ Put on gloves.
➤ Inform the patient that you're going to touch his rectal area.
➤ Spread the gluteal fold and examine the external anal structure; observe for fissures, bleeding, or pus.
➤ Instruct the patient to bear down as if having a bowel movement; observe for hemorrhoids or prolapse of rectal tissue.
➤ Apply lubricant to your index finger and perform a digital rectal examination. Rotate your finger inside the rectum and note irregularities in the contour of the vault.
➤ Lubricate the anoscope.
➤ Instruct the patient to take slow, deep breaths to relax the anal sphincter.
➤ Insert the anoscope, gently angling it toward the umbilicus.
➤ Remove the obturator.
➤ Visualize the rectal mucosa (normal mucosa appears pink with visible vessels).
➤ If fecal matter obstructs the view, remove it with a large cotton-tipped applicator.
➤ Remove the anoscope gently and observe the mucosa on withdrawal for abnormalities and potential trauma from the anoscope.

## PATIENT TEACHING

➤ Tell the patient he can resume normal activity after the procedure.
➤ If he feels light-headed or nauseous, instruct him to remain in the left lateral position for several minutes before sitting up.

➤ Inform him that slight bleeding is normal because of the possibility of trauma from an abrasion, tearing of the mucosa, or hemorrhoids.

➤ Urge him to notify you if bleeding lasts for more than 2 days or becomes heavy with clots.

➤ Advise him that sitz baths twice daily relieve rectal pain and swelling.

## COMPLICATIONS

➤ *Bleeding* can occur if a fissure or thrombosed hemorrhoid is irritated during the procedure. Such bleeding warrants ice application, analgesics, and follow-up care to ensure resolution. Heavy bleeding or other unresolved symptoms may require collaboration with a physician or gastroenterologist.

## SPECIAL CONSIDERATIONS

➤ Use a topical anesthetic lubricant, such as 2% lidocaine, if the patient has evidence of a fissure or can't tolerate the discomfort of anoscope insertion.

 **CULTURAL TIP** Many cultural groups consider touching the anal region embarrassing or taboo. State your intentions matter-of-factly before touching the patient in a private area. By using a professional demeanor and effective distraction techniques, you can minimize the patient's discomfort and reduce muscle tension. Conversely, humor or unnecessary touching during the examination may offend the patient or increase his discomfort.

 **CULTURAL TIP** Gender may play a role during a rectal examination, especially in cultural groups in which women are subordinate. For instance, a female practitioner may need a male health care professional to convey the importance of the examination to a male from a culture that considers women to be inferior. An Asian or Muslim woman may feel uncomfortable being undressed in front of others; use drapes to provide privacy.

## DOCUMENTATION

➤ Record the date and time of the anoscopy, the depth of visualization, the appearance of mucosa and abnormalities (such as pus, hemorrhoids, and fissures), and the patient's tolerance of the procedure.

➤ Use clock referents (such as 12:00 for ventral midline and 6:00 for dorsal midline) to describe abnormal findings.

# Sigmoidoscopy, flexible

CPT CODES
*45330  Sigmoidoscopy, flexible; diagnostic, with or without collection of specimens by brushing or washing (separate procedure)*
*45331  Sigmoidoscopy, flexible; with biopsy, single or multiple*
*45332  Sigmoidoscopy, flexible; with removal of foreign body*

## DESCRIPTION

Flexible sigmoidoscopy is the direct visualization of the distal colon using a fiberoptic or video endoscope. As a colorectal cancer screening technique, it detects 50% to 60% of colon cancers. With flexible sigmoidoscopy, the inner lining of the rectum and the last 2′ (61 cm) of the distal colon can be visualized.

## INDICATIONS

➤ To evaluate rectal bleeding, new onset or persistent diarrhea or constipation, mass on digital examination, lower left quadrant abdominal pain and cramping, anal

or perianal itching or pain, suspected colitis or proctitis, or radiographic lesions identified in the sigmoid region
➤ To screen for colon cancer
➤ To remove a foreign body in the rectum

## CONTRAINDICATIONS

### Absolute
➤ Acute abdomen
➤ Diverticulitis
➤ Cardiovascular or pulmonary disease (acute)
➤ Ileus
➤ Suspected perforation
➤ Megacolon
➤ Pregnancy
➤ Fulminant colitis
➤ Uncooperative patient

### Relative
➤ Recent pelvic or abdominal surgery
➤ Coagulation disorders
➤ Severe inflammatory bowel disease
➤ Change in bowel habits (usually requires colonoscopy)

## EQUIPMENT

Flexible sigmoidoscope, 60 cm ◆ light source ◆ three gloves ◆ water-resistant gown ◆ face shield ◆ suction ◆ suction tubing ◆ water-soluble lubricant (K-Y jelly or 2% lidocaine jelly) ◆ drape ◆ prepared 10% formalin or saline specimen collection jars obtained from pathology laboratory ◆ biopsy forceps

## ESSENTIAL STEPS

➤ Ensure that the patient performed proper bowel preparation before the procedure: clear liquid diet the night before and the morning of the procedure, one bottle of citrate of magnesia the evening before the procedure, and two small-volume hypertonic phosphate enemas (such as Fleet) 60

minutes before the procedure. Alternatively, two Fleet enemas may be given in the office before the procedure if the patient can't complete them at home.
➤ To allay apprehension and anxiety, explain why and how the procedure will be performed. Review the equipment used, the anatomy of the colon to be examined, associated discomforts (cramping and distention), potential complications (perforation, bleeding, and infection), possible findings (polyps, colitis, diverticulosis, and hemorrhoids), and the potential for tissue sampling, biopsy, or photography.
➤ Address the patient's questions and concerns.
➤ Obtain informed consent.
➤ Obtain baseline vital signs.
➤ Complete the patient history and physical examination. Confirm that the patient meets the indications specified for flexible sigmoidoscopy.
➤ Administer enemas if the patient did not do this at home.
➤ Test the sigmoidoscope for light, water, air, and suction.
➤ Drape the rectal area and place the patient in the left lateral decubitus position with the knees bent up toward the chest. (Some practitioners prefer to have the patient's right leg flexed at the hip and knee to facilitate ease of entry.)
➤ Put on a faceshield, a gown, and gloves, including two on the dominant hand.
➤ Using a gloved, lubricated finger, perform a digital examination to dilate the anal sphincter. If stool is present, administer another enema.
➤ Lubricate the anus and the tip of the sigmoidoscope. Be sure not to get gel on the lens because this will distort the view.
➤ Separate the gluteal folds and observe the rectal area for hemorrhoids, fissures, or inflammation.
➤ Insert the scope obliquely by pressing the curved surface of the tip against the

sphincter rather than straight in for 3″ to 4″ (8 to 10 cm).

➤ Remove the contaminated top glove from the dominant hand.

➤ With the dominant hand, advance the scope. With the nondominant hand, work the controls on the scope.

➤ Open the colon by instilling a small amount of air, angulate the tip to locate the lumen, and advance the instrument gently. Note that the tip must be constantly maneuvered to keep the lumen in view as the instrument is passed.

➤ When the lumen is not seen, pull the scope back. Don't advance blindly. If the colon is in spasm, apply gentle bursts of air to open puckered folds. Then continue advancing the instrument toward the dark center of the lumen.

 **ALERT** Don't use too much air; this causes discomfort and can increase the risk of perforation.

➤ Advance the scope using one of the following techniques:

– The *hook and pullout* method straightens the colon. Hook the mucosal fold with the tip of the scope and pull it back gently to straighten the colon.

– The *dither and torque* method shortens the colon. Alternate insertion with slow, partial withdrawal to pleat the colon. Then twist the instrument shaft clockwise or counterclockwise with a forward or backward motion to straighten it before advancing the scope again.

 **ALERT** The goal is to provide a safe, thorough, comfortable examination, not to insert the instrument to its full length.

➤ If the instrument won't advance beyond the rectosigmoid junction (around 6″ [15 cm]), gentle pressure may permit the instrument to pass. This is safe, even if the lumen is not clearly seen, as long as the mucosa slides by. If the patient is uncomfortable or the instrument doesn't advance, withdraw the scope, torque it, and try again.

➤ Also be careful when advancing in a patient with diverticulosis. The mouth of a diverticulum may appear to be the lumen. Inserting the scope into a diverticulum can result in perforation.

➤ Observe for natural landmarks and abnormalities.

➤ Take a biopsy of all abnormal-appearing areas or polyps. The biopsy forceps can be passed through the biopsy channel of the scope. When the forceps are visible and in the area of interest or pathology, open the forceps and grasp a small sample of tissue with the prongs. Close the forceps and, with a tugging motion, retrieve the tissue sample. Remove the forceps through the channel. Place the tissue sample in a specimen jar for pathology and label it according to your laboratory's guidelines, particularly noting location either anatomically or numerically (in centimeters).

 **ALERT** Polypectomy or removal of colon lesions should be performed during a colonoscopy to minimize complications from the procedure. For example, the combination of electrocautery and incomplete bowel preparation has caused explosions.

➤ On reaching 60 cm (or the greatest distance tolerated by the patient), withdraw the sigmoidoscope slowly, reinspecting the mucosa. This provides the best view of the mucosa. Be sure to examine behind each mucosal fold.

➤ When in the rectal vault, retroflex the tip of the scope to visualize the distal rectum (twisting the knob until the tip of the scope flexes 180 degrees). Retroflection is used to diagnose and stage internal hemorrhoids or other pathology in the distal rectum.

➤ Straighten the tip and gently withdraw the scope.

➤ Cleanse, sterilize, and store the sigmoidoscope according to the manufacturer's instructions.

## PATIENT TEACHING

➤ Review the findings with the patient.
➤ Tell him that he can resume normal activity shortly after the procedure (in 5 to 15 minutes) and that no special diet is needed.
➤ Review common complications, such as abdominal cramping with air insufflation (relieved with passage of flatus or suction from scope); feeling of fullness, distention, or flatus; lack of bowel movement for several days; and minor bleeding (if a biopsy is taken in the low rectum). For a vasovagal reaction, such as vertigo, diaphoresis, hypotension, and mild malaise, tell the patient to remain supine and monitor his vital signs until the feeling passes.
➤ Urge the patient to promptly report signs of infection (elevated temperature, diarrhea, or increased or prolonged abdominal pain), bloody diarrhea, or bleeding that persists for more than 2 days.

## COMPLICATIONS

➤ Complications are rare. Their incidence is higher in the patient with previous abdominal surgery or irradiation, which can cause adhesions. *Bowel adhesions* can fixate the bowel and cause tethering, which predisposes the colon to perforation.
➤ *Bowel perforation* requires emergency surgical referral.
➤ *Bleeding* may require referral or collaboration with a gastroenterologist.
➤ *Abnormal distention and pain* require evaluation and treatment, depending on findings.
➤ *Infection* may require antibiotics and referral, depending on whether the infection is local or systemic.
➤ *Vasovagal symptoms* are treated with rest, with the patient in a supine position until symptoms resolve.
➤ *Undetected disease* is minimized with periodic screening.

## SPECIAL CONSIDERATIONS

➤ GI discomfort usually resolves in 24 to 48 hours. A feeling of pressure is generally greatest immediately after the procedure. The patient may feel a need to evacuate stool with no results or may experience increased flatulence for a few days after the procedure.
➤ Provide the patient with written instructions to reinforce your teaching (see *Preparing for a sigmoidoscopy or a colonoscopy*).
➤ The American Cancer Society recommends the use of flexible sigmoidoscopy to screen the patient at average risk for colon cancer. The current recommendation is that males and females age 50 and over should have a flexible sigmoidoscopy every 3 to 5 years and participate in yearly fecal occult blood testing. Average-risk individuals are those without a family history of colon cancer, personal history of adenoma polypectomy, history of pancolitis within the previous 8 years and currently without anemia, heme-positive stools, or change in bowel habits. Because only 60% of colon cancer can be detected with a sigmoidoscopy, the patient with a family history of colon cancer or colon polyps, blood mixed in his stool, or a change in the pattern or characteristic of his stools should undergo a complete colonoscopy rather than a sigmoidoscopy.

 **CULTURAL TIP** Many cultural groups consider touching the anal region embarrassing or taboo. State your intentions matter-of-factly before touching the patient in a private area. By using a professional demeanor and effective distraction techniques, you can minimize the patient's discomfort and reduce muscle tension. Conversely, humor or unnecessary touching during the examination may offend the patient or increase his discomfort.

*(Text continues on page 134.)*

## PREPARING FOR A SIGMOIDOSCOPY OR A COLONOSCOPY

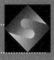

### DEAR PATIENT:

The practitioner wants you to undergo either a flexible sigmoidoscopy or a colonoscopy. If you're scheduled for a colonoscopy, read on because the two tests are similar. Differences are listed at the end of this patient-teaching aid.

A sigmoidoscopy allows the practitioner to see inside the lower part of the large bowel, which includes the sigmoid colon, rectum, and anus. To do this, she'll gently insert a flexible fiber-optic tube called an endoscope into the rectum.

### Why is this test necessary?

Sigmoidoscopy allows careful examination of the lower bowel and rectum for bowel disease. (These areas are difficult to visualize in X-rays.) If needed, this test will also enable the practitioner to take a biopsy specimen for further testing or to remove polyps.

### Will I need to prepare for the test?

Yes. Make sure to follow the practitioner's directions for diet and bowel preparation. Stay on a liquid diet for 48 hours beforehand. You may drink broth, tea, gelatin, water, and clear juices without pulp, and you may continue to take prescription medicine.

Take a laxative the evening before the test and give yourself an enema (for example, a Fleet enema) the morning of the test. If the test is scheduled for early morning, don't consume anything past midnight.

Just before the test, you'll take off your clothes and put on a hospital gown. Leave your socks on for warmth. Also, empty your bladder.

### What can I expect during the test?

The test is performed by the practitioner and an assistant in an office or a special procedures room. It will last about 15 to 30 minutes. Before the test begins, the assistant will help you lie on your left side with knees flexed. Next, she'll drape you with a sheet.

Once you're in position, the practitioner will gently insert a well-lubricated, gloved finger into the anus to examine the area and dilate the rectal sphincter.

Next, the practitioner will gently insert the endoscope through the anus into the rectum. As it passes through the rectal sphincters, you may feel some lower abdominal discomfort and the urge to move your bowels. Bear down gently as the endoscope is first inserted. Also breathe slowly and deeply through your mouth to help you relax. This will help ease the passage of the endoscope through the sphincters. The practitioner will gradually advance the endoscope through the rectum into the lower bowel.

Sometimes air is blown through the endoscope into the bowel to distend it and permit better viewing. If you feel the urge to expel some air, try not to control it and don't be embarrassed. The passing of air is expected and necessary. You may hear and feel a suction machine removing any liquid that obscures the practitioner's view during the test. This machine is noisy, but painless.

The practitioner will advance the endoscope slowly about 24″ (61 cm) into the lower bowel. Continue to breathe slowly and deeply through your mouth to help the test go smoothly.

*(continued)*

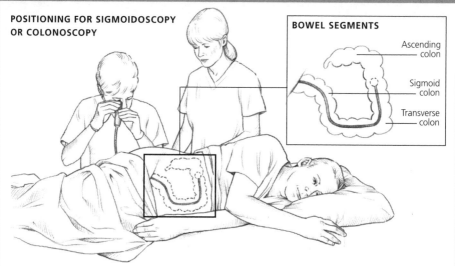

POSITIONING FOR SIGMOIDOSCOPY
OR COLONOSCOPY

BOWEL SEGMENTS

Ascending colon

Sigmoid colon

Transverse colon

The practitioner may remove biopsy specimens or polyps from the lining of the bowel at any time during the test. These procedures are also painless because the bowel lining doesn't sense pain.

Toward the end of the test, the practitioner may insert a rigid anoscope into the lower rectum. This instrument will provide a clearer view of the anal wall, revealing any abnormalities that the flexible endoscope might miss.

### What can I expect afterward?

The assistant will monitor your vital signs for about an hour afterward. Because air was introduced into your bowel, you'll begin to pass large amounts of gas. Also, you may expect to have slight rectal bleeding if the practitioner removed tissue specimens. Notify the practitioner immediately if you experience heavy, bright red bleeding; fever; abdominal swelling; or tenderness after the test.

### How does a colonoscopy differ from a sigmoidoscopy?

The two tests are similar, except a colonoscopy allows the practitioner to visualize *all* of your large bowel, not just the lower portion.

To prepare for this test, follow the practitioner's directions for a clear liquid diet and bowel preparation. The bowel preparation is one of two kinds: You may be instructed to drink a large amount of an electrolyte solution (such as GoLYTELY or Co-Lyte). This solution will clear your bowel in about 4 hours, so plan to stay at home after drinking it. Or you may be asked to take a laxative for 2 nights before the test and give yourself enemas the morning of the test.

Just before a colonoscopy, you'll receive a sedative to help you relax and ease any discomfort you may experience as the practitioner advances the endoscope past the curves of the bowel.

## SAMPLE DOCUMENTATION FORM FOR FLEXIBLE SIGMOIDOSCOPY

### OFFICE FLEXIBLE SIGMOIDOSCOPY

DATE: _4/21/00_     CHART #/ID #: _82995150_

PATIENT NAME: _Ian Mansfield_

DOB: _08/14/49_     AGE: _50_

### SIGNS AND SYMPTOMS

FOBT RESULTS: _Positive_     DATE: _4/10/00_

PREVIOUS SIGMOIDOSCOPY: _None_     DATE:

### PMH

ALLERGIES: _PCN_

MEDICATIONS: _Denies_

BACTERIAL ENDOCARDITIS PROPHYLAXIS: _NO_

BLOOD PRESSURE: _136/88_

### BOWEL PREPARATION USED

- [✓] CLEAR LIQUIDS / CITRATE OF MAGNESIA
- [✓] 2 FLEET ENEMAS AT HOME
- [ ] 2 FLEET ENEMAS IN OFFICE

**ADEQUACY OF PREPARATION:** _Optimal cleansing_

**TYPE OF SCOPE:** _Flexible 35-cm scope with video pathway system_

**DEPTH OF VISUALIZATION:** _35 cm_

**PREOPERATIVE DIAGNOSIS:** _N/A_

**POSTOPERATIVE DIAGNOSIS:** _Internal hemorrhoids_

**FINDINGS:** _Lining of sigmoid colon, rectal mucosa, rectum, and anus appear normal in color, texture, and size except for painless, bluish, engorged veins near anus seen on retroversion._

**LOCATION OF BIOPSIES:** _N/A_

**PLAN:** _Advised patient to engage in physical activity for 30 minutes daily. Recommended increasing intake of low-fat and high-fiber foods (at least five servings of fruits and vegetables daily plus six servings of other high-fiber foods, such as whole-grain breads, rice, and pasta). Discussed smoking cessation._

SIGNATURE: _Megan Frenz, CRNP_     CC: _Rick Gill, FNP_

**CULTURAL TIP** Gender may play a role during a rectal examination, especially in cultural groups in which women are subordinate. For instance, a female practitioner may need a male health care professional to convey the importance of the examination to a male from a culture that considers women to be inferior. An Asian or Muslim woman may feel uncomfortable being undressed in front of others; use drapes to protect her privacy.

## DOCUMENTATION

➤ Document findings in the patient's chart. (See *Sample documentation form for flexible sigmoidoscopy*, page 133.)
➤ Be sure to document the type and adequacy of bowel preparation, type of scope used, depth of visualization, appearance of mucosa, biopsy locations (if taken), complications, the patient's tolerance of the procedure, and instructions given to the patient for follow-up and treatment (if required).

## Urea breath test

### CPT CODES
*83013* Helicobacter pylori; *breath test analysis*
*83014* H. pylori; *breath test analysis; drug administration and collection*

## DESCRIPTION

The urea breath test is used to diagnose *Helicobacter pylori* infection of the stomach. It's a noninvasive test based on the hydrolysis of urea by *H. pylori* to produce carbon dioxide ($CO_2$) and ammonia. A carbon isotope is labeled and given to the patient by mouth; the *H. pylori* then releases the tagged $CO_2$, which is collected in a breath sample.

The American College of Gastroenterology recommends a urea breath test as the best nonendoscopic test for documenting *H. pylori* infection. Other noninvasive tests used to confirm *H. pylori* infection include serology testing, which uses enzyme-linked immunosorbent assay testing to detect immunoglobulin G antibodies. Numerous studies suggest, however, that the accuracy of serum testing ranges only from 83% to 90%. Stool antigen assay is also used. The stool antigen assay appears comparable in accuracy to the urea breath test.

## INDICATIONS

➤ To diagnose suspected *H. pylori* infection
➤ To screen patients with active peptic ulcer disease or a history of documented peptic or duodenal ulcer or of mucosa-associated lymphoid tissue lymphoma
➤ To document eradication in patients who have undergone treatment for *H. pylori*

## CONTRAINDICATIONS

### Absolute
➤ Use of bismuth or antibiotics within 30 days of testing (can produce false-negative result)
➤ Use of sucralfate or proton-pump inhibitors within 14 days of testing (can suppress *H. pylori* and produce false-negative result)
➤ Patient's failure to fast for 6 hours before testing
➤ Pregnancy

 **ALERT** Although the dose of radiation contained in the 14C–urea breath test is small, it isn't currently recommended for use in children or pregnant women. A nonradioactive 13C test may be used instead.

## EQUIPMENT

PYtest capsule ◆ two 30-ml medicine cups
◆ timer ◆ collection balloon ◆ straw

## ESSENTIAL STEPS

➤ Confirm that the patient has not had
bismuth or antibiotics in the past 30 days,
sucralfate or proton-pump inhibitors in
the past 14 days, and food in the past 6
hours.
➤ Explain the purpose of the test and review the procedure. Perform a dry run of
the test to ensure his understanding.
➤ Give him one PYtest capsule and 20 ml
of water. Instruct him to swallow the capsule without chewing, using the 20 ml of
water to wash the capsule down.
➤ After he swallows the capsule, begin
timing for 10 minutes.
➤ After 3 minutes, refill the medicine cup
with 20 ml of water and instruct the patient to swallow this additional water to
ensure that the capsule has passed completely into the stomach.
➤ Label the collection balloon with the
patient's name and date of birth. Insert a
straw into the balloon opening in preparation for the collection.
➤ After 10 minutes have elapsed, give the
balloon with the straw in place to the patient. (See *Using a PYtest balloon*.)
➤ Instruct him to inhale deeply, hold his
breath for 10 seconds, and then fully inflate the balloon through the straw. Tell
him not to overinflate the balloon.
➤ Process the sample following the manufacturer's guidelines or forward it to the
laboratory for processing.

## PATIENT TEACHING

➤ Inform the patient that the test will help
confirm the presence or absence of *H. pylori* infection, which will help determine
whether treatment is necessary. Reassure

### USING A PYTEST BALLOON

A PYtest balloon and straw are needed to
collect the exhaled specimen. Instruct the
patient to inhale deeply, hold his breath
for 10 seconds, then blow into the straw
until the balloon is fully inflated. Reinforce
that he doesn't need to fully exhale and
shouldn't overinflate the balloon.

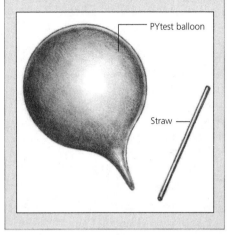

him that he won't experience discomfort
or adverse reactions from the procedure.
➤ Tell him he may leave once the test is
complete.
➤ Review and give the patient preprinted
patient-teaching supplements from the
manufacturer.
➤ Tell him to schedule a follow-up in 1
week to discuss test results and necessary
treatments, if any.

## COMPLICATIONS

None known

## SPECIAL CONSIDERATIONS

Testing for *H. pylori* in patients with nonul-
cer dyspepsia and without history of peptic ulcer disease is controversial, although
some practitioners examine the patient for
infection. In general, testing should be

done only in the patient who will be treated only if the test result is positive.

## DOCUMENTATION

➤ Record the test date, the time the sample was collected, and the patient's name, date of birth, and identification number.
➤ Note the patient's referring physician, if appropriate. (Practitioners can order this procedure without supervision in most states.)
➤ Document your confirmation that the patient did not have bismuth or antibiotics in the past 30 days, sucralfate or proton-pump inhibitors in the past 14 days, and food in the past 6 hours.
➤ Note the patient's history of partial gastrectomy, if applicable.
➤ Record test results, whether positive, negative, or indeterminate.

# Paracentesis, abdominal

CPT CODES
*49080    Abdominal paracentesis, initial*
*49081    Abdominal paracentesis, subsequent*

## DESCRIPTION

Abdominal paracentesis is one of the quickest and most cost-effective methods for diagnosing the cause of ascites. It involves inserting a needle into the peritoneal space of a patient with ascites and withdrawing a fluid sample. Samples of the fluid are sent to the laboratory for diagnosis. In the patient with large-volume ascites, therapeutic paracentesis helps relieve the pressure in the abdominal wall, makes him feel more comfortable, and avoids the complications of respiratory compromise, abdominal pain, and abdominal hernias.

## INDICATIONS

➤ To relieve intra-abdominal pressure causing respiratory distress
➤ To evaluate ascites fluid for signs of infection

## CONTRAINDICATIONS

### Absolute

➤ Acute abdomen requiring immediate surgery
➤ Disseminated intravascular coagulation
➤ Inability of practitioner to demonstrate presence of ascites on physical examination

### Relative

➤ Coagulopathy that can't be corrected with fresh-frozen plasma or vitamin K
➤ Bowel distention or intestinal obstruction
➤ Infection or surgical scar at the needle entry site
➤ History of multiple abdominal surgeries
➤ Poor patient cooperation (patient movement could lead to serious injury)

## EQUIPMENT

Commercially prepared paracentesis kit or the following supplies: Skin cleansing solution (povidone-iodine) and alcohol ◆ gown ◆ mask ◆ eyeshield ◆ sterile gloves ◆ sterile marking pen ◆ sterile drapes ◆ 1% or 2% lidocaine with or without epinephrine (epinephrine helps decrease unwanted abdominal wall bleeding) ◆ 10-ml syringe ◆ 50-ml sterile syringe ◆ 18G 1½" needle ◆ 1 L vacuum bottles ◆ sterile specimen tubes (optional if infection is suspected) ◆ two blood culture bottles ◆ I.V. tubing and 22G needle ◆ adhesive bandage

# ESSENTIAL STEPS

➤ Obtain a recent prothrombin time/partial thromboplastin time to assess for coagulopathy.
➤ Explain the procedure to the patient, including its risks, benefits, and alternatives.
➤ Obtain written or verbal informed consent.

 **ALERT** When obtaining informed consent, assess whether the patient has hepatic encephalopathy; in this case, the individual to whom the patient has given power of attorney will need to sign for consent.

➤ Ask the patient to empty his bladder immediately before the procedure.
➤ Obtain baseline vital signs.
➤ Place the patient in the supine position, with the head of the bed slightly elevated. (Patients with less ascites can be placed in the lateral decubitus position.)
➤ Identify the site of paracentesis and mark it with a sterile pen. You may use the lower left or right quadrant, about ¾″ to 1¼″ (2 to 3 cm) lateral to the rectus muscle border for large-volume paracentesis. This site offers a thin abdominal wall. The linea alba, 1¼″ to 1½″ (3 to 4 cm) below the umbilicus, is an alternative site. The midline site is avascular and has less risk of bleeding. Place midline needles caudal to the umbilicus.

Avoid the following areas:
– rectus muscle, which has an increased risk of hemorrhage from epigastric vessels
– surgical scars because of the increased risk of perforation caused by adhesion of the bowel wall to the wall of the peritoneum
– areas of skin infection because of the increased risk of intraperitoneal infection
– areas cephalic to the umbilicus in a patient with portal hypertension because a large venous collateral is usually located midline.

➤ Don gloves, a gown, a mask, and an eyeshield.
➤ Cleanse the area with povidone-iodine followed by alcohol; then drape the abdomen.
➤ Using 1% to 2% lidocaine, anesthetize the puncture site by infiltrating the skin and deeper tissues down to and including the peritoneum.
➤ Attach a #18G needle to a 10-ml syringe. In patients with a large adipose panniculus, spinal needles (3½″) may be necessary.
➤ Retract the skin at the site caudally (Z-track technique). Insert the needle, attached to a sterile syringe, initially at a 45-degree angle, then perpendicular to the skin; advance the needle slowly in 5-mm increments. You'll feel a "pop" as the needle advances through the anterior and posterior muscular fasciae and a "give" when the needle enters the peritoneal cavity.

 **ALERT** A slow, incremental insertion allows you to observe for a flash of blood if entering a blood vessel and to withdraw the needle to avoid further damage. (See *Tapping the peritoneal cavity,* page 138.)

➤ When ascites fluid returns freely, hold the needle in place. Don't advance the needle further to avoid bowel perforation.
➤ Gently aspirate 10 ml of fluid; then attach the 50-ml syringe. Aspirate further quantities of fluid as needed for analysis (usually 100 to 200 ml).
➤ Obtain fluid for diagnostic purposes. Common tests include lactate dehydrogenase, glucose, albumin, protein, specific gravity, complete blood cell count and differential, Gram stain, cytology (requires 50 ml), amylase, lipase, pH, cholesterol, triglycerides, carcinoembryonic antigen, and special cultures for tuberculosis by acid-fast bacillus, bacteria, viruses, or fungi.
➤ After removing the fluid needed for pathology, remove additional fluid as needed to alleviate symptoms. To do this, attach

## TAPPING THE PERITONEAL CAVITY

After administering a local anesthetic to numb the area near the patient's navel, insert the needle (about ¾" [2 cm]) through the skin and subcutaneous tissues of the abdominal wall. Then advance the needle slowly into the pelvic midline until it enters the peritoneum (feeling for a little pop as it enters the peritoneum and carefully watching for a flash of blood, which would indicate inadvertent entry into a blood vessel).

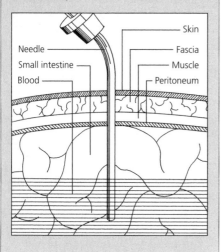

Using a syringe attached to the catheter, aspirate fluid from the peritoneal cavity and look for blood or other abnormal findings.

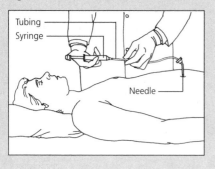

the I.V. tubing to the needle and place a second needle on the opposite end. Insert the free needle end into the vacuum bottle, and fluid will collect spontaneously.

➤ If no fluid returns after several attempts, use ultrasound-directed aspiration.

 **ALERT** When performing therapeutic paracentesis in a patient with significant peripheral edema, remove no more than 6 L of fluid. In a patient without peripheral edema, remove no more than 1,500 ml. If paracentesis is strictly for diagnostic purposes, 100 ml of fluid should be adequate.

➤ When the desired amount of fluid has been collected, withdraw the needle in a quick motion and release the skin retraction. This technique forms a Z-track and helps minimize leakage.

➤ Apply pressure to the site for several minutes and apply an adhesive bandage. If fluid leaks from the site, keep the patient supine with the site upward until leakage stops.

➤ If a large-volume paracentesis was performed (4 to 6 L), monitor the patient's vital signs according to your facility's protocol (usually, every hour for 2 to 4 hours).

➤ Label all samples for analysis according to your facility's policy. Send to the laboratory for analysis.

➤ Review results. (See *Interpreting peritoneal drainage results.*)

## PATIENT TEACHING

➤ Assure the patient that he'll probably feel little if any pain after the procedure. Explain that breathing will be easier if a significant amount of fluid is withdrawn, because it will relieve pressure on the diaphragm.

➤ Tell him to remain on his back with the site facing upward until fluid stops leaking and you tell him he can stand.

➤ Teach him to monitor for and immediately report signs of infection, such as elevated temperature, increased or prolonged abdominal pain, and bleeding.

➤ Have him schedule a follow-up appointment within 48 hours for review of fluid analysis results.

## COMPLICATIONS

➤ *Persistent leakage of ascitic fluid* can be treated by having the patient lie flat while you apply pressure to the site. Place a suture if leakage persists.

➤ *Hypotension and shock* require monitoring and fluid management. Transport to an acute care center may be required if the condition doesn't stabilize.

➤ *Perforated bowel* requires urgent surgical referral and immediate surgery. This rarely occurs; the risk is 0.8%.

➤ *Abscess formation at the puncture site* may require antibiotic therapy and collaboration with a specialist in infectious diseases.

➤ *Peritonitis* may require collaboration with a specialist in infectious diseases and a surgical consult.

➤ *Abdominal wall hematoma* must be monitored. Risk of hematoma requiring transfusion is 0.2% to 1.6% despite coagulopathy.

## SPECIAL CONSIDERATIONS

➤ If you performed large-volume paracentesis (4 to 6 L), monitor the patient's vital signs frequently to detect possible hypotension. If vital signs remain stable, have the patient ambulate as tolerated.

➤ Colloid replacement with albumin is recommended after large-volume paracentesis (4 to 6 L), at a rate of 6 to 8 grams of albumin per liter of ascitic fluid removed.

➤ Bare steel needles are preferable to plastic sheathed cannulas because plastic sheaths tend to kink or collapse after the metal trocar is removed.

### INTERPRETING PERITONEAL DRAINAGE RESULTS

The most common abnormal findings associated with peritoneal drainage include:
➤ unclotted blood, bile, or intestinal contents in aspirated peritoneal fluid (20 ml in an adult or 10 ml in a child)
➤ bloody or pinkish-red fluid, dark enough to prevent the reading of newsprint through it (If you can read newsprint through the fluid, test results are considered negative, although more testing may be indicated.)
➤ green, cloudy, turbid, or milky peritoneal fluid return (Normal peritoneal fluid appears clear to pale yellow.)
➤ red blood cell count over 100,000/µl
➤ white blood cell count exceeding 500/µl
➤ bacteria in fluid (identified by culture and sensitivity testing or Gram stain).

If the patient's condition is stable, borderline positive results may suggest the need for additional tests, such as ultrasonography and arteriography. If test results are questionable or inconclusive, consider leaving the catheter in place to repeat the procedure.

## DOCUMENTATION

➤ Review documentation by other health team members; then initial their notes to signify you're aware of their findings. This doesn't signify agreement with their comments or reduce your responsibility to complete your own history and physical examination. Document abnormal physical findings. (The preprocedural and postprocedural note must include an evaluation of respiratory and GI function.)

➤ Note indications for the procedure and the amount and appearance of fluid removed.

➤ Record laboratory requests regarding specimens sent for diagnostic paracentesis.

➤ Note the patient's vital signs and tolerance of the procedure.

➤ Record any complications, actions taken, and final outcome.
➤ Record albumin replacement per facility guidelines.

# Routine Procedures

## Feeding tube insertion and removal

CPT CODE
*91100    Intestinal feeding tube passage, positioning, and monitoring*

## Description

Inserting a feeding tube nasally or orally into the stomach or duodenum allows a patient who can't or won't eat to receive nourishment. The feeding tube also permits supplemental feedings in a patient who has very high nutritional requirements, such as an unconscious patient or one with extensive burns. The preferred feeding tube route is nasal, but the oral route may be used for patients with such conditions as deviated septums or head or nose injuries.

Feeding tubes differ somewhat from standard nasogastric tubes. Made of silicone, rubber, or polyurethane, feeding tubes have small diameters and great flexibility. This reduces oropharyngeal irritation, necrosis from pressure on the tracheoesophageal wall, distal esophageal irritation, and discomfort from swallowing. To facilitate passage, some feeding tubes are weighted with tungsten, and some need a guide wire to keep them from curling in the back of the throat. These small-bore tubes usually have radiopaque markings

and a water-activated coating, which provides a lubricated surface.

## Indications

➤ To permit feeding of patients who are at high risk for aspiration with gastric feeding or who otherwise can't tolerate it
➤ To permit short-term nutrient replacement

## Contraindications

### Absolute
➤ Absence of bowel sounds
➤ Possible intestinal obstruction
➤ Intractable vomiting
➤ Upper GI bleeding

## Equipment

*For insertion*: Feeding tube (#6 to #18 French, with or without guide wire) ◆ linen-saver pad ◆ gloves ◆ hypoallergenic tape ◆ water-soluble lubricant ◆ skin preparation (such as tincture of benzoin) ◆ facial tissues ◆ penlight ◆ small cup of water with straw, or ice chips ◆ emesis basin ◆ 60-ml syringe ◆ stethoscope
*For removal*: Linen-saver pad ◆ tube clamp ◆ bulb syringe

## Preparation of Equipment

➤ Have the proper size tube available (usually the smallest-bore tube that will allow free passage of the liquid feeding formula). Read the instructions on the tubing package carefully because tube characteristics vary according to the manufacturer. (For example, some tubes have marks at the appropriate lengths for gastric, duodenal, and jejunal insertion.)
➤ Examine the tube to make sure it's free of defects, such as cracks or rough or sharp edges.

➤ Next, run water through the tube. This checks for patency, activates the coating, and facilitates removal of the guide.

## ESSENTIAL STEPS

➤ Explain the procedure to the patient. Show him the tube so he knows what to expect and can cooperate more fully.
➤ Provide privacy.
➤ Wash your hands and put on gloves. Assist the patient into semi-Fowler's or high Fowler's position. Place a linen-saver pad across the patient's chest to protect him from spills.
➤ Determine the tube length needed to reach the stomach by first extending the distal end of the tube from the tip of the patient's nose to his earlobe. Coil this portion of the tube around your fingers so the end stays curved until you insert it. Then extend the uncoiled portion from the earlobe to the xiphoid process. Use a small piece of hypoallergenic tape to mark the total length of the two portions.

### Inserting the tube nasally

➤ Using the penlight, assess nasal patency. Inspect nasal passages for a deviated septum, polyps, or other obstructions. Occlude one nostril, then the other, to determine which has the better airflow. Assess the patient's history of nasal injury or surgery.
➤ Lubricate the curved tip of the tube (and the feeding tube guide, if appropriate) with a small amount of water-soluble lubricant to ease insertion and prevent tissue injury.
➤ Ask the patient to hold the emesis basin and facial tissues in case he needs them.
➤ Insert the curved, lubricated tip into the more patent nostril and direct it along the nasal passage toward the ear on the same side. When it passes the nasopharyngeal junction, turn the tube 180 degrees to aim it downward into the esophagus. Instruct the patient to lower his chin to his chest to close the trachea. Then give him a small cup of water with a straw or ice chips. Direct him to sip the water or suck on the ice and swallow frequently. This will ease the tube's passage. Advance the tube as he swallows.

### Inserting the tube orally

➤ Have the patient lower his chin to close his trachea, and ask him to open his mouth.
➤ Place the tip of the tube at the back of the patient's tongue, give water, and instruct the patient to swallow, as described above. Remind him to avoid clamping his teeth down on the tube. Advance the tube as he swallows.

### Positioning the tube

➤ Keep passing the tube until the tape marking the appropriate length reaches the patient's nostril or lips.
➤ To check tube placement, attach the syringe filled with 10 cc of air to the end of the tube. Gently inject the air into the tube as you auscultate the patient's abdomen with the stethoscope about 3" (7.6 cm) below the sternum. Listen for a whooshing sound, which signals that the tube has reached its target in the stomach. If the tube remains coiled in the esophagus, you'll feel resistance when you inject the air, or the patient may belch. If you can't hear verification of placement, the tube may be in the esophagus. You'll need to advance the tube or reinsert it before proceeding.
➤ After confirming proper tube placement, remove the tape marking the tube length.
➤ Tape the tube to the patient's nose.
➤ Verify tube placement in the stomach by X-ray as needed; then remove the guide wire.
➤ To advance the tube to the duodenum, especially a tungsten-weighted tube, position the patient on his right side. This lets gravity assist tube passage through the pylorus. Write orders for the tube to be advanced 2" to 3" (5 to 7.6 cm) hourly for a total of about 8" (20 cm) until X-ray studies confirm duodenal placement. (An

X-ray must confirm placement before feeding begins because duodenal feeding can cause nausea and vomiting if accidentally delivered to the stomach.)

➤ Apply a skin preparation to the patient's cheek before securing the tube with tape. This helps the tube adhere to the skin and also prevents irritation.

➤ Tape the tube securely to the patient's cheek to avoid excessive pressure on his nostrils.

### Removing the tube

➤ Protect the patient's chest with a linen-saver pad.

➤ Flush the tube with air, clamp or pinch it to prevent fluid aspiration during withdrawal, and withdraw it gently but quickly.

➤ Promptly cover and discard the used tube.

## PATIENT TEACHING

➤ Explain to the patient and his significant others why the patient needs a feeding tube and how long it is expected to be in place. Explain that the tube must move into the intestine by gravity. Therefore, small amounts of tubing will be advanced periodically for about 6 to 12 hours if the patient is ambulatory or 12 to 24 hours if the patient is on bed rest. Then an X-ray will be taken to verify the location of the tube.

➤ Advise the patient that the tube will cause some discomfort. (Minimize such discomfort by secondarily fastening the tube so it doesn't pull as the patient moves, after it's positioned in the duodenum. To do this, place tape around the tube; then place a safety pin through the tape and pin this to the patient's clothing. Emphasize that he'll need to unpin the tube before changing clothing.)

➤ Detail the goals that the patient must achieve before the tube can be removed (such as a positive gag reflex or cessation of food pocketing as he eats), and outline how he can actively participate in achieving them, as indicated.

➤ Teach the patient and caregivers how to use and care for a feeding tube if the patient will go home with the feeding tube in place. Teach them how to obtain equipment, insert and remove the tube, prepare and store feeding formula, and solve problems with tube position and patency.

➤ Instruct the patient or caregiver to contact you immediately if the tube moves or if the patient experiences abdominal pain or cramping or difficulty breathing.

➤ Teach the patient or caregiver to retape the tube at least daily and as needed. Alternate taping the tube toward the inner and outer side of the nose to avoid constant pressure on the same nasal area. Inspect the skin for redness and breakdown.

➤ Teach the patient or caregiver how to perform nasal hygiene using the cotton-tipped applicators and water-soluble lubricant to remove crusted secretions.

➤ Advise the patient or caregiver to brush his teeth, gums, and tongue with mouthwash or a mild saltwater solution at least twice daily.

## COMPLICATIONS

➤ *Pulmonary aspiration* is a life-threatening complication. Reduce the risk for pulmonary aspiration by ensuring tube placement well below the pyloric sphincter.

➤ *Skin erosion at the nostril, sinusitis, esophagitis, esophagotracheal fistula, gastric ulceration, and pulmonary and oral infection* are associated with prolonged intubation.

## SPECIAL CONSIDERATIONS

➤ Write orders to flush the feeding tube every 8 hours with up to 60 ml of normal saline solution or water to maintain patency.

➤ If the patient can't swallow the feeding tube, use a guide wire to aid insertion.

➤ Always compare the potential risks and benefits for the patient. For instance, supplementing nutrition through tube feeding may not improve or prolong the life of a patient with end-stage dementia, but it's likely to cause significant discomfort and distress.

 **ALERT** Precise feeding-tube placement is especially important because small-bore feeding tubes may slide into the trachea without causing immediate signs or symptoms of respiratory distress, such as coughing, choking, gasping, or cyanosis. However, the patient will usually cough if the tube enters the larynx. To be sure that the tube clears the larynx, ask the patient to speak. If he can't, the tube is in the larynx. Withdraw the tube at once and reinsert.

➤ If the feeding tube needs to be repositioned after the guide wire has been removed, fluoroscopic guidance is required.

➤ If your patient will use a feeding tube at home, write orders for home care services. Include the anticipated start and end date of services, the number and duration of skilled nursing visits, and include an as-needed visit for problems related to the tube. Note the amount and frequency of feedings, any durable medical equipment and supplies needed, frequency of laboratory studies such as electrolytes and creatinine, and daily or weekly weighing of the patient.

## DOCUMENTATION

➤ Record the date, time, tube type and size, insertion site, area of placement, and confirmation of proper placement.

➤ For tube removal, record the date and time and the patient's tolerance of the procedure.

# Nasogastric tube insertion and removal

CPT CODES
*91100    Intestinal feeding tube, passage, positioning, and monitoring*
*91105    Gastric intubation for aspiration and treatment (separate procedure)*

## DESCRIPTION

Intended for short-term use, a nasogastric (NG) tube has many clinical indications ranging from gastric evacuation to enteral feeding and medication administration. Made of rubber or plastic, NG tubes are passed into the stomach through the nose. Orogastric tubes inserted through the mouth are an option; however, the nose is the preferred route because it minimizes discomfort related to the gag reflex. A patient with a head injury or known septal deviation or who recently had nasal surgery should have the tube inserted orally.

The Levin tube is a single-lumen catheter used for feeding. The Salem sump tube is a double-lumen tube with a separate port for air ventilation. This is commonly used for gastric decompression and lavage. The air vent allows for a constant flow of air to prevent suction of the gastric mucosa. Nasoduodenal tubes (such as the Dobhoff tube) and other soft feeding tubes are available for long-term use. Feeding tubes differ from NG tubes in that the lumens are smaller and more flexible. This helps prevent oropharyngeal and esophageal irritation and pressure necrosis.

## INDICATIONS

➤ To prevent nausea and vomiting and to facilitate gastric decompression after surgery

➤ To provide a route for feeding and medication administration

➤ To remove stomach contents for laboratory analysis
➤ To assess GI bleeding
➤ To facilitate decompression for paralytic ileus or intestinal obstruction

## CONTRAINDICATIONS

### Absolute
➤ Comatose or obtunded patient with unprotected airway
➤ Facial fractures or basilar skull fracture with cribriform plate injury
➤ Hypothermic patients (insertion may cause myocardial irritability leading to ventricular fibrillation)

### Relative
➤ History of known caustic ingestions
➤ Recent gastrectomy, esophagectomy, or oropharyngeal, gastric, or nasal surgery
➤ Known coagulopathies or anticoagulant therapy

## EQUIPMENT

Gastric tube (14F to 18F) ◆ lidocaine gel and benzocaine spray ◆ water-soluble lubricant ◆ phenylephrine spray ◆ basin filled with warm water or ice (optional) ◆ 20- to 50-ml syringe with adapter ◆ cotton-tipped applicators ◆ emesis basin ◆ 1″ hypoallergenic tape ◆ tincture of benzoin ◆ suction setup ◆ penlight ◆ safety pin and elastic band ◆ bib or towel ◆ glass of water and drinking straw ◆ tissues ◆ stethoscope ◆ gloves

## PREPARATION OF EQUIPMENT

➤ Inspect the NG tube for defects, such as rough edges or partially closed lumens.
➤ Check the tube's patency by flushing it with water.
➤ To ease insertion, increase a stiff tube's flexibility by coiling it around your gloved fingers for a few seconds or by dipping it into warm water. Stiffen a limp rubber tube by briefly chilling it in ice.

## ESSENTIAL STEPS

### Inserting the tube
➤ Explain the procedure to the patient. This will promote cooperation and reduce anxiety. Explain possible complications and alternative treatments, if available.
➤ Explain that she may feel some discomfort, such as gagging or tearing of the eyes. Request that she cooperate as much as possible with swallowing while the tube is inserted. Give her a glass of water with a drinking straw to assist with swallowing the tube.
➤ Agree on a signal for the patient to use when she wants to pause before continuing the procedure.
➤ Place an emesis basin and tissues within her reach.
➤ Cover her clothing or gown with a towel or linen-saver pad to protect from spillage.
➤ Provide privacy and maintain clean technique.
➤ Assist the patient into a high Fowler's position and support her head with a pillow, if available. This position helps decrease the gag reflex, promotes patient swallowing, and allows gravity to assist with tube insertion.
➤ Check for deformity or obstruction of the nostrils. Ask the patient to hyperextend her neck and observe the nostrils either by using a penlight or by having the patient breathe in while occluding the other nostril. Select the most patent naris for tube insertion.
➤ If the patient is unconscious, place her in the left lateral position with her head turned downward and to the side to prevent aspiration.
➤ Apply topical lidocaine to the nares with a cotton-tipped applicator and spray benzocaine into the throat.

➤ Have the patient blow her nose to clear her nasal passages. If she has a lot of nasal congestion, spray a vasoconstrictor such as phenylephrine into each nostril.

➤ Determine how far to insert the tube. (See *Determining the length of an NG tube.*) Mark the tube with adhesive tape if the tube doesn't have printed markings on it.

➤ Curl 4″ to 6″ (10 to 15 cm) of the end of the tube around your finger and then release it. This gives a natural curve to the tube before insertion.

➤ Generously lubricate the tip of the tube with water-soluble gel or lidocaine gel to decrease mucosal irritation. Unlike a lipid-soluble lubricant, a water-soluble lubricant reduces the risk of aspiration pneumonia if the tube enters the trachea.

➤ With the patient's neck hyperextended (if cervical spine is unaffected), insert the tube with its natural curve toward the patient into the selected nostril and gently advance the tube toward the nasopharynx. (See *Positioning for NG tube placement,* page 146.)

➤ Direct the tube along the floor of the nostril and toward the ear on the same side. If you meet resistance, withdraw and relubricate the tube and insert into the other nostril.

➤ Once the tube reaches the oropharynx (throat), you'll meet resistance. At this point, have the patient tilt her head forward and continue to pass the tube steadily. (Tilting the head forward helps pass the tube through the esophagus rather than the larynx.) Encourage the patient to swallow water to assist with passing of the tube.

➤ If the patient continues to gag, have her rest, take a few deep breaths, and drink water.

➤ If the tube doesn't advance with each swallow, withdraw it slightly and inspect the patient's mouth. If the tube is coiled in the back of the mouth or throat, withdraw it until it's straight and then resume insertion.

## DETERMINING THE LENGTH OF AN NG TUBE

To determine how long a nasogastric (NG) tube must be to reach the stomach, hold the end of the tube at the tip of the patient's nose. Extend the tube to the patient's earlobe and then down to the xiphoid process, as shown here.

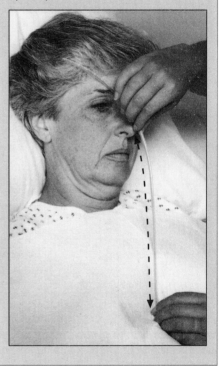

 **ALERT** If the patient is coughing, choking, or otherwise showing signs of respiratory distress, withdraw the tube until symptoms subside. Once the patient recovers, try again to pass the tube. If you can't pass the tube to the measured length, the tube is probably in the trachea. Pull back and try again.

➤ When the tube is inserted to the measured length, verify tube placement by one of these methods, as appropriate:

– Always use radiographic confirmation of tube placement before starting any feed-

## POSITIONING FOR NG TUBE PLACEMENT

Instruct the patient to hold her head straight and upright. Grasp the nasogastric (NG) tube with the end pointing downward, curve it if necessary, and carefully insert it into the nostril. Aim the tube downward and laterally toward the chosen nostril.

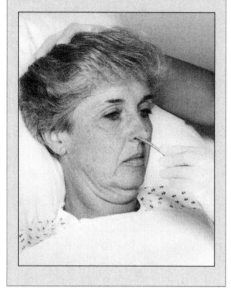

ings or medication administration, except in patients undergoing gastric lavage or in an emergency.

– Aspirate contents with a syringe. Gastric contents help determine tube placement.

– Using a stethoscope, listen over the edge of the epigastric area and inject 10 to 30 cc of air. You'll hear a "whoosh" sound if the tube has been placed correctly.

– Ask the patient to talk and hum. If the tube is in her stomach, she'll be able to talk freely.

➤ After you've confirmed placement, secure the tube with hypoallergenic tape.

➤ Apply benzoin or some type of skin preparation to the patient's face before taping.

➤ Use adhesive tape to secure the tube to the bridge of the patient's nose. (See *Securing the NG tube*.)

➤ Wrap an elastic band around the tube and pin it to the patient's gown, over her shoulder, to prevent her from inadvertently moving the tube.

### Inserting the tube via the mouth

➤ Place the tube over the patient's tongue instead of through the nasopharynx, if nasal insertion is contraindicated.

➤ Remove any dentures before inserting the tube.

➤ Ask the patient to lower her chin and open her mouth.

➤ Place the tip of the tube on the back of the patient's tongue, give her a cup of water, and tell her to swallow.

➤ Advance the tube as she swallows.

➤ Follow the steps above for advancing the tube.

### Removing the tube

➤ Explain the procedure to the patient. Inform her that she may experience discomfort and gagging with tube removal.

➤ Assess bowel sounds.

➤ Turn off the suction and disconnect the patient from it.

➤ Assist her into an upright position and drape a towel over her gown or clothing.

➤ Flush the NG tube with air to remove irritating stomach contents before removing the tube.

➤ Remove adhesive tape and unpin the tube from the patient's gown.

➤ Clamp the tube by folding it in half.

➤ Have her take a deep breath and hold it.

➤ Gently but quickly remove the tube to avoid complications, such as aspiration. Tell the patient she can breathe freely. Dispose of the tube appropriately.

➤ Provide tissues for the patient to blow her nose.

➤ Record tube removal, the patient's response, and the amount and characteristics of gastric contents.

## PATIENT TEACHING

➤ Caution the patient that she'll feel some discomfort from having the NG tube in her nose. Explain that this is common and that the discomfort will be alleviated when the tube is removed.

➤ Tell her to avoid food and drink for several hours after the tube is removed to avoid aspiration. (Some practitioners recommend following a soft, bland diet for 12 to 24 hours.)

➤ Urge her to report nausea, vomiting, abdominal distention, or increased pain occurring within 48 hours after tube removal.

## COMPLICATIONS

➤ *Epistaxis* can be minimized through gentle handling.

➤ *Pneumothorax* requires immediate evaluation and X-ray, possible chest tube placement, and referral to a physician or pulmonologist.

➤ *Aspiration leading to pneumonia* requires evaluation, including X-rays, antibiotics, and supportive therapy.

➤ *Perforation of the esophagus and creation of a false passage* requires referral to an ear, nose, and throat specialist.

➤ *Intracranial tube placement* has been documented with known head trauma and requires immediate referral to a neurosurgeon.

➤ *Tube displacement*, more common with long-term use, requires reevaluation of the patient's need for the tube. In most cases, another tube is inserted.

➤ *Necrosis of nasal mucosa or erosion of the esophagus or stomach* can occur with long-term placement. Because of this, softer tubes are indicated for long-term therapy.

## SECURING THE NG TUBE

To secure the nasogastric (NG) tube to the patient's nose, you'll need about 4" (10 cm) of 1" tape. Split one end of the tape up the center about 1½" (4 cm). Make tabs on the split ends. Stick the uncut tape end on the patient's nose so that the split in the tape starts about ½" to 1½" (1.5 to 4 cm) from the tip of her nose. Crisscross the tabbed ends around the tube. You may apply another piece of tape over the bridge of the nose to secure the tube.

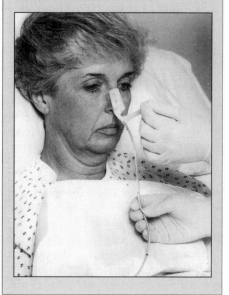

## SPECIAL CONSIDERATIONS

➤ The nose is the preferred route for temporary gastric tube insertion unless contraindicated by head injury or known nasal deformity.

➤ Be aware of respiratory changes during tube insertion. Cyanosis in an unconscious patient and coughing or choking in a conscious patient indicate that the tube may be in the trachea. Withdraw the tube immediately, and try to reinsert it when the patient has recovered.

➤ For the unconscious patient, tilt the head forward to close the epiglottis while inserting the tube. Be sure the patient has been evaluated and that she doesn't have a cervical spine injury. Advance the tube gently between respirations to avoid passage of the tube into the airway.

 **CULTURAL TIP** The Chinese consider it impolite to touch any part of the head. For this reason, explain the procedure and exactly what you'll be doing beforehand. Be sure to state that you intend to touch the patient before extending your hand toward her face. This is a good practice to use with all patients.

## DOCUMENTATION

➤ Review documentation by other health team members; then initial their notes to signify you're aware of their findings. This doesn't signify agreement with their comments or reduce your responsibility to complete your own history and physical examination. Document abnormal physical findings. (The preprocedural and postprocedural note must include an evaluation of neurologic, respiratory, and GI function.)
➤ Record indications for the procedure, the type and size of the NG tube used, and the patient's response to tube insertion.
➤ Document any known trauma during tube insertion. If the tube is attached to suction equipment, document the amount of suctioning and whether it is continuous or intermittent. Describe characteristics of aspirated secretions, such as color, amount, consistency, and odor.
➤ Record the date and time of tube insertion and removal and the patient's tolerance of the procedure.

# EMERGENCY PROCEDURE

## Gastric lavage

CPT CODE
*91105    Gastric intubation or lavage for treatment*

## DESCRIPTION

Gastric lavage flushes the stomach and removes ingested substances through a gastric lavage tube. It's performed after poisoning or a drug overdose, especially in a patient with central nervous system depression or an inadequate gag reflex.

A patient who presents with complaints of melena, hematemesis, or hematochezia must be evaluated with gastric lavage to help assess the extent of bleeding. Lavage also helps prepare the patient for endoscopy; however, it doesn't help stop the hemorrhage.

In cases of known or suspected toxic ingestion and overdose, the goal of GI lavage is to evacuate the stomach of the ingested substance and reduce the potentially life-threatening effects by limiting absorption of the poison. Gastric lavage is most effective when used within 1 hour and shouldn't be used if 4 hours have passed since ingestion. Lavage may be accompanied by administration of ipecac syrup or activated charcoal with a cathartic. Some practitioners argue that charcoal is more effective when used alone. However, it's still widely acceptable to follow lavage with charcoal unless either is contraindicated.

Insertion of a wide-bore nasogastric (NG) or orogastric tube with multiple openings at the distal end is essential for removing pill fragments and large blood clots, which may obstruct a smaller NG tube. The larger size is also preferred because it allows for higher flow rates during lavage. Wide-bore tubes should be inserted orally to promote patient comfort and limit trauma to the nasal passage. (See *Using wide-bore gastric tubes*.) In adults, it's recommended to lavage 3 L of fluid for gastric decontamination. In children, the recommendation is 15 ml/kg of body weight until gastric returns are clear.

A closed system (such as lavage with an Ewald tube) is an active system that uses rapid instillation and evacuation to generate a significant amount of turbulence, which effectively clears the stomach. This method is preferred for large-volume lavage in cases of poisoning and toxic overdose.

Open systems can be active or passive. The active system requires you to manually instill, agitate, and remove fluid using a syringe. The passive system uses gravity to drain the stomach after the gastric tube is in place.

## INDICATIONS

➤ To remove blood and enhance visualization of upper GI bleeding by endoscopy
➤ To flush the stomach after recent drug overdose or ingestion of a highly toxic substance when ipecac-induced emesis is either contraindicated or has failed
➤ To flush the stomach after ingestion of a substance that isn't well absorbed by activated charcoal (such as lithium, iron, lead, and alcohol)
➤ To treat severe hyperthermia

## CONTRAINDICATIONS

### Absolute
➤ Known ingestion of a nontoxic substance or an inconsequential amount of a toxic substance

### USING WIDE-BORE GASTRIC TUBES

If you need to deliver a large volume of fluid rapidly through a gastric tube (for example, when irrigating the stomach of a patient with profuse gastric bleeding or poisoning), a wide-bore gastric tube usually serves best. Typically inserted orally, these tubes remain in place only long enough to complete the lavage and evacuate stomach contents.

**Ewald tube**
In an emergency, using this single-lumen tube with several openings at the distal end allows you to aspirate large amounts of gastric contents quickly.

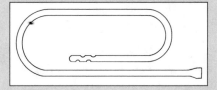

**Levacuator tube**
This tube has two lumens. Use the larger lumen for evacuating gastric contents; the smaller, for instilling an irrigant.

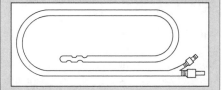

**Edlich tube**
This single-lumen tube has four openings near the closed distal tip. A funnel or syringe may be connected at the proximal end. Like the Ewald tube, the Edlich tube lets you withdraw large quantities of gastric contents quickly.

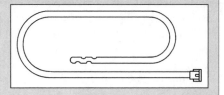

➤ Ingestion of caustic substances (such as corrosives and hydrocarbons) or sharp objects
➤ Conscious, alert patient who hasn't ingested a substance that will lead to rapid change in mental or physiologic status
➤ Comatose or obtunded patient without airway protection
➤ Ingestion of substance more than 4 hours before patient arrival
➤ Passage of NG tube in patients with known or suspected facial or skull fractures (permissible through oral passage)
➤ Known or suspected esophageal varices

### Relative

➤ Vagal stimulation with overdose of beta-adrenergic blockers (This may produce arrhythmias; administration of atropine before the procedure may help prevent bradycardia.)
➤ Recent abdominal surgery (This may place the patient at increased risk for GI hemorrhage or perforation.)
➤ Ingestion of caustic poisons (Tracheal intubation is recommended before gastric lavage.)

## EQUIPMENT

Wide-bore gastric tube (36F to 40F for adults; 24F to 28F for children under age 12) with multiple holes at distal end (closed kits include the Ewald or Levacuator tube set) or an irrigation kit for manual lavage (with 30- to 50-ml syringe) ◆ towel or pads ◆ intubation equipment (with cuffed endotracheal tube) ◆ activated charcoal for poison ingestion or overdose ◆ bite block ◆ tissues ◆ tongue blade ◆ emesis basin ◆ water-soluble gel (such as K-Y jelly) or 2% lidocaine gel ◆ benzocaine spray ◆ phenylephrine spray ◆ stethoscope ◆ soft limb restraints ◆ 200 to 250 ml of tap water for adults; 10 to 15 ml/kg of body weight normal saline solution for children ◆ suction setup ◆ adhesive tape ◆ eye protection ◆ face mask ◆ gown ◆ gloves

## ESSENTIAL STEPS

➤ Explain the procedure to the patient, when possible, to increase his cooperation and reduce anxiety. Review possible complications and alternative treatments, if available. Explain that he may feel some discomfort, such as gagging and tearing of the eyes.
➤ Agree on a signal for the patient to use when he wants to stop for a minute before continuing the procedure.
➤ Check the comatose or obtunded patient for presence of the gag reflex, using a tongue blade. For a patient with diminished reflexes, consider endotracheal intubation and mechanical ventilation because he may not be able to protect his airway.

 **ALERT** A cuffed endotracheal tube doesn't preclude aspiration. Monitor the patient for possible aspiration throughout the procedure and for 15 minutes after lavage.

➤ Place the patient in the left lateral decubitus position with the head elevated 20 degrees. This position decreases the passage of gastric content into the duodenum, preventing further absorption of ingested chemicals, and also helps prevent aspiration. If the patient is awake and somewhat alert, however, have the patient sit upright (high Fowler's position) with his head tilted forward during the procedure.
➤ Drape a towel or pad over the patient to protect his clothing or gown from spillage.
➤ Place tissues and an emesis basin within the patient's reach.
➤ Restrain the patient with soft wrist restraints only when absolutely necessary. Remember not to restrain the patient in a "spread eagle" position. This may prevent him from turning to the side and thus can place him at risk for aspiration.
➤ Provide privacy and maintain aseptic technique.

➤ Put on gloves, gown, face mask, and eye protection to avoid contact with body secretions.

➤ Estimate tube length by measuring the distance from the nose to the earlobe then to the middle of the epigastrium. Measuring before placement minimizes the risk of curling or kinking of extra tubing in the stomach.

### For NG tube placement

➤ Before inserting the tube, spray both nostrils with phenylephrine. (Although not the preferred method, nasal placement of an 18F or smaller tube has been used.)

➤ Check for deformity or obstruction of the nostrils. Ask the patient to hyperextend the head and observe each nostril by using a penlight or having the patient breathe in while occluding the other nostril. Select the most patent nostril for tube insertion.

➤ Lubricate the tube tip well for insertion with water-soluble gel or lidocaine gel. Lubricating the tube decreases mucosal irritation. Lidocaine gel can also be administered via a tube syringe and slowly instilled into the more patent nostril. Unlike a lipid-soluble lubricant, using a water-soluble lubricant decreases the risk of aspiration pneumonia if the tube enters the trachea.

 **ALERT** If the patient was involved in a trauma or was unconscious at any time, you must evaluate for cervical spine injury before hyperextending the head and neck.

➤ With the neck hyperextended, insert the tube into the selected nostril with its natural curve toward the patient and gently advance it toward the nasopharynx.

➤ Direct the tube along the floor of the nostril and toward the ear on that side. If resistance is met, withdraw, relubricate the tube, and insert it into the other nostril.

➤ As the tube enters the nasopharynx, instruct the patient to swallow. This helps to advance the tube.

➤ Advance the tube to the premeasured distance when the mark is at the nostril.

### For oral placement

➤ Spray the posterior pharynx with topical benzocaine.

➤ Introduce an airway protector or bite block to prevent the patient from biting down or chewing on the tube.

➤ Ask the patient to flex his head forward as much as possible (chin on chest) and open his mouth.

➤ Using a tongue blade over the base of the patient's tongue, insert the lubricated tube into the throat as the patient swallows. If he gags, advance the tube immediately after he stops gagging.

➤ When the tube reaches the oropharynx, you'll meet resistance. Ask the patient to keep his head forward and continue to pass the tube steadily. Encourage him to swallow to assist passing of the tube. (Tilting the head forward helps pass the tube through the esophagus rather than the larynx.)

➤ If the patient continues to gag, tell him to rest and take a few deep breaths. Be prepared to remove the tube immediately if vomiting occurs. Have a suction device available to assist the patient in clearing his mouth and airway.

➤ If the patient coughs, chokes, or otherwise shows signs of respiratory distress, withdraw the tube until symptoms subside. This may mean the tube is in the trachea. When the patient recovers, try to pass the tube again. If you can't pass the tube to the measured length, the tube is probably in the trachea. Partially withdraw the tube and try again.

➤ If the patient continues to gag and the tube doesn't advance with each swallow, withdraw it slightly and inspect the patient's mouth. If the tube is coiled in the back of his mouth or throat, withdraw it until straight and then continue inserting it.

➤ When the tube is inserted to the measured length and the mark is at the patient's lip, verify tube placement.

## To assess placement of NG or orogastric tube

➤ Gently aspirate the contents of the tube with a syringe. Return of gastric contents may occur spontaneously on tube insertion.

➤ Auscultate over the stomach while injecting 10 to 30 cc of air; you'll hear a "whoosh" sound if placement is correct.

➤ Ask the patient to talk and hum. If the tube is in the stomach, the patient will be able to talk freely.

➤ Secure the tube with adhesive tape to prevent migration.

➤ After securing the tube, aspirate stomach contents before instilling any fluid. If you're using a closed system, open the drainage port and allow stomach contents to empty by gravity. This helps confirm tube placement and reduces the risk of overfilling the stomach with irrigant and inducing vomiting or forcing toxic contents into the duodenum.

➤ Assess an unconscious patient for cyanosis before proceeding with lavage.

## For a closed system (Ewald)

➤ Be sure that clamps on both the infusion and drainage bags are closed. Fill the fluid bag with at least 3 L of tap water or normal saline solution and hang it from the I.V. pole. Attach the drainage bag to the lower side rail of the bed.

➤ Connect the lavage setup to the Ewald tube and open the drainage port. Drain gastric contents using gravity before initiating lavage. Close the drainage bag clamp.

➤ Begin gastric lavage by opening the inflow clamp and instilling 150 to 200 ml of fluid, with a minimum of 100 ml in children. Close the inflow clamp.

 **ALERT** Don't overfill the stomach. This may cause gastric distention and induce vomiting, which increases the risk of aspiration.

➤ Open the clamp to the drainage bag and begin to drain gastric contents. Assess for bleeding, blood clots, or pill fragments. Alternate installation and drainage until 3 L have been lavaged. In gastric decontamination, continue lavaging until clear to a maximum of 4 L if contents are not clear after 3 L.

## For an open system (active)

➤ Using a tube syringe, begin instilling tap water in small amounts (50 ml) up to 200 ml to assess the patient's tolerance. Instilling larger amounts may trigger vomiting and force toxic chemicals into the duodenum.

➤ Using the syringe, gently aspirate contents and empty into a calibrated container to determine whether the amount returned at least equals the amount instilled. Manual agitation of the stomach may help with retrieval of contents.

➤ Repeat this cycle until at least 3 L are instilled or return is clear. Lavage may return a small amount of clear fluid before it's actually complete. Repositioning the patient and the tube and massaging the epigastric area may help retrieve more pill fragments or blood clots even after lavage appears clear.

➤ When lavage is complete, administer a slurry of activated charcoal in a 20 to 150 ml bolus through the orogastric or NG tube. Then pinch or clamp the tube and remove it. Pinching the tube prevents the spillage of charcoal or gastric contents into the lungs.

➤ Keep the patient intubated for at least 15 minutes after the procedure to prevent aspiration if vomiting occurs.

## PATIENT TEACHING

➤ Caution the patient that he'll feel some discomfort from having the lavage tube in place. Explain that this is common and the discomfort will be alleviated when the tube is removed.

➤ Caution an alcoholic patient that bleeding can recur if he continues to use alcoholic beverages. Refer him for counseling and give him information on detoxification and rehabilitation programs.

➤ Teach the patient who has experienced poisoning or drug overdose about proper management of chemicals and poisons in the home and distribute poison control center information.

➤ Instruct the patient to contact his primary care provider if he experiences recurring bleeding, difficulty breathing or swallowing, melena, or a change in mental status.

## COMPLICATIONS

➤ *Pulmonary aspiration* requires evaluation and referral or collaboration with a physician or pulmonologist.

➤ *Inadequate removal of gastric contents and pill fragments* can be avoided by repositioning the tube and the patient before removing the tube.

➤ *Vomiting and aspiration* can be caused by overfilling the stomach. Instill only a small amount of water, and drain before beginning lavage again.

➤ *Fluid and electrolyte imbalance in children* can be prevented by using normal saline solution (not hypotonic solution).

➤ *Epistaxis* can be avoided by using orogastric intubation rather than an NG tube.

➤ *Mucosa damage* can be avoided by gentle suction or aspiration of stomach contents.

➤ *Esophageal rupture or perforation* requires immediate evaluation by an ear, nose, and throat specialist.

## SPECIAL CONSIDERATIONS

➤ Patients who have undergone gastric lavage will generally be admitted to the facility for observation. A patient with GI bleeding may be sent for endoscopy or surgery when lavage is complete.

➤ In the trauma patient with upper GI bleeding, obtain radiographic evidence to rule out a gastric or esophageal perforation before performing gastric lavage.

➤ Ipecac syrup continues to be useful at home in telephone management of poisoning of children if the offending agent is known and treatment can be initiated within 1 hour after ingestion. Consult a poison control center first. Follow ipecac syrup with water to increase the efficacy of gastric emptying.

– Dosing is as follows: Infants age 6 to 12 months, 10 ml followed by 5 to 15 ml/kg of water; children age 1 to 12, 15 ml followed by 4 to 6 oz of water; adolescents over age 12, 30 ml followed by 6 to 8 oz of water.

– Ipecac syrup is contraindicated in children less than age 6 months; patients who are already vomiting; those with altered mental status, inability to protect airway, or absent gag reflex; and those who have ingested a corrosive substance or sharp object.

➤ Activated charcoal absorbs most toxins (with the exception of lithium, iron, and toxic alcohols). Absorption of toxin in the GI tract prevents absorption into the systemic circulation and usually follows lavage if ingestion occurred within 2 hours. If more than 2 hours have elapsed since ingestion, activated charcoal is more likely to be administered before initiating lavage.

– Dosing is as follows: adults, 50 to 100 g; children, 1g/kg. If you aren't using a premixed solution, mix the charcoal with 4 to 8 parts of water. This is usually given as a single dose and may be combined with a cathartic, such as sorbitol (2ml/kg), to enhance gastric elimination of a toxic-laden charcoal.

– Multiple dosing may be used with ingestion of phenytoin (Dilantin), phenobarbital, carbamazepine (Tegretol), digoxin (Lanoxin), and theophylline (Theo-Dur). Cathartics should be given only with the first dose to prevent alterations in fluid and electrolyte balance.

– Complications associated with charcoal administration include nausea, vomiting, bowel obstruction, and pulmonary aspiration.

– Don't use charcoal in patients with decreased bowel sounds or an ileus. Charcoal is also contraindicated for acetaminophen overdose until the need for N-acetylcysteine (NAC) is determined. Charcoal interferes with the action of NAC and can delay necessary treatment if given first. If charcoal has already been given, either use lavage to remove it or increase the first dose of NAC.

➤ Poison control centers can help guide treatment based on the chemical ingested and the time of ingestion. These trained professionals can help professional staff and laypersons determine the most appropriate action. All medical facilities should post the number of their local poison control center.

➤ Provide social services contact information as needed. Most patients presenting to emergency departments are stabilized medically and then referred to a crisis response center. Further evaluation by a psychiatrist or psychologist will help determine appropriate follow-up care.

➤ Community education is vital to prevent and effectively treat accidental poisonings.

## DOCUMENTATION

➤ Review documentation by other health team members; then initial their notes to signify you're aware of their findings. This doesn't signify agreement with their comments or reduce your responsibility to complete your own history and physical examination. Document abnormal physical findings. (The preprocedural and postprocedural note must include GI, neurologic and respiratory findings.)

➤ Record the initial patient presentation, complaint, vital signs, and level of consciousness. Note the date and time of lavage and the size and type of tube used. Describe the gastric contents, the volume of fluid aspirated in returns, and the patient's tolerance of the procedure. Record drugs or medications given through the tube, the time the tube was removed, and the patient's response to the procedure. Document teaching and follow-up instructions given to the patient and family. Note whether a poison control center was contacted and, if so, the name of the person contacted.

# MUSCULOSKELETAL PROCEDURES 4

Musculoskeletal diseases and injuries rank first among conditions that alter a patient's quality of life. About 1 out of 7 persons in the United States suffers from some sort of musculoskeletal disorder and its resultant activity limitations, disability, or impaired function.

Disorders of the musculoskeletal system include systemic diseases (such as rheumatoid arthritis and systemic lupus erythematosus) and acute and chronic local conditions (such as strains, sprains, tendinitis, fractures, bursitis, and osteoarthritis).

Musculoskeletal defects rank first among workers' compensation and occupational injuries. Among all occupational injuries, lower back pain is the most common cause of temporary or permanent disability.

Estimates indicate that problems related to the musculoskeletal system rank second in the number of office visits. Although not usually fatal, these disorders can significantly affect quality of life because of associated changes in function, limited range of motion, and pain.

As a nurse practitioner, you must be able to diagnose and treat these disorders in the office or in an acute-care setting. The procedures outlined in this chapter will enhance the skills you need to manage these patients. Patient education should focus on care and management of the disorder, follow-up measures, and prevention of future injuries. When discussing ways to prevent reinjury, be sure to review proper exercise techniques, personal protective equipment, ergonomics, lifting techniques, and appropriate fitting of equipment. Finally, you'll need to make appropriate referrals to specialists when the patient's condition warrants it.

 **CULTURAL TIP** Various cultural groups respond to pain in various ways. For instance, Native Americans may complain of pain in general terms, such as "something doesn't feel right." Furthermore, if the patient reports pain but gets no pain relief, he's unlikely to repeat the complaint to the practitioner. Egyptians and Palestinians fear pain and cope better if the source of and prognosis for pain is understood. Other cultural groups, including Brazilians, Puerto Ricans, Cubans, Gypsies, Haitians, and Central Americans, freely express pain by moaning or crying. Still other groups, including Cambodians, Chinese, Japanese, Mexicans, Ethiopians, Russians, and Samoans, are very stoic in communicating pain and may require additional evaluation. Muslims may refuse narcotics for all but severe pain because narcotics are forbidden by their religion. Brazilians, Ethiopians, Iranians, and Haitians are less accustomed to the numerical pain scale and may describe pain qualitatively or only in general terms. Some cultural groups, particularly Asians, may use acupressure and acupuncture to treat pain or illness.

# DIAGNOSTIC TESTING

## Arthrocentesis

### CPT CODES

*20600   Arthrocentesis, aspiration, or injection of small joint or bursa (for example, fingers or toes)*
*20605   Arthrocentesis, intermediate joint or bursa (for example, temporomandibular; acromioclavicular; wrist, elbow, or ankle; or olecranon bursa)*
*20610   Arthrocentesis, major joint or bursa (for example, shoulder, hip, knee joint, or subacromial bursa)*

### DESCRIPTION

Arthrocentesis, a joint puncture, is used to collect fluid for analysis to identify the cause of pain and swelling and to relieve painful joints by draining effusions or instilling medication. When done correctly, it's a simple, safe procedure that causes few complications.

Joint fluid analysis allows differentiation of nontraumatic joint disease (septic joint or crystal-induced arthritis), ligamentous or bony injury (blood or fat globules, or both, in the joint), and hemarthrosis.

Often performed simultaneously with arthrocentesis, intra-articular corticosteroid injection can provide immediate relief from pain and swelling in the affected joint. Such injections typically provide only temporary symptomatic relief. The underlying cause of the problem still needs to be identified and treated. Corticosteroids used for injection include betamethasone, hydrocortisone, methylpredinosolone, and triamcinolone. No one corticosteroid has proven more effective than another in joint infection so medication is dependent on prescriber's preference, cost, and previous injection history. High corticosteroid doses and repeated injections cause serious local and systemic complications so judicious use of the procedure for purposes of corticosteroid administration is essential.

### INDICATIONS

➤ To analyze joint fluid
➤ To treat overuse injuries and rheumatoid arthritis
➤ To relieve painful, swollen joints

### CONTRAINDICATIONS

#### Absolute

➤ Bleeding diathesis
➤ History of fracture, joint surgery, osteoporosis, or sickle cell anemia
➤ Infection or broken skin present in the overlying area
➤ Sepsis
➤ Unavailability of emergency equipment

#### Relative

➤ Anticoagulant therapy
➤ Age (children or adolescents)
➤ Diabetes
➤ Lack of response to previous injections
➤ Prosthetic joints
➤ Recent joint injury (unless infection must be ruled out)

### EQUIPMENT

Povidone-iodine and alcohol sponges ◆ sterile gloves ◆ sterile drapes ◆ 1% or 2% lidocaine solution without epinephrine or vasocoolant spray ◆ sterile syringes (3, 5, 10, 20, or 30 ml [up to 50 ml for larger joints]) ◆ 25G ⅝" needle ◆ 18G, 20G, or 22G needles ◆ hemostat ◆ sterile 4" × 4" gauze pads ◆ appropriate laboratory collection tubes ◆ corticosteroid

## ESSENTIAL STEPS

➤ Explain the procedure to the patient, obtain informed consent, check for allergies, and gather equipment before starting. Place the patient in a comfortable position that allows you to easily access the involved joint, and tell him to slightly flex the joint to be aspirated. Carefully identify landmarks and mark the exact injection site by indenting the skin with the blunt end of a ballpoint pen or a deeply embedded fingernail. Such a marking won't readily wash away. (See *Choosing an intra-articular injection site*.)

➤ Prepare the area using 4" × 4" gauze pads and povidone-iodine solution and let it dry; repeat this three times. Just before injecting, wipe the area with an alcohol sponge. Povidone-iodine solution in the joint can cause a local inflammatory response.

➤ Put on gloves.

➤ Using sterile technique, drape the area and anesthetize it with vasocoolant spray. If appropriate, use the 25G ⅝" needle to infiltrate the subcutaneous skin with the lidocaine solution. Lidocaine may distort landmarks in smaller joints, making aspiration more difficult.

➤ After applying a local anesthetic, quickly insert the needle through the skin to minimize patient discomfort. Avoid moving the needle from side to side as it enters the joint. For smaller joints, use a 22G needle with a 3- to 5-ml syringe. For larger joints, use an 18G needle and as many large syringes as necessary.

➤ Aspirate as the needle advances into the joint space or bursal sac until fluid flows freely. Continue aspirating fluid until the joint is empty.

➤ To change syringes for continued aspiration or for joint injection, use the two-

## CHOOSING AN INTRA-ARTICULAR INJECTION SITE

To avoid injury to adjacent structures during intra-articular injection, you need to identify an appropriate injection site at the target joint. Appropriate sites for finger (A) and toe (B) joints include lateral, medial, or dorsal aspect of the joint.

Before puncturing the joint, flex it slightly to open the joint space. Then direct the needle to enter just medial or lateral to the extensor tendon. Avoid deep lateral or medial penetration of the joint to avoid damaging the nerves or blood vessels.

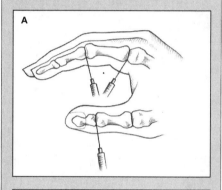

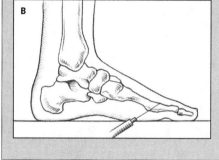

syringe technique. (See *Using the two-syringe technique*, page 158.) Attach the hemostat at the needle hub and stabilize the needle while removing the first syringe (to prevent needle rotation while detaching or attaching a syringe). When you've finished collecting fluid, remove the first sy-

## USING THE TWO-SYRINGE TECHNIQUE

When you're performing joint injection with arthrocentesis, the two-syringe technique can prove valuable. Insert a syringe into the joint and aspirate joint fluid (top illustration). Then attach a hemostat at the needle hub and stabilize the needle while removing the syringe (middle illustration). Replace the syringe containing the joint aspirate with a second syringe containing a corticosteroid (bottom illustration), and inject the drug into the joint space. When the injection is finished, remove the needle and apply pressure and a sterile dressing.

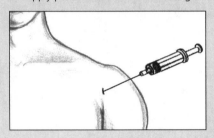

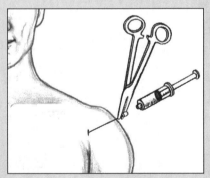

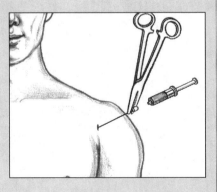

ringe, replace it with the second syringe that contains the medication, and inject into the joint space.

➤ Place the fluid in the appropriate laboratory tubes and send them for analysis. (See *Understanding synovial fluid analysis*.)

➤ When you've finished, remove the needle and apply pressure and a sterile dressing.

➤ As appropriate, perform passive range-of-motion exercises on the joint to help distribute the corticosteroid throughout the joint space.

➤ Immobilize the joint and provide adequate analgesia to control pain.

## PATIENT TEACHING

➤ Explain to the patient that arthrocentesis is typically performed in an office or emergency department and that he can go home after the procedure. Reassure him that pain is minimal once the procedure is completed. Pain relief may be immediate because of decreased fluid pressure or may occur 12 hours later with steroid injection.

➤ Tell him to apply ice, compress the area with an elastic wrap, and elevate the joint to reduce swelling and pain.

➤ Remind him to take acetaminophen and anti-inflammatory analgesics as prescribed.

➤ Instruct him to rest and immobilize the joint for 24 hours after treatment. Tell him that he can remove the dressing and elastic bandage 24 hours after the procedure. An immobilization device and crutches may encourage him to avoid overuse and weight-bearing activities on the affected joint.

➤ Instruct him to return for a follow-up visit within 1 week.

 **ALERT** Urge the patient to report signs of infection (increasing redness, swelling, pain, and warmth; unusual drainage; opening of wound; foul odor; red streak from wound area; or fever)

## UNDERSTANDING SYNOVIAL FLUID ANALYSIS

Analysis of synovial fluid helps identify the underlying cause of pain and swelling in a joint. This chart outlines various tests conducted on synovial fluid, common observations or results of those tests, and what each observation or result indicates.

| TEST | OBSERVATIONS | INDICATIONS |
|---|---|---|
| Color and clarity | ➤ Clear (straw-colored) | ➤ Normal finding or degenerative joint disease |
| | ➤ Cloudy | ➤ Inflammation |
| | ➤ Purulent | ➤ Infection |
| | ➤ Bloody | ➤ Traumatic injury |
| Mucin clot test for viscosity | ➤ Good mucin clot | ➤ Normal |
| | ➤ Denatured mucin | ➤ Inflammation |
| Gram stain | ➤ Positive | ➤ Septic arthritis |
| White blood cell count | ➤ 2,000 to 50,000 cells/μl | ➤ Inflammation |
| | ➤ More than 50,000 cells/μl | ➤ Septic joint |
| Glucose level | ➤ Decreased | ➤ Inflammation |
| Microscopy | ➤ Strong negative birefringence (quality of transmitting light unequally in different directions) with needle-shaped crystals (monosodium urate) | ➤ Gout |
| | ➤ Weakly positive birefringence with box-shaped crystals (calcium pyrophosphate dihydrate crystals) | ➤ Pseudogout |
| Culture | ➤ Positive culture | ➤ Infection |

and warmth or increased pain and stiffness within the joint.

## COMPLICATIONS

➤ *Infection,* the most serious complication, may occur if aseptic technique isn't followed or if the needle passes through an infected area. The patient shouldn't receive a corticosteroid injection if you suspect infection. Repeated intra-articular corticosteroid injections also can result in necrosis of the joint space and the juxta-articular bone, with subsequent joint destruction and instability. Other complications include *tendon rupture, local soft-tissue atrophy, hemarthrosis, and transient nerve palsy.* High-dose or repeated corticosteroid injections might have long-term systemic effects.

➤ *Trauma to the joint* may produce hemarthrosis (bleeding into the joint). Arthrocentesis can help identify this condition, but it can also cause it (rarely) in a patient with a bleeding disorder such as hemophilia. A small amount of blood-tinged fluid may result when the joint has been emptied. Grossly bloody arthrocentesis requires further investigation.

➤ *Improper needle placement or obstruction of the needle lumen or misdiagnosis* may result in failed arthrocentesis, or dry tap. If a needle is improperly placed, try repositioning it without removing it from the joint. If this doesn't help, you will need to insert the needle in another site. If debris or anatomic structures obstruct the needle lumen, limiting access to fluid try adjusting the position of the needle or injecting a small amount of the synovial fluid back into the joint to dislodge the obstructing material. Purulent fluid from an infected joint may be too thick to pass through the lumen, requiring the use of a large-lumen needle. Misdiagnosis of an effusion can occur when a chronically inflamed joint undergoes fat replacement and appears distended.

➤ An *allergic reaction* may result from the local anesthetic; a complete history can reduce this risk.

➤ Fluid may recollect in the joint space (arthrocentesis can only provide temporary relief for an acute condition); identification and treatment of the underlying condition can reduce flare-ups.

➤ *Corticosteroid arthropathy*, a condition in which relief from symptoms results in the patient's overuse of the joint, can cause further injury.

## SPECIAL CONSIDERATIONS

➤ Drain the joint completely. If the flow stops, the joint may be empty or the needle lumen obstructed. To ensure the joint is empty, retract the needle slightly, decrease the pressure applied for aspiration and, if you suspect obstruction, reinject a small amount of fluid into the joint to remove obstruction from the needle lumen itself.

➤ The patient shouldn't receive corticosteroid injections more than three times a year; more frequent injections may cause cartilage damage, systemic effects, and avascular necrosis.

➤ When performing arthrocentesis for culture and sensitivity studies, make sure you don't introduce lidocaine into the joint space because it kills bacteria, possibly altering test results. Change needles between lidocaine injection and joint penetration.

➤ If the patient may have gouty arthritis, examine the fluid for crystals under polarized light.

➤ The presence of fat cells in joint fluid indicates a fracture.

➤ For corticosteroid injection, avoid direct contact with the skin or subcutaneous tissue to prevent skin atrophy. For an intrabursal injection, inject the corticosteroid around — not into — the tendon or ligament. Because direct injection can lead to tendon or ligament rupture, reposition the needle if it meets resistance.

## DOCUMENTATION

➤ Before performing this procedure, document any abnormal physical findings on the consent form and have the patient initial the comments as well as sign the form to signify acknowledgment of preprocedural abnormalities. In the chart, the preprocedural and postprocedural note must include an evaluation of function, range of motion, and neurosensory testing, such as two-point discrimination.

➤ Provide a detailed description of the site before and after the procedure, name of the anesthetic used and dosage administered, the appearance and amount of fluid removed, whether a culture was sent, the patient's reaction to the procedure, medications ordered, time frame for follow-up evaluation, and instructions given to the patient.

# Compartment syndrome pressure testing

## CPT CODE
*20950   Monitoring of interstitial fluid pressure in defection of muscle compartment syndrome*

## DESCRIPTION

Compartment syndrome occurs when pressure within a muscle compartment increases to a level that impairs blood supply to the nerve and muscle tissue. Acute compartment syndrome can occur in various areas of the body, but it occurs in a lower extremity about 80% of the time.

There are two types of compartment syndrome: acute compartment syndrome (ACS) and exertional compartment syndrome (ECS). (See *Comparing acute and exertional compartment syndromes,* page 162.) ACS may result from various internal and external factors but is usually related to trauma. ECS is an overuse injury of the lower extremity characterized by intermittent episodes of increased compartment pressure sufficient to cause ischemic pain and impaired neuromuscular function of the extremity. (See *Potential causes of compartment syndrome,* page 163.)

Compartmental pressures have been tested using various techniques. The more recently developed hand-held fluid pressure monitor is as accurate as the conventional method (which uses a sphygmomanometer, tubing, and a bag of normal saline solution), while having the advantages of greater convenience, versatility, sterility, portability, easy and rapid assembly, and use by a single clinician. Sterile disposable components prevent cross-contamination and allow for repeated use of the transducer, thus decreasing costs. Single measurements using a side-port needle are more often performed for ACS. Continuous monitoring can be done using a slit catheter with a breakaway 14G needle and taping the device to the patient's leg.

## INDICATIONS

➤ To confirm diagnosis of suspected ACS
➤ To diagnose ECS and monitor the effectiveness of treatment
➤ To permit ongoing monitoring of injuries associated with an increased risk of developing ACS

## CONTRAINDICATIONS

### Absolute
➤ Infected tissues

## EQUIPMENT

Intracompartmental pressure monitor system (such as Stryker) ◆ sterile, disposable components: side-ported, noncoring, 18G needle 2½" long; indwelling slit catheter with breakaway needle; diaphragm chamber; luer-lock syringe prefilled with 3 ml normal saline solution; povidone-iodine swabs; 1% lidocaine; needle and syringe; I.V. extension tubing; film dressing (such as Opsite), tape, or nonadhesive elastic wrap (such as Coban)

## ESSENTIAL STEPS

➤ Obtain a detailed history and physical examination, checking for the five "P's" associated with compartment syndrome. Of the five (pain, paresthesia, paresis, pulselessness, and pressure), pain with passive stretching of the affected muscles is the most sensitive diagnostic test finding. Pressure within the tissues is often felt as a hardness to touch but may not be evident in the early stages.

## COMPARING ACUTE AND EXERTIONAL COMPARTMENT SYNDROMES

The chart below compares characteristics of acute compartment syndrome (ACS) and exertional compartment syndrome (ECS).

| CHARACTERISTIC | ACS | ECS |
|---|---|---|
| **Incidence** | ➤ Infrequent<br>➤ Any age | ➤ More common<br>➤ Mostly in young, well-conditioned athletes or others who begin exercising very strenuously |
| **Site** | ➤ Any space enclosed<br>➤ Fascia<br>➤ Most common sites: Anterior compartment of lower leg and volar compartment of forearm<br>➤ Unilateral | ➤ Lower extremities: Anterior and lateral compartments most commonly involved<br><br>➤ Frequently bilateral |
| **Onset of symptoms** | ➤ 3 to 64 hours after injury<br>➤ Rapid progression | ➤ Weeks to months<br>➤ Progresses more slowly |
| **Pain** | ➤ Deep, burning, intractable<br>➤ Progressive<br>➤ Intensity disproportionate to degree of injury<br>➤ Occurs with passive stretch of muscles of involved compartment | ➤ Deep aching<br>➤ Intermittent<br>➤ Induced by intense exercise<br><br>➤ Sustained postexercise intra-compartmental pressure that slowly resolves when extremity at rest |
| **Paresthesia** | ➤ Loss of vibratory sensation and two-point discrimination | ➤ Transitory loss of or decrease in sensation |
| **Paralysis** | ➤ Inability to voluntarily contract involved muscle | ➤ Weakness of involved muscles |

➤ Explain the procedure to the patient, and obtain informed consent.

➤ Test all potentially affected muscular compartments (muscle groups encased in fibrous tissue called fascia).

➤ Assist the patient to a position in which the extremity is in the same plane as the heart.

➤ Prepare the skin at the puncture site by scrubbing in a circular motion from the site outward with povidone-iodine swabs.

➤ Open sterile components.

➤ Turn the unit on (the pressure display frame should read between 0 and 9 mm Hg).

➤ Place the needle on the tapered stem of the chamber. (See *Assembling an intra-compartmental pressure monitor,* page 164.) Use the indwelling slit catheter with breakaway needle and extension tubing for continuous or frequent testing.

 **ALERT** Don't push the catheter beyond the tip of the needle; the sharp needle tip may damage the tip of the catheter during insertion.

➤ Inject the saline to purge the system of air. Don't allow the saline to run back down the needle into the transducer well.

➤ Inject a small amount of local anesthetic under the patient's skin at the planned puncture site.

➤ Hold the unit at the same level or intended insertion site and press the "zero" button. The catheter tip must be at the same height as the diaphragm chamber. The display frame must read "00."

➤ Insert the needle (or needle with catheter) into the desired muscle compartment. Push the catheter (if used) forward while withdrawing the needle.

➤ Tape the catheter in place, remove the breakaway needle, and apply the film dressing.

➤ Hold the monitor with the chamber at the same height as the tip of the catheter in the body.

➤ Slowly inject 0.1 to 0.2 ml of saline into the compartment.

➤ Wait for the system to reach equilibrium (when the numbers stop fluctuating) and read the pressure in the display frame after it stabilizes.

➤ Press the "zero" button each time to reset the device to read "00."

➤ For continuous use, attach the monitor with tape or nonadhesive elastic wrap so the chamber in the monitor is at the same height as the slit tip of the catheter in the body.

### Testing for ECS

➤ Perform this test before the patient exercises and at 1 and 5 minutes after exercise.

➤ Ensure that the exercise is sufficiently intense to reproduce the patient's symptoms (for example, use of a treadmill or repeated dorsiflexion and plantar flexion against resistance).

➤ Ensure that the patient's ankle is always held in the same degree of dorsiflexion during testing. The degree of ankle flexion affects compartment pressure.

## POTENTIAL CAUSES OF COMPARTMENT SYNDROME

Although most commonly a complication of trauma, compartment syndrome can result from various physiologic disruptions, such as those listed here.
➤ Fractures
➤ Blunt trauma
➤ Overuse injuries of the muscle
  – Exercise
  – Seizures
  – Tetany
➤ Muscle hypertrophy due to anabolic steroid abuse
➤ Burns
➤ Snakebite, insect bite, or frostbite
➤ Vascular and bleeding disorders
  – Hemophilia
  – Hematoma
  – Venous occlusion
  – Coagulation disorders and anticoagulant therapy
  – Deep venous thrombi
  – Major vascular injury
  – Cardiac catheterization
  – I.V. infiltration
➤ Orthopedic surgery
➤ Excessive traction on fractured limbs
➤ Baker's cyst
➤ Prolonged external pressure on a limb
  – Constrictive casts, splints, or dressings
  – Surgical positioning (lithotomy)
  – Pressure on head or torso in an unconscious patient

➤ Use the same test procedure outlined above. If possible, use an indwelling catheter to avoid repeated needle insertions, pain, and risk of infection.

➤ Resting pressures above 15 mm Hg and 5-minute postexercise pressures above 20 mm Hg are diagnostic for ECS.

## PATIENT TEACHING

➤ Explain to the patient that test results will determine the need for emergency fasciotomy. If he has ACS, tell him that fail-

## ASSEMBLING AN INTRACOMPARTMENTAL PRESSURE MONITOR

An intracompartmental pressure monitor kit comes with a disposable syringe filled with 3 ml of normal saline solution and a sterile needle. To use the monitor, first verify that batteries are fresh. Then assemble the syringe, needle, and monitor as shown below. Now turn the monitor on and press the syringe until a drop of saline solution exudes from the needle tip to prime the unit and ensure an accurate pressure measurement. Press the "zero" button to clear the unit.

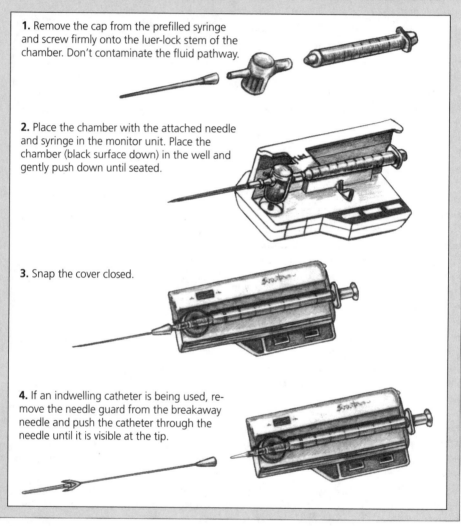

**1.** Remove the cap from the prefilled syringe and screw firmly onto the luer-lock stem of the chamber. Don't contaminate the fluid pathway.

**2.** Place the chamber with the attached needle and syringe in the monitor unit. Place the chamber (black surface down) in the well and gently push down until seated.

**3.** Snap the cover closed.

**4.** If an indwelling catheter is being used, remove the needle guard from the breakaway needle and push the catheter through the needle until it is visible at the tip.

ure to treat it in a timely fashion may result in permanent deformity and disability.

➤ Reassure the patient with ECS that the condition is rarely associated with permanent disability and that it can usually be managed conservatively with rest, ice, compression, and elevation. Note, however, that fasciotomy may be required if the patient's response to conservative treatment is inadequate.

➤ Advise him to decrease the intensity of his exercise and to stop exercising entirely if he experiences pain.

➤ Instruct him not to elevate the extremity above the level of the heart; doing so may decrease arterial pressure and tissue perfusion.

➤ Tell him to contact you if he experiences swelling, weakness, or a change in sensation in the extremity or if he feels unusual pain in the extremity after trauma or exercise.

## COMPLICATIONS

➤ *Local infection* is treated topically if limited to superficial dermal layers. More extensive infection requires systemic antibiotics.

➤ *Injury to adjacent blood vessels, nerves, or tendons* requires referral to an orthopedist, a neurologist, or a neurosurgeon.

## SPECIAL CONSIDERATIONS

➤ A large volume of subcutaneous fat may make it difficult to access the deep posterior compartment, thereby increasing the risk of infection and injury to adjacent structures.

 **CULTURAL TIP** Evaluating the patient's pain level can be difficult. Patients from Asian cultures, for instance, don't like to call attention to themselves and tend to downplay pain or silently withstand it; as a result, they may delay seeking treatment, especially for ECS. Patients of Mediterranean cultures may be more vocal about their pain. In some African cultures, the significant other may vocalize or demonstrate their partner's pain.

➤ Referrals to a sports medicine facility may be indicated because use of a personal trainer to develop gradual and progressive individual training or exercise program may be helpful.

➤ Loss of sensation in the web space between the hallux and second toe suggests involvement of the anterior compartment; over the dorsum of the foot, the lateral compartment; on the lateral side of the foot, the posterior superficial compartment; and on the sole, the deep posterior compartment.

➤ Rapid diagnosis of ACS and appropriate treatment are essential. Tissue necrosis with permanent disability can develop within as little as 4 to 8 hours. (See *Timetable for pathologic tissue changes*, page 166.)

➤ The critical symptoms of ACS are pain, paresthesia, and paralysis. Pain occurs with passive stretching of the muscles of the involved compartment; full extension of the fingers will stretch muscles of the forearm and plantar flexion of the toes will stretch muscles of the lower leg. The inability to actively contract the involved muscles indicates paralysis. Loss of vibratory sensation or two-point discrimination is an early sign of paresthesia. Swelling and palpable tenseness of the involved part of the limb are important diagnostic signs in unconscious patients. Pulse deficits indicate vascular injury, not compartment syndrome. However, vascular trauma and ACS may occur concomitantly. Pallor, temperature, delayed capillary refill, and absence of distal pulses are late and ominous signs for both trauma and ACS.

➤ A compartment pressure of up to 10 mm Hg is considered normal. Tissue necrosis can begin at levels of 30 mm Hg. Thus, the generally accepted critical pressure is 30 mm Hg for intervening (such as referring for an emergency fasciotomy). Other practitioners maintain that the arterial-compartmental pressure difference should be considered as well.

➤ Complications of inadequately treated ACS are permanent deformity (Volkmann's contracture), decreased sensation and disability of the affected extremity, infection, gangrene, rhabdomyolysis, hyperkalemia, metabolic acidosis, myoglobinuria, and re-

## TIMETABLE FOR PATHOLOGIC TISSUE CHANGES

In acute compartment syndrome, pathologic tissue changes due to ischemia occur and progress rapidly.

| TIME | PATHOLOGIC CHANGES |
|---|---|
| 30 minutes | ➤ Nerve changes: paresthesia, anesthesia, hypoesthesia |
| 2 to 4 hours | ➤ Impaired motor strength |
| 3 hours | ➤ Disruption of capillary integrity with resultant swelling |
| 4 hours | ➤ Myoglobinuria due to muscle necrosis<br>➤ Hyperkalemia as damaged muscles release potassium<br>➤ Renal failure caused by myoglobin retention and hyperkalemia |
| 4 to 12 hours | ➤ Irreversible muscle deterioration |
| After 12 hours | ➤ Formation of muscle contracture |

nal failure. The potential for irreversible damage depends on the level of intra-compartmental pressure reached and the duration of pressure elevation.

## DOCUMENTATION

➤ Review recent or pertinent documentation by other health team members; then initial their notes to signify you're aware of their findings. This doesn't signify agreement with their comments or reduce your responsibility to complete your own history and physical examination.

➤ Before performing this procedure, document abnormal physical findings on the consent form and have the patient initial the comments as well as sign the form to signify acknowledgment of preprocedural abnormalities. In the chart, the preprocedural and postprocedural note must list clinical examination findings, including the presence of other injuries; pain response to passive range of motion; ability to actively contract involved muscle groups; response to two-point discrimination, vi-

bration, or light touch; presence or absence and quality of pulses; capillary refill time; degree of visible and palpable swelling; and skin color and temperature.

➤ Record the patient's history, including mechanism of injury, chronic diseases, current medications, and surgeries. Document the patient's description of pain (degree, location, precipitating and alleviating factors), complaints of paresthesia, loss of function of extremity, and decreasing skin temperature or swelling.

➤ Document that informed consent was obtained before the procedure and indicate the patient's level of understanding. Include language barriers and use of an interpreter when indicated.

➤ Record consultations (if any), preparation of the patient and equipment, the procedure itself (including compartments tested), and test results. Also document any referrals, transports, or follow-up visits resulting from the test.

# Lumbar puncture

CPT CODE
*62270   Spinal puncture, lumbar, for diagnostic purposes*

## DESCRIPTION

Lumbar puncture involves the insertion of a sterile needle into the subarachnoid space of the spinal canal, usually between the third and fourth lumbar vertebrae. This procedure is used to detect increased intracranial pressure (ICP) or the presence of blood in cerebrospinal fluid (CSF), to obtain CSF specimens for laboratory analysis, and to inject dyes or gases for contrast in radiologic studies. It's also used to administer drugs or anesthetics and to relieve ICP by removing CSF.

Before performing a lumbar puncture in a patient with papilledema and focal neurologic deficits, computerized tomography (CT) or magnetic resonance imaging (MRI) must be performed first to help rule out a mass, an abscess, or a lesion. Performing lumbar puncture in the presence of any of these conditions could worsen the patient's neurologic condition or precipitate herniation.

## INDICATIONS

➤ To rule out suspected meningitis or encephalitis (Any patient presenting with fever and altered mental status, severe headache, or nuchal rigidity should undergo a lumbar puncture to rule out these potentially life-threatening infections.)
➤ To screen a fever of unknown origin in immunocompromised patients and in neonates under 8 weeks
➤ To identify suspected subarachnoid hemorrhage with negative CT scan

➤ To diagnose certain neurologic disorders, such as multiple sclerosis, Guillain-Barré syndrome, or tertiary syphilis

## CONTRAINDICATIONS

### Absolute
➤ Cellulitis or evidence of infection over proposed injection site
➤ Known supratentorial mass or lesion

### Relative
➤ Coagulopathy or blood dyscrasia

## EQUIPMENT

Two pairs of sterile gloves ◆ sterile gown ◆ mask ◆ spinal needles, 20G and 22G ◆ manometer ◆ three-way stopcock ◆ sterile fenestrated drapes ◆ 1% lidocaine without epinephrine in a 5-ml syringe with a 22G ⅝″ needle and a 25G 1½″ needle ◆ betadine or povidone-iodine ◆ sterile gauze pads (4″ × 4″) ◆ adhesive bandage ◆ sterile collection tubes

Disposable lumbar puncture trays contain most of the sterile equipment needed.

## PREPARATION OF EQUIPMENT

➤ Assemble all equipment at the bedside.
➤ Wash hands thoroughly.
➤ Prepare the equipment or open the disposable lumbar puncture tray, being careful to maintain the sterile field.

## ESSENTIAL STEPS

➤ Explain the procedure to the patient to promote his cooperation and reduce his anxiety. Review possible complications. Discuss the possibility of discomfort during lidocaine administration as the needle is introduced into the subarachnoid space. Stress the importance of remaining still during the procedure.

➤ Obtain written consent from the patient, if he's oriented to person, place, and time. (When a patient's mental status deteriorates and no family member is available, consent may be implied. Be sure to document steps taken to procure consent and indications necessitating the procedure if consent is not obtained.)
➤ Place the patient in either the lateral decubitus or sitting position as desired.
– For the lateral decubitus position, instruct the patient to lie down on the edge of the bed with his back to you. Place him in the knee-chest position, with the knees and hips flexed maximally. Flex his head and shoulders downward as much as possible. Rest his head on a pillow to maintain shoulder and pelvis alignment, parallel to the bed.
– For the sitting position, instruct the patient to sit down and flex his head and arms over a bedside table.
➤ Put on sterile gloves and gown and the mask.
➤ Prepare the puncture site with sterile gauze pads soaked in betadine or povidone-iodine, moving in a circular motion outward from the proposed puncture site.
➤ Drape the area with the fenestrated drape to provide a sterile field.
➤ Remove gloves and put on another pair of sterile gloves to avoid introducing povidone-iodine into the subarachnoid space with the lumbar puncture needle.
➤ Locate the insertion site (L4-L5 interspace).
➤ Palpate the posterior aspect of the iliac crest bilaterally and palpate the L4 spinous process. The L3-L4 interspace should fall along a line connecting the two iliac crests. Use either this interspace or the one below it. Mark the spot with a deeply embedded fingernail.
➤ Anesthetize the skin and subcutaneous tissue with the 1% lidocaine, using the 25G needle. Change to a 22G needle before anesthetizing between the spinous process.

➤ Insert the spinal needle in the midline of the interspace, with the needle parallel to the floor and the point directed toward the patient's umbilicus. Maintain midline alignment. If the patient experiences a tingling or an electric shock down one of the extremities, the needle may have migrated from a midline position. If this occurs, remove the needle as far as the subcutaneous tissue and redirect it.
➤ Advance the needle very slowly about ¾" (2 cm) or until you hear a "pop" (piercing a membrane of the dura). Then withdraw the stylet with every 1- to 2-mm advance of the needle to check for CSF return. If the needle meets the bone or if blood returns, withdraw to the skin and redirect the needle. Bloody return indicates that the needle has entered the venous plexus in the anterior spinal wall. If you can't obtain CSF, don't aspirate. The nerve root may be trapped against the needle, and forceful aspiration will cause injury. Instead, try performing the procedure one disk space below.
➤ As CSF begins to flow from the needle, discard the first few drops.
➤ Attach the stopcock and manometer to the hub of the needle and record the CSF pressure (normal pressure: supine, 80 to 150 mm $H_2O$; sitting, 80 to 120 mm $H_2O$). Allow the patient to relax and check for good respiratory variation of the fluid level in the manometer to ensure that the needle is properly positioned.
➤ Remove the manometer and allow 2 to 3 ml of CSF to flow into each of the sterile tubes. Collection tubes should be filled as follows:
– 2 to 3 ml for cell count and differential
– 2 to 3 ml for glucose and protein
– 2 to 3 ml for culture and sensitivity and Gram stain
– 2 to 3 ml for viral titer or cultures, India ink preparation, cryptococcus antigen, Venereal Disease Research Laboratory test, or cytology.

➤ After the tubes are collected, remove the needle. (See "Special considerations" later in this entry for information on the controversy over replacing the stylet before removing the needle.)

➤ Place an adhesive bandage and apply slight pressure over the area. Tell the patient to lie in bed for 1 to 2 hours after the procedure.

## PATIENT TEACHING

➤ Emphasize the importance of maintaining a flexed position throughout the procedure (see *Preparing for a lumbar puncture*, page 170).

➤ Reassure the patient that discomfort should ease immediately after the procedure ends.

➤ Instruct him to lie supine for 2 hours.

➤ Instruct him to notify you and return to the clinic if he experiences severe headache, nausea, vomiting, or signs of infection at the injection site (erythema, increased warmth, fever, swelling, or purulent drainage).

➤ Tell him to contact you about any additional symptoms that concern him.

## COMPLICATIONS

➤ *Spinal headache* following the procedure is the most common complication. Usually this is a frontal headache that can be quite severe. Using a small-gauge spinal needle and having the patient lie flat for several hours after the procedure can minimize headache incidence. Administration of fluids and a mild analgesic also may help.

➤ *CSF leakage* is suspected if the patient returns within 36 hours after the procedure with complaints of headache. This can be managed with an epidural blood patch placed by an anesthesiologist.

➤ *Infection* can be minimized by preparing the skin with an antiseptic solution and observing strict sterile technique.

➤ *Herniation of the spinal cord and brain stem* are more serious complications that require immediate referral to a neurosurgeon.

## SPECIAL CONSIDERATIONS

➤ Normal CSF is clear and colorless. Any changes in color or consistency must be investigated. Yellow or cloudy fluid indicates an increased concentration of cells in the fluid, signifying infection, jaundice, or increased protein. When bacterial meningitis or encephalitis is suspected, initiate antibiotic therapy as soon as possible. Delaying treatment to wait for the procedure to be performed or results to become available can be more detrimental to the patient.

➤ Bloody cerebrospinal fluid on lumbar puncture has several indications. In the event of a traumatic tap, fluid will be bloody initially and gradually clear. If a subarachnoid hemorrhage is present, fluid will remain uniformly bloody throughout collection. Lumbar puncture can precipitate rebleeding and should be used cautiously with subarachnoid hemorrhage.

➤ CT or MRI should be the first-line diagnostic tools used to evaluate patients who are potential candidates for lumbar puncture. Lumbar puncture should be performed only if these tests are negative and symptoms persist.

➤ Controversy exists over whether the stylet should be reinserted before the needle is removed to prevent headache after the procedure. According to one theory, a piece of the arachnoid tissue enters the needle during outflow of CSF. If the needle is removed without reinserting the stylet, this strand may thread back into the dura, creating a CSF leak, which is known to cause headache. By reinserting the stylet,

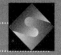

## DEAR PATIENT:

The practitioner has scheduled you for a lumbar puncture. This test is sometimes called a spinal tap because a small amount of fluid is removed from your spine. The cells in the fluid are studied to identify any problems.

Lumbar puncture takes about 15 minutes. Here is what you'll need to do during the test.

**1** Lie on your side at the edge of your bed or the examining table. Draw your knees up as close to your chest as possible. Then, bend your head forward so that your chin touches your chest. As shown in the picture, an assistant will help you stay in this position by standing in front of you and placing one of her arms around your knees and the other around your neck.

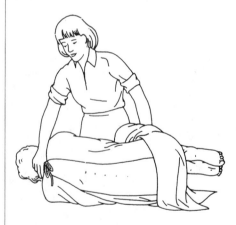

**2** The practitioner will wipe your lower back with a special sterilizing solution. Expect this to feel cold.

**3** Next, the practitioner will inject a local anesthetic through a tiny needle to numb the skin on your back. This may sting.

**4** The practitioner will insert a long needle to collect spinal fluid between the third and fourth lumbar vertebrae (the bones of your spinal column). You may feel some pressure but no pain.

### NEEDLE INSERTION SITE

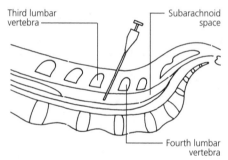

Third lumbar vertebra — Subarachnoid space

Fourth lumbar vertebra

**5** While the fluid drips out of the needle and into a tube, you must lie very still.

**6** After removing the needle, the practitioner will cleanse your back with alcohol and apply a small bandage.

**7** After the test, you may need to lie flat for several hours and drink lots of fluids to prevent a headache.

this strand is cut off or removed and may reduce incidence of headache. Practitioners continue to take opposing sides to this argument. A study conducted by Strupp and Brandt in 1997 demonstrated that only 5% of 300 patients had a postprocedure headache with stylet reinsertion; 16% experienced a headache when the stylet was not reinserted.

## DOCUMENTATION

➤ Review any recent or pertinent documentation by other health team members; then initial their notes to signify you're aware of their findings. This doesn't signify agreement with their comments or reduce your responsibility to conduct your own history and physical examination.

➤ Before performing this procedure, document any abnormal physical findings on the consent form and have the patient or guardian initial the comments as well as sign the form to signify acknowledgment of preprocedural abnormalities. In the chart, the preprocedural and postprocedural note should include an evaluation of function, range of motion, and neurosensory testing.

➤ Record all presenting symptoms and indications for lumbar puncture. Be sure to document any and all allergies to medication or food before administration of antibiotics, contrast dye, or lidocaine for local anesthesia.

➤ Describe the patient's tolerance of the procedure and response to medications, appearance of the injection site, and results of neurovascular checks. Record the CSF pressure, describe the color and characteristics of the CSF, and note which tests were ordered for analysis.

# Bone X-ray interpretation

### CPT CODES
*Codes for X-ray examinations of major anatomic sites are listed here. For more options, refer to a CPT coding manual.*

| | |
|---|---|
| 70250 | *Skull* |
| 71015 | *Chest* |
| 71101 | *Ribs* |
| 72010 | *Spine* |
| 73020 | *Shoulder* |
| 73110 | *Wrist* |
| 73120 | *Hand* |
| 73500 | *Hip* |
| 73590 | *Lower leg* |
| 73600 | *Ankle* |
| 73650 | *Heel* |

## DESCRIPTION

Plain X-rays are the most common initial screening technique and the most useful diagnostic tool for evaluating structural or functional changes in musculoskeletal diseases. X-rays obtained in multiple views, for example, will reveal most dislocations and fractures. They are also the main technique for detecting and monitoring scoliosis. X-rays record levels of brightness or shadow that reveal details about internal structures. (See *Indications of brightness level on X-ray,* page 172.) They also assist in identifying pathologic processes, such as arthritis, bone lesions, and fractures.

Classified by shape and location, bones may be long (humerus, radius, femur, and tibia), short (carpals and tarsals), flat (scapula, ribs, and skull), irregular (vertebrae and mandible), or sesamoid (patella). Bone tissue is of two basic types: compact and spongy (cancellous). Compact bone is dense and looks smooth and uniform. Spongy bone is composed of small needlelike or flat pieces of bone called tra-

## INDICATIONS OF BRIGHTNESS LEVEL ON X-RAY

As emitted photons (commonly called X-rays) pass through the patient, they are deflected by body tissues and absorbed into film on the opposite side. The film is darkened by interaction with the X-rays. Therefore, darker areas indicate less X-ray absorption by the body and more film exposure.

X-rays are deflected and absorbed to different degrees by different body tissue types. The amount of absorption depends on the tissue composition. For example, dense bone tissue absorbs many more X-rays than soft tissues, such as muscle, fat, and blood. The amount of deflection depends on the density of electrons in the tissues. Tissues with high electron density cause more X-ray scattering than those of lower density. The table below shows levels of brightness associated with specific density levels.

| SHADE | GROSS IDENTIFICATION | EXAMPLES |
| --- | --- | --- |
| Bright white | Metal | Jewelry, teeth fillings |
| Almost as white as metal | Bone tissue | Bone |
| Medium brightness | Fluid and muscle tissue | Organs, blood vessels |
| Gray black | Adipose tissue | Breast tissue, fat deposits |
| Black (radiolucent) | Air | Air in lungs, emphysema |

beculae. Spongy bone has large amounts of open space.

The long axis of a bone, called the shaft or diaphysis, is made of a thick collar of compact bone that surrounds a medullary cavity. In adults, the medullary cavity contains fat (yellow marrow) and is called the yellow bone marrow cavity. This long shaft merges into a broader, necklike portion called the metaphysis, composed of spongy bone. The end of the bone, the epiphysis, has a thin layer of compact bone on the outside and red marrow on the inside. In young bones, cartilage at the end of the shaft, where the metaphysis and the epiphysis meet, allows space for the long bone to lengthen as the body grows. (See *Internal structures of bone.*)

The periosteum helps protect the bone. The outer layer of the periosteum is made of dense, irregular connective tissue; the inner layer, abutting the bone surface, consists primarily of bone-forming cells, or

osteoblasts. The periosteum is densely laced with nerve fibers, lymphatic vessels, and blood vessels, which enter the bone. The junctions of long bones that articulate, or move, are covered with a smooth articular cartilage that cushions the bone ends and absorbs stress during joint movement.

## INDICATIONS

➤ To confirm suspicion of bone injury, deformity, or disease
➤ To investigate pain of unknown etiology
➤ To evaluate multiple trauma or any laceration, hematoma, angulation, or edema in long bone or joint

## CONTRAINDICATIONS

### Relative
➤ Pregnancy, particularly in the first trimester

## INTERNAL STRUCTURES OF BONE

To interpret X-ray studies accurately, you must have a thorough understanding of gross and microscopic anatomy. This illustration identifies the internal structures of bone.

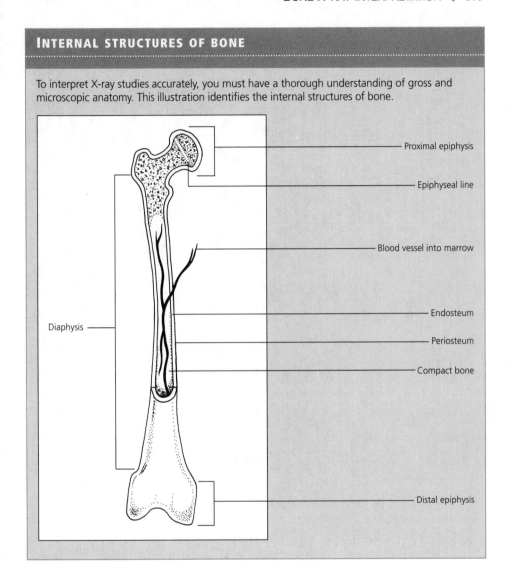

- Proximal epiphysis
- Epiphyseal line
- Blood vessel into marrow
- Endosteum
- Periosteum
- Compact bone
- Distal epiphysis

Diaphysis

## EQUIPMENT

X-ray view box or bright light to examine specific areas of the X-ray

## ESSENTIAL STEPS

➤ Verify the patient's name and the date and time of the X-ray study.
➤ Complete a thorough history and physical examination, focusing on the suspected mechanism of injury. Any suspected frac-

ture requires complete evaluation of adjacent joints.
➤ Verify that a female patient is not pregnant before ordering X-rays.
➤ If you're unsure about the best X-ray view to order, write the site to be X-rayed and identify what you expect to find or rule out.
➤ Request that the patient's previous films be retrieved for comparison.
➤ Verify the position of the X-ray in the view box: Check right and left markers

## RHEUMATOID ARTHRITIS OF THE HANDS

This is the X-ray film of a mature male with rheumatoid arthritis. The X-ray reveals periarticular soft tissue swelling (as indicated by ➤➤) and many erosions involving the distal ulna, carpals, metacarpals, and phalanges (as indicated by ➔). Narrowing of the joint spaces is also apparent. Also note the periarticular osteoporosis around the metacarpal and phalangeal joints (as indicated by ✱).

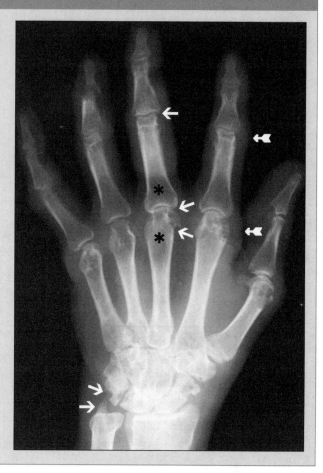

to ensure that your view is as if you were facing the patient (your left should be the X-ray study's right).

➤ Confirm that the view is unobstructed (for example, by jewelry or a medication patch).

➤ Follow a system for viewing that reduces the risk of missing abnormal findings. For example, consistently view the film from left to right, top to bottom, or external to internal.

➤ Verify anatomic alignment and positioning. Knowledge of normal anatomy is essential to X-ray interpretation.

➤ Evaluate bone age. Epiphyseal growth plates (called epiphyseal lines on X-ray film) may be visible in females younger than age 20 and males younger than age 23. These plates can be seen as thin, dark lines between the epiphysis and the metaphysis. In mature adults, decreased density associated with osteoporosis may be visible.

➤ Assess bone density. This is generally consistent over the entire bone; inconsistencies indicate fractures, tumors, and sclerosis. In addition, loss of joint spaces, kyphosis, and stress fractures may be in-

## OSTEOARTHRITIS OF THE KNEE

This is the X-ray film of a mature male with pain in his right knee. The X-ray reveals medial joint space narrowing (as indicated by ➤) and mild osteophyte formation (as indicated by ➔).

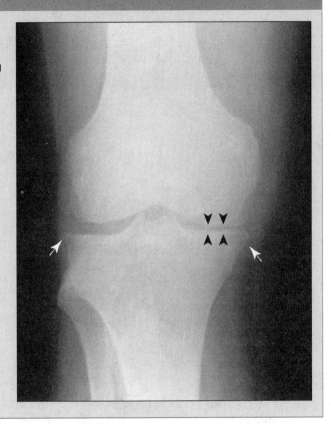

cidental findings. A common finding in mature adults is the degenerative changes and calcifications that bridge the joint spaces between bones associated with arthritis.

➤ Evaluate continuity. Assess the entire perimeter of the bone and then the internal bone structures for disruption in continuity that would reveal fractures or soft tissue inflammation. Check the bone perimeter and then the outer layer (also called the cortex or periosteum) for discontinuities or increased opacity. Increased opacity associated with a fracture may be due to bone impaction, fragment rotation, or callus formation. While cortex thickness decreases with age, loss of 50%

of the cortex or a bony lesion greater than 1″ (2.5 cm) in diameter warrants referral to an orthopedic surgeon. Conversely, thickening indicates stress fractures or inflammation.

➤ Look for lucency in a linear fashion that is common between bone fragments after a fracture. Mottled areas that have both lucent and dense areas suggest neoplasms with metastasis, congenital disorders, infection, or metabolic diseases.

➤ Examine the periosteum. Check the size and shape of bones. Contour abnormalities or excess calcification may indicate either a chronic disorder, such as metabolic disease, or a congenital disorder.

## BONE TUMOR

This is the leg X-ray film of an adolescent female. The X-ray reveals a well-defined, eccentric, bubbly expansile lesion (as indicated by ⇨) in the distal femoral diaphysis.

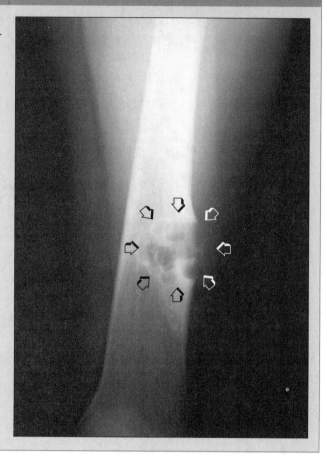

## PATIENT TEACHING

➤ Advise the patient that he may feel slight discomfort or pain, either from touching cold metal surfaces or from positioning the body part to be X-rayed. Reassure him that any discomfort should resolve within minutes after the procedure is completed.

➤ Emphasize the importance of following directions closely to avoid adversely affecting the quality of the X-ray.

➤ Explain that radiation from individual X-ray studies is minimal and that the reproductive organs of children and patients of reproductive age are covered with lead shields.

## COMPLICATIONS

None known

## SPECIAL CONSIDERATIONS

➤ In children, the epiphysis may be evident if bones have not finished growing. Order films of bilateral extremities so you can compare the patient's injured extremity to the uninjured one.

## LEG FRACTURES

This is the X-ray film of the lower leg a young adult male involved in a motor vehicle accident. The X-ray reveals an oblique, comminuted fracture of the tibia (as indicated by ➤) with lateral displacement of distal parts. It also reveals a comminuted avulsion-type fracture of the medial malleolus (as indicated by ➤➤).

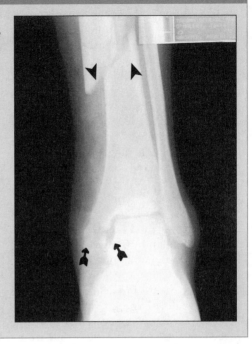

➤ When viewing cervical spine X-rays, be sure to count the vertebrae for proper identification of abnormalities. Follow each rib to its lateral edges to detect subtle fractures.

➤ A pelvic fracture can be hard to detect because it's commonly nondisplaced and because its appearance differs only slightly from a normal pelvis.

➤ In advanced rheumatoid arthritis, the bone atrophies and the joint becomes misaligned, deformed, and fused, resulting in fibrous ankylosis. X-rays reveal:
– loss of joint space and cartilage, periarticular bone erosion, and joint subluxation (See *Rheumatoid arthritis of the hands,* page 174.)
– soft tissue swelling
– bones appearing as osteoporotic and more radiolucent before erosion can be seen, with misalignment of the affected joints often apparent as the disease progresses
– joint fusion in advanced disease.

➤ The following plain X-ray findings indicate osteomyelitis:
– erosions
– aggressive bone destruction
– periostitis
– soft-tissue swelling
– osteosclerosis (chalky or opaque appearance with obliteration of distinct borders between cortex and trabeculae [outer and inner layers])
– bone fragmentation
– fractures
– subluxation
– ill-defined bone contours.

➤ The following plain X-ray findings indicate osteoarthritis:
– joint narrowing and bone sclerosis (See *Osteoarthritis of the knee,* page 175.)
– presence of osteophytes

– bony overgrowths that give the bone a lumpy or irregular contour, a hallmark of osteoarthritis

– cystlike lesions in the subarticular area, which appear as small, radiolucent, circular, or piriform areas that may extend to the joint surface.

➤ X-ray findings that indicate skeletal tumor include:

– osteopenia (scarcity of bone substance), which appears as bone more radiolucent than normal

– lytic lesions, which may appear as radiolucent, "punched out" areas of bone destruction

– pathologic fractures, common in the ribs and vertebrae

– an area of destroyed bone that appears to have been eaten by moths

– indistinct borders merging into normal tissue

– abundant periosteal reaction appearing as irregular new bone growth on bone edges (See *Bone tumor*, page 176.)

– ragged, irregular bone defects that are mottled or radiolucent

– absence of sclerosis along the margin

– foci of dense areas or a diffuse density involving a large area in the bone.

➤ X-ray findings that indicate fracture include:

– displacement of bone fragments

– radiolucent breaks in bone continuity

– misalignment of joints

– associated soft tissue edema. (See *Leg fractures*, page 177.)

➤ Because X-ray interpretation is a skill that requires much experience, have your collaborating physician and radiologist review X-rays.

## DOCUMENTATION

➤ Record the purpose of the X-ray study.
➤ Compare clinical findings with current and previous radiologic findings.

➤ Record any referrals made or collaborative communication with other health professionals.
➤ Note any instructions you gave to the patient, including when to follow up with you.

# SUPPORT PROCEDURES

## Clavicle immobilization

**CPT CODE**
*23500    Closed treatment of clavicle fracture without manipulation*

## DESCRIPTION

A fractured clavicle is one of the most common skeletal injuries among all patients and the most commonly fractured bone in children. About 80% of fractures occur at the middle third of the clavicle, 15% occur at the distal site, and 5% occur proximally. The most common mechanisms of injury are a fall on the outstretched arm or hand or a direct blow or fall to the shoulder. Fracture can also result from high-energy direct blows sustained in motor vehicle accidents or contact sports, such as football, hockey, or wrestling. Clavicular fractures are classified according to location, degree of displacement, and involvement of articular surfaces or ligaments. (See *Subclassification of clavicular fractures*.) Most middle third fractures can be managed appropriately by immobilization with a figure-eight bandage or sling.

Treatment includes immobilizing and stabilizing the fracture site to reduce pain and risk of additional injury, to maintain correct alignment during healing with min-

## SUBCLASSIFICATION OF CLAVICULAR FRACTURES

Distal clavicular fractures may be minimally displaced (type I), displaced due to a fracture medial to the coracoclavicular ligaments (type II), or an articular surface fracture (type III).

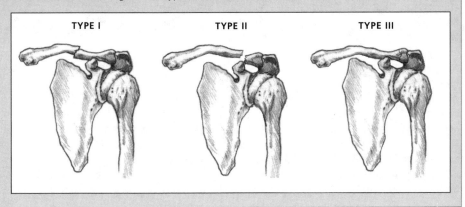

TYPE I    TYPE II    TYPE III

imal residual deformity or loss of function, to reduce the risk of nonunion, and to promote the patient's comfort.

## INDICATIONS

➤ To treat fractures of the middle third and medial third of the clavicle

## CONTRAINDICATIONS

### Absolute
➤ Fractures likely to require surgery, such as open fractures or fractures of the distal third of the clavicle with displacement
➤ Fractures in which neurovascular or respiratory compromise is suspected
➤ Fractures in which shortening of clavicular length is ½" (1.3 cm) or more, with attendant increased risk of postoperative pain and dysfunction

## EQUIPMENT

### For clavicle strap immobilization
Various commercial products are available.

### For figure-eight immobilization
Bandage, 6" wide and 4' to 6' long (length varies with size of patient; may substitute stockinette filled with padding) ◆ 4 to 6 large safety pins

### For sling-and-swathe immobilization
Sling (size based on size of patient) ◆ bandage, 6" wide and 4' to 6' long ◆ 2 to 3 large safety pins

## ESSENTIAL STEPS

➤ Take a complete history and perform a physical examination. Include mechanism of injury or degree of trauma, onset and location of pain, and degree of movement or functioning after the injury.
➤ Examine the clavicle for asymmetry and the ipsilateral shoulder for downward medial position. The proximal fragment of the clavicle will be positioned upward and posteriorly, causing tenting of the skin. The patient will frequently splint the affected side. Gentle palpation over the site will produce pain and crepitus.

➤ Auscultate the lungs for symmetrical breath sounds. Verify absence of underlying neurovascular injury. Evaluate pulses, skin temperature, and sensation and reflexes of the ipsilateral arm.
➤ Obtain upright anteroposterior view X-rays to verify distal and middle third clavicle fractures. Also note the appearance of the lungs and the position of the trachea. A CT scan may be be necessary to clearly visualize medial fractures. Anteroposterior and lateral views of the thoracic spine may be indicated to rule out associated fracture of the first rib.
➤ Explain the procedure and its purpose to the patient (and parent or other family member when applicable), and obtain appropriate consent.

## For application of clavicle strap
➤ Assist the patient to a comfortable sitting position.
➤ Place the straps over his shoulders and under his arms.
➤ Standing behind and slightly above the patient, gently pull the straps toward the middle of his back, pulling both of his shoulders upward, laterally and backward.
➤ Maintain this position as you fasten the straps. (See *Clavicle strap immobilization.*)
➤ Palpate the fracture for alignment and reevaluate neurovascular status.
➤ Repeat the X-ray to confirm proper alignment.

## For figure-eight immobilization
➤ Assist the patient to a comfortable sitting position.
➤ Standing behind and slightly above the patient, hold one end of the long, wide bandage at the center of his back.
➤ Place the bandage over the top of one shoulder, bringing it down and under the axilla.

➤ Bring the bandage diagonally across the back, over the opposite shoulder, and under the axilla.
➤ With the bandage in place, gently tighten the ends until the shoulders are pulled slightly upward, laterally and backward.
➤ Pin the bandage in place.
➤ Palpate for alignment. Assess neurovascular status.
➤ Repeat X-ray to confirm proper alignment.

## For sling-and-swathe immobilization
➤ Assist the patient to a comfortable sitting position.
➤ Select a sling size appropriate to the patient's size, and place the sling on the ipsilateral arm.
➤ Wrap a 6″ bandage around the patient's torso and upper arm on the affected side, holding the arm against the chest wall to stabilize it. Fasten the bandage with safety pins.
➤ Palpate the fracture site for alignment. Assess neurovascular status.
➤ Repeat X-ray to confirm proper alignment.

## PATIENT TEACHING

➤ Reassure the patient that pain is usually greatly reduced after the fracture is immobilized. Explain that a "bump" may persist over the fracture site and won't impair function. Tell him when to expect full healing (4 to 6 weeks in adults, 3 to 4 weeks in children).
➤ Remind the patient that he must wear the immobilizer constantly for 1 week. After that time, if he has no complications, he can remove it briefly for hygiene purposes. In any case, he must wear it until there is clinical evidence of union of the bone and until he can abduct the arm without pain.
➤ Tell a caregiver (such as a spouse or a parent) to frequently check the fit of the

# CLAVICLE STRAP IMMOBILIZATION

To promote healing and comfort, you'll need to immobilize the patient's clavicle properly. Remember to use equipment that can be easily tightened and repositioned because the bandages and straps tend to loosen over time.

Clavicle immobilization is frequently achieved with tube stockinettes (shown below) arranged in a figure-eight pattern (shown below) and secured with safety pins. To increase patient comfort and compliance, pad the stockinette where it fits around the back of the neck and under the axillae.

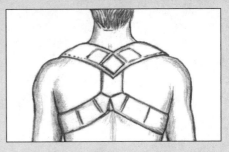

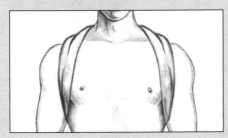

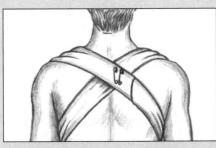

Ready-made figure-eight clavicle immobilization straps use Velcro closures to permit a snug fit (see below). They can be adjusted to maintain proper positioning. Because the straps are thick, additional padding is not usually necessary.

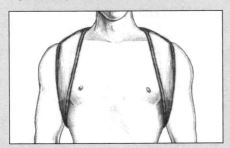

Whether you devise your own immobilization system or use a ready-made one, be sure the patient's shoulders are pulled upward and backward to allow the bones to knit in proper alignment, as shown below in this overhead view.

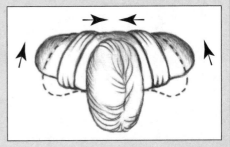

Some patients, particularly children or those with dementia, might be more compliant in a sling-and-swathe position. Immobilizing the arm on the affected side (as shown below) reminds the patient to limit movement, and this position also may cause less discomfort.

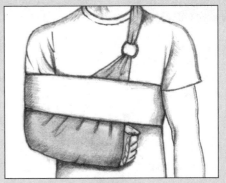

(continued)

## CLAVICLE STRAP IMMOBILIZATION (continued)

The sling-and-swathe method (shown at right) may also be more comfortable for a bedridden or chairbound patient because it doesn't require bulky strap connections along the middle of the patient's back.

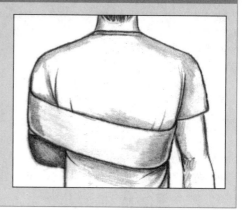

immobilizer or sling. If it feels too loose, it should be tightened. Instruct the patient to stand with his shoulders back in a "military position" while the caregiver tightens the immobilizer.

➤ Instruct the patient (or a responsible caregiver) to frequently check for swelling, color changes, or paresthesia of the hand and fingers. If any of these reactions occur, tell him to loosen the strap or sling until circulation and sensation are restored, and then to reapply it.

➤ Ask the patient to frequently flex all his fingers, his wrist, and his elbow on the affected side to maintain flexibility and function.

➤ Tell him not to raise the affected arm above the shoulder for 6 weeks.

➤ Promote his active participation in rehabilitation exercises, which should begin when the bone has fully healed. These exercises should include:

– the pendulum swing (Bend over from the waist. With the affected arm held down, gently swing it forward and backward in an arc, like a pendulum.)

– internal and external rotation (While lying down, use the unaffected arm to gently pull the affected arm across the chest; then push it out laterally away from the affected side.)

– wall climbing. ("Walk" the fingers of the affected hand up a wall as far as they will comfortably go.)

➤ Instruct him to use his unaffected hand to raise his affected arm forward in front of his chest.

➤ If the patient is an athlete, urge him not to resume play until full range of motion (ROM) and strength are restored (usually about 3 months). After that, special braces or splints are generally not needed for play.

➤ Urge him to contact you if he experiences persisting or worsening pain; numbness, tingling, or lack of sensation or decreasing function in the affected arm or hand; or any unusual swelling or coldness of the arm or hand.

➤ Tell him to schedule a follow-up appointment in 1 week (sooner if he experiences problems).

## COMPLICATIONS

➤ *Nonunion,* although rare, may occur with associated pain, deformity, and dysfunction; it requires referral to an orthopedist or a neurologist.

➤ *Malunion* — with resultant clavicular deformity, compression of underlying structures, shortening of the clavicle, and impaired function — is also possible and requires referral to an orthopedist or a neurosurgeon.

➤ *Arthritis* may result in fractures that involve articular surfaces; they require long-term management and referral to a rheumatologist.

➤ *Excess callus formation* may put pressure on the brachial plexus or subclavian artery, causing thoracic outlet compression and paresthesia; these require referral to a neurologist or a neurosurgeon.

## SPECIAL CONSIDERATIONS

➤ Some children will complain of discomfort and be uncooperative with the figure-eight or clavicle strap immobilizers. In this case, a simple sling or a sling-and-swathe immobilizer may be better tolerated.

➤ Include the patient's major caregiver and support persons in patient teaching.

➤ Refer the patient to physical therapy for more intensive rehabilitation.

 **CULTURAL TIP** Individuals from many Asian cultures don't wish to call attention to themselves. Therefore, they may not comply with wearing a splint, a clavicle strap, or especially a sling unless it can be discreetly concealed. They also may not comply with treatments that impede their ability to perform their usual job functions. Additionally, they may be less vocal or demonstrative regarding their degree of pain, whereas individuals of other cultures, such as Hispanics and Italians, may be much more demonstrative. In Middle Eastern cultures, the male rather than the female commonly communicates with the health care provider. Don't assume that this indicates an abusive relationship.

## DOCUMENTATION

➤ Review recent or pertinent documentation by other health team members; then initial their notes to signify that you're aware of their findings. This does not signify agreement with their comments or reduce your responsibility to conduct your own history and physical examination.

➤ Before performing this procedure, document any abnormal physical findings on the consent form and have the patient initial the comments and sign the form to signify acknowledgment of preprocedural abnormalities. In the chart, the preprocedural and postprocedural note must include an evaluation of function, ROM, and neurosensory testing (like two-point discrimination) along with a respiratory status evaluation. The differential diagnosis list or evaluation should indicate consideration of injury to the lung.

➤ Record the mechanism of injury, any asymmetry or inability to raise the arm, presence of pain, and radiologic verification of fracture and of alignment postreduction.

➤ Record the patient's understanding of instructions after the procedure, particularly in the event of potential language barriers.

## Splinting

CPT CODES
*29105    Application of long arm splint*
*29125    Application of short arm splint, static*
*29130    Application of finger splint, static*
*29505    Application of long leg splint*
*29515    Application of short leg splint*
*29550    Strapping: toes*
*99070    Splinting: supplies and material beyond those usually included for the office visit or service rendered*

## DESCRIPTION

Splinting can temporarily stabilize and immobilize acute injuries and provide symptomatic relief of chronic conditions, increasing patient comfort and preventing further injury. Acute injuries — such as sprains, strains, and fractures — typically require immediate joint stabilization; at the scene of the trauma, any rigid object can function as a splint. A temporary measure, splinting is initially preferred over circumferential casting for acute injuries because increased swelling within a circumferential cast can lead to vascular compromise, compartment syndrome, and distal swelling.

Inversion injuries with plantar flexion, the most common cause of acute ankle injuries, typically occur in young adults who take part in recreational activities and sports. Fractures are more common in older adults. Sprains vary based on the level of injury, disability, pain, and swelling.

Chronic conditions typically occur in the upper extremities and can usually be managed in a primary care setting or by an orthopedic specialist. Chronic injuries typically affect the wrists and hands and usually result from tenosynovitis and can occur with repetitive-motion injuries, such as carpal tunnel syndrome and tennis elbow. Splints increase the patient's comfort by keeping the joint immobilized and in proper alignment.

Consider referrals for an unstable joint, a fracture, potential limb loss, suspected internal derangement (indicated by clicking, popping, or locking of the joint), persistent pain, or unresolved injury.

## INDICATIONS

➤ To stabilize an acute strain, sprain, or fracture
➤ To relieve repetitive-motion disorders and overuse disorders
➤ To immobilize a joint after dislocation reduction

## CONTRAINDICATIONS
### Absolute
➤ Neurovascular compromise
➤ Soft-tissue compression
➤ Open injury

## EQUIPMENT

Tube stockinette in various diameters ◆ casting material in various widths ◆ 4" or 6" elastic wraps ◆ bucket of water ◆ soft padding ◆ scissors (optional) ◆ 1" to 2" adhesive tape (optional) ◆ sling (optional) ◆ aluminum splints (optional) ◆ wrist and finger splints (optional) ◆ knee immobilizer (optional)

## ESSENTIAL STEPS

➤ Take a complete history and perform a physical examination. Obtain a description of the injury and the joint involved, how and when it occurred, the patient's level of activity right after the injury and at the time of evaluation, and previous history of injury to the joint. Physical assessment should focus on the joint involved and its physical appearance, including swelling, obvious deformity, bleeding, and ecchymosis, possibly including a comparison with the other uninjured extremity. Also assess the patient's neurovascular status and ask if he can move the extremity.

### Ankle splinting
➤ Perform X-rays as appropriate to rule out fracture. Use the Ottawa ankle rules, listed here, to determine if X-rays are needed. If the patient is between ages 18 and 55 and can walk four steps immediately after the injury or when being evaluated, X-rays aren't required.
– If the patient feels pain on ambulation immediately after the injury and on evaluation, plus tenderness within 2½" (6.3 cm) of the posterior edge of the malleoli, order ankle X-rays.

–If the patient feels pain on ambulation immediately after the injury and on evaluation, plus tenderness of the fifth metatarsal or navicular, order foot X-rays.

➤ After the X-ray has been read and fracture has been ruled out, prepare the patient for immobilization. Place him in a comfortable position that permits splinting. The joint must be in a neutral position while ensuring adequate stretching of the tendons.

➤ Measure the casting material against the patient and then add about 1½″ (3.8 cm) to the length of the splint to ensure a proper fit. After measuring out 10 to 15 lengths of material and cutting it, fold the material into overlapping layers to form the desired length.

➤ Put on the stockinette; it should be approximately 2″ to 3″ (5 to 7.5 cm) above and below the area to be splinted.

➤ Alternatively, apply a soft cotton padding such as Webril to the extremity to protect the skin (with extra layers over bony prominences as needed) before applying the splint. Make sure the material doesn't bunch up and cause a pressure area.

➤ Holding the ends of the overlapping layers of material, submerge the material for 5 to 10 seconds in cool water. Shear off excess water before applying to the patient and molding to the limb.

➤ Allow the casting material to harden for 10 minutes. Then fold over the edge of the stockinette, and wrap an elastic bandage around the extremity and splint while maintaining the extremity in the proper position.

➤ Secure the elastic bandage with tape or clips.

## Finger splinting

➤ Although several types of finger splints exist, the aluminum finger splint is most commonly used for isolated proximal and distal interphalangeal joint injuries. Place it on both sides of the injured finger and secure it with tape.

➤ If this isn't the first injury to the finger, incorporate the finger splint into a volar arm splint.

## Arm splinting

➤ Obtain a volar arm splint for grades 2 and 3 wrist sprains.

➤ Have the patient extend his wrist slightly, with the metacarpophalangeal joint flexed 60 to 70 degrees and the fingers flexed 10 to 20 degrees.

➤ Put on the stockinette; it should be at least 3″ longer than the intended casting area. Cut a hole for the thumb.

➤ Cut the casting material to the length needed; then submerge the material for 5 to 10 seconds in cool water.

➤ Maintain this position as you mold the casting material and as it hardens. Fold the excess stockinette over the casting material. Secure it with an elastic bandage. The splint should extend from the tip of the fingers to about 1¼″ to 1½″ (3 to 4 cm) distal to the elbow joint.

## Thumb splinting

➤ Obtain an aluminum thumb splint.

➤ Flex the thumb slightly at the distal interphalangeal joint.

➤ Measure the aluminum splint to fit 1″ to 2″ (2.5 to 5 cm) beyond the wrist.

➤ Bend the splint to the position of the thumb, and apply it to the dorsal side of the thumb.

➤ Wrap the splint with an elastic wrap; include the thumb in the wrap.

## Below-the-knee splinting

➤ Obtain an ankle fracture brace for injury to the tibiofibular, lateral collateral, or deltoid ligament to limit inversion and eversion.

➤ Place the patient in a prone position (if possible), making sure the knee and ankle are flexed 90 degrees. Help him maintain this position as you apply the splint, which should extend from the metatarsal joint to about 1½″ below the popliteal fossae.

Secure the splint with an elastic bandage (usually 4″ to 6″ [10 to 15 cm] wide).

➤ Alternatively, you can use a stirrup ankle splint for such injuries. Place a 5″ (12.7 cm) plaster splint over the plantar aspect of the foot and up both the medial and the lateral sides of the foreleg to the level of the fibula head.

### Toe splinting

➤ Obtain hard-sole shoes that lace.

➤ To "buddy tape" the injured toe, use 1″ (2.5 cm) of silk tape to tape the toe to the neighboring toe; this stabilizes and immobilizes the fracture or sprain.

➤ Help the patient put the shoe on and lace it securely to provide support and immobilization.

## PATIENT TEACHING

➤ Teach the patient the RICE regimen — rest, ice, compression, and elevation.

➤ Tell him to apply ice every 2 to 3 hours for 20 to 30 minutes for the first 24 hours. Then he can switch to moist heat (without wetting the dressing) for the next 24 to 48 hours.

➤ Tell him to wear the splint except when sleeping or showering until he's reevaluated and to avoid activities that cause pain.

➤ Instruct him to watch for signs of neurovascular compromise, such as coolness, swelling, pain, darkness, or pallor in the area around the splint or tape. If he notes any, he should rest at once with the extremity elevated above his heart. Emphasize that swelling can occur swiftly with activity but will take much longer to subside. Urge him to contact you if swelling doesn't improve within 30 minutes.

➤ Tell him to take acetaminophen, a nonsteroidal anti-inflammatory drug, or both to relieve pain as directed.

➤ Instruct the patient to follow up with you 48 hours after the initial taping or splinting and then as indicated.

➤ Tell him to remove the splint or tape and immediately call you if he experiences signs of neurovascular compromise (peripheral pallor or blue-purple color, pain, coldness, swelling, or numbness and tingling) that don't resolve.

## COMPLICATIONS

➤ *Vascular compromise, ischemia, and compartment syndrome of the affected extremity* can result from a splint that is wrapped too tightly. To prevent this, make sure the elastic bandage is snug but not tight, and use a linear splint rather than a circular splint.

➤ *Pressure ulcers* can result from the splint rubbing against bony prominences. Soft cotton padding applied directly to the skin beneath the splint can help minimize this complication.

## SPECIAL CONSIDERATIONS

➤ For chronic injuries, consider taping to stabilize and support the joint, particularly for an athlete. Taping immobilizes the area and provides supports, allowing the athlete to continue activities with minimal interference. Make sure the tape isn't too tight, and keep in mind that most taping loosens after activity, placing the joint at risk for further injury. Several methods of taping exist; a skilled professional (such as a trainer or sports medicine clinician) should perform such taping.

➤ As appropriate, refer the patient to an orthopedic specialist for a custom-made splint; such a splint may be more comfortable than standard-sized splints.

## DOCUMENTATION

➤ Review recent or pertinent documentation by other health team members; then initial their notes to signify you're aware of their findings. This doesn't signify agreement with their comments or reduce your responsibility to conduct your own history and physical examination.

➤ Before performing this procedure, document any abnormal physical findings on the consent form and have the patient initial the comments as well as sign the form to signify acknowledgment of preprocedural abnormalities. In the chart, the preprocedural and postprocedural note must include an evaluation of function, range of motion, and neurosensory testing, such as two-point discrimination.

➤ Record indications for and details of the procedure, including a detailed description of the site, the type of splint used, the patient's reaction to the procedure, medications ordered, the time frame for follow-up evaluation, and any instructions given to the patient.

## Crutch walking and cane walking

### CPT CODE
No specific code has been assigned.

## DESCRIPTION

Ambulation aids such as crutches and canes remove full or partial weight from one or both legs, enabling the patient to support himself with his hands and arms. These aids protect injured legs from further injury and can help a patient with lower extremity weakness to walk.

To use ambulation aids successfully, the patient must have balance, stamina, control of his trunk, and upper-body strength. The patient's condition will determine the type of aid and the gait to use. Ambulation aids require use of the abdominal and paraspinous muscles of the trunk, the muscles of the upper extremities, and those of the unaffected lower extremity. Canes are used for partial weight-bearing reduction.

Crutches may be used for partial or full weight-bearing reduction. The patient who can't use crutches may be able to use a walker.

Three types of crutches are commonly used. Standard aluminum or wooden crutches are used by the patient with a sprain, strain, or cast. They require stamina and upper-body strength. The paraplegic or other patient using the swing-through gait may use aluminum forearm crutches. These have a collar that fits around the forearm and a horizontal handgrip that provides support. Platform crutches are used by the arthritic patient who has an upper-extremity deficit that prevents weight bearing through the wrist. They provide padded surfaces for the upper extremities.

## INDICATIONS

➤ To aid ambulation in patients with sprains or strains, stress fractures, fractures of a lower extremity requiring partial or no weight bearing, or neuromuscular deficits or injuries

## CONTRAINDICATIONS

### Relative
➤ Upper extremity injury or weakness
➤ Balance abnormality

## EQUIPMENT

Crutches with axillary pads, handgrips, and rubber suction tips ♦ cane with handgrip and rubber suction tip (such as walking cane, quad cane, or platform crutch cane) ♦ walking belt (optional)

## ESSENTIAL STEPS

➤ After choosing appropriate crutches for the patient, adjust their height with the patient standing or, if necessary, lying down.

➤ To fit a patient for crutches, position each crutch so that it extends from a point

4" to 6" (10 to 15 cm) to the side and 4" to 6" in front of the patient's feet to 1½" to 2" (4 to 5 cm) below the axillae (about the width of two fingers). Adjust the handgrips so that the patient's elbows are flexed at a 15-degree angle when he's standing with the crutches in the resting position.

➤ To fit a patient for a cane, have him hold the cane in the hand opposite the injured leg. The cane's length should be such that the patient's elbow is flexed at about 20 degrees with the rubber tip resting 3" to 4" (7.5 to 10 cm) lateral to the patient's shoe.

➤ Consult with other health care professionals (physical therapists, orthopedists) as needed to coordinate rehabilitation and teaching to optimize patient outcomes.

➤ If needed, place a walking belt around the patient's waist to help prevent falls. Tell him to position his crutches and to shift his weight from side to side. To facilitate learning and coordination, place the patient in front of a full-length mirror.

➤ Describe the gait you will teach and the reason for your choice. Demonstrate the gait as necessary. Tell the patient to perform a return demonstration.

## PATIENT TEACHING

➤ Provide the patient with written aids as appropriate. (See *Learning to use crutches*.)

➤ Teach the four-point gait to the patient who can bear weight on both legs. Although this is the safest gait, because three points are always in contact with the floor, it requires greater coordination than others because of its constant shifting of weight. Teach this sequence: right crutch, left foot, left crutch, right foot. Suggest counting to help develop rhythm, and make sure each short step is of equal length. If the patient gains proficiency at this gait, teach the faster two-point gait. This approach is used when weight bearing of a combination of extremities must be reduced (for example, in a patient with rheumatoid arthritis in both upper and lower extremities).

➤ Teach the two-point gait to the patient with weak legs, but good coordination and arm strength. This is the most natural crutch-walking gait because it mimics walking, with alternating movement of the arms and legs. Instruct the patient to advance the right crutch and left foot simultaneously, followed by the left crutch and right foot. This approach only partially relieves weight bearing of legs.

➤ Teach the three-point gait to the patient who can bear only partial or no weight on one leg. Instruct him to advance both crutches 6" to 8" (15 to 20 cm) along with the involved leg. Tell him to bring the uninvolved leg forward and to bear the bulk of his weight on the crutches. The patient may at this time place partial weight on the involved leg if allowed and pain-free. Stress the importance of taking steps of equal length and duration with no pauses. This approach completely eliminates weight bearing of one extremity. The energy cost of this gait is twice as great as normal.

➤ Teach the swing-to or swing-through gaits — the fastest ones — to the patient with complete paralysis of the hips and legs. Instruct him to advance both crutches simultaneously and to swing his legs parallel to (swing-to) or beyond (swing-through) the crutches. Caution him that this gait requires much energy.

➤ If the patient will be using a cane, teach him to place it in the hand opposite the affected leg. Tell him to practice so that the cane and the heel of the injured leg strike the ground simultaneously.

➤ Teach the patient who uses crutches how to get up from a chair. Instruct him to hold both crutches in one hand, with the tips resting firmly on the floor. Then tell him to push up from the chair with his free hand, supporting himself with the crutches.

➤ Teach him to reverse this process to sit down. Tell him to support himself with the crutches in one hand and to lower himself with the other.

*(Text continues on page 193.)*

## LEARNING TO USE CRUTCHES

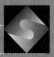

DEAR PATIENT:

Learning to use crutches requires time and patience. Practice the techniques described below to make sure you're using your crutches properly.

### Crutch walking with partial weight on your injured leg

The practitioner may allow you to place some of your weight on the injured leg. To do this, look over the diagrams below. They show how to walk with crutches if your right leg is injured. (If your left leg is injured, place most of your weight on your right leg, and adapt the instructions. You may want to draw the step patterns for yourself.)

**1** Stand straight, with your shoulders relaxed and your arms slightly bent. Lean your body slightly forward, distributing your weight between the crutches and your uninjured leg. You can put some weight on your injured leg (shown as the patterned foot).

**2** Move the crutches forward. Then move your injured leg up to meet them.

**3** Put some weight on your injured leg as you move your uninjured leg ahead of the crutches.

**4** Now repeat these steps to keep walking.

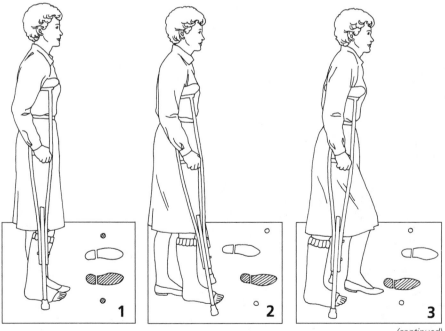

*(continued)*

### Crutch walking with no weight on your injured leg

If the practitioner says you shouldn't put any weight on your injured leg while walking with crutches, use this method.

The step patterns below show how to walk with crutches if your left leg is injured. (If your right leg is injured, rest your weight on your left leg, and adapt the instructions. You may want to draw the step patterns for yourself.)

**1** Stand straight, with all your weight on your uninjured leg. Relax your shoulders. Hold the foot of your injured leg off the floor, flexing your knee slightly.

Balancing all your weight on the crutches, position the uninjured leg's foot so it's even with the crutch tips, slightly in front of you. Use the uninjured leg and the crutches to support your weight as you lean your body slightly forward.

**2** Shift all your weight to the uninjured leg and move the crutches forward together, swinging the injured leg along with them. Don't put any weight on your injured leg!

**3** Now shift all your weight back to the crutches to your hands and wrists, swing your uninjured leg forward, and again place all your weight on this leg, using the crutches to keep your balance.

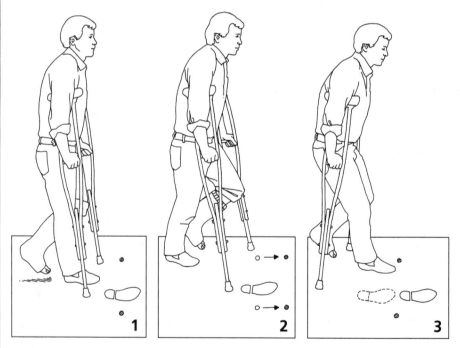

PATIENT-TEACHING AID

## LEARNING TO USE CRUTCHES *(continued)*

### Climbing and descending stairs

If the banister is on your left side and your right leg is injured, follow the directions below.

**1** Standing at the bottom of the stairs, shift both crutches to your right hand. Then grasp the banister firmly with your left hand. Using your right hand, carefully support your weight on the crutches.

**2** Next, push down on your crutches and hop onto the first step, using just your uninjured leg. Lift your injured leg as you go.

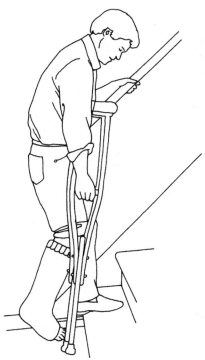

**3** Support your weight on that leg as you continue to grasp the banister tightly. Then swing the crutches up onto the first step. Now hop onto the second step, using your uninjured leg. Repeat this procedure, but go slowly.

**4** To get down the stairs, reverse these maneuvers. But always advance the crutches and your injured leg first. Remember: Your strong leg goes up first and comes down last.

*(continued)*

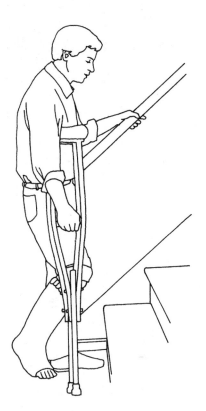

## Sitting down

**1** Using your crutches, walk over to the chair. Turn around, and step backward until the back of your uninjured leg touches the chair's front edge.

**2** Keeping your weight on your uninjured leg, transfer both crutches to the hand on the same side as your injured leg. Support most of your weight on your crutches. Next, reach back with your other hand and grasp the chair arm.

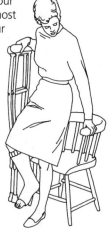

**3** Carefully sit down, making sure to keep your weight off your injured leg. Keep your crutches next to the chair.

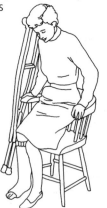

## Getting up

**1** Move your uninjured leg backward until it touches the back of the chair's front edge. While you're still sitting, take the crutches and stand them upright.

**2** Using the hand on the same side as your injured leg, hold onto the handgrips. With your other hand, hold onto the chair arm.

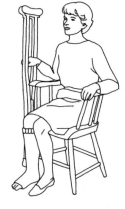

**3** Slide forward, with your uninjured leg slightly under the chair. Push yourself up onto your uninjured leg. Once you're standing, transfer a crutch to your uninjured side. Or push yourself up while grasping the handgrip of a crutch in each hand.

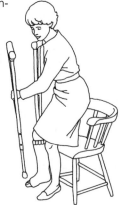

➤ Teach the patient to ascend stairs using the three-point gait. Tell him to lead with his uninvolved leg and then follow with both crutches and the involved leg. To descend stairs, he should lead with the crutches and the involved leg and follow with the uninvolved leg.

## COMPLICATIONS

➤ *Atrophy of the hips and legs* can occur if a patient who uses the swing-to or swing-through gait for a prolonged period neglects to perform appropriate therapeutic exercises routinely.

➤ *Brachial nerve palsy* can develop in a patient who habitually leans on his crutches, causing prolonged pressure on the axillae. Instruct the patient to return to the clinic for reevaluation of gait and fitting if he feels tingling or numbness in the side of his chest, axillae, or upper arms.

## SPECIAL CONSIDERATIONS

➤ Encourage arm- and shoulder-strengthening exercises to prepare the patient for crutch walking. If possible, teach two techniques — one fast and one slow — so he can alternate between them to prevent excessive muscle fatigue and can adjust more easily to various walking conditions.

## DOCUMENTATION

➤ Before conducting patient teaching, document any abnormal physical findings and have the patient initial documentation of pre-existing alterations in function or neurosensory findings.

➤ Record the patient's level of understanding. Include language barriers and use of an interpreter when indicated.

➤ Describe the patient's condition and your assessment of his function, range of motion, and neurovascular status (paresthesia, pulses, pain, and pallor).

➤ Record consultations (as indicated), preparation of the patient and equipment, and the gait trained.

➤ Note any referrals, follow-up visits, and reasons that the patient should contact you.

➤ Record the type of gait the patient is to use, his ability to perform a return demonstration, his tolerance of the procedure, and anticipated duration of use.

➤ Review recent or pertinent documentation by other health team members; then initial their notes to signify you're aware of their findings. This doesn't signify agreement with their comments or reduce your responsibility to conduct your own history and physical examination.

➤ Record the quality and duration of the patient's ambulation (for instance, the patient can ambulate 30′ [9.1 m] without resting and can navigate a flight of stairs) and the use of proper technique independently, thus making the patient safe for discharge per facility protocol.

# TREATMENTS

## Dislocation reduction

CPT CODES
*23650    Closed treatment of shoulder dislocation, with manipulation*
*24600    Closed treatment of elbow dislocation*
*26700    Closed treatment of metacarpophalangeal dislocation, single, with manipulation*
*26770    Closed treatment of interphalangeal joint dislocation, single, with manipulation*
*27550    Closed treatment of knee dislocation*

## DESCRIPTION

Dislocation is the partial or complete displacement of one bone from another. It can occur spontaneously due to structural defect, traumatic injury, or joint disease. A dislocated joint is reduced when normal position is returned. Reduction decreases pain, helps prevent structural defects and lost or decreased use of the joint, and facilitates healing.

## INDICATIONS

➤ To alleviate pain and promote healing of a dislocated shoulder, elbow, finger, patella, or toe

## CONTRAINDICATIONS

### Absolute
➤ Fracture of the joint
➤ Separation of the acromioclavicular joint
➤ Fracture of the joint capsule
➤ Abnormal neurovascular status of the extremity
➤ Dislocation of the hip or knee

## EQUIPMENT

Cleaning solution, such as povidone-iodine or alcohol ◆ 3 ml lidocaine without epinephrine ◆ 5-ml syringe with 25G needle

## ESSENTIAL STEPS

➤ Take a complete history and perform a physical examination.
➤ Obtain radiographic confirmation to rule out fractures and to determine the direction of dislocation. If a fracture is found, immobilize the joint and refer the patient to an orthopedic specialist.
➤ If necessary, use an assistant to help stabilize the patient. (For a pediatric patient,

the parents usually provide the best assistance and can help calm the child.)
➤ As needed, use an oral narcotic or muscle relaxant or both, but have naloxone (Narcan) available and monitor the patient's vital signs and airway patency during and after the procedure for signs of overdose.

### Finger or toe reduction
➤ Use a digital nerve block. Clean the digit with povidone-iodine or alcohol. Infiltrate up to 3 ml of lidocaine (without epinephrine) using a 25G needle for field anesthesia.
➤ Grasp and stabilize the proximal segment in one hand.
➤ With your other hand, grasp and apply firm and steady longitudinal traction to the distal segment in the direction of angulation.
➤ Slowly move the distal segment in the opposite direction of the angulation while continuing to apply steady traction and pressure to the dorsal side.
➤ Continue moving the distal segment toward the neutral position until reduction occurs.
➤ Check joint stability.
➤ Apply an aluminum finger splint with tape to maintain the joint in position of function; you can tape a stable joint to the adjacent finger.
➤ As needed, obtain an X-ray to confirm positioning of the joint.

### Shoulder reduction
*Manual reduction*
➤ With the patient supine, grasp and support his upper arm above the elbow with both hands, and support the forearm under your own arm against your body. Make sure the arm is adducted, externally rotated, and flexed.
➤ Apply firm, steady, distracting axial traction to the arm, pulling it distally. ("Distracting" in this context means to pull away from the skeletal attachment.)

➤ While maintaining traction, slowly ease the arm into the shoulder until reduction occurs. You may also need to provide some internal or external rotation or slight pressure directed anteriorly from beneath the upper arm.

➤ As needed, ask an assistant to apply countertraction to stabilize the patient. Do this by wrapping a bed sheet around the patient's upper torso and having the assistant apply countertraction from the side opposite the affected shoulder.

➤ Obtain anteroposterior and axillary lateral X-rays to confirm reduction.

➤ Apply a sling and swathe to prevent shoulder external rotation and abduction.

*Passive reduction (Stinson's method)*
➤ Use this method for patients with recurrent dislocations. Place the patient in a prone position on the examination table with the involved extremity hanging off the table toward the floor.

➤ Place a folded towel under the shoulder.

➤ Apply steady traction to the distal extremity, either manually or with a 10- to 15-lb (4.5- to 6.8-kg) weight attached to the patient's wrist. Allow weights to pull on the arm for 15 to 20 minutes. Reduction should occur spontaneously. If it doesn't, immobilize the extremity and call an orthopedist. You may need to provide some rotation or flexion of the extremity.

## Patella reduction
➤ Place the patient in the supine position. Apply steady manual pressure to the lateral aspect of the patella with one hand while slowly extending the knee with the other hand until reduction occurs.

➤ Rule out patella fracture or rupture of the patellar or quadriceps tendon.

➤ Apply a knee immobilizer to prevent knee flexion.

## Radial head subluxation in children (nursemaid's elbow)
➤ Rule out elbow, shoulder, and clavicle fracture or dislocation.

➤ Seat the child in the parent's lap. Explain to the parent that the child may experience brief pain with the procedure but then should experience immediate relief of symptoms once reduction occurs.

➤ Grasp the patient's wrist and distal forearm in one hand, and support the elbow with the opposite hand, with the thumb over the radial head.

➤ Supinate the forearm, rotating the hand palm up.

➤ Flex the elbow until you feel a snap over the radial head, indicating that the orbicular ligament has reduced. The child shouldn't require a sling or immobilization.

## PATIENT TEACHING

➤ Explain that the joint will probably swell for 24 to 48 hours after the injury and that keeping the joint elevated and applying ice for 20 minutes intermittently should minimize pain and swelling.

➤ Promote use of an anti-inflammatory medication, which will help decrease pain and swelling.

➤ Tell the patient with a patella or shoulder dislocation — especially a patient under age 30 — that the risk of recurrence is high. After reduction, refer him to an orthopedic surgeon for evaluation within 1 week. Rest the joint until evaluated by the surgeon.

➤ Tell the patient to call or return at once if he experiences redislocation, loss of normal sensation of the limb (numbness and tingling), or increased pain.

## COMPLICATIONS

➤ *Malposition or failure to maintain reduction, vascular compromise, and neurologic compromise* require collaboration with or referral to other health care professionals.

➤ *Narcotic overdose* can be reversed with naloxone. Monitor the patient for several hours, and repeat naloxone administration as needed.

## SPECIAL CONSIDERATIONS

 **ALERT** Don't attempt reduction of a large joint or a joint with a concurrent fracture if acute vascular or neurologic compromise threatens the limb. Refer this patient immediately to an orthopedist or send him to the emergency department for reduction. Dislocations of the elbow, hip, knee (femorotibial), and ankle also require an emergency referral unless acute neurovascular compromise exists.

## DOCUMENTATION

➤ Review recent or pertinent documentation by other health team members; then initial their notes to signify that you're aware of their findings. This doesn't signify agreement with their comments or reduce your responsibility to conduct your own history and physical examination.

➤ Before performing this procedure, document any abnormal physical findings on the consent form. Have the patient initial the comments and sign the form to signify acknowledgment of preprocedural abnormalities. In the chart, the preprocedural and postprocedural note must include an evaluation of function, range of motion, and neurosensory testing, such as two-point discrimination.

➤ Record indications and details of the procedure, the patient's reaction to it, medications ordered, the time frame for follow-up evaluation, and any instructions given to the patient.

# Transcutaneous electrical nerve stimulation

CPT CODE
*64550    Application of surface (transcutaneous) neurostimulator*

## DESCRIPTION

Transcutaneous electrical nerve stimulation (TENS) is based on the gate theory of pain, which proposes that painful impulses pass through a "gate" in the brain.

A portable, battery-powered device transmits painless electrical current to peripheral nerves or directly to a painful area over relatively large nerve fibers. This treatment effectively alters the patient's perception of pain by blocking painful stimuli traveling over smaller fibers. A TENS device reduces the need for analgesic drugs and may allow the patient to resume normal activities. Typically, a course of TENS treatments lasts 3 to 5 days. Some conditions, such as phantom limb pain, may require continuous stimulation; other conditions, such as a painful arthritic joint, require shorter periods (3 to 4 hours).

## INDICATIONS

➤ To alleviate postoperative or chronic pain

## CONTRAINDICATIONS

### Absolute
➤ Cardiac pacemakers
➤ Pregnant patients
➤ Senility

### Relative
➤ Cardiac disorders
➤ Vascular disorders or seizure disorders (TENS electrodes should not be placed on

## POSITIONING TENS ELECTRODES

In transcutaneous electrical nerve stimulation (TENS), electrodes placed around peripheral nerves (or an incisional site) transmit mild electrical pulses to the brain. Clinicians think the current may block pain impulses. The patient can influence the level and frequency of his pain relief by adjusting the controls on the device.

Typically, electrode placement varies even though patients may have similar complaints. Electrodes may be placed to cover the painful area or surround it (as with muscle tenderness or spasm or painful joints) or to capture the painful area between electrodes (as with incisional pain).

In peripheral nerve injury, electrodes should be placed proximal to the injury (between the brain and the injury site) to avoid increasing pain. Placing electrodes in a hypersensitive area also increases pain. In an area lacking sensation, electrodes should be placed on adjacent dermatomes.

The accompanying illustrations show combinations of electrode placement (black squares) and areas of nerve stimulation (shaded) for lower back and leg pain.

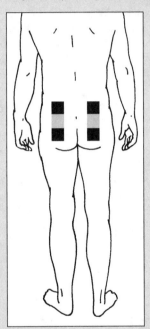 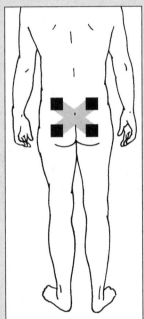 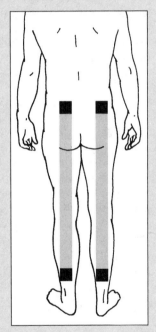

the head or neck. See *Positioning TENS electrodes*.)

## EQUIPMENT

TENS device ◆ alcohol sponges ◆ electrodes ◆ electrode gel ◆ warm water and soap ◆ leadwires ◆ charged battery pack ◆ battery recharger ◆ adhesive patch or nonallergenic tape (optional: commercial TENS kit that includes the stimulator, lead-wires, electrodes, spare battery pack, battery recharger, and sometimes the adhesive patch)

## PREPARATION OF EQUIPMENT

➤ Before beginning the procedure, always test the battery pack to make sure that it's fully charged.

## ESSENTIAL STEPS

➤ Maintain aseptic technique. Provide privacy. If the patient has never seen a TENS unit before, show him the device and explain the procedure.

➤ With an alcohol sponge, thoroughly clean the skin where the electrode will be applied. Then dry the skin.

➤ Apply electrode gel to the bottom of each electrode.

➤ Place the electrodes on the proper skin area, leaving at least 2″ (5.1 cm) between them. Then secure them with the adhesive patch or nonallergenic tape. Tape all sides evenly so the electrodes are firmly attached to the skin.

➤ Plug the pin connectors into the electrode sockets. To protect the cords, hold the connectors, not the cords themselves, during insertion.

➤ Turn the channel controls to the "off" position or to the position recommended in the operator's manual.

➤ Plug the leadwires into the jacks in the control box.

➤ Turn the amplitude and rate dials slowly, as the manual directs. (The patient should feel a tingling sensation.) Then adjust the controls on the device to the prescribed settings or to settings that are most comfortable. Most patients select stimulation frequencies of 60 to 100 Hz.

➤ Attach the TENS control box to part of the patient's clothing, such as a belt, pocket, or bra.

➤ To make sure the device is working effectively, monitor the patient for signs of excessive stimulation (such as muscular twitches) or inadequate stimulation (the patient's inability to feel a mild tingling sensation).

### After TENS treatment

➤ Turn off the controls and unplug the electrode leadwires from the control box.

➤ If another treatment will be given soon, leave the electrodes in place; if not, remove them.

➤ Clean the electrodes with soap and water and clean the patient's skin with alcohol sponges. (Don't soak the electrodes in alcohol because it will damage the rubber.)

➤ Remove the battery pack from the unit and replace it with a charged battery pack.

➤ Recharge the used battery pack so it's always ready for use.

## PATIENT TEACHING

➤ Tell the patient that TENS involves placement of small electrodes on his body, usually near the pain site. The electrodes are connected to a small, battery-powered generator, which electrically stimulates nerve fibers, inhibiting or blocking pain sensations. Add that TENS treatments also help stimulate endorphin production. Mention, too, that they help to distract the patient from his pain.

➤ Advise the patient that he may feel varying degrees of pain relief. Some patients report relief only when the unit is on; others report prolonged pain relief. (See *Learning about TENS*, page 199.)

➤ Inform the patient that TENS effectively treats both acute and chronic pain. In particular, it may benefit the patient concerned about adverse effects of drug therapy for such conditions as headache syndromes, chronic or acute musculoskeletal disorders, or menstrual cramps. Add that TENS is most effective for localized mild to moderate pain. It's contraindicated only in patients with pacemakers or loss of sensation. Tell the patient that it can be used indefinitely (without adverse effects) to control pain. However, skin breakdown is possible either from prolonged use or an allergic reaction to the adhesive on the electrodes.

➤ Explain that treatment will begin with a TENS trial of at least 1 week, usually conducted by a physical therapist, a nurse, a nurse practitioner, or a physician. The trial will help determine the best placement of the electrodes and the optimal settings for amplitude frequency and pulse

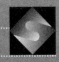

## LEARNING ABOUT TENS

DEAR PATIENT:

Your practitioner has ordered transcutaneous electrical nerve stimulation (also called TENS) to help relieve your pain.

### How TENS works
A small, battery-operated device sends safe electrical signals through wires and into your body by way of electrodes, which you attach to your skin.

### Where to place the electrodes
Your practitioner will show you where to attach the electrodes. Ask her to label the sites with a marker. If necessary, use a mirror to help you see them. Ask a friend or a family member to note the sites, too. That way he can give you reassurance if you feel nervous the first few times you use the TENS unit. Or, if needed, he can help you place the electrodes another time.

If your electrodes require conductive jelly, spread it in a thin layer across each electrode before applying the electrode.

Placing your electrodes on the wrong sites probably won't harm you, but avoid placing them on your belly if you are pregnant, on the sides of the neck, or on the voice box area.

### Using TENS
The knobs on your unit are adjustable:
➤ Set the AMP/A at ____.
➤ Set the rate at ____.
➤ Set the pulse-width at ____.

➤ Turn your TENS unit on for _____ minutes and off for _____ minutes throughout the day.

You should feel a pleasant sensation while the machine is working. If you develop muscle spasms, contact the practitioner. The AMP may be set too high, or you may have placed the electrodes in the wrong places.

If your pain is increasing, follow the directions your practitioner gave you to change the settings on your TENS unit.

### Safety tips
Follow your practitioner's instructions carefully for the amount of time you should leave your TENS unit on. Don't get into water with the unit on, and don't sleep with it on.

### Skin care
Take good care of your skin. Prevent local skin irritation — redness and rash — by cleaning your skin before attaching the electrodes. Watch for signs of irritation.

If your skin becomes irritated, don't place electrodes on those areas. Keep the skin clean and dry until it heals. If it's still irritated after a week, contact the practitioner.

If you repeatedly develop local skin irritation from the electrodes, contact your practitioner to discuss an alternate wearing schedule or another type of electrode.

### Caring for the TENS unit
Clean your TENS unit weekly by lightly wiping it with rubbing alcohol.

width. It will also give the patient practice in using the TENS unit at home.

➤ If appropriate, allow the patient to study the operator's manual. Teach him how to place the electrodes properly and how to take care of the TENS unit.

## COMPLICATIONS

None known

## SPECIAL CONSIDERATIONS

➤ If you must move the electrodes during the procedure, turn off the controls first. Incorrect placement of the electrodes will result in inappropriate or inadequate pain control.

➤ Setting the controls too high can cause pain; setting them too low will fail to relieve pain.

➤ Never place the electrodes near the patient's eyes or over the nerves that innervate the carotid sinus or laryngeal or pharyngeal muscles to avoid interference with critical nerve function.

➤ If TENS is used continuously for postoperative pain, remove the electrodes at least daily to check for skin irritation and provide skin care.

## DOCUMENTATION

➤ Before performing this procedure, document any abnormal physical findings on the consent form. Have the patient initial the comments and sign the form to signify acknowledgment of preprocedural abnormalities. In the chart, the preprocedural and postprocedural note must include an evaluation of function, range of motion, and neurosensory testing, such as two-point discrimination.

➤ On the patient's medical record, note the electrode sites and control settings used, document the patient's tolerance of the procedure, and evaluate the effectiveness of pain control.

# Trigger point injections

CPT CODE
*20550    Injection of tendon sheath, ligament, trigger points, or ganglion cyst*

## DESCRIPTION

A trigger point is a highly localized sensitive spot in a taut band of myofascial muscle fibers. It produces local and referred pain when pressure is applied. Trigger point injections interrupt the pain cycle, allowing other pain relief measures (such as dry needling, stretch and spray, and transcutaneous electrical nerve stimulation) and the body's natural healing process a chance to work. Trigger point injections cause the release of chemicals that dilate local arterioles and restore circulation to the trigger point, relax the motor end plates, release calcium and thus decrease muscle rigidity, and extend the peripheral nerve refractory period. This is referred to as insertional activity.

## INDICATIONS

➤ To treat myofascial pain syndromes of cervical, thoracic, and lumbar back and extremities; fibromyalgia syndrome; and temporomandibular disorders

➤ To alleviate chronic pelvic pain (rare)

## CONTRAINDICATIONS

### Absolute
➤ Cellulitis or broken skin at injection site
➤ Anticoagulant therapy or coagulopathy
➤ Septicemia or suspected bacteremia
➤ Unavailability of emergency equipment

### Relative
➤ Lack of response to previous two or three injections

# EQUIPMENT

Alcohol wipes ◆ gloves ◆ drape ◆ marking pen ◆ 0.5% to 1% lidocaine (without epinephrine) or bupivacaine 0.125% to 0.25% (single-dose vials to avoid preservative or precipitation problems) ◆ methylprednisolone, 10 to 20 mg ◆ 25G or 27G 1¼″ needles ◆ 3-, 5-, and 10-ml syringes ◆ emergency resuscitation equipment

# ESSENTIAL STEPS

➤ Explain the procedure to the patient, and obtain written consent before beginning.
➤ Lay all equipment on a tray within easy reach.
➤ Put on gloves.
➤ Position and drape the patient for privacy, comfort, and safety.
➤ Expose the area surrounding the injection site.
➤ Identify the exact location of the trigger point by palpating the maximal point of tenderness with your thumb or forefinger.
➤ Mark the area by drawing a circle around your finger.
➤ Clean the skin with alcohol wipes.
➤ Draw up the desired amount (usually from 1 to 5 ml) of lidocaine or bupivacaine, depending on the site to be used. If using methylprednisolone, draw the local anesthetic first and change the needle to prevent dulling or contamination; then draw up 0.5 to 1 ml of the steroid.
➤ Proceed with the trigger point injection, using one of two techniques:
– Insert the needle at a 90-degree angle until it reaches the trigger point. Aspirate for blood. Inject 0.5 to 2 ml, withdraw slightly but not totally from the skin, and then reinject at a 60-degree angle both to the left and to the right of the original injection. (See *Choosing an angle for trigger point injection,* page 202.)
– Insert the needle at a 50- to 70-degree angle into the subcutaneous tissue adjacent to the trigger point region. Aspirate for blood. Using about three needle insertions, inject 0.5 to 2 ml with each insertion into the trigger point without removing the needle from the skin.
➤ If the procedure is done correctly, the patient will experience immediate relief.
➤ Remove the needle and place an adhesive bandage over the injection site.

 **ALERT** Observe for reactions to the local anesthetic: light-headedness, tinnitus, peripheral numbness, slurring of speech, drowsiness, or seizure activity. Treatment includes general supportive measures and drug discontinuation. Maintain a patent airway and carry out other respiratory support measures immediately. Administer diazepam or thiopental to treat seizures. Administer vasopressors (including dopamine and norepinephrine) to treat significant hypotension.

# PATIENT TEACHING

➤ Inform the patient that he may feel a burning sensation for a few seconds as the medication is injected. Explain that the area may become numb for up to 3 hours and that pain relief generally lasts for several days.
➤ Tell him he can apply heat to the site before exercising the muscle.
➤ Ask him to move the muscles passively or actively to enhance the effectiveness of the injection and to begin restoring normal function and range of motion (ROM) to the area. Within 4 hours of injection, he can start working on ROM and stretching exercises; then gradually add weight-bearing exercises over the following days to weeks. Encourage him to progress to exercising at least five times daily (frequency is crucial to symptom relief).
➤ Urge the patient to avoid isometric exercises, such as weight lifting, and excessively quick, jerky movements because these tend to exacerbate pain and injury.

## CHOOSING AN ANGLE FOR TRIGGER POINT INJECTION

When injecting trigger points, you'll commonly use either a 90-degree angle or a 50- to 70-degree angle, depending on your preference and the depth and location of the trigger point.

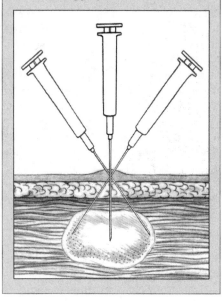

➤ Advise the patient not to constrict muscles in the trigger point area, such as by carrying a heavy knapsack.

➤ Tell him to observe for edema and ecchymosis, which may indicate bleeding into the muscle. Instruct him to apply ice to the site to minimize these symptoms, which will resolve over a few days.

➤ Tell him to report signs and symptoms of infection (increased pain after 24 hours, elevated temperature, redness, swelling, yellow or green discharge, and foul odor).

## COMPLICATIONS

➤ *Vasovagal syncope or a reaction to the local steroid* may require use of emergency equipment.

➤ *Skin infection* can be treated with topical or oral antibiotics.

➤ *Hematoma formation* can be treated by applying ice to the affected site for 15 to 20 minutes.

➤ *Neuritis* may require supportive care and physical therapy.

## SPECIAL CONSIDERATIONS

➤ Patients with myofascial pain are likely to experience pain reduction and increased ROM.

➤ Patients with fibromyalgia may initially experience increased ROM without pain relief, and pain relief may be delayed up to 2 weeks after the injection.

➤ Trigger point injections with a local anesthetic can be repeated every 3 to 4 days; if steroids are used, injections should be 6 weeks apart. Research suggests that the specific medication injected is less important than the actual piercing of the muscle with a needle.

➤ Apply heat for 20 to 30 minutes after the injection to increase permeability into the trigger point area.

## DOCUMENTATION

➤ Before performing this procedure, document any abnormal physical findings on the consent form. Have the patient initial the comments and sign the form to signify acknowledgment of preprocedural abnormalities. In the chart, the preprocedural and postprocedural note must include an evaluation of function, ROM, and neurosensory testing, such as two-point discrimination.

➤ Record an accurate history of the trigger point area, the patient's ROM, and strength of affected muscles.

➤ Specify the type and amount of local anesthetic and steroid used, the exact location of the injection (draw a picture of the muscle group area), and the appearance of the injection site.

➤ Note the patient's pain perception before and after the injection.

# DERMATOLOGIC PROCEDURES

5

From 50% to 70% of all dermatologic problems are treated in the primary care office. As a practitioner, therefore, you must develop confidence in treating skin disorders and skill in performing dermatologic procedures. In addition, because of the visual nature of dermatologic problems, sensitivity and compassion are also important.

Besides helping to shape a patient's self-image, the skin performs many physiologic functions. For instance, it protects internal body structures from the environment and from potential pathogens. It also regulates body temperature and homeostasis and serves as an organ of sensation and excretion. As a result, meticulous skin care is essential to overall health. When skin integrity is compromised by pressure ulcers, burns, or lesions, you'll need to take steps to prevent or control infection, promote new skin growth, control pain and itching, and provide emotional support.

Because the skin is the body's first line of defense against infection, any damage to its integrity increases the risk of infection, which could delay healing, worsen pain, and even threaten the patient's life. Most burn deaths, for example, result from complications of infection rather than from the burns themselves.

Infection control requires aseptic technique to avoid introducing new pathogens into an already contaminated wound. You can achieve this by maintaining aseptic technique throughout dermatologic procedures and by using antiseptic agents and sterile equipment during invasive procedures.

To enhance natural healing, skin wounds need regular dressing changes (extra changes for soiled dressings); thorough cleaning; and, if necessary, debridement to remove debris, reduce bacterial growth, and encourage tissue repair. Using warm solutions for wound cleaning increases circulation to the site, which promotes delivery of oxygen and the nutrients required to support tissue repair.

To control pain effectively, you need to evaluate each patient's response to pain and adapt your treatment plan accordingly. If the patient has minor to moderate pain or skin discomfort such as pruritus, an analgesic or topical medication, reassurance, distraction, comfortable positioning, and ample rest may be adequate. However, if the patient has severe pain, only strong narcotic analgesics may provide relief. An awareness of cultural differences also may be crucial in guiding your treatment plan.

 **CULTURAL TIP** Various cultural groups respond to pain in various ways. For instance, Native Americans may complain of pain in general terms, such as "Something doesn't feel right." Furthermore, if the patient reports pain but gets no pain relief, he's unlikely to repeat the complaint to you. Egyptians and Palestinians fear pain and cope better if the source of and prognosis for pain is understood. Other cultural groups, including Brazilians, Puer-

203

to Ricans, Cubans, Gypsies, Haitians, and Central Americans, freely express pain by moaning or crying. Still other groups, including Cambodians, Chinese, Japanese, Mexicans, Ethiopians, Russians, and Samoans, are very stoic in communicating pain and may require additional evaluation. Muslims may refuse narcotics for all but severe pain because narcotics are forbidden by their religion. Brazilians, Ethiopians, Iranians, and Haitians are less accustomed to the numerical pain scale and may describe pain qualitatively or only in general terms. Some cultural groups, particularly Asians, may use acupressure and acupuncture to treat pain or illness.

 **CULTURAL TIP** Many cultural groups, including Mexicans, may use alternative health practices that they may not readily disclose to you. These include applying onions to the skin (similar to a poultice), taking herbal baths, and drinking herbal preparations — all of which may confound your findings or treatments. A Mexican patient may also attribute a sudden physical condition to *mal de ojo* (evil eye) caused by "admiration" (jealousy). Green-eyed persons are thought to be especially capable of inflicting *mal de ojo*. To admire an infant without touching it supposedly puts an infant at increased risk. Keep such cultural beliefs in mind as you provide dermatologic care to your patients.

Finally, remember that a patient with a painful and disfiguring skin disorder may also have to deal with depression, frustration, and anger. Along with physical support, such a patient needs continuing emotional support as he develops coping mechanisms to accommodate an altered self-image. Severe disfigurement — common in a burn patient — may require emotional support and psychological or psychiatric referral throughout the slow and painful recovery period. Scars or other evidence of skin injury or disease can influence the patient's self-acceptance as well as his acceptance by others. Sensitivity to the patient's needs and respect for his man-

ner of coping are among your most important challenges.

# DIAGNOSTIC TESTING

## Skin scraping

### CPT CODES
*87210    Specimen smear with interpretation; wet mount with simple stain for bacteria, fungi, or ova and parasites*
*87220    Tissue examination for fungi*

### DESCRIPTION

A skin scrape involves the gentle removal of a skin specimen that is then placed on a microscope slide for evaluation. This procedure is commonly performed to confirm a diagnosis of superficial fungal infection or arthropod infestation.

### INDICATIONS

➤ To verify the presence of a superficial fungal infection or arthropod infestation

### CONTRAINDICATIONS

None known

### EQUIPMENT

Surgical blade such as #15 Bard-Parker blade (if unavailable, use the edge of a glass microscope slide) ◆ gloves ◆ alcohol pad ◆ microscope slide and coverglass ◆ 5% to 20% potassium hydroxide (KOH) solution ◆ match ◆ lens paper

## ESSENTIAL STEPS

➤ Explain the procedure to the patient, and answer any questions he has.
➤ Position the patient comfortably, leaving the area to be scraped easily accessible.
➤ Put on gloves.
➤ Clean the area with an alcohol pad.
➤ Lightly run the surgical blade perpendicular to the skin. When the blade has collected enough of the superficial skin layer, wipe it across the microscope slide. Make sure you use a gentle technique; the patient shouldn't bleed or experience pain.
➤ Place the coverglass on the slide.
➤ If you suspect a dermatophyte infection, apply KOH to the edge of the coverglass, allowing capillary action to draw the solution under it.
➤ Gently heat the slide with a match until bubbles begin to expand.
➤ Blot excess KOH solution with lens paper.
➤ Look for hyphae (septated, tubelike structures), dermatophytes, pseudohyphae (tubelike structures without septa), and budding yeast forms to identify candidiasis.

## PATIENT TEACHING

➤ Just before scraping, tell the patient that you're about to scrape the skin but that the scraping shouldn't cause pain.
➤ Explain that the scraping will help ensure proper diagnosis and treatment.
➤ Tell him when to schedule a follow-up appointment based on the diagnostic findings.

## COMPLICATIONS

None known

## SPECIAL CONSIDERATIONS

➤ If KOH results are negative, collect a culture specimen and send it to the microbiology laboratory for growth and species identification.

## DOCUMENTATION

➤ Record indications for testing, the location and appearance of the specimen site, results of testing, and the patient's tolerance for the procedure.
➤ Note the prognosis, patient instructions given, and follow-up appointment information.

## Skin lesion biopsy and removal

CPT CODES
*Note:* Precise code depends on lesion size.
*11200    Removal of skin tags or multiple fibrocutaneous tags on any area less than or equal to 15 lesions*
*11201    As above, for each additional 10 lesions after the first 15 lesions (code may be listed as many times as needed)*
*11300 to 11303    Shaving of epidermal or dermal lesion on trunk, arms, or legs*
*11305 to 11308    Shaving of epidermal or dermal lesion on scalp, neck, hands, feet, or genitalia*
*11400 to 11406    Excision of benign lesions on trunk, arms, or legs*
*11420 to 11426    Excision of benign lesions on scalp, neck, hands, feet, or genitalia*
*11600 to 11606    Excision of malignant lesions on trunk, arms, or legs*
*11620 to 11626    Excision of malignant lesions on scalp, neck, hands, feet, or genitalia*

## DESCRIPTION

A skin biopsy is performed to obtain material for pathologic evaluation or to remove a precancerous lesion or one causing the patient discomfort. It can be either incisional (removing only part of a lesion) or excisional (removing the entire lesion). The entire lesion is generally removed if doing so will permit proper healing and an aesthetically acceptable outcome.

There are three types of skin biopsy: shave, scissor, and punch. In a shave biopsy, the specimen doesn't extend deep into the dermis. It's a quick, easy way to remove superficial lesions and is ideal for raised lesions in the epidermis or superficial dermis; if necessary, the procedure can extend down to the subcutis. The procedure is faster than a punch biopsy, generally requires only local anesthesia and topical aluminum chloride to control bleeding, has a favorable cosmetic outcome, and can provide a relatively large specimen. However, a shave biopsy can leave a depressed scar if the biopsy goes too deep. Most practitioners remove lesions with a sterilized razor blade; some prefer a surgical blade such as the #15 Bard-Parker blade. The inexpensive, sharp, flexible razor blade allows you to curve the blade to match the surface of the lesion by applying pressure with your index finger and thumb. You can then advance the blade across the base of the lesion with a steady sawing motion.

The scissor biopsy, a variant of the shave biopsy, allows removal of small, superficial growths, such as skin tags and filiform warts. It usually doesn't require local anesthesia.

For a punch biopsy, a specialized instrument is used to remove a cylindrical, full-thickness skin specimen. It's performed to obtain material for pathologic evaluation and to remove small cutaneous lesions quickly and effectively. Punches are available in sizes ranging from 1.5 to 10 mm and can be permanent or disposable. Disposable punch biopsy instruments are preferable because they're sterile and inexpensive, and they don't get dull from repeated use. Because the instrument can

only go as deep as the length of the cylinder, a biopsy that must include deeper fat or fascia may require two complete punches. The resulting wound may require suturing. Punch biopsies generally produce an acceptable cosmetic result, provide a deep specimen, and heal rapidly when sutured. However, they require sterile technique and local anesthesia, specimen size is limited by the width and depth of the punch, and the wound may require extra time for suturing.

## INDICATIONS

➤ To remove a precancerous skin lesion or one causing discomfort
➤ To obtain material for pathologic evaluation

## CONTRAINDICATIONS
### Absolute
➤ Suspected cancerous lesion
➤ Unknown diagnosis
➤ Infection at the biopsy site

## EQUIPMENT

Antiseptic such as 70% isopropyl alcohol or povidone-iodine ◆ gloves ◆ sterile drape (optional)

### For shave biopsy
Local anesthesia ◆ 25G to 30G ½" to 1" needles and 3- to 5-ml syringe ◆ razor blade or surgical blade such as #15 Bard-Parker blade ◆ aluminum chloride (20% to 40%) or electrocautery ◆ cotton-tipped applicators ◆ triple antibiotic ointment with adhesive dressing

### For scissor biopsy
Forceps ◆ sterile sharp scissors ◆ aluminum chloride (20% to 40%) ◆ triple antibiotic ointment with adhesive dressing

## For punch biopsy

Local anesthesia ◆ 25G to 30G ½″ to 1″ needles and 3- to 5-ml syringe ◆ punch, skin hook, blade (such as P2 or P3 blade), or needle ◆ sterile sharp scissors ◆ suture equipment ◆ sterile adhesive strips such as Steri-Strips or monofilament nylon sutures ◆ three-layer pressure dressing with antibiotic ointment ◆ adhesive dressing

## ESSENTIAL STEPS

➤ Obtain a detailed history, and perform a physical examination.
➤ Verify that the patient is not allergic to iodine preparations or local anesthetics.
➤ Explain the procedure to the patient, and answer any questions he has.
➤ Obtain informed consent.
➤ Place the patient in a comfortable position that leaves the skin lesion and surrounding area easily accessible.
➤ Clean the skin lesion and a 3″ (7.6 cm) area around it with antiseptic solution.
➤ Drape the area if appropriate.
➤ Put on gloves.

## For shave biopsy

➤ Inject the local anesthetic under the lesion, using the 25G or 30G needle to create a wheal.
➤ Secure the lesion and the surrounding tissue with your nondominant hand while passing the razor blade or scalpel under the lesion. Control the depth of the biopsy with the appropriate angle of entry. (See *Performing a shave biopsy*, page 208.)
➤ To control bleeding, apply 20% to 40% aluminum chloride directly to the wound with a cotton-tipped applicator or use electrocautery.
➤ Apply triple antibiotic ointment and an adhesive dressing.

## For scissor biopsy

➤ To perform a scissor biopsy, use forceps to gently grasp and apply traction to the lesion.
➤ Using the sterile sharp scissors, cut the lesion at its base.
➤ Apply aluminum chloride and pressure to control any bleeding.
➤ Apply triple antibiotic ointment and an adhesive dressing.

## For punch biopsy

➤ Inject the local anesthetic under the lesion, using the 25G or 30G needle to create a wheal.
➤ Position the punch vertically over the area. Using your nondominant hand, apply perpendicular tissue traction. This results in an oval rather than a circular defect. (A circular defect may result in a redundant cone of skin, called a "dog-ear," on closure.)
➤ Push the punch against the skin with firm, steady pressure, and simultaneously twist it clockwise. Continue this until you feel the punch advance slightly, indicating the descent of the punch into the fat layer.
➤ Withdraw the punch with the column of tissue. Remove the specimen gently to avoid histologic artifacts.
➤ Use a skin hook or local anesthesia needle to elevate the plug of tissue, and transect the base with a pair of sharp scissors.
➤ To obtain the best cosmetic result and fastest healing, suture the biopsy site using simple interrupted or vertical mattress sutures. Typically, a 2-mm punch requires one suture, a 4- to 6-mm punch requires two sutures, and a 7- to 10-mm punch requires three to four sutures. Using 4-0 monofilament nylon sutures and a P2 blade is best for wounds on the extremities and trunk, and using 5-0 and 6-0 monofilament nylon sutures with a P3 blade is best for biopsies taken from the face and anterior neck. If necessary, reinforce the

## PERFORMING A SHAVE BIOPSY

When performing a shave biopsy, hold the scalpel so that it's almost parallel to the skin surface.

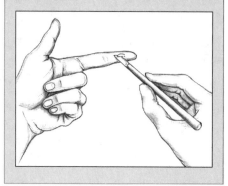

sutures on a wound under tension with sterile adhesive strips.

➤ Place a three-layer pressure dressing that contains triple antibiotic ointment (Polysporin) on the wound, followed by a nonadherent pad, gauze, and an adhesive dressing overlay.

### PATIENT TEACHING

➤ Advise the patient how long the pain will last and how long the wound will take to heal. Pain may be minimal to moderate, and resolution of pain varies with the size of the wound and progression of healing. Tell him to expect bloody to clear yellow drainage in the first 24 to 48 hours.

➤ Teach him how to care for the wound. He should gently clean the biopsy site daily with tap water and soap (with no rubbing or scrubbing) and then apply a small amount of antibiotic ointment, preferably Polysporin rather than an ointment that contains neomycin, which carries a higher risk of allergic reaction. Tell him to continue wound care until the area completely heals.

➤ Explain that the wound will appear uniformly pink or red when epithelialization

is complete. Emphasize that keeping the wound covered and occluded promotes rapid healing and reduces the risk of scarring.

➤ Advise the patient to minimize activity to prevent bleeding and wound dehiscence, if the punch biopsy site is in an area of tension.

➤ Teach the patient to examine his skin frequently to detect new or changing lesions. (See *How to examine your skin*.)

➤ Instruct the patient to make a follow-up appointment in 2 days so that you can evaluate wound healing and conduct a neurosensory examination, as indicated by depth of injury. Emphasize that even superficial wounds must be evaluated.

 **ALERT** Instruct the patient to notify you promptly if he develops signs of infection (increasing redness, swelling, pain, and warmth; cloudy yellow, green, or brown drainage; opening of the wound; foul odor; a red streak leading from the site; or fever after 24 hours).

## COMPLICATIONS

➤ *Infection* may be treated with local or systemic antibiotics and antiseptic soaks. You also may need to refer the patient to a physician, a dermatologist, or an infectious disease specialist.

➤ *Scarring* can be minimized with gentle handling and with the use of skin adhesives and such techniques as undermining.

➤ *Pain* is minimized with local anesthesia and over-the-counter medications, such as acetaminophen or ibuprofen.

## SPECIAL CONSIDERATIONS

 **ALERT** For deeper lesions, suspected neoplasms, and facial or penile lesions, consult with a dermatologist or refer the patient to one.

➤ Deeper shave biopsies can result in permanent depression at the biopsy site.

PATIENT-TEACHING AID

## HOW TO EXAMINE YOUR SKIN

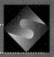

**DEAR PATIENT:**

It's a good idea to examine your skin every month. That is because persistent sun exposure or photosensitivity reactions can lead to skin cancer. See your practitioner if you notice suspicious-looking changes in the size, texture, or color of a mole or if you have a sore that doesn't heal. Detected early, most skin cancers are curable.

Check your skin right after a bath or shower. Stand before a full-length mirror in a well-lighted room. Keep a small mirror handy for seeing behind you and for examining hard-to-see spots. Note any freckles, moles, blemishes, and birthmarks, remembering where they are and what they look like. Then proceed.

**1** Standing unclothed in front of the mirror, check the front of your body. Turn to each side and look over your shoulder to see behind you. Use your hand mirror also. Then lift your arms and examine the sides of your body.

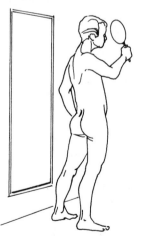

**2** Inspect your arms and hands. Check the backs of your hands, your palms, your fingers, and both sides of your forearms and upper arms.

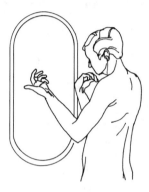

**3** Examine your legs, checking the fronts, backs, and sides. Look between your buttocks and around the genital area.

**4** Next, move close to the mirror to look carefully at your neck, face, lips, eyes, ears, nose, and scalp. Part your hair with a comb to see better.

**5** Now, sit down. Bend your knees to bring your feet close to you. Examine your soles, insteps, ankles, and between your toes.

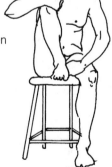

➤ If the patient has an atypical-appearing melanocytic lesion, don't remove it with the shave procedure. Instead, obtain a good specimen for pathology by performing a deep punch biopsy. If unsure of the diagnosis, consider referral before biopsy to minimize the cost and the number of painful procedures that the patient will experience.

➤ Don't keep removing the punch from the biopsy site to check your progress; if you do, the specimen may have histologic artifacts.

➤ The pathologist needs an adequate specimen for diagnosis (for instance, a specimen that includes the dermis for a dermal lesion). If the pathologist also needs a portion of adjacent normal skin (for example, if the patient has a more complex skin disease, such as panniculitis), a wedge-shaped section can provide the larger and deeper specimen needed. You should also provide as much detail about the site as possible.

➤ If you can't identify a lesion or don't plan to treat it, don't biopsy it. Instead, refer the patient to someone who may be able to recognize the lesion, possibly saving the patient the discomfort and cost of biopsy.

➤ If a patient has a lesion that you suspect is skin cancer, refer him to a dermatologist. The dermatologist has the background needed to choose the most appropriate treatment (including excision, radiation therapy, and chemotherapy).

## DOCUMENTATION

➤ Before performing this procedure, document any abnormal physical findings on the consent form. Have the patient initial the comments and sign the form to signify acknowledgment of preprocedural abnormalities. In the chart, the preprocedural and postprocedural note must include an evaluation of potentially affected function, range of motion, and sensation.

➤ Record the indications for and details of the procedure, including a thorough description of the site before and after the procedure, the patient's reaction to the procedure, medications ordered, patient instructions given, and the time frame for follow-up evaluation.

## Wood's light examination

### CPT CODE
No specific code has been assigned.

### DESCRIPTION

The Wood's light is used in many observational assessments, ophthalmologic procedures, and dermatologic presentations to enhance visibility and aid diagnosis. The lamp converts ultraviolet light into visible light. A fluorescein stain and a magnifying lens are sometimes used to help increase visibility of the area being examined. In ophthalmologic procedures, the fluorescein stain allows the injured area in the cornea or sclera to present as a bright yellow-green color. In dermatologic presentations, the light allows the practitioner to see many lesions and parasites that might otherwise go undetected.

### INDICATIONS

➤ To aid differential diagnosis of bacterial, fungal, and pigmented skin lesions and to delineate borders of suspicious lesions
➤ To enhance visualization of corneal abrasions, ulcers, and foreign objects in the cornea and conjunctiva
➤ To detect porphyria

### CONTRAINDICATIONS

None known

## UNDERSTANDING WOOD'S LIGHT FINDINGS

A Wood's light is commonly used with a fluorescein stain and a magnifying glass to aid in the differential diagnosis of dermatologic problems (such as fungal infections) and ophthalmologic conditions (such as corneal abrasions). You'll make your diagnosis only after reviewing the patient history and physical findings; the following table can help you narrow your focus. The listed findings pertain to the skin, unless otherwise noted.

| WOOD'S LIGHT FINDINGS | POTENTIAL DIAGNOSES |
|---|---|
| Cold bright white | Albinism or loss of pigmentation |
| Blue-white | Tuberous sclerosis (genetic), hypopigmentation, leprosy, vitiligo |
| Blue-green to green | *Pseudomonas* |
| Pale green to brilliant green | Dermatophytosis (tinea) |
| Off-white or yellow to deep green | Tinea versicolor |
| Bright yellow to green (conjunctiva) | Corneal abrasion |
| Darker, sometimes a purple brown | Hyperpigmentation |
| Orange-red to pink-red (urine) | Porphyria (genetic) |
| Pink to coral red | Erythrasma (bacteria) |
| Bright red | Squamous cell carcinoma |
| Enhanced visualization of tunneling beneath the skin and mites | Scabies (parasite) |
| Enhanced visualization of lice | Pediculosis (parasite) |

## EQUIPMENT

Wood's light apparatus ◆ magnifying lens, if necessary, for increased visibility ◆ fluorescein stain (optional)

## ESSENTIAL STEPS

➤ Explain the procedure to the patient, and answer any questions he has.
➤ Place him in a comfortable position that fully exposes the area to be examined.
➤ Stain the area, if indicated.
➤ Darken the room.

➤ Turn on the Wood's light to examine the area. Use a magnifying lens if necessary. Hold the light approximately 6″ to 8″ (15 to 20 cm) away for maximum effectiveness.
➤ Note findings (see *Understanding Wood's light findings*).

## PATIENT TEACHING

➤ Explain the purpose of the Wood's light examination.
➤ Assure the patient that the procedure is painless.

## COMPLICATIONS

None known

## SPECIAL CONSIDERATIONS

➤ Question the patient about any treatments, lotions, or ointments previously applied to the skin. Use of these items could confound your findings.

## DOCUMENTATION

➤ Include in your procedural documentation the use of the Wood's light in aiding and establishing your diagnosis.

# EMERGENCY PROCEDURES

## Mammal bite care

CPT CODES
*12001 to 12007   Simple repair of superficial wounds of scalp, neck, axillae, external genitalia, trunk, and extremities*

## DESCRIPTION

Although seldom fatal, bites from animals or humans can cause injuries ranging from bruises and superficial scratches to severe crush injuries, deep puncture wounds, tissue loss, and severe damage to blood vessels. In the United States, most mammalian bites involve dogs, with cat bites second and human bites third. Surprisingly, human bites are the most to be feared because of the great variety of infectious bacteria and viruses normally present in the oral cavity.

A dog bite may cause muscle, tendon, and nerve damage, dislocation of involved joints, and crush injuries; infection occurs only 2% to 10% of the time. A cat's sharp teeth can cause deep puncture wounds that damage muscles, tendons, and bones; because these tissues have a limited blood supply, the risk of developing infection from a cat bite is 30%.

Infection is more likely to occur if the wound isn't treated promptly, if there is a crush injury, or if the hand is involved. Clenched-fist injuries are the most serious because damaged joint capsules increase the risk of developing osteomyelitis and septic arthritis.

Unfortunately, many animals—usually wild ones—carry the rabies virus in their saliva and can transmit it by biting or licking an open wound. Rabies is rare in the United States, but it's fatal unless treated. The risk of getting rabies from a dog is low. Bats cause nearly all cases of rabies in the United States.

Human bites can infect other humans with diseases such as herpes simplex virus, cytomegalovirus, syphilis, tuberculosis and, possibly, acquired immunodeficiency syndrome.

Animal bites commonly occur when a sick or injured animal is trying to protect itself or when an animal is protecting its food, territory, or offspring. Human bites most often result from fights among school-age children and young adults.

## INDICATIONS

➤ To prevent infection after trauma

## CONTRAINDICATIONS

### Relative
➤ Clenched-fist injuries requiring X-rays and, possibly, referral to a plastic surgeon or hand surgeon

➤ Facial wounds requiring referral to a plastic surgeon

## EQUIPMENT

Sterile basin ◆ antiseptic solution (such as Hibiclens or povidone-iodine) ◆ sterile saline solution ◆ sterile gloves ◆ 5- to 10-ml syringe, 60-ml syringe ◆ 27G needle ◆ 18G to 20G needle ◆ 1% or 2% lidocaine ◆ scissors (sterile) ◆ curved hemostat (sterile) ◆ hemostat (sterile) ◆ #3-0 to #5-0 nylon suture material ◆ 4" × 4" gauze pads ◆ topical antibiotic (such as bacitracin) ◆ culture swab with transport medium (optional)

## ESSENTIAL STEPS

➤ Obtain a detailed history, and conduct a physical examination.
➤ Explain the procedure to the patient, and answer any questions he has.
➤ Obtain written informed consent.
➤ Obtain a wound culture if the bite occurred at least 3 days ago. Insert the culture swab to the wound base, and rotate it to collect as much exudate as possible.
➤ If the wound is new and isn't bleeding heavily (as with a puncture wound), wash it vigorously with soap and water for 5 to 10 minutes. Let it bleed a bit to help flush out pathogens. You can use a syringe and catheter to create a high-pressure water stream to clean the wound.

 **ALERT** Don't scrub a bite wound; you could bruise the tissue. Also, don't tape the wound or seal it in any way — doing so increases the risk of infection. Apply an ice pack to the wound site for 20 minutes to reduce edema and pain.
➤ Verify that the patient is not allergic to iodine or local anesthetics.
➤ If the wound involves an arm or a leg, place the extremity in an antiseptic bath for 15 to 20 minutes with warm water and antiseptic solution. For other areas, generously irrigate with equal parts of povidone-iodine and sterile saline solution. (The saline solution reduces the harmful effects of the povidone-iodine on healthy tissue.)
➤ Draw up lidocaine in the smallest syringe, using a 27G needle.
➤ Insert the needle at a 45-degree angle.
➤ Ask the patient if he notices any change in sensation. If he reports pain, indicating direct contact with the nerve, withdraw the needle 1 mm.
➤ Aspirate to make sure there is no blood return. If there is, the needle is in a blood vessel. Withdraw the needle slightly and reinsert in another area.
➤ Inject 1 to 2 ml of lidocaine while partially withdrawing the needle. Then redirect the needle across the surface, advance it, and inject another 0.5 ml while withdrawing the needle. This method distributes the anesthetic uniformly, providing the optimal effect in 5 to 15 minutes.
➤ Clean the wound using antiseptic solution and 4" × 4" gauze pads.
➤ Irrigate the wound with copious amounts of sterile saline solution, using a 60-ml syringe and a large-gauge (18G or 20G) needle.
➤ Put on sterile gloves and have the patient replicate the moment of injury, if a joint may be involved, to evaluate internal structures for damage. Then place the affected area in extension. Use the curved hemostat to separate the wound edges and the straight hemostat to thoroughly expose the wound for visualization of potential damage and debris, removing any devitalized tissue and foreign objects.
➤ Suture the wound as indicated. (Suturing is not indicated for initial treatment of human bites or if infection is suspected.)
➤ Apply topical antibiotic ointment and a dry sterile dressing.
➤ Administer tetanus prophylaxis as indicated: 0.5 ml of tetanus toxoid I.M. for a patient who has been immunized before but who hasn't had a booster within the past 5 years; 0.5 ml of tetanus toxoid and

## TREATING RABIES

When making decisions about how to treat rabies, you'll need to consider several factors, including the details of the exposure, the animal's species and vaccination status, and the prevalence of rabies in your region. The first step is to clean the wound thoroughly with soap and water. The table below provides general guidelines for which actions to take next. Note that the Food and Drug Administration (FDA) considers all three rabies vaccines equally safe and effective.

| SPECIES | ANIMAL'S CONDITION | TREATMENT |
| --- | --- | --- |
| **WILD** | | |
| Skunk<br>Raccoon<br>Bat<br>Other carnivores | Considered rabid unless proven negative (the animal should be killed and the head tested immediately; observation is not recommended) | Rabies immune globulin (RIG), human RIG* and human diploid cell vaccine (HDCV) or rabies vaccine (RVA), absorbed RVA** |
| **DOMESTIC** | | |
| Cat<br>Dog | Healthy and available: 10 days of isolation and observation | None |
| | Unknown (escaped) | Consult public health officials; if treatment is indicated, RIG* and HDCV or RVA** |
| **OTHER** | | |
| Livestock<br>Gnawing animals (such as hamsters, rabbits, and beavers) | Rabies suspected or known | RIG* and HDCV or RVA** (Consider individually.) |

*RIG should be administered at the beginning of treatment. Administer 20 IU/kg. Infiltrate the wound and then inject the rest I.M.

**HDCV and RVA are equally effective. Administer 1 ml of vaccine I.M. on days 0, 3, 7, 14, and 28. If using HDCV, divide the dose in half, giving one-half I.M. and one-half infiltrated thoroughly around the wound. HDCV is the only rabies vaccine approved by the FDA for intradermal use.

tetanus immune globulin for a patient who has never been immunized.

➤ Administer rabies prophylaxis, if rabies is possible, without delay after consulting with a physician. (See *Treating rabies*.)

➤ Prescribe antibiotics to nullify infection, as indicated.

## PATIENT TEACHING

➤ If the bite results in a puncture wound or a tear, advise the patient that bleeding may occur immediately, and bruising and swelling may appear later.

➤ Teach him that signs and symptoms of infection usually appear after 24 hours. Instruct him to call his practitioner for fever higher than 101° F (38.3° C); redness; increased swelling; cloudy, yellow, or green drainage; red streaks in the skin; or a lump in the wound that grows.

➤ Urge him to schedule and keep a follow-up appointment in 2 days so that you can evaluate his progress and check for infection.

➤ If he has a hand or foot injury, advise him that the follow-up visit is especially important because you'll need to check his neurovascular status. Tendon injuries aren't always apparent at initial presentation.

➤ Instruct the patient to urge any witness to the incident to report it to the authorities. (If the animal is wild, the authorities will try to capture it and confine it for 10 days for observation. If it appears rabid, it will be killed and its brain tissue tested for rabies.)

## COMPLICATIONS

➤ *Infection* is treated with antiseptic soaks and antibiotics four times a day.

➤ *Neurovascular compromise* may require surgical referral, and repair is possible up to 5 to 7 days after injury.

➤ *Bleeding, pain, tenderness, swelling, and decreased sensation at the injury site* are minimized by ice and elevation.

## SPECIAL CONSIDERATIONS

➤ Consult with a physician whenever you suspect that rabies is involved.

➤ For temperature elevations, request a complete blood count, erythrocyte sedimentation rate and, possibly, blood cultures.

➤ Over-the-counter analgesics (such as acetaminophen and ibuprofen) are usually adequate for pain relief.

➤ If puncture wounds are simple and don't involve the hands, no other treatment is necessary. Debride moderate to severe wounds, and give the patient phenoxymethylpenicillin for 3 to 5 days. If no signs or symptoms of infection appear after 2

days, close the wound with sutures or tape strips.

➤ For all human bites, obtain a wound culture to rule out gram-negative organisms. The patient should receive penicillin and a beta-lactamase-resistant penicillin-like anti-infective such as amoxicillin. Delay wound closure for 2 days; then close the wound if no infection is evident.

➤ Splint clenched-fist injuries, elevate them, and order X-rays to rule out fractures. Visualize the wounds fully to detect damage to internal structures and debris, such as tooth fragments. Because tendons can retract significantly, the patient must replicate the positioning of the hand when the injury occurred (tight fist). Once damage is ruled out, clean the wound with the hand in extension.

## DOCUMENTATION

➤ Before performing this procedure, document any abnormal physical findings on the consent form. Have the patient initial the comments and sign the form to signify acknowledgment of preprocedural abnormalities.

➤ Describe in detail the injury site before and after the procedure, including its location. Record your evaluation of any potentially affected function, range of motion, and sensation. Include the anesthetic type and amount used, any culture taken, the patient's reaction to the procedure, medications ordered, the time frame for follow-up evaluation, and any patient instructions given.

## Suturing of simple lacerations

### CPT CODES
*Note:* Precise code depends on wound size.

## USING A SKIN ADHESIVE

Many lacerations can be treated without sutures, using a skin adhesive such as Dermabond. It's quicker and less painful than suturing and may achieve better cosmetic results.

To use a skin adhesive, you must approximate the wound edges. While maintaining well-approximated closure, apply thin layers (usually three) of adhesive, with light brushstrokes of the applicator. Moisture on the skin's surface activates the adhesive. Full strength is achieved in about 2½ minutes.

Be sure to review appropriate wound care with the patient. Instruct him not to rub or scrub the wound area. Tell him to wet the site only briefly during showering and to pat it dry. If you applied a protective dressing, remind the patient not to let the tape touch the site or adhesive. Advise him to avoid prolonged sunlight and tanning lamps, particularly while the wound is fresh and the adhesive is in place. Similarly, advise him to avoid activities or environments likely to cause heavy perspiration and to refrain from applying other medications, lotions, or creams to the site; these actions can cause premature separation of the adhesive.

Follow up with the patient to check for infection and neurovascular compromise. Urge him to contact you if the wound edges separate. Advise him that the adhesive will wear off by itself in 5 to 10 days.

*Note:* Don't apply a skin adhesive if the wound involves subcutaneous approximation or if the patient has an infection, pressure sores, or hypersensitivity to cyanoacrylate or formaldehyde. Also consider a different method if the patient has deep wounds (the adhesive can penetrate below the dermal layer), wounds involving tension areas (such as the knuckles, elbows, and knees), or wounds of the scalp, mucosa, or periorbital area.

*12001 to 12007    Simple repair of superficial wounds on the scalp, neck, axillae, external genitalia, trunk, and extremities*

*12011 to 12018    Simple repair of superficial wounds on the face, ears, eyelids, nose, lips, and mucous membranes*
*12020    Treatment of superficial wound dehiscence and simple closure*
*12031 to 12037    Intermediate repair with layered closure of wounds of the scalp, axillae, trunk, and extremities (excluding hands and feet)*
*12041 to 12047    Intermediate layered closure of wounds of the neck, hands, feet, and external genitalia*
*12051 to 12057    Intermediate repair with layered closure of wounds of face, ears, eyelids, nose, lips, and mucous membranes*

## DESCRIPTION

Wounds may require the use of absorbable and nonabsorbable sutures, such as polypropylene (for example, Prolene) and nylon (for example, Monosof). Usually placed deep within a wound, absorbable sutures are absorbed into the body over time; nonabsorbable sutures are used at the wound surface and require removal. Some wounds may be closed with a skin adhesive (such as DERMABOND), which can reduce pain, shorten the time spent on wound closure, and provide a more aesthetically pleasing outcome. (See *Using a skin adhesive.*)

Suturing typically starts with a dermal layer of interrupted absorbable sutures. Such sutures are especially important in high-tension areas, where the risk of pulling apart is greatest.

Nonabsorbable sutures are used on the epidermal layer; these sutures allow for improved approximation and eversion of the wound edges, producing optimal cosmetic results.

A simple interrupted suture for the epidermal layer completely closes the wound. This type of suture offers the advantages of properly everting skin edges so that the wound lies flat when it spreads, lining up unequal wound edges, and allowing for regional variations of tension. It takes longer to close a wound with this suture than with a running suture, however.

Wounds closed by approximation of the skin edges heal by primary intention. Wounds heal faster under an occlusive or semiocclusive dressing, which prevents crust formation.

## INDICATIONS

➤ To repair surgical and traumatic disruptions of skin or tissue that won't heal naturally

## CONTRAINDICATIONS

### Relative
➤ Clinical risk factors for poor healing
➤ Dirty and infected wounds
➤ Contaminated wounds
➤ Malnutrition
➤ Diabetes
➤ Sepsis
➤ Chemotherapy
➤ Immunosuppression
➤ Peripheral vascular disease
➤ Obesity
➤ Radiation therapy
➤ Edema
➤ Foreign bodies
➤ Tension on wound edge
➤ Pressure over a bony prominence
➤ Dog and cat bites
➤ Human bites

## EQUIPMENT

20- to 60-ml syringe with a 20G plastic I.V. cannula ◆ sterile saline solution ◆ antiseptic solution (such as povidone-iodine) ◆ smooth or multitooth forceps ◆ needle holder ◆ scissors ◆ scalpel, if needed ◆ sterile gloves ◆ sutures ◆ needles (round and tapered for mucosa, fascia, and muscle) ◆ injectable anesthetic (such as lidocaine) ◆ 4″ × 4″ gauze dressings ◆ non-adherent dressing ◆ antibiotic ointment ◆ tape

## ESSENTIAL STEPS

➤ Explain the procedure to the patient, and address his questions or concerns.
➤ Obtain informed consent.
➤ Place the patient in a comfortable position that allows full wound visualization.
➤ Wash your hands and put on gloves.
➤ Verify that the patient is not allergic to iodine or local anesthetics.
➤ Clean the wound with povidone-iodine solution in a circular pattern from the wound edges outward.
➤ Anesthetize the skin along each side of the wound. First on one side, and then the other, insert the needle containing the anesthetic at a 45-degree angle. Ask the patient if he notices any change in sensation. If he reports pain, indicating direct contact with the nerve, withdraw the needle 1 mm. Aspirate to make sure there is no blood return. If there is, the needle is in a blood vessel. Withdraw the needle slightly and redirect it to another area. Inject lidocaine slowly along the length of the wound as you partially withdraw the needle. Then redirect the needle across the surface, advance it, and inject while withdrawing the needle. This method distributes the anesthetic uniformly, providing the optimal effect in 5 to 15 minutes.
➤ Examine the wound to its base for foreign bodies or injury to underlying structures, such as a tendon or joint capsule.
➤ Use the syringe and I.V. cannula to irrigate the wound with antiseptic or sterile saline solution. Some practitioners recommend equal parts antiseptic and sterile saline solution to decrease tissue toxicity except for very dirty wounds.
➤ Trim and undermine wound edges as needed to provide effective approximation.
➤ Using your dominant hand, grasp the suture needle securely with the needle holder. Use a toothed forceps in your other hand

to stabilize the wound edge in a slightly everted position.

➤ Insert the needle at a right angle through the skin about ¼″ to ¾″ (0.5 to 2 cm) from the wound edge. Grasp the needle from the exterior with the needle holder. Before inserting the needle again, be sure the tissue layers are well approximated with minimal tension.

➤ Repeat the process and then tie the suture, being careful not to pull the suture edges too taut.

➤ Use scissors to trim jagged edges from the wound.

➤ As appropriate, place a vertical mattress suture in the middle of the wound and bisect each half sequentially with vertical mattress sutures. (See *Choosing a suture technique*.)

➤ After approximating skin edges, fill in the remaining gaps with simple interrupted stitches.

➤ Remove redundant cones of skin (called "dog ears") to optimize the cosmetic result. Excise the residual skin by making a small ellipse that extends the defect or by making an incision that lifts the dog ear with the skin hook and drapes excess tissue over the side of the wound.

➤ To help equalize tension on wound edges, make a "hockey stick" incision, an angled incision that extends one end of the wound in the shape of a hockey stick. This incision creates a curvilinear line that allows for approximation of skin edges without placing undue tension on any specific point along the line.

➤ After suturing the wound, compress the wound gently and look for residual bleeding. Use direct pressure for 5 minutes to minimize swelling and bleeding from the wound edge.

➤ Cover the site with a three-layer pressure dressing by applying a thin layer of antibiotic ointment, a nonadherent dressing, and 4″ × 4″ gauze pads with tape to secure it. Apply pressure to the site. Leave this in place for 24 hours.

➤ Splint if necessary.

➤ Prescribe an antibiotic, such as cephalexin, if the area is infected.

➤ Administer tetanus prophylaxis if the patient hasn't been immunized within the past 5 years.

## PATIENT TEACHING

➤ Instruct the patient to keep the sutures dry.

➤ Tell him to remove the initial dressing in 24 hours.

➤ Teach him to clean the wound site twice daily with soap and water (no rubbing or scrubbing of the wound) and to cover it with antibiotic ointment.

➤ Teach him how to apply the nonadherent dressing, the 4″ × 4″ gauze pads, and the tape to form a pressure dressing.

➤ Tell him to switch to a thin layer of antibiotic ointment and a smaller gauze bandage when drainage no longer appears on the large dressing. Caution him not to place the gauze itself directly over the wound. (Fibers in the gauze can get trapped in the wound edge, become matted, and delay healing.)

➤ Advise him to use over-the-counter analgesics, such as acetaminophen or ibuprofen, to manage pain.

➤ Instruct him to notify you promptly if he experiences signs and symptoms of infection (increasing redness, swelling, pain, and warmth; cloudy yellow, green, or brown drainage; opening of wound; foul odor; a red streak from wound area; or fever).

➤ Have him schedule a follow-up appointment so that you can remove the sutures and check for signs of infection or nerve damage.

## CHOOSING A SUTURE TECHNIQUE

The most commonly used suture techniques include the simple continuous, simple interrupted, and horizontal and vertical mattress sutures. The type of suture technique used depends on the site, shape, size, and depth of the wound.

The space left between sutures also varies, according to the wound's location or the amount of tension applied to the wound. For instance, the space between sutures in most wounds is about 0.25 cm, but you should place sutures even closer for facial wounds or those associated with high tension, such as those on the elbow or knee.

The four common suture techniques and their advantages are shown here.

### Simple continuous
Simple continuous sutures provide even tension across the incision and are used for quick repair.

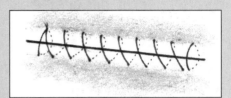

### Simple interrupted
Simple interrupted sutures allow precise approximation of wound edges.

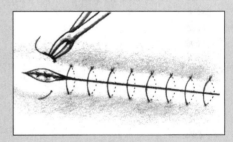

### Horizontal mattress
Horizontal mattress sutures reduce dead space within the wound and reinforce subcutaneous tissue.

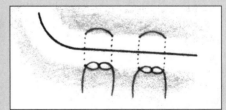

### Vertical mattress
Vertical mattress sutures also reduce dead space within the wound and reinforce subcutaneous tissue. They're used in thick skin, such as in the palms or the soles, and in lax skin, but they're difficult to approximate and take more time to place.

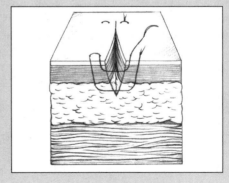

## SELECTING NONABSORBABLE SUTURE MATERIALS

Nonabsorbable suture materials are commonly chosen based on the type of tissue surrounding the wound site. The following chart shows which type of suture works best in each type of tissue.

| TISSUE TYPE | SUTURE MATERIAL |
| --- | --- |
| Skin | Nylon (Ethilon), polypropylene (Prolene), silk, or polyester fiber (Mersilene) |
| Subcutaneous tissue | Chromic gut or polyglycolic, polylactic acid (such as Dexon or Vicryl) |
| Subcuticular tissue | Nylon (Ethilon) |
| Fascia | Polyglactin 910 (coated Vicryl) or silk |
| Mucosa | Plain gut |

## COMPLICATIONS

➤ *Infection* may be treated with local or systemic antibiotics and antiseptic soaks. It may also require consultation with a physician, a dermatologist, or an infectious disease specialist.

➤ *Scarring and keloids* are minimized with gentle handling and the use of such techniques as undermining and layered suturing.

## SPECIAL CONSIDERATIONS

 **ALERT** Refer the patient to a plastic surgeon for debridement or if the wound has a large amount of dead space (expect drain placement).

➤ Lidocaine with epinephrine at a concentration of 1:100,000 may be used, except in wounds involving an appendage (such as the nose, the penis, or a digit).

➤ Scalp sutures should be removed in 6 to 8 days; face sutures, in 3 to 5 days; abdomen and chest sutures, in 7 to 10 days; upper-extremity sutures, in 7 to 8 days; lower-extremity sutures, in 7 to 14 days; and back sutures, in 10 to 14 days.

➤ To avoid infection, the wound should be closed within 6 hours of injury.

➤ For embedded sutures, absorbable material is required because it dissolves over time. Absorption rate varies according to the material selected, based on the patient's needs: plain gut (7 to 14 days), chromic gut (20 to 40 days), and polyglycolic acid synthetic and polyglactin 910 (60 to 90 days).

➤ For nonabsorbable sutures, selection is usually based on the suture site (see *Selecting nonabsorbable suture materials*).

## DOCUMENTATION

➤ Before performing this procedure, document any abnormal physical findings on the consent form. Have the patient initial the comments and sign the form to signify acknowledgment of preprocedural abnormalities. In the chart, the preprocedural and postprocedural notes must include an evaluation of potentially affected function, range of motion, and sensation.

➤ Record indications for and details of the procedure. Describe the wound site before and after the procedure, any preprocedural abnormalities in function, the type and amount of anesthetic used, the patient's reaction to the procedure, medications ordered, the time frame for follow-up evaluation, and any patient instructions given.

# Ring removal

CPT CODE
*26989 Unlisted procedure, hands or fingers*

## DESCRIPTION

Many patients come to the office, clinic, or emergency department for removal of a ring or other constricting band from an edematous finger or toe when they can't remove the object at home. Trauma, weight gain, fluid retention, arthritic changes, I.V. infusion infiltration, general soft-tissue swelling from sunburn, dependent edema, or allergic reaction may cause a ring to constrict the digit, resulting in pain, hypoxia, and neurovascular compromise. Children may also cause neurovascular compromise by placing circular or oval objects, such as pull tabs or toys, on a finger or toe.

The least invasive means of ring removal remains lubrication and circular traction. If this method fails, the string wrap method may be attempted; although this procedure can be painful and is time-consuming, it does retain the integrity of the ring. If all other attempts fail, the ring should be removed by cutting the band with a ring cutter, orthopedic pin cutter, or hand-operated circular saw. All cutting methods pose an additional risk to the patient, involving potential cuts or abrasions from the equipment and the possibility of metal shavings, which may lead to foreign-body granuloma if left undetected.

## INDICATIONS

➤ To relieve chronic or acute edema and prevent vascular compromise in a finger or toe constricted by a ring or other metal band

## CONTRAINDICATIONS

### Relative

➤ Open wound or finger fracture
➤ Deeply embedded ring erosion
➤ Lack of appropriate cutting tools

## EQUIPMENT

2% lidocaine without epinephrine (optional) ◆ water-soluble lubricant (optional) ◆ 3-ml syringe and 27G needle (optional) ◆ 3' (0.9 m) of string (polyester fiber strip such as no. 1 Mersilene, umbilical tape or 1-0 silk suture) ◆ small hemostat ◆ manual or electric ring cutter with new blade ◆ two large hemostats ◆ 20-ml syringe filled with water

## ESSENTIAL STEPS

 **ALERT** Even if the patient tells you he has tried to remove the object from the finger at home, it's generally worthwhile to attempt removal with a water-soluble lubricant before trying other techniques. The pain from constriction often prevents the patient from applying adequate circular traction to remove the ring. Having the patient place his finger or toe in a cup of icy water for 10 minutes may reduce the edema enough to effect removal with lubrication and circular traction.

➤ Explain the procedure to the patient. If the ring is to be cut off, obtain written consent for cutting and removing the ring. Lubrication and string removal don't require written consent.

 **ALERT** Some practitioners advocate using a digital block before these procedures to reduce pain and make the patient more comfortable and cooperative. Remember, though, that lidocaine will cause additional edema. If it's necessary to use a digital block, use the least amount of lidocaine necessary to obtain anesthesia. *Never* use any product containing epineph-

## USING THE STRING METHOD

If lubrication and circular traction are ineffective in removing a patient's ring, your next option is to use the string method. Forewarn the patient that this procedure will be uncomfortable; injecting an anesthetic can cause additional problems due to vasoconstriction.

Lubricate the ring finger lightly with water-soluble lubricant. Grasp one end of the string in the jaws of the hemostat. Slide the tip of the hemostat under the ring on the palmar surface with the jaws pointing proximally. Pull enough string through so that you can grasp it firmly later. Tape the string in place.

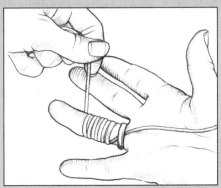

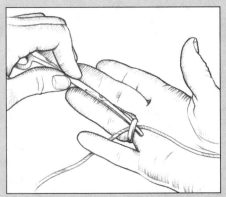

Wrap the string firmly around the finger, beginning adjacent to the ring margin. Wrap the string in a smooth, single layer, progressing from proximal to distal until it covers the area of greatest swelling, compressing the edematous tissue as you progress.

Place a small amount of lubricant over the string to facilitate sliding the ring. Remove the tape from the proximal end and pull the string distally, sliding the ring over the wrapped string and off the finger. If the ring hasn't traversed the entire area of edema, repeat the string wrapping process until the ring is removed.

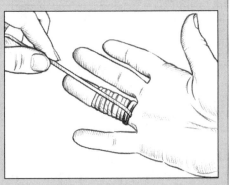

---

rine in a finger or toe because epinephrine exerts a vasoconstrictive effect.

### String wrap method
➤ Lubricate the ring finger lightly with water-soluble lubricant.
➤ Use the string wrap method to remove the ring. (See *Using the string method.*)
➤ Reassess neurosensory and neurovascular function.

### Ring cutter removal
➤ Place the small hook of the ring cutter (called the ring cutter guard) under the ring on the palmar surface (see *Using a ring cutter*).
➤ Hold the ring cutter firmly in your nondominant hand and apply steady, firm, downward pressure on the handle while turning the cutter blade with your dominant hand.

## USING A RING CUTTER

Whether you use a manual, a battery-operated, or an electric ring cutter, you'll follow the same procedure. Place the ring cutter guard under the ring on the palmar surface of the patient's hand to protect the tissue from the cutting blade. Then turn the "key" that causes the blade to cut through the ring, as shown.

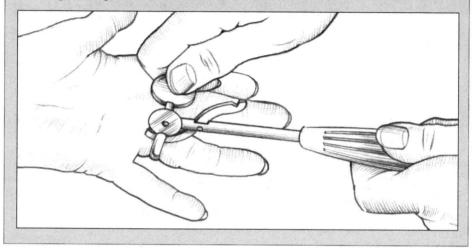

 **ALERT** Inexpensive rings are generally the most difficult to cut because they are composed of a number of alloys and very little silver or gold. They usually require extensive cutting and may require more than one blade to complete the job.

 **ALERT** Some very hard rings require extensive cutting. The friction caused by the cutting may produce an uncomfortable amount of heat in the ring and the patient's hand. Ask the patient if he's comfortable, and regularly check the temperature of the ring and cutter blade with your own fingers. Stop briefly to allow the ring and cutter to cool down if necessary.

➤ When cutting is complete, grasp each of the cut ends with a large hemostat and spread the ring edges with a steady opposing force.

➤ Irrigate the skin with high-pressure water to remove any metal particles.

➤ Reassess neurovascular and neurosensory function.

## PATIENT TEACHING

➤ Warn the patient that either method will cause some pain due to the edema in the digit and the nature of the removal technique.

➤ Tell the patient that pain should resolve within 1 to 2 hours and edema should resolve within 24 hours or as indicated by initial trauma to the digit. All symptoms should resolve within 48 hours.

➤ Tell the patient that no follow-up is needed unless complications arise.

➤ Instruct the patient to apply an ice pack to the digit for 20 minutes four times daily for 36 to 48 hours to relieve edema and pain.

➤ Advise the patient to take ibuprofen or acetaminophen for pain relief every 4 to 6 hours as needed.

➤ Caution the patient to avoid constricting objects on fingers and toes and to remove rings from digits when edema is possible.

➤ Instruct the patient to contact you promptly if he experiences signs and symptoms of infection (such as warmth, increased edema, and pain).

## COMPLICATIONS

➤ *Infection* may be treated with an appropriate topical antibiotic. Soak the area in warm salt water four or five times daily. Oral antibiotics may be needed for extensive infection.
➤ *Skin abrasion or a cut from a cutting tool* may be treated by washing with an antimicrobial and then applying an antibiotic ointment.

## SPECIAL CONSIDERATIONS

 **ALERT** Inability to remove a ring requires immediate referral to emergency care. Have the patient hold an ice pack over the digit and elevate it as much as possible while in transit.
➤ Explain to the patient that the cut in the ring is a straight line that a jeweler can usually repair. Carefully clean the ring and store it safely in a container, and return it to the patient or significant other as soon as possible. Most rings (such as wedding bands, family heirlooms, and gifts from loved ones) hold great sentimental value to patients. Treat the cutting and removal with respect.
➤ When removing rings or other objects from children, use age-appropriate language. Allow the parent to stay with and hold the child during the procedure. Allow the child to examine the equipment if appropriate.
➤ When you suspect a fracture, order X-ray studies as indicated, to be performed before or after the ring removal.
➤ The patient may request that the ring not be removed. If edema is expected to be transient and vascular compromise isn't expected, conservative management may be tried. Instruct the patient to elevate the affected area and intermittently apply ice or cold compresses to the site until able to slide the ring off. Review signs and symptoms that indicate vascular compromise and the risk for losing his finger.

## DOCUMENTATION

➤ Before performing this procedure, document any abnormal physical findings on the consent form. Have the patient initial the comments and sign the form to signify acknowledgment of preprocedural abnormalities. In the chart, the preprocedural and postprocedural notes must include an evaluation of potentially affected function, range of motion, and sensation. Be certain to document evidence of skin breakdown or concomitant injury.
➤ Note that you obtained written consent for removal with a cutter and that you discussed the options and risks at length.
➤ Indicate the disposition of the ring.
➤ If the patient declines ring removal, document that you informed him of the risks of losing his finger, the warning signs and symptoms indicating he should seek emergency ring removal, and care measures for his finger.

## Topical hemostasis

CPT CODE
No specific code has been assigned.

## DESCRIPTION

Topical hemostatic agents are used to rapidly control and stop bleeding from capillaries and small surface vessels. Application of a hemostatic agent is a quick, easy, and usually painless procedure that can be performed in the office or in an acute care setting without the use of electrocautery.

Various hemostatic agents are available; your selection will depend on product availability, the area of the body involved, the patient's sensitivity to the product, and the degree of tissue staining possible.

Products commonly used to control bleeding include silver nitrate, aluminum chloride 30%, Monsel's solution (ferric subsulfate), and epinephrine (topical and injectable). All are fast-acting, very effective, and inexpensive. However, the likelihood of staining and necrosis is low to moderate with aluminum chloride 30%, moderate with Monsel's solution, high with larger doses of epinephrine (topical or injectable), and highest with silver nitrate.

## INDICATIONS

➤ To stop bleeding from skin lesions, superficial tissue lacerations, broken capillaries, or small blood vessels

## CONTRAINDICATIONS

### Relative

➤ History of cardiovascular disease
➤ Highly visible area (if staining likely)
➤ Potential for development of ischemia and necrosis resulting from vasoconstriction of a finger or toe

## EQUIPMENT

Topical hemostatic agent of choice ◆ field drape ◆ gloves ◆ sterile 4″× 4″ gauze pads ◆ large cotton-tipped applicator ◆ tape

## ESSENTIAL STEPS

➤ Verify that the patient is not allergic to topical medications.
➤ Explain all steps to the patient to ensure cooperation and relieve anxiety.
➤ Obtain informed consent, if applicable.
➤ Prepare the field and set up the equipment.

➤ Place the patient in a comfortable position that fully exposes the site.
➤ Assess the type of lesion or laceration, direct and surrounding skin tissue responses, estimated blood loss, and the patient's mental status.
➤ Select an appropriate hemostatic product based on your assessment of the wound site and the advantages and disadvantages of the product to the skin site and surrounding tissue area.
➤ Drape the area.
➤ Put on gloves.
➤ Apply direct pressure to the site with 4″× 4″ sterile gauze pads; blot the site.
➤ Apply the topical hemostatic product, using direct pressure with a cotton-tipped applicator or sterile gauze (depending on the wound site) for approximately 15 seconds.
➤ Clean off excess blood at the site and surrounding tissue.
➤ Repeat the application, if necessary to complete hemostasis.
➤ Assess the wound site.
➤ Apply sterile 4″× 4″ gauze and tape, if necessary.
➤ If appropriate, give a tetanus immunization before the patient leaves the office. Administer tetanus prophylaxis for a deep, dirty wound if the patient hasn't had one in the past 5 years and for a clean, superficial wound if the patient hasn't had one in the past 10 years.

## PATIENT TEACHING

➤ Advise the patient that bleeding should stop immediately after application of the hemostatic agent. Assure him that he should feel little if any pain or discomfort. Explain that the site may be red for the first 24 to 48 hours.
➤ Tell the patient to call you if he experiences recurrence of bleeding, increased pain or discomfort, or signs of infection (such as fever, red surrounding tissue,

swelling, and colored drainage from the site).

➤ Advise the patient to use a mild analgesic such as ibuprofen, if necessary, for site pain or discomfort.

➤ Inform him that site tissue staining may not resolve and could be permanent.

## COMPLICATIONS

➤ *Tissue staining* is possible, depending on the hemostatic agent used.

## SPECIAL CONSIDERATIONS

➤ Evaluate potentially negative cosmetic effects that could occur when using a particular agent with staining possibilities.

➤ Because of its high vasoconstrictive potential with epinephrine, don't use topical hemostasis on body appendages (such as the fingers and nose) if permanent damage can occur from ischemia or necrosis.

## DOCUMENTATION

➤ Before performing this procedure, document any abnormal physical findings on the consent form. Have the patient initial the comments and sign the form to signify acknowledgment of preprocedural abnormalities. In the chart, the preprocedural and postprocedural notes must include an evaluation of potentially affected function, range of motion, and sensation.

➤ Note that informed consent was received, if necessary; consent should indicate that options and risks (specifically for staining and necrosis) were discussed and that the patient agreed to treatment.

➤ Record the results of the site assessment before and after the procedure, the type of hemostatic agent used, the patient's response to the procedure, and the patient's understanding of your instructions.

# ROUTINE PROCEDURES

## Anesthesia: topical and local

CPT CODE
No specific code has been assigned. (Usually included as part of procedure being performed.)

## DESCRIPTION

Anesthesia causes loss of sensation and is beneficial in many situations, such as surgery. Factors that affect the type, amount, and duration of anesthetic needed include the local blood supply, the presence of infection, the effects of certain chronic diseases, the size of the affected area, the diameter and conduction of nerve fibers, and psychological factors, such as anxiety and pain threshold.

## INDICATIONS

➤ To render the patient incapable of feeling pain during surgical repair (such as incision and drainage), laceration repair, biopsy, foreign-body removal, and dislocation reduction

## CONTRAINDICATIONS

### Absolute
➤ Allergy (to a specific anesthetic)
➤ History of hypersensitivity reaction to a specific anesthetic

### Relative
➤ Cellulitis
➤ Compromised circulation

## EQUIPMENT

Anesthetic such as eutectic mixture of local anesthetic (EMLA), ice, ethyl chloride, or anesthetic such as 1% to 2% lidocaine with or without a vasoconstricting agent ◆ antiseptic skin cleaner such as povidone-iodine solution ◆ normal saline solution ◆ gloves ◆ appropriate-sized syringe for site ◆ 25G to 30G ½" to 1" needle ◆ occlusive dressing (optional) ◆ soap (optional) ◆ acetone or rubbing alcohol (optional)

## ESSENTIAL STEPS

➤ Verify that the patient is not allergic to iodine, topical medications, or local anesthetics.
➤ Place the patient in a comfortable position with the affected area fully exposed.
➤ Put on gloves.
➤ Remove visible debris by irrigating the area with normal saline solution.
➤ Clean the site and surrounding area with povidone-iodine solution.

### For topical anesthesia of intact skin

➤ Remove oils from the skin with soap, acetone, or alcohol.
➤ Apply EMLA and an occlusive dressing for 1 to 2 hours.

### For topical short-term anesthesia of intact skin

➤ Rub the skin firmly with ice for 10 seconds, or spray with ethyl chloride for no longer than 2 seconds (to reduce the risk of blistering).

### For local anesthesia

➤ Draw up the anesthetic into the syringe, using the appropriate-sized needle.
➤ Identify the appropriate injection site. For digital anesthesia, use anterior and posterior web spaces of the digit, close to the bone.

➤ Insert the needle at a 45-degree angle.
➤ Ask the patient if he notices any change in sensation. If he reports pain, indicating direct contact with the nerve, withdraw the needle 1 mm.
➤ Aspirate to make sure there is no blood return. If there is, the needle is in a blood vessel. Withdraw the needle slightly and reinsert it in another area.
➤ Inject 1 to 2 ml of lidocaine while partially withdrawing the needle. Then redirect the needle across the surface, advance it, and inject another 0.5 ml while withdrawing the needle. This method distributes the anesthetic uniformly, providing the optimal effect.
➤ Wait for the local anesthetic to work before beginning the procedure. The maximum effect should occur in 5 to 15 minutes.

## PATIENT TEACHING

➤ Tell the patient that full sensation usually returns within 2 hours.

 **ALERT** Urge the patient to contact you if he experiences changes in sensation lasting longer than 2 hours or notices signs or symptoms of infection (increasing redness, swelling, pain, and warmth; cloudy yellow, green, or brown drainage; opening of wound; foul odor; red streak from wound area; or fever).

## COMPLICATIONS

➤ *Ice or ethyl chloride blistering* is prevented by avoiding excessive freezing.

## SPECIAL CONSIDERATIONS

➤ EMLA is indicated for use on intact skin when required penetration is less than or equal to 5 mm. EMLA penetrates more quickly in diseased tissues and is contraindicated for use on mucous membranes and genitalia. The duration of action of EMLA is 2 hours after removal of the agent.

➤ Ice or ethyl chloride is useful for such procedures as skin tag clipping and before injecting a local anesthetic as its duration of action is less than 3 seconds.

➤ An anesthetic without a vasoconstrictor is used for poorly vascularized, infected areas and for immunocompromised patients. The addition of sodium bicarbonate (1 mg/ml:10 ml of a 1% concentration of anesthetic) will significantly reduce the anesthetic's initial burning sensation.

➤ An anesthetic with a vasoconstrictor such as epinephrine is best used for a clean wound in a highly vascular area to reduce bleeding and systemic absorption.

 **ALERT** A vasoconstrictor is contraindicated for use in extremities (such as the digits, nose, ear, and penis); in patients with vascular disorders, diabetes, or thyrotoxicosis; and in areas with compromised blood flow (such as a skin flap).

➤ Topical anesthesia is indicated for nosebleeds and eye injuries and before painful procedures on mucous membranes.

➤ Topical lidocaine starts working in under 5 minutes. A dose of 1 to 2 drops of tetracaine (0.5%) is indicated before examination of an eye injury and has an onset of action of 5 to 8 minutes. These drugs readily penetrate mucous membranes. Topical phenylephrine can also cause vasoconstriction. Most topical anesthetics have a duration of action of 30 to 45 minutes.

➤ Duration of anesthesia for a nerve block is 30 minutes to 1 hour. The duration of action increases if a vasoconstrictor (such as epinephrine) is also used.

## DOCUMENTATION

➤ Before performing this procedure, document any abnormal physical findings on the consent form. Have the patient initial the comments and sign the form to signify acknowledgment of preprocedural abnormalities. In the chart, the preprocedural and postprocedural notes must include an evaluation of potentially affected function, range of motion, and sensation.

➤ Record the type and amount of anesthetic used.

# Abscess incision and drainage

**CPT CODES**
*10060   Incision and drainage of abscess, single or simple*
*10061   Incision and drainage of abscess, multiple or complicated*
*10080   Incision and drainage of pilonidal cyst, simple*
*10081   Incision and drainage of pilonidal cyst, complicated*

## DESCRIPTION

An abscess is a local collection of pus in a cavity formed by tissue breakdown and surrounded by inflamed tissue. The pressure, tissue damage, and pain can be relieved by incising and draining the abscess. Abscesses typically result from *Staphylococcus aureus* or a streptococcal infection. Males and children have a higher incidence of abscess formation than adult females.

Specific types of abscesses include furuncles, pilonidal cysts, and perianal cysts. Furuncles, or boils, occur in hair follicles or sweat glands. Pilonidal cysts result from ingrown hairs close to the anus and may have sinus openings. Perianal cysts typically result from a rectal fistula.

## INDICATIONS

➤ To relieve the pressure and pain associated with an abscess (furuncle, pilonidal cyst, perianal cyst) that doesn't resolve with application of warm compresses

# CONTRAINDICATIONS

## Relative

➤ Cellulitis
➤ Coagulopathies
➤ Facial furuncles located within the triangle of the nose and the corners of the mouth
➤ Diabetes
➤ Immunosuppression

# EQUIPMENT

Antiseptic skin cleaner (such as povidone-iodine) ◆ topical anesthetic (such as ethyl chloride or a tissue freezing kit) ◆ 1% to 2% lidocaine with or without epinephrine or 50 mg/ml diphenhydramine (Benadryl) ◆ 3- to 10-ml syringe ◆ 25G to 30G ½" needle ◆ 16G to 18G needle ◆ 4" × 4" sterile gauze pads ◆ #11 scalpel ◆ sterile drape ◆ sterile gloves ◆ sterile curved hemostat ◆ iodoform gauze ◆ culture swab (optional) ◆ sterile scissors ◆ tape ◆ protective eyewear (optional)

# ESSENTIAL STEPS

➤ Explain the procedure to the patient, and answer any questions he has.
➤ Obtain informed consent.
➤ Position the patient comfortably, with the abscess exposed.
➤ Verify that the patient is not allergic to iodine.
➤ Clean the site and surrounding area with an antiseptic skin cleaner.
➤ Wear protective eyewear if abscess contents appear under pressure.
➤ Apply the sterile drape and put on sterile gloves.
➤ Anesthetize the area by spraying the surface with a topical anesthetic until it appears frosted or by injecting the perimeter with lidocaine solution, using a small gauge (25G to 30G ½") needle on a 3-ml syringe.

➤ With the scalpel, make an incision deep and wide enough to allow purulent material to drain easily and to prevent premature closure.
➤ Insert the culture swab deep into the wound to collect material for culturing if culture is indicated. (Alternatively, you can use a 16G or 18G needle and a syringe to withdraw fluid for culturing before incising.)
➤ Use curved hemostat to explore the cavity and break down membranes leading to other fluid-filled compartments.
➤ After expressing all purulent material, pack the cavity with iodoform gauze, leaving at least ¼" (0.6 cm) of gauze extending outside the wound.
➤ Dress the wound with sterile gauze and tape.
➤ Prescribe broad-spectrum antibiotic prophylaxis, such as cephalexin or cefadroxil.
➤ Prescribe a narcotic analgesic (such as Tylenol #3) the first day.
➤ Prescribe a nonsteroidal anti-inflammatory drug (such as ibuprofen) to be used after the first day.

# PATIENT TEACHING

➤ Tell the patient that he can expect immediate pain relief when the abscess is drained.
➤ Advise him of alternatives to abscess incision and drainage, such as application of warm compresses.
➤ Emphasize the importance of thorough hand washing and appropriate changing of the site dressing.
➤ Have him return for a follow-up visit in 2 days.
➤ Explain that healing can take up to 3 weeks.
➤ Instruct the patient with a pilonidal cyst to take a sitz bath four times a day. Tell him to clean and irrigate the area with a flexible shower hose or water from a squeeze bottle and to leave the wound open

to air to promote drainage and healing. Explain that the wound must heal from the inside outward, which can take an additional 2 months.

 **ALERT** Urge the patient to notify you promptly if he experiences signs and symptoms of infection (increasing redness, swelling, pain, and warmth; cloudy yellow, green, or brown drainage; opening of wound; foul odor; a red streak from the wound area; or fever).

## COMPLICATIONS

➤ *Recurrence or worsening of symptoms, cellulitis, and gangrene* warrant collaboration with or referral to a physician, a surgeon, or an infectious disease specialist. Extensive debridement and I.V. antibiotics may be required.
➤ *Pain and scarring* are minimized by use of pain medications, antibiotics, aseptic technique, and skilled wound closure.
➤ *Chronic anal fistula* is common after perianal abscess incision and drainage and requires a referral to a surgeon for fistulectomy.
➤ *Hand, joint, or facial involvement* warrants referral to a specialist.
➤ *An abscess close to blood vessels, nerves, or tendons* warrants referral to a specialist.

## SPECIAL CONSIDERATIONS

➤ Don't inject lidocaine into the abscess; lidocaine loses its effectiveness in an acidic environment.
➤ Breast abscesses, excluding those in the subareolar area, are rare and should be biopsied to rule out malignancy. Local breast infection introduced through the nipple during breast-feeding is the only common cause of subareolar abscess.
➤ For paronychia under the nail, use a hot needle to bore through the nail and facilitate drainage. Partial removal of the nail may be necessary.
➤ For a pilonidal cyst, position the patient in the left lateral or lithotomy position.

Probe the sinus tracts with a cotton-tipped applicator. If the abscess is more than 5 mm deep, refer the patient to a surgeon. For a pilonidal cyst less than 5 mm in depth, perform elliptical excision.
➤ Certain patient populations require more stringent observation after the procedure. A history of diabetes, a compromised immune system, or a debilitating disease indicates a need for increased vigilance. Consider sending an aspiration or swab specimen for culture and sensitivity testing to help you detect and efficiently treat unusual organisms.

## DOCUMENTATION

➤ Before performing this procedure, document any abnormal physical findings on the consent form. Have the patient initial the comments and sign the form to signify acknowledgment of preprocedural abnormalities. In the chart, the preprocedural and postprocedural notes must include an evaluation of potentially affected function, range of motion, and neurosensory testing (such as two-point discrimination).
➤ Note whether a culture was sent to the laboratory.
➤ Describe the site before and after the procedure, the type and amount of anesthetic used, the characteristics of the drainage, the patient's reaction to the procedure, medications ordered, the time frame for follow-up evaluation, and any instructions given to the patient.

# Cyst injection, ganglion

### CPT CODES
*20550   Injection, tendon sheath, ligament, trigger point, or ganglion cyst*
*20600   Arthrocentesis, aspiration, or injection of a small joint, bursa, or ganglion cyst (leg, fingers, toes)*

*20605   Arthrocentesis, aspiration, or injection of an intermediate joint, bursa, or ganglion cyst (temporomandibular, acromioclavicular, wrist, elbow, ankle, olecranon bursa)*

## DESCRIPTION

A ganglion cyst is a tumor that develops on or in a tendon sheath. The most common cause is chronic or recurrent inflammation from frequent strains or contusions at the site. Joints contain a thick, gel-like material. When this gel leaks from the joint into the weakened tendon sheath, it forms a cyst that not only is cosmetically unappealing but also may inhibit function and cause discomfort. Injection of an anesthetic with or without a steroid into the ganglion cyst provides pain relief and often increases range of motion. These benefits may not be permanent, however.

## INDICATIONS

➤ To relieve discomfort and joint mobility interference caused by a ganglion cyst

## CONTRAINDICATIONS

### Absolute
➤ Cellulitis
➤ Infection

### Relative
➤ Coagulopathies

## EQUIPMENT

Antiseptic skin cleaner such as povidone-iodine ◆ sterile drape ◆ sterile gloves ◆ 3- and 10-ml syringes ◆ 18G 1½″ needle ◆ 22G or 25G 1½″ needle ◆ 1% lidocaine ◆ culture tube ◆ corticosteroid: short-acting (such as hydrocortisone 20 mg), intermediate (such as methylprednisolone 4 mg), or long-acting (such as dexamethasone 0.6 mg) ◆ sterile 4″ × 4″ gauze pads ◆ tape

## ESSENTIAL STEPS

➤ Verify that the patient is not allergic to iodine.
➤ Explain the procedure to the patient, and answer any questions he has.
➤ Obtain informed consent.
➤ Position the patient comfortably, with the cyst clearly exposed.
➤ Clean the site and surrounding area with povidone-iodine solution and gauze pads.
➤ Apply the sterile drape and put on sterile gloves.
➤ Use a 22G or 25G needle with the 3-ml syringe to draw up 2.5 ml of 1% lidocaine and 0.5 ml of corticosteroid. Agitate gently.
➤ Using the 10-ml syringe with the 18G needle, insert the needle into the cyst and aspirate. If the aspirate appears cloudy, send the specimen for culture and sensitivity testing and continue the procedure; if the return is bloody, remove the needle, apply a dressing, and end the procedure.
➤ Unscrew the syringe and replace it with the second syringe that contains lidocaine and corticosteroid, and aspirate for blood. If no blood appears, inject the medications.
➤ Remove the needle and apply a pressure dressing.

## PATIENT TEACHING

➤ Instruct the patient to leave the dressing on for 12 hours.
➤ Explain that some redness, oozing, swelling, and warmth are normal.
➤ Advise him to rest and elevate the joint for 24 hours.
➤ Recommend a nonnarcotic analgesic, such as acetaminophen or ibuprofen, for pain.
➤ Have the patient schedule a follow-up appointment in 1 week.

➤ Urge the patient to call you promptly if he experiences signs and symptoms of infection (rapidly increasing redness, swelling, pain, and warmth; cloudy yellow, green, or brown drainage; opening of wound; foul odor; red streak from wound area; or fever).

## COMPLICATIONS

➤ *Recurrence* is possible. Before giving a second injection, consider the effectiveness of the first one. Refer the patient to a surgeon if warranted.
➤ *Corticosteroid flare (increased pain after cyst injection)* is rare but very painful. Manage the patient's pain with ice application and nonsteroidal drug administration. If fever occurs or the condition doesn't resolve within 72 hours, however, corticosteroid flare is an unlikely cause of symptoms.
➤ *Atrophy of subcutaneous tissue and depigmentation* may occur. The risk increases with the number of injections and may be more of an issue for aesthetically conscious patients.
➤ *Adverse drug reactions* generally require no action but are contraindications for use of the same drug in further treatments. To minimize the risk of adverse effects, use single-dose vials; many practitioners believe that adverse reactions result from preservatives in multi-dose vials.
➤ *Injection into a vein or artery* can be avoided by aspirating before injecting to check for blood.
➤ *Infection* is detected as early as possible through follow-up appointments and treated locally or systemically as indicated.
➤ *Trauma to adjacent structures (bone, cartilage, and nerves)* may require physical therapy or referral to an orthopedist or a surgeon; minimize the risk of this complication by limiting steroid injections to three per year.
➤ *Tendon rupture* is usually due to multiple injections or overuse after injection. To minimize this risk, avoid injecting into tendons and against resistance.

## SPECIAL CONSIDERATIONS

➤ If the cyst recurs, consider excising it instead of administering a second injection.

## DOCUMENTATION

➤ Before performing this procedure, document any abnormal physical findings on the consent form. Have the patient initial the comments and sign the form to signify acknowledgment of preprocedural abnormalities. In the chart, the preprocedural and postprocedural notes must include an evaluation of potentially affected function, range of motion, and sensation.
➤ Note whether a culture was sent to the laboratory.
➤ Describe the site before and after the procedure, the type and amount of anesthetic used, the patient's reaction to the procedure, medications ordered, the time frame for follow-up evaluation, and any instructions given to the patient.

## Cyst excision

CPT CODES
*Note:* Precise code depends on lesion size.
*10060    Incision and drainage of abscess (cutaneous or subcutaneous abscess or cyst); simple or single*
*10061    Incision and drainage of abscess (cutaneous or subcutantous abscess or cyst); complicated or multiple*
*11420 to 11426    Excision, benign lesion; diameter 0.5 cm or less; except skin tag, scalp, neck, hands, feet, genitalia*
*26160    Excision of lesion of tendon sheath or capsule, hand or finger*

## DESCRIPTION

A sebaceous or epidermal cyst consists of a small, mobile, superficial sac that contains sebum or keratin. It is commonly found on various areas of the body, such as the neck, back, scalp, and face. Its etiology is unknown. Cysts grow at varying rates, sometimes taking many years.

Cyst excision may be performed in two ways. In the first method, the cyst sac and its contents are removed simultaneously. In the second method, the cyst sac is removed only after expelling the contents. The site, size, and depth of the cyst all help determine which method is used.

Once the cyst is removed, closure is done by suture or by secondary intention with iodoform packing. If the cyst sac can be easily identified and pulled through the incision, this method is preferred because it reduces the chance of recurrence.

## INDICATIONS

➤ To diminish the occurrence of scarring or infection

## CONTRAINDICATIONS

### Relative
➤ Coagulopathies
➤ Anticoagulant therapy
➤ Anticipated complications or postsurgical scarring concerns
➤ Large cyst area

## EQUIPMENT

1% or 2% lidocaine without epinephrine ◆ 3-ml and 10-ml syringe ◆ 27G or 30G ½" needle ◆ 18G 1½" needle ◆ #11 scalpel with handle ◆ sterile suture setup ◆ sterile curved hemostat ◆ sterile normal saline solution ◆ small sterile container with 10% formalin ◆ ¼" to 1" package iodoform gauze ◆ sterile 4" × 4" gauze pads ◆ sterile scissors ◆ tape ◆ antiseptic skin cleaner such as povidone-iodine ◆ sterile gloves ◆ sterile drape ◆ gloves

## ESSENTIAL STEPS

➤ Explain the procedure to the patient, and address any questions or concerns that he has.
➤ Obtain informed consent.
➤ Establish a sterile field and assemble the equipment to be used.
➤ Place the patient in the position that allows the best view of the surgical site.
➤ Assess the surgical site for its size, consistency, redness, drainage, and tenderness.
➤ Put on gloves.
➤ Verify that the patient is not allergic to iodine.
➤ Clean the surrounding site with an antiseptic skin cleaner.
➤ Remove and dispose of gloves.
➤ Put on sterile gloves.
➤ Place the sterile drape appropriately over the cyst site.
➤ Anesthetize the cyst perimeter with 1% or 2% lidocaine *without* epinephrine. Avoid direct injection into the cyst site.
➤ Insert the needle at a 45-degree angle.
➤ Ask the patient if he notices any change in sensation. If he reports pain, indicating direct contact with the nerve, withdraw the needle 1 mm.
➤ Aspirate to make sure there is no blood return. If there is, the needle is in a blood vessel. Withdraw the needle slightly and reinsert it in another area.
➤ Inject 1 to 2 ml of lidocaine while partially withdrawing the needle. Then redirect the needle across the surface, advance it, and inject another 0.5 ml while withdrawing the needle. This method distributes the anesthetic uniformly, providing the optimal effect.
➤ Massage the area gently. The maximum effect should occur in 5 to 15 minutes.
➤ Incise the cyst site lengthwise with a #11 scalpel to allow an easy extraction of the cyst sac and its contents.
➤ Open the incised area with curved hemostat, and pull the sac and contents onto the skin.

➤ Cut the elastic tissue of the sac around the outer edges until it is released. Removal of the entire sac reduces the likelihood of recurrence.

➤ If the sac is already open after incision of the site, apply external pressure, using your fingers to remove its contents. This approach may also extrude the sac, depending on the site area. Never apply external pressure to a cyst on the face or mastoid.

➤ Put the contents into the sterile container with formalin for pathology review.

➤ Irrigate the wound site with normal saline solution, using 18 G needle and syringe.

➤ Depending on the wound, use a suture or packing approach to close the wound.

➤ If you're using a suture approach, close the wound with sutures at this time.

➤ If you're using an iodoform packing approach (other than on a head site), pack the cavity site fully. Leave a small amount of packing outside the wound to facilitate easy removal. If the surgical site is on the head, suture the incision in two areas, loosely enough to facilitate drainage. Leave the ends of the sutures 2″ to 3″ (5 to 7.5 cm) long. Form a gauze roll with sterile 4″ × 4″ gauze pads, and place it on top of the incision. Secure it tightly to the incision by tying the ends of the sutures and forming a pressure dressing.

➤ Apply a pressure dressing to the site with 4″ × 4″ gauze pads and tape.

➤ Assess the need for over-the-counter or prescription-strength medications, depending on the patient's pain tolerance (using a pain scale) and degree of recovery.

## Pᴀᴛɪᴇɴᴛ ᴛᴇᴀᴄʜɪɴɢ

➤ Advise the patient to apply cool compresses to the surgical site to help relieve pain and reduce swelling. Mild analgesics may also be necessary for the first few days after the procedure for pain control.

➤ Explain that healing usually occurs in 10 to 14 days, depending on the surgical site, the size of the wound, complications that arise, and the presence of infection before the procedure.

➤ Inform the patient that his sutures can be removed in 7 to 10 days, depending on the size of the site and the appearance of complications.

➤ Have the patient schedule a follow-up appointment in 48 hours to assess the site and wound status and then again in 7 to 10 days to have the sutures removed.

➤ Instruct the patient to notify you promptly if he experiences increased pain after the first few days, fever, drainage with foul odor, a color change, increased site tenderness, bleeding, or a new opening in wound edges.

## Cᴏᴍᴘʟɪᴄᴀᴛɪᴏɴs

➤ *Infection* may be treated with local or systemic antibiotics and antiseptic soaks. It may also require consultation with a physician, a dermatologist, or an infectious disease specialist.

➤ *Scarring and keloids* are minimized with gentle handling and the use of such techniques as undermining and layered suturing.

## Sᴘᴇᴄɪᴀʟ ᴄᴏɴsɪᴅᴇʀᴀᴛɪᴏɴs

➤ If using the iodoform gauze dressing, remove some of the gauze every 1 to 2 days until it's completely removed (approximately 10 to 14 days).

➤ If the patient has a large cyst area or facial cysts in a highly visible area, if you anticipate complications, or if you have concerns about postsurgical scarring, consider referring the patient to a general surgeon or a plastic surgeon.

## Dᴏᴄᴜᴍᴇɴᴛᴀᴛɪᴏɴ

➤ Before performing this procedure, document any abnormal physical findings on

the consent form. Have the patient initial the comments and sign the form to signify acknowledgment of preprocedural abnormalities. In the chart, the preprocedural and postprocedural notes must include an evaluation of potentially affected function, range of motion, and sensation.
➤ Record when the informed consent was received and confirmed.
➤ Note whether you sent any specimens to the laboratory for analysis.
➤ Describe the surgical site before and after the procedure, the type of wound closure method used (suture or gauze packing), the patient's tolerance for the procedure, complications that arose, and any instructions given to the patient.

## Soft-tissue aspiration

### CPT CODES
*20600   Arthrocentesis, aspiration, or injection: small joint, bursa, or ganglionic cyst (for example, fingers or toes)*
*20605   Arthrocentesis, aspiration, or injection: intermediate joint or bursa (for example, wrist, elbow, ankle, olecranon bursa)*
*20610   Arthrocentesis, aspiration, or injection: major joint or bursa (for example, shoulder, hip, knee joint, subacromial bursa)*

## DESCRIPTION

Soft-tissue aspiration involves removing fluid or exudate from an area of soft tissue for evaluation and palliative care.

## INDICATIONS

➤ To relieve pain or swelling in soft tissue
➤ To evacuate a hematoma resulting from trauma

## CONTRAINDICATIONS

### Absolute
➤ Broken skin at the site

### Relative
➤ Coagulopathies
➤ Swelling of the face
➤ Cellulitis
➤ Prosthetic joint

## EQUIPMENT

Povidone-iodine solution or alcohol swabs ◆ sterile gloves ◆ drape (optional) ◆ hemostat (optional) ◆ 10-ml syringe with 18G to 20G 1″ needle ◆ red-topped collection tube (optional) ◆ elastic bandage ◆ sterile 3″ × 3″ or 4″ × 4″ gauze pads ◆ tape

## ESSENTIAL STEPS

➤ Explain the procedure to the patient, and address any questions or concerns that he has.
➤ Obtain informed consent.
➤ Assemble the equipment before beginning.
➤ Place the patient in as comfortable a position as possible to allow performance of the procedure. Drape as appropriate for the site to be aspirated.
➤ Verify that the patient is not allergic to iodine.
➤ Clean the area with povidone-iodine solution or with an alcohol swab.
➤ Apply gloves and maintain aseptic technique throughout the procedure.
➤ Attach an 18G or a 20G 1″ needle to a 10-ml syringe.
➤ Insert the needle with the bevel (the sloped edge) down into the leading edge of the swelling. Aspirate as you advance the needle.
➤ If the syringe becomes full and needs to be changed, attach the hemostat to the needle hub to avoid needle rotation, re-

move the first syringe, replace it with an empty syringe, and continue aspirating.

➤ Place the aspirated fluid into a red-topped collection tube, and send it to the laboratory for analysis, if indicated.

➤ Apply a pressure dressing and compression device such as an elastic bandage.

## PATIENT TEACHING

➤ Advise the patient that discomfort is minimal after the procedure (except in patients with fibromyalgia).

➤ Urge him to keep the pressure dressing intact for 24 hours and then to remove it.

➤ Suggest applying ice or heat for the first 24 hours to relieve discomfort.

➤ Emphasize the need to rest the affected area to ensure proper healing, even after pain is relieved.

➤ Instruct the patient to notify you promptly if he experiences signs and symptoms of infection (red streaking; increased pain, redness, or warmth at the site; purulent drainage; fever; and chills).

## COMPLICATIONS

➤ *Infection* may be treated with local or systemic antibiotics and antiseptic soaks. It may also require consultation with a physician, a surgeon, or an infectious disease specialist.

## SPECIAL CONSIDERATIONS

➤ Aspiration of cloudy fluid does not necessarily indicate infection; sebaceous fluid will also appear cloudy. As long as no other signs of infection are evident, treatment with antibiotics is not indicated.

## DOCUMENTATION

➤ Before performing this procedure, document any abnormal physical findings on the consent form. Have the patient initial the comments and sign the form to signify

acknowledgment of preprocedural abnormalities. In the chart, the preprocedural and postprocedural notes must include an evaluation of potentially affected function, range of motion, and sensation.

➤ Note whether a culture was sent to the laboratory.

➤ Describe the site before and after the procedure, the characteristics of the aspirated fluid, the patient's reaction to the procedure, medications ordered, the time frame for follow-up evaluation, and any instructions given to the patient.

# Cryotherapy for lesion removal

## CPT CODES

*Note:* Precise code depends on lesion size.
*17000    Destruction by any method (including laser, with and without surgical curettement or local anesthesia) of all benign and premalignant lesions in any location, excluding cutaneous vascular proliferative lesions*
*17003    Destruction of multiple lesions*
*17110    Destruction by any method of less than 14 flat warts, molluscum contagiosum, or milia*
*17260    Destruction of less than 0.5-cm malignant lesion from trunk, arms, or legs*
*17261 to 17266    Destruction of malignant lesions from trunk, arms or legs; varying lesion sizes*
*17270    Destruction of less than 0.5-cm malignant lesion from scalp, neck, hands, feet, or genitalia*
*17271 to 17276    Destruction of malignant lesions from scalp, neck, hands, feet, or genitalia; varying lesion sizes*

## DESCRIPTION

Cryotherapy efficiently removes common skin lesions with minimal scar formation and pain. Pigment changes, which are more noticeable in darker skinned patients, are permanent. Cryotherapy uses freezing temperatures to destroy cells. Temperatures of 14° F (–10° C) to –4° F (–20° C) destroy tissue; a temperature of –58° F (–50° C) destroys malignant cells. In the procedure, a blister forms at the dermal-epidermal junction, and the skin superficial to the blister is left essentially bloodless and without sensation. The time needed for freezing varies with the type of skin lesion and the freezing method used.

## INDICATIONS

➤ To remove verruca vulgaris (common warts), verruca plantaris (plantar warts), actinic keratosis, condylomata acuminata, lentigines, molluscum contagiosum, papular nevi, sebaceous hyperplasia, seborrheic keratosis, and skin tags and polyps

## CONTRAINDICATIONS

### Absolute
➤ Sensitivity or adverse reaction to cryotherapy
➤ Inability of patient to accept the possibility of skin pigment changes
➤ Areas with compromised circulation
➤ Areas with a great deal of hair (cryotherapy destroys hair follicles)
➤ Lesions that require pathologic evaluation

### Relative
➤ History of an exaggerated response
➤ History of collagen disorders, ulcerative colitis, glomerulonephritis, or high cryoglobulin levels (abnormal proteins that dissolve at body temperature but precipitate when cooled)
➤ History of endocarditis, Epstein-Barr virus infection, syphilis, cytomegalovirus infection, or chronic hepatitis B
➤ Patients taking high-dose corticosteroids

## EQUIPMENT

Sterile drapes ◆ sterile gloves ◆ tissue-freezing kit such as the Verruca Freeze unit, nitrous oxide cryotherapy unit, or liquid nitrogen in a foam cup ◆ 4" × 4" gauze pads soaked with water ◆ antiseptic skin cleaner such as povidone-iodine ◆ cotton-tipped applicators ◆ water-soluble lubricating gel ◆ topical antibiotic such as triple antibiotic ointment ◆ dry 4" × 4" gauze pads ◆ tape

## ESSENTIAL STEPS

➤ Explain the procedure to the patient, and address any questions and concerns he has.
➤ Obtain informed consent.
➤ Place the patient in a comfortable position, with the lesion easily accessible.
➤ Verify that the patient is not allergic to iodine.
➤ Clean the area with an antiseptic skin cleaner.
➤ Apply water-soaked gauze pads to the lesion for 5 to 10 minutes.
➤ Drape the lesion.
➤ Put on gloves.

### Verruca Freeze
➤ Choose the smallest size speculum that will cover the lesion and attach it to the cryogun.
➤ Place the speculum firmly against the skin so no liquid can escape.
➤ Depress the trigger gently until the speculum is filled approximately ⅛" to ¼". Hold the unit in place for 25 seconds to allow the fluid to evaporate before removing the speculum.

### Nitrous oxide
➤ Use a cotton-tipped applicator to apply water-soluble lubricant to the lesion.
➤ Choose the cryoprobe that best matches the size, shape, and depth of the lesion

## SELECTING THE PROPER CRYOPROBE

Successfully freezing a lesion depends on selecting the appropriate cryoprobe tip. The shape of the tip determines the width of the freeze area. Applying pressure to the cryoprobe allows the probe to freeze at a greater depth.

The first two illustrations here show the use of appropriately shaped cryoprobes. The final illustration shows an inappropriate cryoprobe. In this example, the probe doesn't cover the lesion sufficiently.

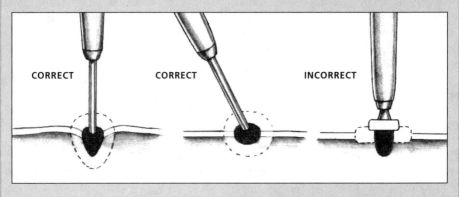

CORRECT    CORRECT    INCORRECT

without being larger than the lesion. (See *Selecting the proper cryoprobe.*).

➤ With the cryogun in your dominant hand, rest the cryoprobe against the lesion and press the trigger. The tip will form an ice ball that will adhere to the skin in 5 to 10 seconds. (See *Freeze time guidelines.*)

### Liquid nitrogen

➤ Soak a cotton-tipped applicator in the liquid.

➤ Apply the liquid to the lesion slowly to avoid splattering. The size of the cotton-tipped applicator and the amount of pressure affect how quickly and how deeply the area will freeze.

➤ Alternatively, you may use a cryogun with a probe or spray-tipped nozzle to deliver the liquid nitrogen.

➤ Stop freezing once you have an ice ball extending 2 mm beyond the lesion's boundaries.

➤ Apply a topical antibiotic.

➤ Cover the area with gauze and tape.

## PATIENT TEACHING

➤ Inform the patient that wart removal will cause a blister to form. After the blister forms, he should remove the top layer of skin from the blister with soap and water, apply a thin coat of antibiotic ointment, and then cover the area with an adhesive bandage.

➤ Inform him that immediate redness, swelling, and blisters are likely in the first 16 to 36 hours, but they decrease within 72 hours. Crusting occurs within 72 hours and resolves within 1 week.

➤ Tell him to make an appointment in 1 week to check for resolution of the blister and in 3 to 4 weeks for evaluation and, possibly, retreatment.

➤ Instruct the patient to keep the skin clean and dry. Explain the role of skin in defending the body against infection. Emphasize hygiene, sparing application of antibiotic ointment to the site, and the importance of keeping the site covered.

➤ Tell the patient that his skin in that area may become lighter or the hair less plentiful but that only minimal scarring should occur. Advise him to wear sunscreen, particularly on that area.
➤ If sensory nerves are affected, reassure the patient that recovery typically occurs within 2 months.
➤ Urge the patient to notify you promptly if he experiences signs and symptoms of infection (increasing redness, swelling, pain, and warmth; cloudy yellow, green, or brown drainage; opening of wound; foul odor; a red streak from the site; or fever after 24 hours).

## COMPLICATIONS

➤ *Pigment changes and increased photosensitivity* are permanent changes to the affected area.
➤ *Ischemia and infection* are rare but require follow-up evaluation and treatment.

## SPECIAL CONSIDERATIONS

➤ Use caution when treating the palmar surface of the hand because cutaneous sensory nerves run superficially in the hands. If a nerve is affected, the patient usually recovers within 6 weeks. When freezing an area adjacent to a nerve, apply traction and advise the patient that temporary sensory loss may occur.
➤ Refer the patient to a dermatologist for mucosal and periorbital cryotherapy because they require shorter freezing times and may produce excessive swelling that may be aesthetically and functionally disabling.
➤ Wart removal generally requires two freeze and thaw cycles, with the thaw time lasting 45 seconds.

## DOCUMENTATION

➤ Before performing this procedure, document any abnormal physical findings on the consent form. Have the patient initial

### FREEZE TIME GUIDELINES

Successful cryotherapy depends on use of the appropriate freeze time for the particular lesion being removed. This table shows the times needed to freeze various types of skin lesions. If the freeze time noted yields insufficient coverage, allow the area to thaw and then refreeze. Subsequent refreezing yields deeper penetration of the cold.

| TYPE OF LESION | FREEZE TIME (IN SECONDS) |
|---|---|
| Actinic keratosis | 90 |
| Condyloma acuminata | 45 |
| Lentigines (freckles) | 10 to 15 |
| Molluscum contagiosum | 25 to 30 |
| Papular nevi | 30 to 45 |
| Sebaceous hyperplasia | 30 to 45 |
| Seborrheic keratosis | 30 |
| Skin tags and polyps | 30 to 45 |
| Verruca plantaris (plantar warts; after debridement) | 30 to 40 |

the comments and sign the form to signify acknowledgment of preprocedural abnormalities. In the chart, the preprocedural and postprocedural notes must include an evaluation of potentially affected function, range of motion, and sensation.
➤ When documenting consent, note that options and risks (particularly pigment changes and scarring) were discussed at length and that the patient wanted the procedure done.
➤ Record indications for cryotherapy, freeze times, the time frame for follow-up evaluation, and any instructions given to the patient.

## Subungual hematoma evacuation

CPT CODE
*11740 Evacuation of subungual hematoma*

### DESCRIPTION

A subungual hematoma is the accumulation of blood between the nail and the nail bed, generally secondary to trauma. The expanding collection of blood causes pain and pressure and, if not relieved, may cause future nail deformity by compressing the underlying nail matrix. The primary indication for release of a subungual hematoma is pain management.

Hematoma release may be effected either by handheld cautery or by a heated paper clip. Although both are equally effective, use of a handheld cautery is preferred when the equipment is available.

### INDICATIONS

➤ To evacuate a visible, painful hematoma involving less than 50% of the nail bed

### CONTRAINDICATIONS

#### Relative

➤ Crushed or fractured nail
➤ Fracture of the distal phalanx without laceration of the nail bed
➤ Already split nail (allows blood to evacuate)
➤ Presence of tumor under the nail
➤ Hematoma involving more than 50% of the nail

### EQUIPMENT

Handheld battery or electric cautery unit or large needle or paper clip ◆ heat source such as matches or a lighter ◆ hemostat to hold the hot paper clip ◆ antiseptic solution such as povidone-iodine ◆ finger splint (optional) ◆ hydrogen peroxide ◆ gloves ◆ alcohol wipes ◆ adhesive bandage ◆ eye protection (optional)

### ESSENTIAL STEPS

➤ Explain the procedure and rationale to the patient, and address any questions or concerns that he has.
➤ Obtain informed consent.
➤ Discuss the fact that the nail has no nerve endings and the procedure should be painless. No anesthesia is required.
➤ Alert the patient to the fact that the burning nail may have an irritating or unpleasant smell.
➤ Put on gloves, then examine the digit and assess neurovascular and neurosensory function.
➤ Consider X-ray of the digit to rule out distal phalanx fracture.
➤ Assess the patient's level of pain, using a pain scale.
➤ Verify that the patient is not allergic to iodine.
➤ Soak the digit in antiseptic solution for 5 minutes.
➤ Clean the nail with an alcohol wipe and allow to dry.
➤ Heat the handheld cautery or the tip of the paper clip until it is red hot.
➤ Apply firm, gentle pressure over the nail, holding the cautery or paper clip at a 90-degree angle to the nail. A hole should develop in the nail almost instantly (see *Subungual hematoma release*).

 **ALERT** A glowing red tip is necessary for rapid, effective evacuation. If a hole doesn't appear in the nail plate within 2 seconds of heat application, the cautery or paper clip isn't hot enough. Reheat the tool and reapply to the nail.

➤ As soon as a hole appears in the nail, quickly withdraw the heat source and observe for fluid drainage. Sometimes a second heat application is necessary to en-

## SUBUNGUAL HEMATOMA RELEASE

Although a cautery needle looks more professional, a heated paper clip is just as effective in subungual hematoma release. The important point is to apply just enough pressure to penetrate the nail, then immediately release and encourage drainage by lowering the extremity and wicking away blood as it appears.

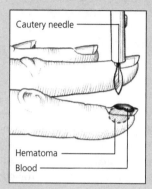
Cautery needle
Hematoma
Blood

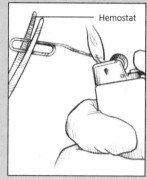
Hemostat

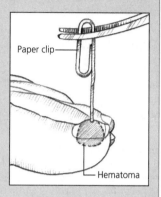
Paper clip
Hematoma

large the hole to a size sufficient for the hematoma to evacuate (1 to 2 mm).

➤ Soak the digit in an antiseptic solution (approximately 50 ml povidone-iodine with 20 ml of hydrogen peroxide) for 5 to 10 minutes to complete evacuation.

➤ Reassess neurovascular and neurosensory function.

➤ Clean the nail with an alcohol wipe, and apply a loose dressing or adhesive bandage.

➤ Optionally, the digit may be splinted for 24 hours for comfort.

## PATIENT TEACHING

➤ Tell the patient to expect almost immediate improvement in his level of pain, with continued resolution over the next 24 hours. Pain and throbbing can be relieved by acetaminophen or ibuprofen (assuming no fracture). The digit will feel normal in 2 to 3 days.

➤ Tell the patient that complete healing of the nail and resolution of the remaining ecchymosis will take 5 to 7 months (the length of time for the new nail to grow out).

➤ Inform him that no follow-up is necessary unless complications develop.

➤ Explain that there is a possibility of nail deformity, even with new nail growth, if the nail matrix was damaged at the time of trauma.

➤ Tell the patient to keep the digit elevated above the level of the heart for 24 hours after the procedure, if possible.

➤ Remind the patient to soak the finger in warm salt water three times a day for the next 3 days.

➤ Advise him to keep the open nail area loosely covered with an adhesive bandage.

➤ Explain that small amounts of serosanguineous drainage are likely for the next 24 to 48 hours.

➤ If a splint was applied, tell the patient to remove it for soaks and then to reapply it; he can use the splint for 24 to 48 hours to promote comfort.

➤ Inform the patient that he can take acetaminophen 650 mg every 4 hours or ibuprofen 600 mg every 6 hours as needed for pain.

➤ Tell the patient that he may return to normal activity as tolerated.

➤ Urge the patient to notify you promptly if he experiences signs and symptoms of infection, such as chills, temperature higher than 101° F (38.3° C), redness, purulent drainage, increased pain, and red streaking of the digit.

## COMPLICATIONS

➤ *Infection* needs to be assessed; the patient may be placed on antibiotic therapy and soaks continued four times a day.

➤ *Edema* resulting in vascular compromise (usually as a result of the trauma, not the subungual hematoma evacuation) requires assessment of neurosensory and neurovascular function and referral to the emergency department immediately for a surgical consultation.

## SPECIAL CONSIDERATIONS

➤ Assess for indications of domestic, elder, or child abuse during the history and physical examination. Remember that striking the hands and nails with a blunt object or compressing the fingers or toes can cause subungual hematoma.

➤ Subungual hematoma evacuation should be a painless procedure that results in immediate pain improvement for the patient. It is important that you make sure you have a very hot cautery or paper clip tip and apply enough pressure for the tip to "pop" through the nail. The release feels very similar to the "pop" of going through a vein wall for venipuncture or I.V. insertion. Beware of a fountain of blood when the nail is penetrated and the hematoma is large. If this is a possibility, wear eye protection.

➤ A subungual hematoma involving more than 50% of the nail may indicate a laceration of the underlying nail bed. Some experts recommend leaving the nail in place to act as a splint; others recommend total nail removal to effect laceration repair. In either case, the patient should be informed that without nail bed examination and possible laceration repair, there may be future nail deformity.

## DOCUMENTATION

➤ Before performing this procedure, document any abnormal physical findings on the consent form. Have the patient initial the comments and sign the form to signify acknowledgment of preprocedural abnormalities. In the chart, the preprocedural and postprocedural notes must include an evaluation of potentially affected function, range of motion, sensation, and evaluation for further injury.

➤ This patient must be assessed for domestic, elder, or child abuse, and you must document notification of appropriate authorities for any suspicion of child or elder abuse. This notification is mandatory. However, you can't report domestic violence without the patient's consent.

➤ Include in your notes that options and risks associated with the procedure were discussed at length and that the patient agreed that the procedure should be done.

➤ Relate the cause of injury, the type of X-rays and results as indicated, the type of heat source used, the size and resultant release of the hematoma, the quantity of blood evacuated, and improvement in the patient's level of pain (pain scale).

➤ Record the patient's understanding of all patient teaching.

## Elliptical excision

CPT CODES
*Note:* Precise code depends on lesion size.
*11400 to 11406   Excision of benign lesions on trunk, arms, or legs*

*11420 to 11426  Excision of benign lesions on scalp, neck, hands, feet, or genitalia*
*11600 to 11606  Excision of malignant lesions on trunk, arms, or legs*
*11620 to 11626  Excision of malignant lesions on scalp, neck, hands, feet, or genitalia*

## DESCRIPTION

In an elliptical excision (also called fusiform excision), the practitioner can remove a skin lesion too large for a cutaneous punch and then suture the area closed, leaving behind a linear scar (larger lesions require a different form of excision and require skin flaps or grafts for closure). The location of the incision usually depends on the location of natural skin tension lines, which correspond with wrinkle lines. If such lines aren't readily apparent, gently pinching the skin in several directions should bring them out (this technique may not work with children and adolescents).

The goal of such surgery is to remove the lesion and leave as small a cosmetic defect as possible by following skin tension lines and, for lesions on the face, facial expressions. When deciding where to make the excision, the practitioner must consider the depth of the skin; the impact of the excision on adjacent structures; the length, width, and orientation of the resulting scar; and the scar's effect on function. Placement of a shoulder incision, for instance, depends more on creating a scar that won't pull apart than on appearance. Ideally, the procedure will transform the oval-shaped wound left by the excision into a thin-line closure.

## INDICATIONS

➤ To excise suspected melanoma
➤ To remove lesions too large for punch biopsy

## CONTRAINDICATIONS

### Absolute

➤ Lesion on eyelid, lip, face, or genitalia
➤ Suspected infection

### Relative

➤ Tension on the incision line (such as on joint or scalp wounds)
➤ Coagulopathy impairing hemostasis
➤ Deep lesions
➤ Allergy to anesthetic

## EQUIPMENT

Marker ◆ sterile gloves ◆ sterile drape ◆ masks ◆ protective eyewear ◆ antiseptic solution ◆ 2" × 2" or 4" × 4" gauze pads ◆ anesthetic ◆ #11 scalpel ◆ straight or curved iris scissors ◆ forceps or hook ◆ specimen container with 10% formalin ◆ electrocautery unit ◆ sutures ◆ suture needles (see *Indications for suture materials*, page 244) ◆ 3-ml syringe ◆ 25G or 27G needle ◆ antibiotic ointment ◆ nonadherent dressing ◆ tape

## ESSENTIAL STEPS

➤ Explain the procedure to the patient, and address any questions or concerns that he has.
➤ Obtain informed consent.
➤ Note the area to be excised in a circle at its clinical margins. Imagine a concentric circle around the first circle that includes the margin for normal skin. Use the marker to draw a final ellipse that is three times as long as it is wide.
➤ Wash and dry your hands, put on sterile gloves and a mask, and use eye protection.
➤ Verify that the patient is not allergic to local anesthetics and iodine.
➤ Clean the area in a circular motion from the site outward with antiseptic solution.
➤ Draw up the anesthetic for injection.

## INDICATIONS FOR SUTURE MATERIALS

Sutures can be absorbable or nonabsorbable. Absorbable sutures eventually dissolve. Nonabsorbable sutures must be removed because the body can't dissolve them. This chart outlines various types of suture material and their indications for use.

| TYPE OF SUTURE | INDICATIONS FOR USE |
|---|---|
| ABSORBABLE | |
| Plain gut | Superficial vessels and rapid-healing subcutaneous tissues (rarely used due to its high tissue reactivity) |
| Chromic catgut | Oral mucosa, vermilion border |
| Polyglycolic acid | Superficial closure of skin and mucosa |
| NONABSORBABLE | |
| Silk | Tying off of blood vessels |
| Nylon | Use and size of suture vary with location of wound: |
| | ➤ 6-0 for eyelids and face |
| | ➤ 5-0 for forehead, neck, and other delicate skin |
| | ➤ 4-0 for neck, scalp, extremities, and back |
| | ➤ 3-0 for running suture of scalp |

➤ Using a syringe and a 25G to 27G needle, inject in a ring to obtain field anesthesia. Insert the needle with the anesthetic agent at a 45-degree angle.

➤ Ask the patient if he notices any change in sensation. If he reports pain, indicating direct contact with the nerve, withdraw the needle 1 mm.

➤ Aspirate to make sure there is no blood return. If there is, the needle is in a blood vessel. Withdraw the needle slightly and reinsert it in another area.

➤ Inject 1 to 2 ml of lidocaine while partially withdrawing the needle. Then redirect the needle across the surface, advance it, and inject another 0.5 ml while withdrawing the needle. This method distributes the anesthetic uniformly, providing the optimal effect. Make sure that you anesthetize beyond the demarcated margins in anticipation of undermining.

➤ Massage the area gently and wait 5 to 15 minutes for the optimal effect to occur.

➤ Use a gauze pad to apply antiseptic to the area, starting at the center and spiraling outward. Then drape the area to allow a clear view of the surgical site.

➤ Hold the scalpel like a pencil at a 90-degree angle, with the anterior belly of the blade in contact with the previously marked line. Apply three-point traction with the other hand, using firm, confident, vertical pressure at the corner of the ellipse. (See *Using three-point traction*.)

➤ Press down gently with the scalpel, and draw it through the skin in one firm, constant stroke, keeping the blade perpendicular to the skin surface (to avoid beveling the wound and margins). You don't have to cut through the skin's full thickness with a single stroke, but make sure you can see upper subcutaneous fat before trying to remove the specimen.

➤ Rarely, you may encounter a highly active blood vessel. If this happens, remove the blade and cauterize the affected site before continuing.

➤ After making the incisions, use a straight or curved iris scissor and forceps or hook and gently elevate one end of the fusiform ellipse.

➤ Insert the scissors through the subcutis and complete the incision through the subcutis along both sides of the specimen. Undermine the base completely and elevate the specimen (see *Mastering the undermining technique,* page 246).

➤ Place the specimen in a specimen container.

➤ Cauterize as needed to stop bleeding, but don't cauterize too much or the wound won't heal as quickly.

➤ Suture the wound closed.

➤ Apply a thin layer of antibiotic ointment, a nonadherent dressing, and 4″ × 4″ gauze pads; tape securely.

## PATIENT TEACHING

➤ Caution the patient to keep the sutures dry.

➤ Tell him to remove the initial dressing in 24 hours and to replace it with a smaller gauze bandage. Advise him not to place the gauze itself directly over the wound (fibers in the gauze can get trapped in the wound edge, become matted, and delay healing).

➤ Teach him to clean the site twice a day with soap and water (no rubbing or scrubbing, just pat on and rinse off) and to cover it with antibiotic ointment and a three-layer dressing (triple antibiotic ointment, nonadherent dressing, and gauze followed by tape covering).

➤ Instruct him to limit his sun exposure, particularly to the affected area. (See *Minimizing sun exposure,* page 247.)

### USING THREE-POINT TRACTION

Making an elliptical incision requires that you maintain firm traction to the skin surface in more than one direction. The illustration below shows how to apply three-point traction to maintain multidirectional traction when making an elliptical incision.

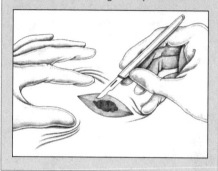

➤ Inform the patient that he must return for suture removal. Have him return in 3 to 6 days for a face wound, 7 to 10 days for an ear wound, or 5 to 10 days for a trunk or an extremity wound.

➤ Urge the patient to notify you promptly if he experiences signs and symptoms of infection (increasing redness, swelling, pain, and warmth; cloudy yellow, green, or brown drainage; opening of wound; foul odor; a red streak from the site; or fever after 24 hours).

## COMPLICATIONS

➤ *Infection* may be treated with local or systemic antibiotics or antiseptic soaks. It may also require consultation with a physician, a dermatologist, or an infectious disease specialist.

➤ *Scarring and keloids* are minimized with gentle handling and the use of such techniques as undermining and layered suturing.

## MASTERING THE UNDERMINING TECHNIQUE

Undermining, the technique of freeing the skin from underlying tissues, can decrease tension on the wound edge and is critical for obtaining acceptable cosmetic results after wound repair. Proper undermining minimizes scarring and keloid formation.

The level of undermining that you should perform depends on the location and natural plane of the wound. In general, you'll undermine an area about the size of the widest part of the wound.

### Blunt undermining
In blunt undermining, advance the scissors with the tips closed and then force them open. This causes blunt dissection of the underlying tissues.

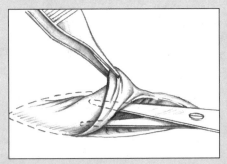

### Sharp undermining
In sharp undermining, a less frequently used technique, use short, cutting strokes with a scalpel to separate the skin from underlying tissues.

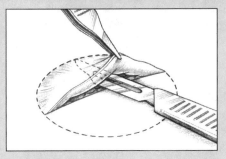

### Undermining level
The proper undermining level is achieved when the skin is carefully separated from the subcutaneous fat.

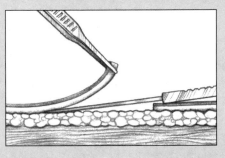

### Undermining tips
➤ Keep in mind that undermining increases bleeding. Make sure you can see the source of bleeding before cauterizing it. Cauterizing blindly may damage the surrounding tissue without stopping the bleeding.
➤ Treat the wound edge gently. Handle it with a single-pronged skin hook instead of forceps, and stay within the subcutaneous fat layer.

## SPECIAL CONSIDERATIONS

**ALERT** Refer the patient to a plastic surgeon for facial lesions greater than ¼" (0.6 cm); refer him to a dermatologist for deep lesions.

➤ Tools for marking the lesion before excision include a skin marker (such as the Devon skin marker). It doesn't leave a very dark mark, however, and tends to dry out when the cap is left off. Because of these drawbacks, many practitioners prefer using an indelible marker, although this can leave a permanent mark if the ink isn't completely removed before wound closure.

➤ Keep in mind that wounds closed by approximation of the skin edges heal by primary intention.

## MINIMIZING SUN EXPOSURE

DEAR PATIENT,

The easiest way to prevent skin cancer is to reduce your exposure to the sun. Although most skin cancers appear after age 50, the sun's damaging effects begin early—in childhood.

Fortunately, it's never too late to start protecting yourself from skin cancer. Here is how.

### Wear sunscreen
Protect your skin with a lotion or cream containing para-aminobenzoic acid (PABA) or another sunscreen.

Sunscreens are related to strength according to sun protection factor (SPF). Choose a sunscreen with an SPF of 15 or higher—especially if you have fair skin and burn easily.

Apply sunscreen at least 15 minutes before you go outside; then reapply it every 2 or 3 hours. Apply sunscreen more frequently if you perspire heavily or after you swim or exercise. Consider using a water-resistant sunscreen.

Get in the habit of applying a sunscreen routinely before you go outside because the sun's rays can damage your skin whether you're on your way to work or lounging at the pool.

Consider storing your sunscreen in a safe place near your front or back door. Keep an extra container in your car.

### Cover up
Wear protective clothing, such as a wide-brimmed hat, long sleeves, and sunglasses.

Keep in mind that flimsy, lightweight clothes may not protect against sunburn because the sun's rays can penetrate them.

Don't rely on a shady tree, an umbrella, or a cloudy day to prevent sunburn. Remember that burning ultraviolet rays penetrate overcast skies and a canopy of leaves as well.

Also keep in mind that sun reflected from water, snow, or sand can burn your skin even more intensely than direct sunlight, so carry a coverup with you when you go out.

### Adjust your schedule
Avoid outdoor activities when the sun's rays shine their strongest—between 10 a.m. and 3 p.m. (11 a.m. and 4 p.m. daylight savings time). Schedule outdoor activities at other times. For example, play tennis in the early morning or mow the lawn in the late afternoon.

### Other tips
Remember: No matter how attractive it is, a suntan isn't healthful.
➤ Don't use oils or a reflector device to promote suntan.
➤ Check with your practitioner or pharmacist about possible phototropic (sensitizing) effects related to any prescription or over-the-counter medications you take.
➤ Avoid artificial ultraviolet light. Steer clear of sunlamps, and stay out of tanning parlors or booths.

➤ To speed healing and prevent crust formation, cover the wound with an occlusive or a semiocclusive dressing (particularly important for wounds created by a procedure).

## DOCUMENTATION

➤ Before performing this procedure, document any abnormal physical findings on the consent form. Have the patient initial the comments and sign the form to signify acknowledgment of preprocedural abnormalities. In the chart, the preprocedural and postprocedural notes must include an evaluation of potentially affected function, range of motion, and sensation.
➤ Note whether you sent a culture to the laboratory for analysis.
➤ Record indications for and details of the procedure. Describe the site before and after the procedure, the type and amount of anesthetic used, the patient's reaction to the procedure, medications ordered, the time frame for follow-up evaluation, and any instructions given to the patient.

# Mechanical debridement

CPT CODES
*11040 Debridement of the skin, partial thickness*
*11041 Debridement of the skin, full thickness*
*11042 Debridement of skin and subcutaneous tissue*

## DESCRIPTION

Debridement involves removing dead or devitalized tissue. Wounds can be debrided enzymatically, mechanically, or autolytically to allow underlying healthy tissue to regenerate. Mechanical debridement procedures include irrigation, hydrotherapy, and excision of dead tissue with forceps and scissors. Excision may be done in the office or in a specially prepared room. Depending on the type of wound, a combination of debridement techniques may be used.

Burn wound debridement removes devitalized tissue. This prevents or controls infection, promotes healing, and prepares the wound surface to receive a graft. Frequent, regular debridement guards against possible hemorrhage resulting from more extensive and forceful debridement. It also reduces the need to conduct extensive debridement under anesthesia.

## INDICATIONS

➤ To remove necrotic or devitalized tissue

## CONTRAINDICATIONS

➤ Closed blisters over partial-thickness burns

## EQUIPMENT

Pain medication (such as morphine) ◆ two pairs of sterile gloves ◆ two gowns or aprons ◆ mask ◆ cap ◆ sterile scissors ◆ sterile forceps ◆ 4″ × 4″ sterile gauze pads ◆ sterile solutions and medications as ordered ◆ hemostatic agent such as silver nitrate sticks ◆ needle holder (optional) ◆ gut suture with needle (optional)

## ESSENTIAL STEPS

➤ Explain the procedure to the patient, and answer any questions he has.
➤ Provide privacy. Administer an analgesic 20 minutes before debridement begins, or give an I.V. analgesic immediately before the procedure.
➤ Keep the patient warm. Expose only the area to be debrided.

➤ Put on the gown or an apron, gloves, a mask, and a cap. Maintain aseptic technique throughout the procedure.

➤ Remove the dressings and clean the wound.

➤ Change your gown or apron and dispose of gloves. Put on a fresh set of sterile apparel.

➤ Lift loosened edges of eschar with forceps. Use the blunt edge of scissors or forceps to probe the eschar. Cut the dead tissue from the wound with the scissors. Leave a ¼" (0.6 cm) edge on remaining echar to avoid cutting into viable tissue.

➤ If bleeding occurs, apply gentle pressure on the wound with sterile 4"× 4" gauze pads. Then apply the hemostatic agent as needed.

➤ Perform additional procedures, such as application of topical medications and dressing replacements, as indicated.

## PATIENT TEACHING

➤ Advise the patient that this procedure is painful. Explain that the intensity of pain will depend on the level of injury and the degree of neurologic compromise. Assure him that pain medication will be prescribed. Have him take it 30 to 60 minutes before the procedure.

➤ Teach the patient distraction and relaxation techniques to ease pain.

➤ Instruct him to schedule a follow-up appointment when you determine, guided by the degree of injury.

## COMPLICATIONS

➤ *Infection* may develop any time the protective skin barrier is broken. The use of sterile technique and equipment is mandatory. If infection occurs, obtain a culture and sensitivity specimen of the wound site, and treat the patient with antibiotics.

➤ *Blood loss* may occur if debridement exposes an eroded blood vessel or if a vessel is cut inadvertently. Apply mild to moderate compression until hemostasis is achieved.

➤ *Fluid and electrolyte imbalances* may result from exudate lost during the procedure; order serum electrolyte levels as indicated.

## SPECIAL CONSIDERATIONS

➤ Because debridement removes only dead or devitalized tissue, bleeding should be minimal. Excessive bleeding or spurting vessels may require ligation using suturing materials (sutures, needle, needle holder).

➤ Refer the patient to a specialist if the wound is greater than 4" (10.2 cm) and deeper than ⅓" (1 cm), if infection is present, or if the wound is on the face, hand, or forearm.

➤ If possible, work with an assistant and complete the procedure within 20 minutes to limit the patient's pain.

➤ Acknowledge the patient's discomfort and provide emotional support throughout the procedure.

## DOCUMENTATION

➤ Before performing this procedure, document any abnormal physical findings on the consent form. Have the patient initial the comments and sign the form to signify acknowledgment of preprocedural abnormalities. In the chart, the preprocedural and postprocedural notes must include an evaluation of potentially affected function, range of motion, and sensation.

➤ Record the date, time, and indications for wound debridement, the area debrided, and solutions and medications used. Describe the wound condition, noting signs of infection or skin breakdown. Record the patient's tolerance for the procedure. Note indications for additional therapy.

## Foot care

**CPT CODES**
*11055 Paring or cutting of benign hyperkeratotic lesion (corn or callus), single lesion*
*11056 As above, for 2 to 4 lesions*
*11057 As above, for more than 4 lesions*
*11719 Trimming of nondystrophic nails, any number*

## DESCRIPTION

The goal of foot care is to improve comfort of the feet. Nails, skin, and circulation must be assessed for abnormalities such as corns, calluses, and plantar warts. Identification and monitoring of these abnormalities reduces the risk of infection and complications of untreated conditions.

Corns are caused by pressure from bony prominences against a shoe, the ground, or another bony prominence. A corn may be hard or soft, but either type requires smoothing and flattening of hyperkeratotic tissue to reduce pressure and pain. Once reduced, the corn has a white core and should be evaluated for a possible sinus tract. If this is present, treatment with an antibiotic such as triple antibiotic cream or ointment may be necessary. Padded and correctly fitted shoes are essential to reduce pressure.

Calluses are caused by excessive friction and pressure, usually on the plantar aspect of the foot. Calluses (diffuse hyperkeratotic tissue) may also be smoothed and flattened with a sanding tool, a pumice stone, or a file to reduce pressure and pain. The underlying tissue is pink, making it easier to identify adequate reduction of hyperkeratotic tissue. Padding is essential to reduce friction. Arch support or other orthotics may be necessary to restore balance to gait.

Plantar warts, caused by a common wart virus, are very painful. Located on the metatarsal head or heel of the foot, they differ from corns or calluses in that they have a soft, central core and are surrounded by a firm hyperkeratotic ring. Multiple tiny black spots on the surface represent coagulated blood. A plantar wart is usually painful when squeezed. This helps distinguish a plantar wart from a callus, which is generally not painful when squeezed. Reduction of hyperkeratotic tissue reduces pain. Surgical removal may lead to deep, painful scarring. Avoid acidic removal preparations, especially in the diabetic patient.

## INDICATIONS

➤ To prevent foot and wound complications, especially in patients with diabetes or peripheral vascular disease
➤ To relieve pressure, pain, or discomfort caused by corns, calluses, or plantar warts
➤ To achieve cosmetic improvements

## CONTRAINDICATIONS

**Absolute**
➤ Open wounds on feet
➤ Infected, ingrown toenails
➤ Injured, ecchymotic feet, toes, or nails
➤ Severe fungal infections
➤ Numbness or tingling

**Relative**
➤ Use of warfarin (Coumadin) or aspirin
➤ Previous surgery

## EQUIPMENT

Foot-soaking basin with disposable liner ◆ bath thermometer ◆ warm water not to exceed 105° F (40.6° C) ◆ mild liquid soap (may use commercial foot bath preparation with antibacterial properties) ◆ towel ◆ paper towels ◆ comfortable chair ◆ gloves ◆ impervious gown ◆ mask (high-efficiency particulate air [HEPA] filter) ◆ protective eyewear ◆ toenail nippers ◆ file ◆ manicure stick ◆ sanding tool with grinder ◆ assorted corn and callus pads ◆ moleskin ◆ lambs' wool ◆ massage oil or lotion ◆ trash bag ◆ assessment tool ◆ topical antibiotic, such as bactroban, neosporin, or polysporin ◆ adhesive bandage ◆ #17 scalpel

## ESSENTIAL STEPS

➤ Assemble all equipment in the room. Seat the patient in a comfortable chair. Before beginning the procedure, decide how you will sit (on a cushion placed on the floor or on a low stool in front of the patient).

➤ Take a brief history per the assessment tool. (See *Foot assessment and care*, page 252.) Specifically ask questions regarding use of warfarin or aspirin, diabetic status, peripheral vascular disease, foot or leg pain, and previous foot or leg surgery.

➤ Verify that the patient is not allergic to iodine (an ingredient in many commercial foot baths).

➤ Explain the procedure to the patient, and answer any questions he has.

➤ Obtain informed consent.

➤ Place a towel on the floor under the patient's feet and chair, and wash your hands.

➤ Fill a lined basin with warm water (less than 105° F) and antibacterial soap or foot bath preparation.

➤ Tell the patient to soak his feet for 10 minutes.

➤ Adjust room lighting as needed.

➤ Put on an impervious gown, protective eyewear, and gloves. Remove the patient's feet from the bath. Using a paper towel, pat the feet dry. Using a second paper towel, dry between toes.

➤ Examine the feet. Use feet maps to record findings, including any abnormalities.

➤ Nip the patient's toenails, taking small nips across the entire nail border. Follow

the shape or contour of the top of the toe. Don't cut deeply into the corners. Run a thumb over the nail and the top of the toe to be sure the nail is short enough. Avoid nipping any skin surfaces. Cut thickened, discolored, or unhealthy nails last to prevent transmission of possible infection to healthy nails.

➤ File rough edges with a nail file.

➤ Use a manicure stick to remove debris around and under the nails.

➤ Check between the toes for nail clippings; remove them with a paper towel.

➤ Use the sanding tool and grinder to flatten and smooth any corns or calluses. Don't exceed the 2 setting on the sanding tool. (*Note:* You and the patient must wear masks and the room must be properly ventilated when grinding and sanding are taking place. *Optional:* Instead of using a sanding tool, you may use a #17 scalpel blade.) Slowly and gently sand the surface of the corn or callus. Avoid abrading the surrounding healthy skin. Apply light pressure while sanding across the entire corn or callus, until the area feels soft and flexible. Don't sand below the level of healthy tissue. Stop if the tissue feels warm or if the patient reports feeling "heat."

➤ Pare corns with a #17 scalpel. Remove the corn core carefully, avoiding damage to healthy skin. Apply topical antibiotic and an adhesive bandage.

➤ Pad bony areas with moleskin, corn pads, or lambs' wool.

➤ Massage the foot, using a light oil (such as almond or baby oil) or a massage lotion without alcohol. Begin with a gentle thumb massage at the Achilles tendon, and circle the malleolus. Hold the foot in the left hand and massage the dorsum with the heel of the right palm. Change hands. Massage the outer aspect of the foot between the thumb and fingers. Massage each toe. Knead the ball of the foot down through the arch, using the flat surface of the fist. Use thumbs and small circles to massage the heel. Reknead the arch.

## FOOT ASSESSMENT AND CARE

**NAME:** _Robert Messer_    **PHYSICIAN:** _K. Diehl_
**AGE:** _72_    **MALE/FEMALE:** _Male_    **INITIAL VISIT:** _10/6/00_
**DATE:** _10/6/00_    **SUBSEQUENT VISIT:** _____

**Medical History:** __Amputation  __Arthritis  __HTN  __Diabetes  _X_ Foot/Leg Pain  _X_ PVD/CAD/CVI  __Smoker  __Stroke  __Previous Surgery  __ Other

**Medications:** _____

**Vascular Status:** Pulses (DP) _+_ R _+_ L  Pulses (PT) _+_ R _+_ L  Temperature _w_ R _w_ L  Color _DR_ R _DR_ L  Edema _+_ R _+_ L

(+) Present  (D) Diminished  (–) Absent  (N) Normal  (W) Warm  (C) Cool  (DR) Dependent Rubor  (EP) Elevation Pallor  (1+–4+) Edema

**Nails:** Excess Length _X_ R _X_ L  Thick _X_ R _X_ L  Discolored__R__L  Ingrown__R _X_ L  Debris__R__L  Incurvated__R__L  Thick Cuticles__R__L  Capillary Refill__R__L

**Skin:** Calluses__R__L  Corns _X_ R _X_ L  Dry__R__L  Fat Padding __R__L  Fissures__R__L  Maceration__R__L  Moist__R__L  Ulcer(s)__R__L

**Deformities:** Bunions __R__L  Crossover Toes __R__L  Hammer Toes __R__L  Flat Foot __R__L  Plantar Wart __R__L

**Sensation:**     _X_ R Comments _Decreased_
         _X_ L Comments _Decreased_

**Nursing Interventions:** _X_ Hygiene  __Clip, 5 or less  _X_ Clip, 5 or more  __Grind, 5 or less  __Grind, 5 or more  _X_ Buff Corns  __Buff Callus  __Apply Lotion  __Instruction

**Recommendations:** _X_ Daily Hygiene  _X_ Daily Foot Inspection  __Footwear  __Nail Care  __Skin Care Stockings (compression)  __Other

**Referral(s):** _____

**Label Feet Below: C**-Callus  **CN**-Corn  **E**-Edema  **M**-Maceration  **P**-Pain  **R**-Redness  **W**-Warmth  **U**-Ulcer(s)  **PW**-Plantar Wart

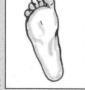
R

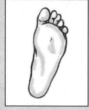
L

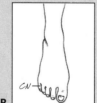
R

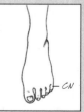
L

Signature: _Paula Smith, CRNP_

____ ✓ Check if narrative is written on reverse side.

➤ Assist the patient with socks and shoes.
➤ With gloves still on, empty the water basin and discard the liner. Discard the paper towels and manicure stick.
➤ Clean equipment per facility policy.
➤ Remove gloves, eyewear, and gown. Dispose of them according to facility policy. Wash your hands. Place the towel in the hamper.
➤ Assist the patient to the waiting area.

## PATIENT TEACHING

➤ Inform the patient that he should experience immediate relief from pressure and pain after the procedure.
➤ Teach him how corns, calluses, bunions, and hammertoes develop, and review ways to prevent their formation.
➤ Review proper foot care with the patient. Instruct him to:
– wash feet daily with lukewarm water and a mild soap and dry feet well, especially between the toes.
– trim toenails straight across, using an emery board to shape the nails even with the toes and to smooth rough edges.
– keep skin supple with a moisturizing lotion or light oil (but tell him not to apply lotion or oil between the toes).
– change socks daily and wear proper-fitting shoes that are free from cracks, pebbles, nails, or anything that can hurt the feet.
➤ Demonstrate the proper way to inspect shoes. (See *Footwear inspection*.)
➤ Caution him not to walk barefoot, indoors or outdoors.
➤ Teach him to check his feet daily for blisters, cuts, sores, and other abnormalities.
➤ Urge him to notify you immediately if he experiences signs or symptoms that persist, worsen, or cause anxiety, such as tingling, numbness, open lesions, dark toes, skin maceration with heavy odor, cracks between toes and on heel (especially if bleeding), drainage, or pain in toenails,

### FOOTWEAR INSPECTION

Many foot problems arise from shoes that fit improperly. You can help the patient avoid unnecessary foot problems by instructing him in proper footwear inspection.
*Proper fit:* Shoes should extend ½" (1 cm) beyond the longest toe. They should also be wide enough to ensure no unnecessary pressure on any part of the foot.
*Quality and type of shoe:* Shoes should be firm and well constructed and should not cause feet to perspire.
*Shoe interior:* Inspect the inside of the shoes for tears in lining or insole; pebbles, nails, or other debris; cracks; holes; or odor indicating moisture. Hold the shoe firmly by the toe and tap the heel on the floor. This will loosen any debris that may have adhered to the shoe lining.

heels, metatarsal pads, or other areas of the foot.
➤ Schedule a follow-up appointment as needed for calluses. Instruct the patient to return to the office in 1 week for a follow-up for corns.
➤ Recommend foot care every 4 to 6 weeks as indicated.

## COMPLICATIONS

None known

## SPECIAL CONSIDERATIONS

➤ A patient should see a podiatrist for treatment of secondary infections, split toenails, or separating nails. Nail removal may be indicated.
➤ As a person ages, the toenails become more yellow and grow slower as the nail plate thickens. Nails may also thicken and develop transverse ridges.
➤ Nails appear pink in whites and may have a bluish hue in dark-skinned people.

## DOCUMENTATION

➤ In the chart, the preprocedural and postprocedural note must include an evaluation of potentially affected function, range of motion, and neurosensory testing, such as two-point discrimination.
➤ Record a brief history, with attention to medication, pain in feet or legs, diabetic status, and peripheral vascular disease.
➤ Note all abnormal findings on the assessment sheet.
➤ Describe the type of care provided (hygiene, padding, massage with oil, and so on), instructions given to the patient and his understanding of them, and his ability to perform return demonstrations of foot and shoe inspections.
➤ Describe referrals, if any, and their purpose.

## Ingrown toenail care

### CPT CODES
*11730    Avulsion of nail plate, partial or complete, simple; single*
*11732    Avulsion of each additional nail plate*
*11750    Excision of nail and nail matrix, partial or complete*

## DESCRIPTION

An ingrown toenail is a common condition that can cause a great deal of disability and discomfort for the patient. It occurs when the proper fit of the toenail into the lateral nail groove is altered. The great toe is generally the only one affected, and the problem may occur on either the medial or lateral aspect of the toe. Causes include:
➤ improperly fitting shoes
➤ toenails cut at an inappropriate angle (rounded instead of flat)

➤ accumulation of debris under the nail
➤ congenital malformation of the great toenail (an autosomal dominant trait)
➤ curling or deformity of the nail due to trauma or excessive length.

A splinter or small piece of the great toenail invades the sulcus and subcutaneous tissue, resulting in inflammation of the surrounding area. This leads to callous formation, edema, and perforation into the nail groove as a result of rubbing. The nail edge becomes embedded in the lateral skin fold, causing pain, erythema, and ultimately infection. Either partial or total removal of the toenail is commonly indicated at this point.

The three stages of this disorder must be understood to develop a sound treatment plan:
➤ Stage I is characterized by tenderness on palpation and when wearing shoes, erythema, and slight swelling at the site (paronychia).
➤ Stage II is associated with erythema, tenderness with associated suppuration, and a small collection of pus.
➤ Stage III is characterized by all of the above signs and symptoms plus hypertrophy of the nail wall and granulation tissue formation.

Each stage requires a different approach to care. Stage I warrants conservative management with toenail elevation and wicking. Stage II may require partial toenail removal in the office (as described in this procedure). Stage III should be referred to a specialist for more aggressive treatment under appropriate sedation or anesthesia.

## INDICATIONS

➤ To treat ingrown toenail, medial or lateral aspect (onychocryptosis); chronic, recurrent inflammation of the nail fold (paronychia); or deformed or curved nail (onychogryposis)

## CONTRAINDICATIONS

### Absolute

➤ Coagulopathies likely to inhibit hemostasis
➤ Allergy to local anesthetics
➤ Use of phenol solution in pregnancy

### Relative

➤ Diabetes mellitus (may refer to specialist)
➤ Peripheral vascular disease
➤ Immunocompromised status
➤ Peripheral neuropathy

## EQUIPMENT

### Conservative management (stage I)

Splinter forceps or disposable tweezers ◆ nail file ◆ cotton for packing (3 mm × 2.5 mm) ◆ tincture of iodine or 60% alcohol solution (optional) ◆ scissors ◆ gloves ◆ antiseptic, germicidal solution (such as povidone-iodine) ◆ a basin for soaking the foot ◆ dressing material and tape ◆ antibiotic ointment

### Partial toenail removal (stage II)

Equipment above plus: narrow periosteal elevator (nail elevator) ◆ english nail splitter or sterile scissors with straight blades ◆ phenol solution (88%) or 60% alcohol solution (optional) ◆ sterile drapes ◆ two sterile straight hemostat ◆ local anesthetic such as lidocaine without epinephrine ◆ rubber band or Penrose drain ◆ 5-ml syringe with 1″ 27G or 25G needle ◆ alcohol wipes

## ESSENTIAL STEPS

➤ Obtain a detailed history, and conduct a physical examination.
➤ Verify that the patient is not allergic to latex and iodine.

➤ Explain the procedure to the patient, and address any questions or concerns that he has.
➤ Obtain written consent for partial toenail removal. (No consent is needed for conservative management.)
➤ Position the patient comfortably on the examination table.
➤ Soak the affected foot in an antiseptic, germicidal solution.

### For conservative management

➤ Have the patient lie comfortably with flexed knees and feet flat on the examination table. Put on gloves.
➤ Thin the middle-third of the nail on the affected side by filing the upper surface until you can see the nail matrix.
➤ Using scissors, cut cotton to proper length. Stretch and roll the cotton to form a wick. (See *Using conservative management,* page 256.)
➤ Optional: Soak cotton in a 60% alcohol or tincture of iodine solution to prevent infection.
➤ Lift the nail edge using forceps and gently push the wick firmly under the distal portion of the affected lateral nail groove.
➤ Apply antibiotic ointment to the infected cuticle edge.
➤ Tape the cotton wick to prevent displacement (tape the lateral edge between the first and second toes to prevent irritation; tape the medial edge to the medial aspect of the toe to prevent rubbing from shoes).
➤ Cover with a dressing.

### For partial toenail removal

➤ Put on gloves and drape the foot with a sterile drape.
➤ Administer a digital block. Wipe the site with an alcohol wipe and insert the needle with the anesthetic agent at a 45-degree angle.
➤ Ask the patient if he notices any change in sensation. If he reports pain, indicating

## USING CONSERVATIVE MANAGEMENT

An ingrown toenail in stage I usually requires conservative management. Using a forceps, lift the nail away from the inflamed soft tissue. Gently push a cotton wick under the nail and leave in place for 1 week; replace as indicated. This allows the edema and inflammation to resolve and the nail to grow out in a normal manner.

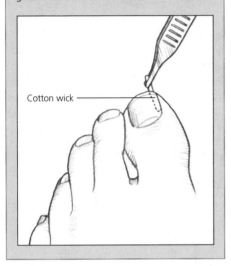

Cotton wick

direct contact with the nerve, withdraw the needle 1 mm.

➤ Aspirate to make sure there is no blood return. If there is, the needle is in a blood vessel. Withdraw the needle slightly and reinsert it in another area.

➤ Inject 1 to 2 ml of lidocaine while partially withdrawing the needle. Then redirect the needle across the surface, advance it, and inject another 0.5 ml while withdrawing the needle. This method distributes the anesthetic uniformly, providing the optimal effect.

➤ Massage the area gently. The maximum effect should occur in 5 to 15 minutes.

 **ALERT** Always ensure that the local anesthetic does not contain epinephrine; failure to do so can lead to vasoconstriction and tissue hypoxia.

➤ When adequate anesthesia is attained (usually in 5 to 15 minutes), wrap a rubber band or Penrose drain securely around the proximal toe as a tourniquet (optional).

➤ Remove the affected portion of the nail. (See *Removing a part of the nail.*)

➤ Examine the nail bed and remove any debris.

➤ Remove the tourniquet, if used.

 **ALERT** Never leave the tourniquet in place for more than 10 minutes.

➤ Apply antibiotic ointment to the nail bed, and then cover with a sterile dressing. Cut to proper size with scissors.

➤ Optional: Use phenol to cauterize the matrix where the nail was removed.

## PATIENT TEACHING

➤ Inform the patient that serosanguineous drainage should be minimal within 24 hours and that pain should be well controlled with nonnarcotic analgesia and elevation of the foot. Explain that sterile exudate may be present for up to 4 weeks, that the toe should be fully healed in 4 to 6 weeks, and that complete nail regrowth takes 8 to 12 months in an adult.

➤ Instruct the patient to rest the foot and elevate it for 24 hours.

➤ Advise him to change the dressing in 24 hours and to observe for signs of infection (redness, swelling, pain, and purulent drainage).

➤ Instruct him to begin ambulation with open-toe shoes or sandals after 24 hours and to wear only this type of shoe for 2 weeks. Have him avoid tight or poorly fitting footwear at all times.

➤ Teach him proper wound care. Tell him to soak the toe in warm water for 20 minutes twice daily for 4 days, to dry the toe and apply a thin layer of antibiotic oint-

## REMOVING A PART OF THE NAIL

Partial nail removal (partial avulsion) is indicated for more advanced cases of paronychia.

Administer a digital block proximal to the toenail on the outer edge of the toe, inserting the needle toward the plantar surface on the affected side.

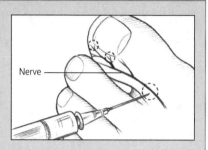
Nerve

Use a gauze pad to separate the toes. Loosen and lift the affected nail edge, using the periosteal elevator or hemostat. Introduce and advance the elevator, applying upward pressure against the nail (freeing the nail sulcus and eponychium from the nail plate) and away from the nail bed to minimize bleeding and injury.

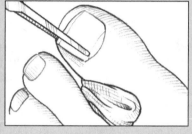

Using the nail splitter or sterile scissors, wedge off a 2- to 3-mm section of the affected nail, and then use the nail elevator to free the wedge from the nail bed. Grasp the nail wedge with a hemostat. In one steady, continuous movement, pull the wedge out while simultaneously twisting toward the affected side of the toe.

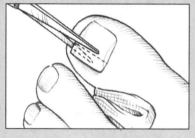

ment to the toe's affected edge, to reapply nail packing (if used) after each soaking, and to keep a bandage on the toe until it heals.

➤ Advise the patient to take acetaminophen or ibuprofen as directed for pain.

➤ Instruct him to avoid running or strenuous activity for 2 weeks.

➤ Urge him to notify you promptly if he experiences chills, fever higher than 100° F (37.8° C), pus, foul-smelling odor, increased warmth or red streaks, bleeding after the first 48 hours, pain unrelieved by acetaminophen or ibuprofen, or a return of symptoms as the nail regrows.

➤ Encourage him to schedule a follow-up appointment in 1 week for evaluation of the wound, including a neurosensory evaluation.

## COMPLICATIONS

➤ *Infection* is treated with antimicrobial soaks and antibiotics.

➤ *Excessive bleeding* may be cauterized with handheld cautery or silver nitrate sticks. Refer the patient to a physician or an acute care center if you can't control the bleeding.

➤ *Nail regrowth with paronychia* is treated with a repeat procedure.

## SPECIAL CONSIDERATIONS

 **CULTURAL TIP** Most Asians find it extremely disrespectful to show one's soles or to extend one's feet in the direction of a respected person. If you note patient reluctance to expose the feet, try changing positions so that you are initially looking at the superior aspect. When possible, avoid sitting with legs crossed or in any other position in which your leg is extended in the direction of a patient, particularly an elder.

 **CULTURAL TIP** Ethiopians and Filipinos may object to cutting nails at night. South Asians may insist that nail parings be thrown into a sink with running water. Native Americans may prefer to have their nail parings returned to them.

➤ Many patients don't realize how long it takes to clear paronychia. They may stop treatment when results aren't evident in 1 or 2 months. Before initiating treatment and with each visit, reinforce that the nail takes a year to regrow.

## DOCUMENTATION

➤ Before performing this procedure, document any abnormal physical findings on the consent form. Have the patient initial the comments and sign the form to signify acknowledgment of preprocedural abnormalities. In the chart, the preprocedural and postprocedural note must include an evaluation of potentially affected function, range of motion, and sensation.
➤ In documenting the patient's consent to the procedure, note that you discussed treatment options, duration of treatment, and the significant risk for recurrence of infection.
➤ If applicable, indicate the type, amount, and placement of local anesthesia administered; the needle gauge used; and the patient's reaction to the injection.
➤ Record the time of tourniquet placement and removal.

➤ Describe the wound appearance (including amount of bleeding) after the procedure.
➤ Note discharge instructions explained to the patient and family.

# Unna's boot application

CPT CODE
*29580    Strapping with Unna's boot*

## DESCRIPTION

Unna's boot is a commercially prepared, medicated gauze compression dressing that wraps around the foot and leg. It's used to treat uninfected, nonnecrotic leg and foot ulcers. Alternatively, a preparation known as Unna's paste (gelatin, zinc oxide, calamine lotion, and glycerin) may be applied to the ulcer and covered with lightweight gauze. The boot's effectiveness results from compression applied by the bandage combined with moisture supplied by the paste.

## INDICATIONS

➤ To treat leg and foot ulcers resulting from venous insufficiency or stasis dermatitis

## CONTRAINDICATIONS

### Absolute
➤ Allergy to any ingredient used in the paste
➤ Presence of arterial ulcers, weeping eczema, cellulitis, suspected infection, or necrosis
➤ Deep vein thrombosis, phlebitis, or arterial insufficiency

## HOW TO WRAP UNNA'S BOOT

After cleaning the patient's skin thoroughly, flex his knee. Then, starting with the foot positioned at a right angle to the leg, wrap the medicated gauze bandage firmly—not tightly—around the patient's foot. Make sure the dressing covers the heel. Continue wrapping upward, overlapping the dressing slightly with each turn. Make sure that the dressing circles the leg at an angle to avoid compromising the circulation. Smooth the boot with your free hand as you go, as shown below.

Stop wrapping about 1" (2.5 cm) below the knee. If necessary, make a 2" (5-cm) slit in the boot just below the knee to relieve constriction that may develop as the dressing hardens.

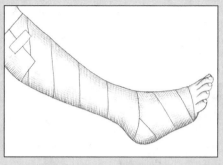

If drainage is excessive, you may wrap a roller gauze dressing over the Unna's boot. As the final layer, wrap an elastic bandage in a figure-eight pattern.

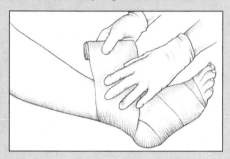

## EQUIPMENT

Scrub sponge with cleaning agent ◆ normal saline solution ◆ commercially prepared gauze bandage saturated with Unna's paste (or Unna's paste and lightweight gauze) ◆ bandage scissors ◆ gloves ◆ elastic bandage to cover Unna's boot ◆ metal clips or tape ◆ extra gauze for excessive drainage (optional) ◆ mineral oil (optional)

## ESSENTIAL STEPS

➤ Explain the procedure to the patient, and answer any questions he has.
➤ Verify that the patient is not allergic to topical medications.
➤ Wash your hands and put on gloves.
➤ Assess the ulcer and the surrounding skin. Evaluate ulcer size, drainage, and appearance. Perform a neurovascular assessment of the affected foot.

 **ALERT** If pulses are undetectable, order Doppler studies immediately. Depending on the patient's condition, consider referring to a physician or surgeon.
➤ Clean the affected area gently with the sponge and cleaning agent. Rinse with normal saline solution.
➤ Some practitioners use mineral oil on the unaffected areas that will be covered with the dressing to decrease pruritus. Don't allow mineral oil onto any compromised skin.
➤ If a commercially prepared gauze bandage isn't available, spread Unna's paste evenly on the leg and foot. Then cover the leg and foot with the lightweight gauze. Apply three to four layers of paste interspersed with layers of gauze. In a prepared bandage, the bandage is impregnated with the paste.
➤ Apply gauze or the prepared bandage in a spiral motion, from just above the toes

to the knee. Be sure to cover the heel. The wrap should be snug but not tight. To cover the area completely, make sure each turn overlaps the previous one by half the bandage width (see *How to wrap Unna's boot*, page 259).

➤ Continue wrapping the patient's leg up to the knee, using firm, even pressure. Stop the dressing 1″ (2.5 cm) below the popliteal fossa. Mold the boot with your free hand as you apply the bandage.

➤ Cover the boot with an elastic bandage, using the same technique.

➤ Secure the bandage with metal clips or tape.

➤ Instruct the patient to remain with his leg outstretched and elevated until the paste dries (approximately 30 minutes). Observe the patient's foot for signs of impairment, such as cyanosis, loss of feeling, and swelling. These signs indicate that the bandage is too tight and must be removed.

➤ Leave the boot on for 3 to 14 days (with an average of 5 to 7 days), depending on the amount of exudate.

➤ Change the boot as indicated to assess the underlying skin and ulcer healing. Remove the boot by unwrapping the bandage from the knee back to the foot.

## PATIENT TEACHING

➤ Advise the patient that the amount of discomfort varies with the degree of neurovascular compromise. Assure him that discomfort will lessen over time.

➤ Explain that resolution of the ulcer also can vary, depending on the ulcer's size and on the coexistence of other conditions, such as diabetes, peripheral vascular disease, and infection.

➤ Emphasize the need to keep the affected leg clean and dry. Remind him to wrap it in plastic to a point above the knee before bathing, and caution him not to submerge the affected leg.

➤ Advise him not to put anything inside the boot or to scratch under the dressing;

doing so increases the risk of infection and additional skin breakdown.

➤ If the patient can change his own dressing, review the proper technique to use, and answer any questions he has. (See *Applying a medicated boot*.)

➤ Instruct the patient to walk on and handle the wrap carefully to avoid damaging it. Tell him the boot will stiffen but won't be as hard as a cast.

➤ Instruct the patient to notify you promptly if he experiences severe itching or signs and symptoms of neurovascular compromise (change in color or temperature, numbness or tingling, swelling, or increased pain) or infection (increasing redness, swelling, drainage, odor, or pain).

➤ Have the patient schedule weekly follow-up appointments so you can evaluate progress.

## COMPLICATIONS

➤ *Contact dermatitis* may result from hypersensitivity to Unna's paste and is treated by immediately removing the Unna's boot.

➤ *Vascular compromise* is minimized by promptly removing and reapplying the boot, as indicated, and by teaching the patient to detect and report signs and symptoms of vascular compromise.

## SPECIAL CONSIDERATIONS

➤ If the boot is applied over a swollen leg, it must be changed as the edema subsides — if necessary, more frequently than every 5 days.

➤ Don't make reverse turns while wrapping the bandage. This could create excessive pressure areas that may cause discomfort as the bandage hardens.

➤ For bathing, instruct the patient to cover the boot with a plastic kitchen trash bag sealed at the knee with an elastic bandage to avoid wetting the boot. A wet boot softens and loses it effectiveness. If the pa-

# APPLYING A MEDICATED BOOT

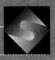

DEAR PATIENT:

A medicated boot (called an Unna's boot) can protect and medicate your leg ulcers while it prevents swelling. The boot is a bandage containing calamine, glycerin, zinc oxide, and gelatin. Here is how to apply it.

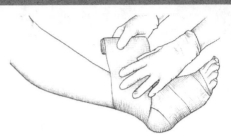

### Getting ready
Gather the equipment that you'll need. This includes a scrub sponge with hexa-chlorophene, normal saline solution, a gauze bandage saturated with medicated paste (Unna's boot), an elastic bandage, paper tape, and moisturizer.

Now, wash your hands thoroughly.

### Cleaning the area
Gently clean the lower half of your leg with the scrub sponge. Rinse with normal saline solution. If the skin of your upper calf is dry, apply moisturizer.

### Wrapping the boot
Place your foot at a right angle to your leg. Begin wrapping the bandage by making a circular turn around your foot. Then slant the bandage over your heel. Cut the bandage and smooth the edges.

Repeat this procedure, making sure to overlap the bandage in spiral fashion as you wrap.

Next, circle the medicated bandage up and around your leg, moving toward your knee. Use less pressure now than you did when wrapping your foot and ankle. Stop wrapping at 1" to 2" (2.5 to 5 cm) below your knee. To cover the area completely as you wrap, make sure you overlap the previous turn by half the bandage's width.

Repeat this procedure twice more so that your bandage has three layers.

Mold the boot as you apply the bandage to make it smooth and even.

### Is the boot too tight?
Wait 30 minutes as the boot dries and hardens. Periodically pinch your toes to make sure they blanch but color returns when you release the pressure. If they don't, the boot may be too tight. (You'll have to unwrap the boot and start over.)

### Fastening the boot
Now wrap the elastic bandage around the boot to cover it. Secure the end of the elastic bandage with paper tape.

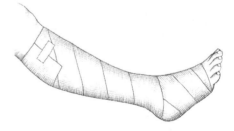

### Follow-up
Remove the boot and repeat this procedure every 5 to 7 days.

tient's safety is a concern, instruct him to take a sponge bath.

## DOCUMENTATION

➤ Record the date and time of application, indications, and the presence of a pulse in the affected foot.
➤ Specify which leg you bandaged.
➤ Describe the appearance of the patient's skin before and after boot application.
➤ Name the equipment used (a commercially prepared bandage or Unna's paste and lightweight gauze).
➤ Describe any allergic reaction.
➤ Note instructions given to the patient and the patient's tolerance for the procedure.

## Suture removal

### CPT CODE
No specific code has been assigned. (Removal is included as part of suture insertion.)

## DESCRIPTION

The goal of suture removal is to remove skin sutures from a healed wound without damaging newly formed tissue. More can be learned about suture technique and final results at the time of suture removal than at the end of the procedure. If sutures are placed too tightly, resulting in ischemic skin margins, the detrimental results of ischemia are readily apparent at the time of suture removal. Only by seeing the wound after suture removal can a practitioner modify techniques that will influence the final result.

## INDICATIONS

➤ To promote complete wound healing and minimize the occurrence of inflammation and scarring

## CONTRAINDICATIONS

### Relative
➤ Skin edges that require support

## EQUIPMENT

Waterproof trash bag ◆ adjustable light ◆ gloves ◆ sterile gloves ◆ sterile forceps or hemostat ◆ normal saline solution ◆ sterile gauze pads ◆ antiseptic cleaning agent ◆ sterile curve-tipped suture scissors ◆ povidone-iodine sponges ◆ adhesive butterfly strips or Steri-Strips (optional) ◆ compound benzoin tincture or other skin protectant (optional) ◆ prepackaged, sterile suture-removal trays (optional) ◆ hydrogen peroxide or sterile water (optional) ◆ cotton-tipped applicators

## PREPARATION OF EQUIPMENT

➤ Assemble all the equipment.
➤ Check the expiration date on each sterile package and inspect for tears.
➤ Open the waterproof trash bag, and place it near the patient. Form a cuff by turning down the top of the trash bag.

## ESSENTIAL STEPS

➤ Obtain a detailed history, and conduct a physical examination as indicated.
➤ Verify that the patient is not allergic to adhesive tape and povidone-iodine or other topical solutions and medications.
➤ Explain the procedure to the patient, and answer any questions he has. Assure him that this procedure is typically painless but that he may feel a tickling sensation as the sutures are removed.

➤ Place the patient in a comfortable position that doesn't put undue tension on the suture line. Because some patients experience nausea or dizziness during the procedure, have the patient recline, if possible.

➤ Adjust the light so that it shines directly on the suture line.

➤ Wash your hands thoroughly. If the patient's wound has a dressing, put on gloves and carefully remove the dressing. Discard the dressing and gloves in the waterproof trash bag.

➤ Observe the wound for gaping, drainage, inflammation, signs of infection, and embedded sutures. Absence of a healing ridge under the suture line 5 to 7 days after insertion indicates that the line needs continued support and protection during healing. Either postpone suture removal for up to 3 days or consider the use of adhesive butterfly strips.

➤ Establish a sterile work area with all the equipment and supplies you'll need for suture removal and wound care.

➤ Put on sterile gloves.

➤ Remove crusts from the wound with cotton-tipped applicators and hydrogen peroxide or sterile water. Then gently lift the suture with the forceps, cut at the edge close to the skin surface, and pull the suture across the wound to remove it. Use gentle traction to avoid breaking the suture material.

➤ Remove the sutures according to the suture type (see *Removing sutures,* page 264).

➤ After removing the sutures, wipe the incision gently with gauze pads soaked in an antiseptic cleaning agent or with a povidone-iodine sponge. Rinse clean with gauze pads and normal saline solution.

➤ Apply a light, sterile gauze dressing or adhesive butterfly strips, if needed (optional).

## PATIENT TEACHING

➤ Inform the patient that discomfort should be minimal unless granulation has occurred over the sutures. Assure him that redness surrounding the incision should gradually disappear, leaving only a thin line.

➤ Teach him how to remove the dressing (if applicable) and care for the wound.

➤ Tell him that he may shower in 1 to 2 days if the incision is dry and heals well.

➤ Instruct him to notify you promptly if he experiences signs and symptoms of infection (increasing redness, swelling, pain, and warmth; cloudy yellow, green, or brown drainage; opening of wound; foul odor; a red streak from the site; or fever).

## COMPLICATIONS

➤ *Infection* may be treated with local or systemic antibiotics and antiseptic soaks. It may also require consultation with a physician, a dermatologist, or an infectious disease specialist.

➤ *Scarring and keloids* are minimized with gentle handling and the use of such techniques as undermining and layered suturing.

➤ *Dehiscence* requires additional wound support and may require referral. If the wound dehisces during suture removal, apply butterfly adhesive strips or Steri-Strips to support and approximate the edges until the wound can be repaired. Repair depends on the extent of the dehiscence. Consult with the collaborating physician as indicated. Options include using Steri-Strips alone or with an elastic bandage to relieve tension on the wound edges or monitoring the wound as it heals by secondary intention.

## SPECIAL CONSIDERATIONS

➤ The blood supply and healing times vary with location, requiring that sutures be re-

## REMOVING SUTURES

The technique you use to remove a suture depends on the suture type.

For all suture types, you should grasp and cut sutures to avoid pulling the exposed — and thus contaminated — suture material through subcutaneous tissue. The illustrations here show how to remove four common suture types.

### Simple interrupted sutures

Using sterile forceps, grasp the knot of the first suture and raise it off the skin. This will expose a small portion of the suture that was below skin level. Place the rounded tip of sterile curved-tip suture scissors against the skin and cut through the exposed portion of the suture. Then, still holding the knot with the forceps, pull the cut suture up and out of the skin in a smooth continuous motion to avoid causing the patient pain. Discard the suture. Repeat the process for every other suture. If the wound doesn't gape, remove the remaining sutures.

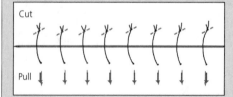

### Mattress interrupted sutures

If possible, remove the small visible portion of the suture opposite the knot by cutting it at each end and lifting the small piece away from the skin to prevent pulling it through and contaminating subcutaneous tissue. Then remove the rest of the suture by pulling it out in the direction of the knot, as shown. If the visible portion is too small to cut twice, cut it once and pull the entire suture out in the opposite direction. Repeat for the remaining sutures. Monitor the incision carefully for signs of infection.

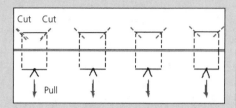

### Simple continuous sutures

Cut the first suture on the side opposite the knot. Next, cut the same side of the next suture in line. Lift the first suture out in the direction of the knot. Proceed along the suture line, grasping each suture where you grasped the knot on the first one.

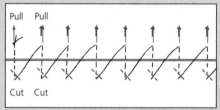

### Mattress continuous sutures

Follow the procedure for removing mattress interrupted sutures. First remove the small visible portion of the suture, if possible, to prevent pulling it through and contaminating subcutaneous tissue. Then extract the rest of the suture in the direction of the knot.

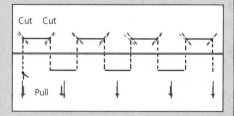

moved at different times in different locations. In general, remove face, neck, and scalp sutures in 3 to 5 days and trunk and extremity sutures in 7 to 14 days.

## DOCUMENTATION

➤ Document indications for and details of the procedure, including a detailed description of the site before and after the procedure, any abnormalities in function before the procedure, the patient's reaction to the procedure, medications ordered, the time frame for follow-up evaluation, and any instructions given to the patient.

## Staple removal

### CPT CODE
No specific code has been assigned. (Removal is included as part of the staple insertion procedure.)

### DESCRIPTION
Skin staples or clips may be used in place of standard sutures to close lacerations and surgical wounds. They can secure a wound more quickly than sutures, making them useful in areas where cosmetic results are less important, such as the abdomen. When properly placed, staples and clips distribute tension evenly along the suture line with minimal tissue trauma and compression, promoting healing and minimizing scarring. Because staples and clips are made from surgical stainless steel, tissue reaction to them is minimal.

### INDICATIONS
➤ To remove staples once a wound is fully healed

### CONTRAINDICATIONS
None known

### EQUIPMENT
Waterproof trash bag ◆ adjustable light ◆ gloves if wound is dressed; otherwise, sterile gloves ◆ sterile gauze pads ◆ sterile staple or clip extractor (prepackaged, sterile disposable staple or clip extractors

are available) ◆ povidone-iodine solution or other antiseptic cleaning agent ◆ sterile cotton-tipped applicators ◆ adhesive butterfly strips or Steri-Strips (optional) ◆ compound benzoin tincture or other skin protectant (optional)

### PREPARATION OF EQUIPMENT
➤ Assemble all equipment.
➤ Check the expiration date on each sterile package and inspect for tears.
➤ Open the waterproof trash bag and place it near the patient, forming a cuff by turning down the top of the bag.

### ESSENTIAL STEPS
➤ Obtain a detailed history, and conduct a physical examination.
➤ Verify that the patient is not allergic to latex and iodine.
➤ Assess the wound and confirm the appropriateness of staple removal.
➤ Explain the procedure to the patient, and answer any questions he has. Inform him that he may feel a slight pulling or tickling sensation but little discomfort during staple removal. Reassure him that because his incision is healing properly, removing the supporting staples or clips won't weaken the incision line.
➤ Position the patient so that he's comfortable without placing undue tension on the incision line. Because some patients experience nausea or dizziness during the procedure, have the patient recline if possible.
➤ Adjust the light so that it shines directly on the suture line.
➤ Wash your hands thoroughly.
➤ If the patient's wound has a dressing, put on gloves to remove and discard the dressing and gloves.
➤ Observe the wound for gaping, drainage, inflammation, signs of infection, and embedded staples. Absence of a healing ridge

## REMOVING STAPLES

Removing a staple from a wound involves changing the shape of the staple before pulling it out of the skin. These illustrations show how to properly remove a staple using a staple extractor.

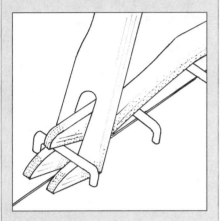

Position the extractor's lower jaws beneath the span of the first staple, as shown above. Squeeze the handles until they're completely closed.

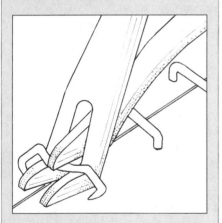

Then lift the staple away from the skin, as shown above. The extractor changes the shape of the staple and pulls the prongs out of the intradermal tissue.

under the suture line 5 to 7 days after insertion indicates that the line needs continued support and protection during healing. Either postpone suture removal for up to 3 days or consider the use of adhesive butterfly strips.

➤ Establish a sterile work area with all the equipment and supplies you'll need for staple removal and wound care. Open the supplies and put on sterile gloves.

➤ Wipe the incision gently with sterile gauze pads soaked in an antiseptic cleaning agent or with sterile cotton-tipped applicators to remove surface encrustations.

➤ Pick up the sterile staple or clip extractor. Then, starting at one end of the incision, remove the first staple or clip. Dislodge an embedded staple by gently rocking it from side to side.

➤ Hold the extractor over the trash bag and release it to discard the staple or clip.

➤ Repeat the procedure for each staple or clip until all are removed (see *Removing staples*).

➤ Apply a sterile gauze dressing, if applicable, to prevent infection or provide comfort and protection from rubbing. Discard gloves.

➤ Make sure that the patient is comfortable.

### PATIENT TEACHING

➤ Inform the patient that he may shower in 1 to 2 days if the incision is dry and healing well.

➤ Teach him how to remove the dressing, if applicable, and care for the wound.

➤ Advise him that the redness surrounding the incision should gradually disappear and that after a few weeks only a thin line should show.

➤ Inform him that Steri-Strips or butterfly strips will fall off in 3 to 5 days, frequently in the shower. Instruct him not to pull them off.

➤ Urge the patient to notify you promptly if he experiences signs of infection (increasing redness, swelling, pain, and warmth; cloudy yellow, green, or brown drainage; opening of wound; foul odor; a red streak from the site; or fever).

## COMPLICATIONS

➤ *Infection* may be treated with local or systemic antibiotics and antiseptic soaks. It may also require consultation with a physician, a dermatologist, or an infectious disease specialist.

➤ *Dehiscence* requires additional wound support and may require referral. If the wound dehisces during staple removal, apply butterfly adhesive strips or Steri-strips to support and approximate the edges until the wound can be repaired. Repair depends on the extent of the dehiscence. Consult your collaborating physician as indicated. Options include using Steri-Strips alone or with an elastic bandage to relieve tension on the wound edges or monitoring the wound as it heals by secondary intention.

➤ *Scarring and keloids* are minimized with gentle handling and the use of such techniques as undermining and layered suturing.

## SPECIAL CONSIDERATIONS

➤ If the incision appears to need additional support, consider removing only alternate staples or clips initially and leaving the others in place for 1 or 2 more days. When removing a staple or clip, place the extractor's jaws carefully between the patient's skin and the staple or clip to avoid pinching the patient. Staples or clips that have been placed too deeply within the skin or left in place too long may resist removal.

➤ If the wound dehisces after staples or clips are removed, apply butterfly adhesive strips or Steri-Strips to approximate and support the edges and repair the

### USING STERI-STRIPS OR BUTTERFLY STRIPS

Steri-Strips are used as a primary means of keeping a wound closed after suture removal. They're made of thin strips of sterile, nonwoven, porous fabric tape.

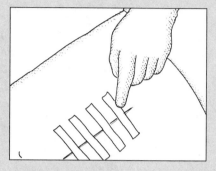

Butterfly closures consist of sterile, waterproof adhesive strips. A narrow, nonadhesive "bridge" connects the two expanded adhesive portions. These strips are used to close small wounds and to assist healing after suture or staple removal.

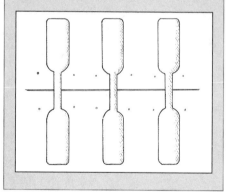

wound (see *Using Steri-Strips or butterfly strips*).

➤ You may also apply butterfly adhesive strips if the wound is healing normally to give added support to the incision and prevent lateral tension from forming a wide scar. Use a small amount of compound benzoin tincture or other skin protectant to ensure adherence. Leave the strips in place for 3 to 5 days.

## DOCUMENTATION

➤ Record the date and time of staple or clip removal, the number of staples or clips removed, dressings or butterfly strips applied, signs of wound complications, and the patient's tolerance for the procedure.
➤ Include a detailed description of the site before and after the procedure; any abnormalities in potentially affected function, range of motion, or sensation before the procedure; medications ordered; the time frame for follow-up evaluation; and any instructions given to the patient.

# Eye, Ear, and Nose Procedures

# 6

As common as they are troublesome, eye, ear, and nose disorders are frequently seen in settings such as a hospital, a clinic, or an extended-care facility. As a practitioner, you may perform eye, ear, and nose procedures in situations ranging from emergencies to routine checkups. Whatever the situation, these procedures call for precision and care to prevent infection and injury and preserve function.

Because the eyes transmit most of the sensory information reaching the brain, vision impairment can severely limit a patient's ability to function independently and to perceive and react to his surroundings. Likewise, untreated hearing loss can drastically impair his communication and social interaction. Inner-ear disorders may disrupt his equilibrium and the ability to move freely. In addition, nasal disorders can interfere with his respiration, reduce vitality, and cause marked discomfort.

A patient with a sensory loss can also experience perceptual impairment. The combined losses significantly alter a patient's daily activity and threaten his security and self-image.

As a practitioner, performing procedures that diagnose, treat, or even briefly cause sensory impairment requires that you give clear, simple instructions and explanations. In an emergency setting, effective communication becomes even more crucial because you'll be dealing with a patient suddenly disoriented by sensory and perceptual impairments.

You make an important contribution to the patient's understanding of eye, ear, and nose disorders. As various procedures are implemented, inform your patient about preventive care measures. Educate him to recognize signs and symptoms of sensory disorders. Encourage regularly scheduled examinations to detect problems early. Stress the importance of using safety equipment at work and, as appropriate, at home. When the patient leaves your care, he should be better able to prevent, cope with, and manage not only the current sensory disorder, but any that could arise in the future.

 **CULTURAL TIP** Touching any part of the head is considered impolite in some cultural groups such as the Chinese. Likewise, the Vietnamese consider the head sacred as it houses the soul, and touching the head can allow the soul to escape. Thus, it's important to explain the test carefully to the patient, then tell him immediately before touching his head.

## EYE PROCEDURES

### Eyelid eversion

CPT CODE
No specific code has been assigned. Usually performed with another procedure.

## EYELID EVERSION

To evert the eyelid, place a cotton-tipped applicator along the upper edge of the eyelid approximately ⅓″ (0.8 cm) above the lid margin. Grasp the upper eyelashes with the thumb and forefinger.

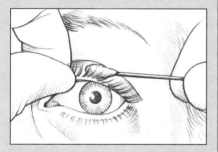

Pull the upper lid down and forward. Press gently downward on the eyelid (but not pressing against the globe) with the cotton-tipped applicator while lifting the eyelashes up. This will evert the eyelid for inspection. Stabilize the everted eyelid with

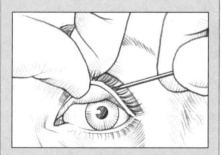

the thumb against the superior orbital ridge.
To release the eyelid, have the patient look up while gently pulling eyelashes outward.

## DESCRIPTION

Eyelid eversion is a technique for manipulating the upper eyelid to allow inspection of the lid and conjunctiva for a foreign body, lesions, or swelling. Careful inspection of the eye must be performed when the patient complains of a foreign body sensation, excessive tearing, blurred vision, light sensitivity, or a history of known foreign body hitting the eye. The foreign body sensation originates from the superficial layer of the cornea and, if left untreated, can lead to a variety of vision disturbances.

## INDICATIONS

➤ To remove known foreign body
➤ To treat eye trauma
➤ To evaluate unexplained eye irritation

## CONTRAINDICATIONS

➤ Uncooperative or combative patient
➤ Penetrating eye injury
➤ Eyelid laceration

## EQUIPMENT

Cotton-tipped applicator ◆ gloves ◆ magnification (such as a slit lamp [optional])

## ESSENTIAL STEPS

➤ Explain the procedure to the patient and explain why it is necessary. Answer any questions he has.
➤ Inform the patient that he may experience some discomfort.
➤ Ask the patient to lie supine for comfort and to facilitate the examination.
➤ Put on gloves.
➤ Instruct the patient to look downward.
➤ Tell him to try to relax the eye.
➤ Without putting pressure on the eyeball, place a cotton-tipped applicator along the upper edge of the eyelid. (See *Eyelid eversion*.)
➤ Examine the under surface of the lid under magnification such as a slit lamp, if necessary. If a foreign body is identified, gently remove it with a dampened cotton-tipped applicator.

➤ To release the eyelid, have the patient look up while gently pulling the eyelashes outward.

## PATIENT TEACHING

➤ Tell the patient that he'll experience minimal discomfort from the procedure. Follow-up may be required.

## COMPLICATIONS

➤ *Trauma* is minimized by gentle handling.
➤ *Infection* is minimized by using standard precautions.

## SPECIAL CONSIDERATIONS

None

## DOCUMENTATION

➤ Document eyelid eversion as part of the eye examination.
➤ Record findings on examination and how the foreign body was removed, if applicable.
➤ Note any and all instructions, medications prescribed, and expected follow-up.

## Corneal abrasion treatment

CPT CODES
65205   *Removal of foreign body, external eye, conjunctival, superficial*
65210   *Removal of foreign body, external eye, conjunctival, embedded*
65220   *Removal of foreign body, external eye, conjunctival, corneal without slit lamp*
99070   *Eye tray: supplies and material provided over and above what is usually included in office visit*

## DESCRIPTION

Corneal abrasion (injury to the covering of the cornea) treatment involves a thorough eye examination, irrigation, and daily follow-up evaluations until the abrasion heals completely, or, if necessary, a referral.

The cornea has five layers: the epithelium (outer), Bowman's layer, stroma (middle), Descemet's layer, and endothelium (inner). An abrasion to the cornea can result from chemical or mechanical injury (trauma), typically a contact lens or other foreign body in the eye. Injury limited to the epithelium heals without scarring; if the injury extends to the Bowman's layer, scar tissue may form. Signs and symptoms include pain, foreign body sensation, photophobia, tearing, blurred vision, and blepharospasm; the conjunctiva may also appear red from vascular response to the injury.

## INDICATIONS

➤ To treat known eye trauma, foreign body sensation, tearing, or unilateral pain on opening or closing of eyelid
➤ To investigate photophobia or exposure to ultraviolet light (arc welding, tanning beds, excessive sunlight) and certain chemicals
➤ To alleviate continuing eye irritation in contact lens wearers

## CONTRAINDICATIONS

### Absolute

➤ Potential high-velocity injury such as from metal fragments from heavy machinery
➤ Practitioner not familiar with treatment recommended by a poison control center
➤ Chemical exposure to a highly acidic, basic, or agent unknown

### Relative

➤ Noncompliant patient

## EQUIPMENT

Snellen's chart ◆ gloves ◆ antibiotic ointment such as tobramycin (optional) ◆ eyelid retractors (optional) ◆ topical ophthalmic anesthetic (such as 0.5% proparacaine unless the patient is allergic to ester anesthetics) ◆ sterile fluorescein sodium strips ◆ sterile cotton-tipped applicators ◆ bright white light source (penlight) ◆ Wood's light or other source of cobalt-blue light ◆ 8- to 10-power magnification (magnifying glass, ophthalmoscope on the +20 to +40 diopter setting) ◆ isotonic irrigant (sterile saline or other ophthalmic irrigation solution, such as Dacriose) ◆ sterile eye patches and 1" paper tape (optional) ◆ cycloplegic drops for severe pain such as one drop of 1% cyclopentolate HCl (2% for heavily pigmented eyes) (optional)

## ESSENTIAL STEPS

➤ Explain the procedure to the patient, answer questions, and obtain informed consent.
➤ Perform a vision screening with a Snellen's chart.
➤ Examine the patient's pupillary reflex, extraocular movements, anterior and posterior chambers, and fundi.
➤ Wash your hands and put on gloves.
➤ Using a magnification source, inspect the eye and eyelid for erythema, drainage, and foreign bodies.
➤ Place the patient in the supine position with his head turned laterally to the affected side.
➤ Open the affected eye and instill one to two drops of topical ophthalmic anesthetic and wait for 1 to 2 minutes.
➤ Inspect the eye using the penlight and compare it with the unaffected eye. The sclera should appear intact, the anterior chamber free of purulent material or blood, the iris and pupil symmetrical in size and shape, and the pupils equally reactive to

light. If signs and symptoms deviate from those findings, refer the patient to an ophthalmologist.
➤ Evert the upper lid by placing a cotton-tipped applicator on the upper lid, grasping the eyelashes, and pulling the upper lid down and forward while pressing gently downward on the eyelid with the cotton-tipped applicator to expose the posterior surface of the upper lid. If available, use eyelid retractors to expose the conjunctiva.
➤ Examine the eye for signs of trauma, foreign bodies, an infection, a stye, or an inverted eyelash.
➤ Moisten a fluorescein strip with one to two drops of normal saline solution; you may also use the patient's own tears. Don't use too much solution because excessive fluorescein staining can adhere to mucus and make it difficult to identify a defect.
➤ Retract the lower lid and touch the fluorescein strip to the conjunctiva.
➤ Instruct the patient to blink to distribute the stain.
➤ Use a Wood's light to examine the entire cornea and to identify areas of bright green concentrated fluorescence on the conjunctiva. The fluorescence indicates the location of the abrasion. (See *Fluorescein staining patterns*.)
➤ If you don't find a defect or if you note vertical streaking on the cornea, it is possible that a foreign body is embedded on the conjunctiva of the eyelid and you should then examine the entire conjunctiva.

 **ALERT** If you still can't find the cause of the patient's signs and symptoms, refer him to an ophthalmologist.

➤ Gently rinse the eye with sterile saline solution to flush the fluorescein stain from the conjunctiva.
➤ Administer cycloplegic drops for severe pain, if indicated. Instill antibiotic ointment for prophylaxis against infection. Administer minimal effective amount of anes-

## FLUORESCEIN STAINING PATTERNS

Abnormalities may be visible to the naked eye, such as the foreign body shown below. However, fluorescein staining may enhance physical findings. Fluorescein staining allows you to differentiate these diagnoses with the sharply demarcated circle or oval common in corneal abrasion.

Foreign bodies may become more visible with fluorescein staining.

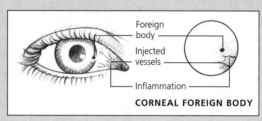

Foreign body
Injected vessels
Inflammation

**CORNEAL FOREIGN BODY**

Fluorescein staining permits the identification of the dendritic pattern of herpes simplex.

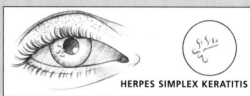

**HERPES SIMPLEX KERATITIS**

Here you can see the geographic appearance of keratitis sicca (dry eyes syndrome).

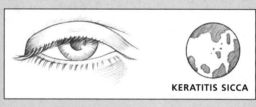

**KERATITIS SICCA**

Fluorescein staining enhances visibility of the band left by a chemical where it has been dragged across the eye's surface.

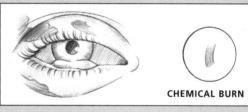

**CHEMICAL BURN**

Note the penetrating lines in this lateral view of corneal erosion.

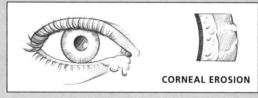

**CORNEAL EROSION**

Note the sharply demarcated circle or oval typical in cases of corneal abrasion.

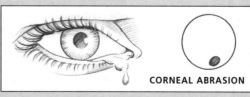

**CORNEAL ABRASION**

thetic because it could decrease the rate of healing, resulting in scarring.

➤ Cover the affected eye with a sterile eye patch to promote patient comfort. Have the patient close both eyes and firmly tape two eye patches (the first patch folded in half prevents the eye from opening) over the affected eye.

➤ Prescribe ophthalmic antibiotics for prophylaxis, such as tobramycin ointment or sulfacetamide ointment for 3 days.

## PATIENT TEACHING

➤ Instruct the patient to schedule a return office visit in 24 hours for reevaluation and for removal of the eye patch, if applicable.

➤ Tell the patient that it's crucial for you to monitor his progress every day until the eye is completely healed to catch complications such as infection at an early, treatable stage. Instruct him to contact you and return in 12 hours if symptoms persist.

➤ Tell him not to rub his eyes; doing so could disrupt new layers of epithelial granulation and delay healing. To alleviate pain, the patient may take pain medicine such as acetaminophen or apply moist compresses if no eye patch was used.

➤ Tell the patient who isn't wearing an eye patch to rest his eye, especially if he is a child or has a history of amblyopia.

➤ Tell the patient to call you for symptoms that persist or recur, acute changes in vision, and signs of infection (rapidly increasing redness, swelling, pain, and warmth; cloudy appearance of the eye; yellow, green, or brown drainage; or fever).

➤ Emphasize to the patient the importance of administering eyedrops as directed. (See *How to administer eyedrops.*)

➤ Encourage the patient to wear protective eyewear for high-risk occupational activities such as arc welding and mixing chemicals.

## COMPLICATIONS

➤ *Infection, scarring, permanent vision impairment, uveitis, and conjunctivitis* are minimized by gentle handling and rapid treatment. However, these conditions may also be unavoidable complications of the original injury. Early referral to a specialist is indicated when complications are suspected or if the patient has no relief within 12 hours of the initial visit.

## SPECIAL CONSIDERATIONS

➤ Cyclopentolate HCl may be repeated in 5 minutes if needed (note that the drug's effects peak in about 45 minutes and have a duration of up to a day, so pupils may be unequal on follow-up examination.)

 **ALERT** Use individually packaged fluorescein sodium strips to avoid chemical preservatives or increased infection risk associated with multiple-use vials.

➤ Refer the patient immediately to an ophthalmologist for acute vision loss, a herpes lesion, an intraocular foreign body, blunt or sharp trauma to the eye, corneal infection, deterioration of vision or acute vision loss, chemical burns (after immediate copious irrigation for 15 minutes with tap water from a shower or hose), a metallic foreign body, possible globe penetration (signs include hyphema, lens opacity, and pupil irregularity), noncompliance (for instance, a child who may need sedation), a foreign body that can't be irrigated out, an abrasion that isn't healing well within 24 hours or completely healed within 48 hours, or signs of infection. Also refer the patient for dendritic, large, or centrally located defects found on fluorescein examination. Inform the ophthalmologist if you've administered cycloplegic drops as dilation may persist through the next day.

➤ The epithelium may become more fragile due to chronic hypoxia associated with wearing hard contact lenses.

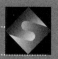

# HOW TO ADMINISTER EYEDROPS

DEAR PATIENT,

Your practitioner has prescribed these eye-drops for you.

---

**Medicine #1:** _____

Use ___ drops ___ times a day in your _____ eye.

---

**Medicine #2:** _____

Use ___ drops ___ times a day in your _____ eye.

---

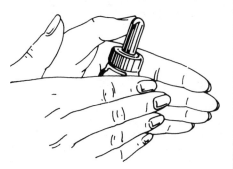

Here is how to instill drops in your eye.

**1** Begin by washing your hands thoroughly.

**2** Hold the medication bottle up to the light and examine it. If the medication is discolored or contains sediment, don't use it. Instead, take it back to the pharmacy and have it examined.

If the medication looks okay, warm it to room temperature by holding the bottle between your hands, as shown in the illustration at the top of the next column. Hold it for 2 minutes.

**3** Moisten a cotton ball or a tissue with water, and clean any secretions from around your eyes. Use a fresh cotton ball or tissue for each eye.

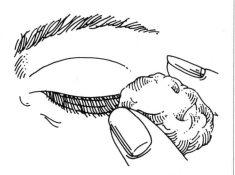

**4** Now, stand or sit before a mirror or lie on your back, whichever is most comfortable for you. Squeeze the bulb of the eyedropper and slowly release it to fill the dropper with medication.

*(continued)*

**5** Tilt your head slightly back and toward the eye you're treating. Pull down your lower eyelid.

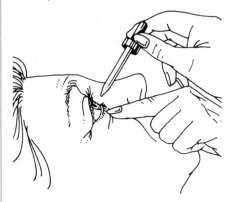

**6** Position the dropper over the conjunctival sac you've exposed between your lower lid and the white of your eye. Steady your hand by resting two fingers against your cheek or nose.

**7** Look up at the ceiling. Then squeeze the prescribed number of drops into

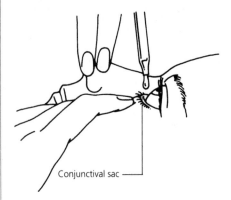

Conjunctival sac

the sac. Be careful not to touch the dropper to your eye, eyelashes, or finger. Wipe away excess medication with a clean tissue.

**8** Release the lower lid. Try to keep your eye open and not blink for at least 30 seconds. Apply gentle pressure to the corner of your eye at the bridge of your nose for 1 minute. This will prevent the medication from being absorbed through your tear duct.

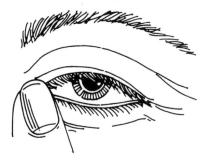

**9** Repeat the procedure in the other eye, if the practitioner orders.

**10** Cap the bottle and store it away from light and heat. If you're using more than one kind of drop, wait 5 minutes before you use the next one.
*Important:* Call your practitioner immediately if you notice any of these side effects: _____
_____
_____
_____

And remember, never put medication in your eyes unless the label reads "For Ophthalmic Use" or "For Use in Eyes."

➤ Look carefully for a foreign body in the cul-de-sac if you note a pattern of multiple vertical lines during conjunctival staining.
➤ If you are unable to rule out the possibility of a penetrating ocular injury, apply a shield to the eye and refer the patient immediately to a nearby emergency department or ophthalmology practice.
➤ Perform a Seidel's test if you suspect leakage of intraocular fluid. To do so, place a fluorescein strip directly over the site and look for a flow of green liquid.
➤ Don't patch the eye in a patient with only a small peripheral defect (less than 5 mm), in children, or in cases of suspected infection.
➤ Don't use topical corticosteroids; they may interfere with healing.
➤ Use a slit lamp for eye examination only if you're skilled in the technique.

## DOCUMENTATION

➤ Record a detailed case history before performing any procedures or treatments. Record the time, place, and type of injury as well as the presenting signs and symptoms.
➤ Note visual acuity of both eyes before the procedure.
➤ Document the size and location of all abrasions. Illustrations can help, but be careful that the illustration doesn't magnify the size of the lesion. During subsequent examinations, document the degree of healing.
➤ List any patient instructions and his understanding.

# Eye irrigation

CPT CODES
65205 *Removal of foreign body, external eye, conjunctival, superficial*
68399 *Unlisted procedure, conjunctiva*

## DESCRIPTION

The goal of this procedure is to flush and eliminate irritants to the eye itself, its cavity, and surrounding tissue. This may include foreign bodies, chemicals, or bodily secretions. The type of irritant (if known) should be identified before irrigation. Some irritants, such as alkali chemicals, are highly damaging to the eye, and patients should be referred for emergency or specialist care.

In an emergency, tap water may serve as an irrigant. The amount of solution needed to irrigate an eye depends on the contaminant. Secretions require a moderate volume; major chemical burns require a copious amount. Usually, an I.V. bottle or bag of normal saline solution (with I.V. tubing attached) supplies enough solution for continuous irrigation of a chemical burn. (See *Three devices for eye irrigation*, page 278.)

## INDICATIONS

➤ To remove chemical irritant or foreign particles and prevent further damage to the eye

## CONTRAINDICATIONS

### Relative
➤ Noncompliant patient
➤ Possibility of orbital fracture

## EQUIPMENT

Gloves ◆ towels ◆ eyelid retractor ◆ cotton balls or 4" × 4" gauze pads ◆ ophthalmoscope ◆ magnifying glass ◆ protective eyewear ◆ reservoir basin

### Optional
Litmus paper ◆ proparacaine hydrochloride topical anesthetic ◆ prepackaged, commercially prepared sterile irrigation

## THREE DEVICES FOR EYE IRRIGATION

Depending on the type and extent of injury, a patient's eye may need to be irrigated using different devices.

### Squeeze bottle

For moderate-volume irrigation — to remove eye secretions, for example — apply sterile ophthalmic irrigant to the eye directly from the squeeze bottle container. Direct the stream at the inner canthus and position the patient so that the stream washes across the cornea and exits at the outer canthus.

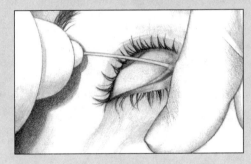

### I.V. tube

For copious irrigation — to treat chemical burns, for example — set up an I.V. bag and tubing without a needle. Use the procedure described above for moderate irrigation to flush the eye for at least 15 minutes.

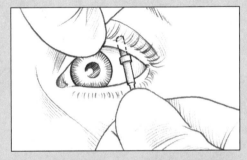

### Morgan lens

Connected to irrigation tubing, a Morgan lens permits continuous lavage and also delivers medication to the eye. Use an adapter to connect the lens to the I.V. tubing and the solution container. Begin the irrigation at the prescribed flow rate. To insert the device, ask the patient to look down as you insert the lens under the upper eyelid. Then tell him to look up as you retract and release the lower eyelid over the lens.

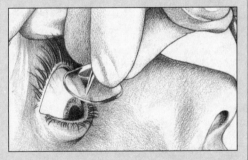

solution ◆ fluorescent stain ◆ prepackaged eye irrigation kit ◆ eye patch ◆ tape

### For moderate-volume irrigation

Sterile ophthalmic irrigant ◆ cotton-tipped applicators ◆ 20-ml sterile syringe

### For copious irrigation

One or more 1,000-ml bottles or bags of normal saline solution ◆ standard I.V. infusion set without needle ◆ I.V. pole

## PREPARATION OF EQUIPMENT

➤ All solutions should be at body temperature: 98.6° F (37° C). Read the label on the sterile ophthalmic irrigant. Double-check its sterility, strength, and expiration date.

### For moderate-volume irrigation

➤ Remove the cap from the irrigant container and place the container within easy reach. (Be sure to keep the tip of the container sterile.)

### For copious irrigation

➤ Use aseptic technique to set up the I.V. tubing and the bag or bottle of normal saline solution. Hang the container on an I.V. pole, fill the I.V. tubing with the solution, and adjust the drip regulator valve to ensure an adequate but not forceful flow. Place all other equipment within easy reach.

➤ Ensure there is adequate lighting for an ophthalmic examination.

## ESSENTIAL STEPS

➤ Wash hands and put on gloves and protective eyewear. Explain the procedure to the patient, and answer any questions he has. If the patient has a chemical burn, ease his anxiety by explaining that irrigation prevents further damage. Obtain history and patient consent when appropriate.

➤ Inspect the eyelids. Assess external and then internal structures with the magnifying glass and the ophthalmoscope.

➤ Assist the patient into a supine position. Turn his head slightly toward the affected side to prevent solution flowing over his nose and into the other eye.

➤ Place a towel under the patient's head, and let him hold another towel against his affected side to catch excess solution.

➤ If the patient has identified the irritant as a chemical, place a piece of litmus paper in the inner canthus area. This will identify if it's an alkali- or acid-based chemical.

➤ Using the thumb and index finger of your nondominant hand, separate the patient's eyelids.

➤ If indicated, instill proparacaine hydrochloride eyedrops as a comfort measure. Use them only once because repeated use retards healing. Wait a few minutes for maximal anesthetic effect.

➤ To irrigate the conjunctival cul-de-sac, continue holding the eyelids apart with your thumb and index finger.

➤ To irrigate the upper eyelid (the superior fornix) use an eyelid retractor. Steady the hand holding the retractor by resting it on the patient's forehead. The retractor prevents the eyelid from closing involuntarily when solution touches the cornea and conjunctiva.

➤ Position the reservoir basin close to the side of the patient's head.

### For moderate-volume irrigation

➤ With your nondominant hand, place your thumb along the lower eyelid and pull down. Place your index finger on the upper eyelid and separate the upper and lower eyelids.

➤ Holding the bottle of sterile ophthalmic irrigant or a sterile 20-ml syringe filled with sterile normal saline about 1" (2.5 cm) from the eye, direct a constant, gentle stream at the inner canthus so that the solution flows across the cornea to the outer canthus.

➤ Evert the lower eyelid and then the upper eyelid to inspect the eye cavity and eye structures for retained foreign particles. Flush the entire area of the cavity and eye structures.

➤ Remove any foreign particles by gently touching the conjunctiva with sterile, wet, cotton-tipped applicators. Don't touch the cornea.

➤ Resume irrigating the eye until it's clean of all visible foreign particles.

### For copious irrigation

➤ Hold the control valve on the I.V. tubing about 1″ above the eye, and direct a constant, gentle stream of normal saline solution at the inner canthus so that the solution flows across the cornea to the outer canthus.

➤ Ask the patient to rotate his eye periodically while you continue the irrigation. This action may dislodge foreign particles.

➤ Evert the lower eyelid and then the upper eyelid to inspect for retained foreign particles. (This inspection is especially important when the patient has caustic lime in his eye.)

➤ At this time, you may place the sterile I.V. tubing tip under the eyelid to hold it in place as irrigation continues.

➤ After eye irrigation, gently dry the eyelids with cotton balls or sterile gauze pads, wiping from the inner to the outer canthus. Use a new cotton ball or pad for each wipe. This reduces the patient's need to rub his eye.

➤ Reassess external and internal eye structures with the magnifying glass and ophthalmoscope.

➤ If corneal abrasion is suspected, apply fluorescent stain and evaluate for color changes.

➤ When you are finished, place an eye patch over the eye, secure it with tape and tell the patient to keep it in place for 24 hours.

➤ Remove and discard your gloves and goggles.

➤ Wash your hands to avoid burning, residual chemical contaminants.

## PATIENT TEACHING

➤ Tell the patient that discomfort should be minimal. Notable relief should be identified after the procedure or within a few hours. Instruct the patient to keep eye patch in place for 24 hours. If further irritation or pain or discomfort is noted, tell the patient to contact you for further evaluation. Generally, no antibiotics or further medications are necessary for this procedure.

➤ Instruct the patient to call if any increase or ongoing discomfort is noted or if any change in vision, eye pain or sensation, or eye drainage is noted. Tell the patient to avoid rubbing his eyes. Reinforce good hand-washing practices. Tell the patient that applying clean, cool compresses to the affected eye may help alleviate any postprocedure discomfort.

## COMPLICATIONS

➤ *Trauma or infection* may be caused secondary to the original injury or procedure and must be evaluated and treated on a case-by-case basis.

## SPECIAL CONSIDERATIONS

➤ If symptoms continue, vision changes are noticed, or irritation is seen on the ophthalmoscopic examination, a fluorescent stain examination should be completed.

➤ If any suspicious findings are noted during the procedure or assessment, refer the patient to an ophthalmologist for evaluation.

➤ Immediate irrigation with normal saline solution is the single best initial treatment for chemical burns to the eye and reduces the ultimate physical damage to the eye.

➤ For chemical burns, irrigate each eye for at least 15 minutes with normal saline solution to dilute and wash away the harsh chemical. (After irrigating any chemical, note the time, date, and chemical for your own reference in case you develop contact dermatitis.)

➤ Most acid burns with mild to moderate stromal haze will get better with time. Alkaline burns may initially look far better than they will appear at day 2 or 3. There-

fore, it's important to refer the patient to a facility or ophthalmologic practice immediately after irrigating the eye.
➤ When irrigating both eyes, have the patient tilt his head toward the side being irrigated to avoid cross-contamination.
➤ Proparacaine hydrochloride ophthalmic anesthetic should be stored tightly closed in its original container and refrigerated. Don't use discolored solution.

## DOCUMENTATION

➤ Record the results of the preprocedure and postprocedure external and internal ophthalmoscopic examinations. Note any abnormal color, drainage, assessment of vision changes, and pain or discomfort before and after irrigation.
➤ Document if ophthalmic anesthetic was used and how much.
➤ Note the type of irritant seen, removed, or irrigated. If litmus paper was used, document the findings.
➤ Record the type of irrigating procedure used.
➤ List what patient instructions were given and the patient's understanding of those instructions.
➤ Note the duration of irrigation, the type and amount of solution, and characteristics of the drainage. Record your assessment of the patient's eye before and after irrigation. Also note his response to the procedure.

## Foreign body removal from the eye

CPT CODES
65205   Removal of foreign body, external eye, conjunctival, superficial
65210   Removal of foreign body, external eye, conjunctival, embedded
65220   Removal of foreign body, external eye, corneal without slit lamp
65222   Removal of foreign body, external eye, corneal with slit lamp
99070   Eye tray: supplies and materials provided over and above what is usually included in office visit

## DESCRIPTION

Foreign body removal from the eye involves removing foreign matter through irrigation or dislodgment without causing further injury. A patient who complains of eye pain, burning, and the feeling that he has something in his eye may have a foreign body in the eye — typically dust, dirt, or a particle of metal, plastic, or wood. If the patient also displays photophobia and a tearing eye, he may have a corneal abrasion. People who take part in such activities as digging, drilling, hammering, welding, and woodworking without appropriate eye protection are at increased risk for injury to the eye.

The practitioner should evaluate a patient who complains of eye pain for one or more foreign bodies in the eye as some types of injuries can scatter fragments across the cornea. The foreign body typically lodges underneath the upper eyelid or in the superior temporal cul-de-sac, where the upper lid attaches to the eyeball; foreign bodies can also lodge in the inferior cul-de-sac below the lower lid.

## INDICATIONS

➤ To treat foreign body sensation, photophobia, tearing, or unilateral pain on opening or closing eyelid
➤ To remove extraocular foreign bodies

## CONTRAINDICATIONS

### Absolute
➤ High-velocity injury
➤ Hyphema

## EXTRACTION WITH A NEEDLE

If other methods are unsuccessful, you may gently attempt to dislodge the object with a small-gauge needle attached to a syringe for stability. Under magnification, approach the object from the side rather than from the front to avoid scratching the cornea.

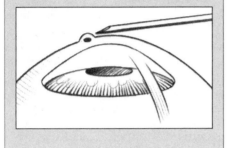

➤ Lens opacity
➤ Pupil irregularity
➤ Penetrating object or injury

### Relative
➤ Metallic object

## EQUIPMENT

Short-acting ophthalmic anesthetic solution (0.5% proparacaine) ◆ vision-screening device such as a Snellen's chart ◆ gloves ◆ cotton-tipped applicators or eyelid retractor ◆ ophthalmoscope ◆ sterile fluorescein stain strips ◆ sterile saline solution ◆ ophthalmic antibiotic solution or ointment (such as gentamicin, tobramycin, and ciprofloxacin) ◆ eye patches or eye shield and adhesive tape (if indicated) ◆ binocular loupe or slit lamp (if available) ◆ small-gauge needle (may be attached to a syringe for stability) (optional) ◆ 3-ml syringe ◆ small burr drill (if you are skilled in this procedure)

## ESSENTIAL STEPS

➤ Explain the procedure to the patient, answer questions, and obtain patient consent when appropriate.
➤ Inspect the eye and lid for erythema, drainage, and hemorrhage. If you suspect intraocular perforation or open globe injuries, refer to an ophthalmologist at once.
➤ Perform a vision screening using a Snellen's chart.
➤ Examine the pupillary reflex, extraocular movements, anterior and posterior chambers, and fundi.
➤ Wash your hands and put on gloves.
➤ Open the affected eye and instill one or two drops of short-acting ophthalmic anesthetic.
➤ While the patient looks down, evert the upper lid by placing a cotton-tipped applicator on the upper lid, grasping the eyelashes, and pulling the upper lid down and forward while pressing gently downward on the eyelid with the cotton-tipped applicator to expose the inner surface of the upper lid; you can also use an eyelid retractor to expose the conjunctiva.
➤ Examine the entire cornea, including the cul-de-sac, with an ophthalmoscope, slit lamp, or binocular loupe to locate and determine the depth of a foreign body.
➤ Locate the foreign body, assess if it is embedded or not, and determine the best technique of removal.
➤ If the foreign body is lying on the surface, use an oblique stream of sterile saline solution to flush the eye or use a saline-moistened, cotton-tipped applicator to gently attempt to remove the foreign body without embedding it or scratching the conjunctiva.
➤ If you can't remove the object with the applicator, gently attempt to dislodge the object with a small-gauge needle attached to a syringe for stability. (See *Extraction with a needle.*)
➤ Gently irrigate the eye with sterile saline solution to clean the area.

➤ Stain the conjunctiva with fluorescein to assess for corneal abrasion.

➤ Apply ophthalmic antibiotic solution or ointment.

➤ Cover the affected eye to promote patient comfort and protect the eye. Have the patient close both eyes and tightly tape two eye patches or an eye shield over the affected eye.

## PATIENT TEACHING

➤ Tell the patient to schedule a return office visit within 24 hours for reevaluation of the eye and restaining of the cornea as indicated.

➤ Encourage the patient to wear protective eyewear for high-risk occupational and recreational activities like arc welding, mixing chemicals, and lighting fireworks.

## COMPLICATIONS

➤ *Corneal ulcer or abrasion, intraocular foreign body, uveitis, conjunctivitis (viral or bacterial)* may resolve with time and antibiotics, such as gentamicin, tobramycin, or ciprofloxacin. If any of these conditions don't resolve, refer the patient to an ophthalmologist.

## SPECIAL CONSIDERATIONS

➤ If the patient complains of increased pain during the procedure, stop at once.

➤ If the patient has a metallic object in his eye — especially from a high-velocity injury — an X-ray should be taken or a computed tomography scan of the orbit should be performed to make sure no object penetrated the eye itself. The patient shouldn't undergo magnetic resonance imaging if there is a metal object in the eye, although this type of scan may be indicated for a nonmetallic foreign body.

➤ Use an ophthalmic magnet to remove metallic foreign bodies.

➤ Use a syringe or small burr drill to remove rust rings *only* if you are skilled in the procedure.

➤ Signs of intraocular perforation include softness of the orbit on gentle palpation, any change in pupillary size or reaction, abnormality of the anterior chamber, and leakage of fluid from the chamber. If any of these signs are present, cover the eye with a patch and protective shielding, instruct the patient to rest the eye and elevate his head, and refer him to an ophthalmologist. Call to ensure the patient will be seen immediately.

➤ Refer the patient to an ophthalmologist if there is a metallic injury with rust rings that can't be removed, a corneal ulceration that won't heal, signs of uveitis, or vision loss.

➤ Don't apply a topical corticosteroid or pain medication because they may mask changes or interfere with healing.

## DOCUMENTATION

➤ Document the indications for the procedure, any visual or cosmetic defects, and note that you have discussed with the patient at length the potential for vision loss due to unavoidable scarring, particularly when a corneal foreign body encroaches on the visual axis.

➤ Record the type, number, and location of foreign bodies. Note the removal procedure used.

➤ List any patient instructions and his understanding.

➤ Record if the patient was referred to an opthalmologist.

## Eye trauma stabilization

CPT CODE
No specific code has been assigned.

## Description

Eye trauma stabilization procedures are dependent on the type of injury and commonly include chemical burns, and blunt and sharp trauma. Ocular trauma is a major cause of monocular blindness, vision impairment, and disfiguring disability. There is a rare amount of statistical data on the incidence, type, severity, and etiology of eye trauma. A 1993 study by the National Center for Health Statistics, Centers for Disease Control and Prevention, found that males sustained more ocular injuries in all diagnostic categories and were more likely to be injured by a foreign body during a fight, a sporting event, or a motor vehicle accident. The sports most frequently associated with ocular injuries were basketball (with another player coming in contact with the eye), racquetball, ice hockey, and squash. Ocular injuries in women are more often the result of assaults and falls. Severe injuries include chemical and thermal burns of the globe, lacerations and open wounds of the globe, avulsions and severe burns of the periorbital tissues and eyelids, and extensive orbital fractures. Penetrating injuries in the past had the worst prognosis until the advent of current microsurgical techniques. A patient presenting with ocular trauma frequently will have sustained other trauma, particularly to the head and neck. In the event of potentially life-threatening trauma, evaluation and treatment of the eye is delayed until the patient is stabilized.

Chemical burns to the eye are most likely to occur in the occupational setting or as a result of accidents. (See *Chemical burns: Sources, presentation, and effects.*) Radiation injury of the eye commonly occurs secondary to prolonged exposure to bright sunlight or blinding snow, sun lamps, tanning booths, and welders' arcs.

## Indications

➤ To prevent further trauma to the eye while transporting or preparing for eye surgery
➤ To minimize duration of exposure to chemical irritant
➤ To prevent or minimize risk of permanent vision loss or cosmetic disfigurement
➤ To alleviate ocular pain

## Contraindications

None known

## Equipment

Equipment depends on the nature of the injury.
Eye lavage basin ◆ gloves ◆ sterile saline solution, lactated Ringers solution, or sterile water ◆ Morgan or Medi-flow irrigation lens (optional) ◆ I.V. tubing ◆ standard Snellen's chart or near-vision card ◆ large metal or plastic eye shield or paper or styrofoam drinking cup ◆ 4" × 4" gauze bandage and tape ◆ ophthalmic anesthetic agent (such as pontocaine) and antibiotic (such as gentamicin) ◆ sterile pH strips ◆ eye patches

## Essential Steps

### Stabilization for ocular trauma: Chemical burns

 **ALERT** Irrigation of lens is contraindicated if a deep corneal injury, penetrating foreign body, orbital fracture, or rupture of globe is suspected.
➤ Obtain history and patient consent when appropriate.
➤ Position the eye lavage basin close to the side of the patient's head.
➤ Put on gloves. Begin immediate eye lavage using an I.V. bag, tubing, and copious amount of sterile normal saline, lactated Ringers solution, or sterile water, di-

## CHEMICAL BURNS: SOURCES, PRESENTATION, AND EFFECTS

| TYPE | SOURCE | PRESENTATION | EFFECTS |
|---|---|---|---|
| **ACIDS** | | | |
| Acetic acid | Vinegar and household cleaners | ➤ Decreased visual acuity | ➤ Penetration limited |
| | | ➤ Corneal erosion | ➤ Damage immediate and limited to area of contact |
| Hydrochloric acid | Household cleaners | ➤ Conjunctiva inflamed | ➤ Posterior of eye rarely suffers injury |
| Sodium hypochlorite | Bleach | ➤ Necrosis of cornea and conjunctiva | ➤ Delayed damage possible |
| Sulfuric acid | Toilet cleaners and battery acid | | ➤ Necrosis of cornea and conjunctiva; outcome related to concentration and duration of exposure |
| Hydrofluoric acid | Etching and gasoline production | | |
| **ALKALI** | | | |
| Magnesium hydroxide | Fireworks | ➤ Painless vision loss | ➤ Exposure more serious than acid exposure |
| | | ➤ Few symptoms initially | ➤ Damage proportionate to pH, concentration, and time elapsed before lavage is initiated |
| Calcium hydroxide | Lime, plaster, mortar, and cement | ➤ Conjunctival chemosis | |
| Potassium hydroxide | Drain cleaners | ➤ Corneal erosion | ➤ Can penetrate deeply and continue penetration for hours to days |
| Sodium hydroxide | Drain cleaners, lye, and automobile air bags | ➤ Whitened or blanched appearance of cornea, sclera, or conjunctiva due to necrosis | ➤ Potential outcomes: blindness; glaucoma; chronic inflammation of iris and ciliary body (iridocyclitis) and globe, lens, and iris; scarring; lid deformity; cataract formation |
| | | ➤ Degree of opacification of cornea and ischemia of limbus indicative of the degree of damage and prognosis | |

recting flow from inner to outer canthus and under the lid.

➤ Identify chemical causing injury. If chemical is unknown, use pH strip to determine presence of acid or alkali.

➤ If chemical is a known alkali, irrigate continuously without stopping to check pH until the patient reaches the emergency department. Otherwise, irrigate continuously for 15 to 20 minutes and then check pH. Place pH strip in conjunctival sac of lower lid. Do not touch the cornea. Continue lavage until pH reaches at least 7. (Normal pH of tears is 7.3 to 7.7.)

➤ Instill ophthalmic anesthetic and place Morgan or Medi-flow lens to facilitate irrigation and examination, if necessary.

➤ If the chemical is hydrofluoric acid, mix five 10-ml vials of 10% calcium gluconate in 1,000 ml of sterile water and flush eye continuously until in the emergency department.

➤ Assess visual acuity with Snellen's chart or near-vision card.

### Ocular trauma: Blunt or sharp injury

➤ First, rule out life-threatening trauma.
➤ Perform a neurologic examination to rule out possible accompanying head or cervical spine injuries. Stabilize these injuries first.
➤ Obtain history and patient consent for treatment, if possible.
➤ In a conscious, stable patient, first test visual acuity with Snellen's chart or near-vision card.
➤ Perform an eye examination, taking special note of critical signs and symptoms. If rupture of globe is suspected or present, defer the rest of the examination.
➤ If retinal tears or detachment are suspected, place the patient in supine position if possible.
➤ Don't attempt to remove any penetrating foreign body.
➤ If eyelid is lacerated and the globe is injured, apply cool saline compress using 4″ × 4″ gauze and protective shield.
➤ Provide protective cover for the eye during transport to the emergency department. (See *Protective eye covering.*)
➤ If eyelid is avulsed, locate lid fragments and place on sterile saline gauze and in sterile container. Transport it with the patient.

## PATIENT TEACHING

➤ Generally, patient instruction is dependent on the type of trauma.
➤ Instruct the patient not to remove the eye patch.
➤ Tell the patient to keep his head still during transport.
➤ Make sure the patient doesn't bend or lift his head.
➤ Inform the patient that further evaluation and education will be performed after the crisis is resolved.

## COMPLICATIONS

➤ *Eye trauma necrosis, blindness, glaucoma, adhesions, cataracts, deformity, and infection* can result but are minimized by emergency evaluation and treatment by a specialist.

## SPECIAL CONSIDERATIONS

 **ALERT** If life-threatening trauma, head injury, or cervical spine injury is present, stabilization of these injuries takes priority. In the event of potential chemical injury, lavage of the eye takes priority, even before the nature of the chemical is determined.

Do not attempt to open the eyelid of a severely traumatized eye if the patient is uncooperative.

Fluorescein staining is contraindicated if injury to the globe is suspected.
➤ Pain and tearing from a corneal abrasion or chemical exposure may result in an inaccurate visual acuity assessment. If the patient is unable to read the eye chart, assess his ability to see finger movement or light discrimination.
➤ Avoid pressure on the globe in case of blunt or penetrating injury to reduce the risk of globe rupture and loss of vision.
➤ With corneal lacerations, less interference is better. Assess the injury, arrange for immediate referral and evaluation, and then shield the eye gently for protection while the patient is in transit.
➤ Immediate irrigation is the single best initial treatment for chemical burns to the eye and reduces the ultimate physical damage to the eye.
➤ Most acid burns with mild to moderate stromal haze will get better with time. Alkaline burns may initially look far better than they will appear at day 2 or 3. Therefore, it's important to refer the patient as soon as the eye is irrigated.

## PROTECTIVE EYE COVERING

Provide a protective cover for the eye during transport to the emergency department. To do this, make padding by wrapping gauze loosely around your hand several times to form a "donut" with a central opening diameter large enough to avoid any pressure on the globe. Secure with over and under wrap of gauze to form a firm edge.

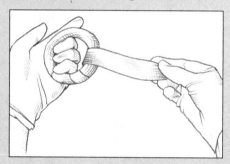

Apply the "donut" over the orbit of eye, avoiding contact with the globe.

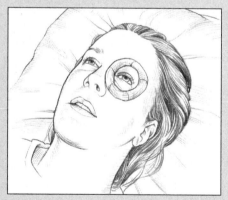

Lay an eye shield (or styrofoam cup) on top of the donut.

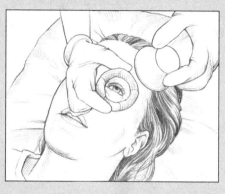

Apply an eye patch to the unaffected eye to prevent consensual movement of and further trauma to the affected eye. Secure the eye patch and the eye shield by wrapping 4" gauze around the head several times.

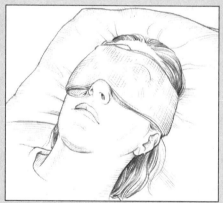

**CULTURAL TIP** Many Asians believe that the eyes are a link to the soul. Blindness is a disability that could prevent the patient from carrying out his duty to care for his family. He may feel he has no value and thus may be particularly distressed.

➤ Don't deny that the current level of visual acuity may be permanent or make promises. Although vision may improve significantly, it's best to foster conservative expectations because the outcome is unknown.

## DOCUMENTATION

➤ Document history, including a detailed description of the event, such as the object causing trauma, direction and force of the blow, and type of foreign body or chemical involved.

➤ Note if the patient was using protective gear or safety goggles at the time of the accident.

➤ Record pretrauma visual acuity and function; other symptoms, such as flashes, floaters, pain, and diplopia; and previous ocular disease.

➤ List current medications, allergies (especially to local anesthetics or PABA sunscreen lotions), and the use of over-the-counter preparations.

➤ Document current visual acuity, symptoms, and physical findings.

➤ Note pupil size and reactivity, extraocular movements, symmetry of facial and orbital bones, tissue integrity (lids and globe), color, swelling, presence of foreign body, and neurologic examination findings if head injury also occurred.

➤ Record any informed consent obtained. Document the patient's level of understanding.

➤ List treatments or stabilization procedures initiated and document patient response to treatments.

➤ Note patient disposition (referrals or transport to emergency department) and patient status when discharged from immediate care.

## Chalazion and hordeolum therapy

CPT CODE
No specific code has been assigned.

## DESCRIPTION

A chalazion is a focal inflammation of the meibomian glands, which are sebaceous follicles located between the tarsi and the conjunctiva of the eyelid. This may result from a chronic hordeolum or a chronic granuloma from an obstructed meibomian gland. A hordeolum, also called a stye, is usually caused by the *Staphylococcus aureus* organism. It is a localized, purulent, inflammatory infection that plugs one or more sebaceous glands of the eyelids and usually projects from or localizes on the lid border. When a patient presents with an inflammatory disorder that affects the eye, prompt assessment, diagnosis, and treatment is imperative along with an ophthalmic referral (if necessary) for incision and drainage. However, in general, asymptomatic chalazia and hordeola normally resolve with periodic application of warm moist compresses in under a weeks' time and don't require invasive treatment.

## INDICATIONS

➤ To treat the presence of chalazia or hordeola

## CONTRAINDICATIONS

### Relative
➤ Suspected infection

## EQUIPMENT

Ophthalmoscope ◆ Snellen's chart ◆ topical antibiotics (such as gentamicin, tobramycin, or ciprofloxacin) ◆ warm moist 4″ × 4″ compresses ◆ eye patch ◆ sterile swab with medium and transport tube such as Culturette (optional)

## ESSENTIAL STEPS

➤ Explain the procedure to the patient, and answer any questions he has.
➤ Assess the external and internal eye structures using the ophthalmoscope and visual fields examination.
➤ Assess the external structure for any abnormal masses or localized area of the eyelid or eyelash borders. Look for any redness, swelling, drainage, or pustular areas. If desired, obtain a culture specimen at this time with a Culturette. If these symptoms are present, apply warm 4" × 4" compresses for 15 minutes to provide comfort and clean the eyelid and eyelash area.
➤ Assess visual acuity with the Snellen's chart.
➤ Reassess the external and internal eye structures.
➤ Prescribe an antibiotic ointment, such as gentamicin, tobramycin, or ciprofloxacin, if indicated.
➤ If palliative treatment isn't successful and the patient complains of severe pain, if a large pustule is present, or if vision is impaired, an ophthalmic referral should be made for chalazion removal or incision and drainage.
➤ Apply an eye patch before discharge for comfort, if necessary.

## PATIENT TEACHING

➤ Inform the patient that temporary pain relief should be noted with the application of the warm compresses. Most discomfort should fully resolve within 7 to 10 days of therapy.
➤ Tell the patient to follow up with you in 7 to 10 days if no relief is noted; otherwise, in 2 to 3 weeks.
➤ Inform the patient that pain relief can also be achieved by systemic analgesics, if necessary.

➤ Teach the patient that no eye makeup should be used until the eye is clinically resolved. Instruct the patient to discard old eye makeup to prevent reinfection.
➤ Instruct the patient to use an eye patch over a gauze pad between compress applications to collect any drainage and promote comfort until the eye feels better.
➤ Tell the patient to apply warm compresses several times a day (four to five) for approximately 15 to 20 minutes at a time. Also tell the patient not to squeeze the site but to allow it to open and drain spontaneously.
➤ If you prescribe antibiotics, instruct the patient to apply a thin layer to the affected area with a cotton swab.

## COMPLICATIONS

➤ *Cellulitis or corneal abrasion* may occur if a chronic chalazion is large enough or grows to a large size. *An induced astigmatism* may persist until the nodule is removed. An ophthalmology consult should be made for evaluation and treatment of these cases.
➤ *Recurrent infections* may indicate immunocompromise and require systemic evaluation.

## SPECIAL CONSIDERATIONS

➤ Ophthalmic referral should be considered because up to one-half of adults with chalazia may have rosacea, and meibomian gland carcinoma presentation is similar to that of chalazia.
➤ Topical antibiotics (such as gentamicin, tobramycin, or ciprofloxacin) may be prescribed for 7 to 10 days to eliminate any microorganisms.

## DOCUMENTATION

➤ Document the pretreatment ophthalmic assessment.
➤ Record the visual acuity results with Snellen's chart.

➤ Note the appearance, color, and amount of wound drainage.

➤ Record the patient's understanding of any instructions given.

➤ Document whether ophthalmic referral is necessary. When referring a patient, include name, address, and phone number of the specialist and that you discussed the patient's need to go for further evaluation and treatment at length.

## Vision evaluation

### CPT CODE

No specific code has been assigned. Vision evaluation is usually charged as part of the clinical examination.

### DESCRIPTION

The purpose of this procedure is to assess visual acuity, visual field defects, and color vision and to determine the presence or absence of strabismus — all of which must be detected early for intervention to be most effective. Visual acuity is best assessed using the Snellen's eye chart if the patient is able to read or the Illiterate E chart if the patient can't read. Defects of the visual fields are best identified through confrontation testing, and color vision is best assessed using Ishihara's book. Furthermore, to determine and identify the presence or absence of strabismus, the cover-uncover test, corneal light reflex test, or extraocular muscle movement tests are usually performed.

### INDICATIONS

➤ To perform routine screening as part of wellness visit

➤ To evaluate visual function and acuity

➤ To detect visual field defects

➤ To assess vision complaints

➤ To determine the level of ocular trauma

➤ To screen for school or employment

### CONTRAINDICATIONS

None known

### EQUIPMENT

Penlight ◆ Snellen's chart, Illiterate E chart (also called the tumbling E), or a standard near-vision pocket chart ◆ color vision book such as Ishihara's (optional)

### ESSENTIAL STEPS

➤ Obtain a complete history and physical examination.

➤ Explain the procedure to patient or parent and answer any questions he has.

➤ Perform the screening in a well-lit area where the patient can stand 20' (6 m) from the Snellen's chart. If using the near-vision pocket chart, the chart should be 14" (35.6 cm) from the patient's eyes.

#### Test visual acuity

➤ Have the patient cover one eye and ask him to identify all the letters beginning at any line.

➤ Determine the smallest line in which he can identify all the letters and record the visual acuity.

➤ Repeat this step with the opposite eye and then perform the screening with both of the patient's eyes open.

➤ Alternatively, if the patient can't read, use the Illiterate E chart and have him point his finger in the direction of the E on the chart.

#### Test visual fields — confrontation

➤ Standing 2' (0.6 m) away from the patient, have him cover one eye and look into your uncovered eye (for example, if the patient covers his left eye, you should cover your right eye).

➤ Move an object such as a pen or penlight into each of the visual fields and have the patient tell you when he can see the object in each area. The examiner's view and the patient's view should match.

### Test color vision

➤ Using a color vision book, have the patient describe the number he sees on each page. The numbers or figures in the color vision book are distorted by color variances and are unreadable to the person who has abnormal color discrimination ability.

### Test for strabismus

➤ Carefully observe both eyes for any obvious deviation.
➤ Standing 2' directly in front of the patient, shine a light into the eyes and inspect the reflections of the light in each cornea. Following this, ask the patient to follow the light as you move through the six cardinal fields of gaze (making a large H in the air, guide the patient's gaze to the extreme right, to the upper right, to the lower right, to the extreme left, to the upward left, and to the lower left).
➤ Looking directly at the patient's eyes, cover one of his eyes for a brief time. Unveil the eye and observe for any movement of the uncovered eye indicating it had strayed while covered. Repeat the procedure with the opposite eye.

## PATIENT TEACHING

➤ Inform the patient that no pain or discomfort is associated with this procedure.
➤ Explain the results of the testing and the epidemiology, if there is a problem. Discuss choices for therapeutic interventions and expected resolution timetable. Instruct the patient or parent of the need for follow-up care and evaluation and specify the date for each. If deviations from the norm are elicited, refer him to the appropriate professional.

➤ Provide verbal and written instructions. Any referrals should include the provider's name, address, and phone number. Explain the need for prompt evaluation by an ophthalmologist and provide a specific time frame for further evaluation.
➤ If a prescription is written, instruct the patient to take all of the medication that is prescribed and administer it as ordered.
➤ Instruct patient to call you if any vision problems develop.

 **CULTURAL TIP** Many cultural groups believe that illness or disease has a different cause than the typical Western beliefs imply, so it is important to explain the reasons and benefits of screening in relation to the patient's own belief system. Some members of cultural groups, such as Native Americans, Africans, Colombians, Gypsies, Hmong, and Japanese, believe that illness is the result of magico-religious causes (like punishment for improper behavior or the result of voodoo). Others, such as Central Americans, Filipinos, Iranians, Mexicans, and Russians, may attribute illness to naturalistic causes like imbalances (like too much hot or cold, or not taking care of oneself). It's also possible that many cultural groups believe in more than one cause of illness (such as magico-religious, naturalistic, and biomedical combined).

## COMPLICATIONS

None known

## SPECIAL CONSIDERATIONS

➤ If a vision problem is detected, consult with a vision specialist or consider immediate referral.

## DOCUMENTATION

➤ Note the reason for vision testing.
➤ Record the number, type, and frequency of problems.
➤ List any previous treatment modalities.

➤ Record findings of all vision tests performed.

➤ Document referral recommendations, including contact information given and risks of not being further evaluated or treated.

# EAR PROCEDURES

## Audiometry testing

CPT CODES
*92551    Audiologic screening test, pure tone, air only*
*92552    Audiometry, threshold test, pure tone, air only*

## DESCRIPTION

A hearing screening is simply a pass or fail test that gives a general idea if a patient has some type of hearing loss. In audiometry testing, hearing thresholds are also recorded. Audiometry uses a standard pure-tone audiometer to present stimuli through earphones (air conduction testing) or through a bone conduction vibrator (bone conduction testing). The pure-tone threshold measurement finds the lowest level that the person can hear each tone about 50% of the time and uses these data to form an audiogram. By quantifying the patient's ability to hear various intensities and frequencies, the audiogram assists the practitioner in determining the type of hearing disorder that exists and assesses the degree of impairment.

Audiometry requires specialized training, an audiometer, and the cooperation of the patient.

## INDICATIONS

➤ To evaluate hearing loss
➤ To screen patients working in noisy settings
➤ To assess complaints of tinnitus
➤ To assess speech and language developmental delays in children and infants
➤ To assess children who are experiencing poor academic progress
➤ To assess geriatric patients with unexplained behavior changes
➤ To assess infants at high risk for a hearing deficit

## CONTRAINDICATIONS

### Absolute
➤ Cerumen obstruction
➤ Otitis externa

### Relative
➤ Children under age 6 months

## EQUIPMENT

Otoscope ◆ appropriately sized earphone speaker or earplug ◆ audiometry tool with a minimal decibel frequency range of 500 to 4,000 Hz

## ESSENTIAL STEPS

➤ Explain the procedure to the patient or parent.
➤ Perform the screening in a quiet area with the patient sitting comfortably upright but not looking at you or the audiometer.
➤ Have the patient remove any jewelry or glasses that could interfere with earphone application.
➤ Instruct the patient to indicate when a tone is heard by raising a hand.
➤ Using an otoscope, inspect the ear for evidence of infection or obstruction.
➤ Place an earphone speaker over the external os and check to be certain that noth-

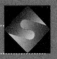

# PREVENTING HEARING LOSS

**DEAR PATIENT:**

A chief cause of hearing loss is overexposure to loud noise. Unfortunately, we're constantly bombarded by noise — from things like motor vehicles, power tools, appliances, televisions, and radios. But we can take steps to protect our hearing. How? We can cover our ears or wear hearing protectors when we expect to be exposed to loud noise and we can avoid loud music or other noisy situations as much as possible.

How much noise is too much? First, consider how sound is measured. It's calculated two ways — by frequency (pitch) and intensity (loudness). Frequency is measured in sound vibrations per second, or hertz (Hz). For example, a boat whistle has a frequency of about 250 Hz, and a bird singing has a frequency of about 4,000 Hz.

Intensity is measured in decibels (dB). A conversational voice measures about 65 dB. A shout measures 90 dB or more. A jackhammer registers 100 to 120 dB. Loud rock music is 120 to 130 dB, and an explosion registers 140 dB or more.

Low-intensity sounds are harmless and often quite pleasant. Sounds at or above the 85 to 90 dB range — called the caution or action zone — are dangerous.

If the noise occurs 3' (1 m) away and you have to raise your voice to be heard, the level is probably about 85 dB. Constant exposure to noise at this level can cause permanent hearing loss. So can short exposure to extremely loud noises (greater than 140 dB), a condition called acoustic trauma.

Hearing loss can occur if you're exposed to a large *dosage* of noise. Dosage = intensity (amount of noise exposure) × duration (over a period of time). When noise is less intense and of shorter duration, hair cells in the inner ear aren't damaged as much, and hearing is affected less.

The Occupational Safety and Health Administration has set the following standards for safe noise levels:

| AMOUNT OF NOISE | MAXIMUM EXPOSURE TIME |
|---|---|
| 90 dB | 8 hours |
| 95 dB | 4 hours |
| 100 dB | 2 hours |
| 105 dB | 1 hour |
| 110 dB | ½ hour |
| 115 dB | ¼ hour |

**Wearing hearing protectors**

Earplugs and earmuffs help prevent hearing loss by decreasing the amount of sound entering the ear. Wear them when you'll be exposed to sounds above the caution zone (for example, when using loud appliances, power tools, lawn mowers, tractors, and jackhammers; when shooting a gun; and when you're around motorcycles, snowmobiles, speedboats, or other noisy vehicles).

Although ear protectors may seem inconvenient or uncomfortable at first, wearing them will preserve your hearing in the future. Here are some tips for choosing hearing protectors.

*(continued)*

*Disposable plugs*
Place disposable plugs inside the ear canal to block out noise. They also help keep dirt from entering the ear. Almost invisible, they're available in several styles. Try different plugs to find the most comfortable kind. Look for pliability and a snug fit. Never break off the tips.

Wash your hands before shaping and inserting plugs. If they're inserted correctly, your own voice should sound louder to you. If they contain wax, dirt, or grease, throw them away and use a new pair.

*Reusable plugs*
Placed inside the ear canal, these plugs block out noise and help keep dirt from entering the ear. They're available in several styles. Some are joined by a string to prevent losing them. Do the plugs fit snugly in the ear canal? Check their fit and whether they're comfortable.

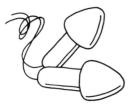

Before inserting the plugs, wash your hands and inspect the plugs for dirt. Wash them if necessary. If you use them all day at work, wash them every day; then rinse, dry, and store them in a plastic case or clean pill bottle. Replace them when they harden or discolor.

*Headband plugs*
Place the plugs in your ears with the headband under your chin. The plugs should fit snugly yet comfortably.

Wash the entire headband often. Don't twist or bend it — this will interfere with the fit of the plugs. Store the headband safely.

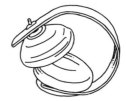

*Earmuffs*
Place earmuffs over your ears with the band over your head. Cushioned muffs form a seal around the ear, completely blocking out noise. Cushions are foam or liquid-filled. Don't loosen the earmuffs — this reduces their effectiveness. They may not fit correctly if you wear glasses.

Remove the cushions for washing often. Inspect them periodically to see if they need replacing (they harden with use). Store them in a safe place.

**Other tips**
Here are some other hearing protection hints:
➤ Run appliances one at a time. When buying appliances, ask about decibel levels.
➤ Cover your ears when near noise, such as that from sirens or subways.
➤ Avoid loud music, and don't listen to music with earphones.
➤ Give your ears an occasional vacation. Turn off the TV and read a book.

ing (including the tragus) covers the opening. The earphone or earplug must have a tight seal.

➤ If using a handheld audiometry tool, gently pull the pinna back (for children) and up and back (for adults) to obtain a good seal.

➤ If one ear is known to have better hearing, begin testing with that ear.

➤ Observe for each tone indicator and the patient's response. Repeat the test in the opposite ear.

➤ Testing is typically repeated four times, until the patient reproduces the same response at least 50% of the time. This is the result entered on the audiogram. *Note*: Some audiometers require the results to be sent to the company and analyzed by specially trained personnel. Typical results are as follows: less than or equal to 20 dB is normal hearing; 21 to 40 dB is a mild hearing loss; 41 to 55 dB is a moderate hearing loss; 56 to 70 dB is a moderately severe hearing loss; 71 to 90 dB is a severe hearing loss; and greater than or equal to 91 dB signifies a profound hearing loss.

 **ALERT** If results are not within normal limits, ask the patient to return for repeat testing. If not persistently within normal limits at that time, the patient should be referred to an audiologist.

➤ Review the results and implications with the patient or parent.

## PATIENT TEACHING

➤ Tell the patient that there should be no discomfort associated with this procedure.

➤ Explain the results of the procedure and the epidemiology if a problem is present. Discuss choices for therapeutic interventions and expected resolution, including a timetable. Instruct the patient or parent of need for follow-up care and evaluation. Be sure to specify the date and practitioner's name, phone number, and address for each needed referral or follow-up evaluation.

➤ Teach the patient how to avoid overexposure to loud noise. (See *Preventing hearing loss*, pages 293 and 294.)

➤ Instruct the patient to call you if any problems develop, although none are expected.

## COMPLICATIONS

None known

## SPECIAL CONSIDERATIONS

➤ This is a good time to review environmental variables that affect hearing, such as allergies and smoke, with the patient or parent.

➤ *Note*: Audiometers range from semi-automatic to fully automatic. Some models, such as the Castle RA500 audiometer, repeat frequencies that evoke an inconsistent response, analyze data as the test is performed, and even provide categorized results to guide the practitioner.

## DOCUMENTATION

➤ Record the reason for audiometry testing.

➤ Provide the number, type, and frequency of problems reported.

➤ Note previous treatment modalities.

➤ Record audiogram findings.

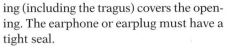

# Tympanometry

CPT CODES
*92567 Tympanometry (impedance testing)*
*92568 Acoustic reflex testing*

## DESCRIPTION

The purpose of tympanometry is to objectively assess the air pressure within the middle ear and the mobility of the tympanic membrane. This provides an objective analysis of middle ear function. Using a tympanometer, positive, normal, and negative air pressures are introduced into the external meatus of the ear to measure the sound energy flow. The sound energy flow is then traced on a graph called a tympanogram.

This procedure is useful in determining resolution of otitis media and serous otitis media through the assessment of middle ear function and in identifying dysfunction that could result in hearing loss or repeated infections.

## INDICATIONS

➤ To determine eustachian tube patency
➤ To evaluate hearing loss or ear pain
➤ To detect perforations of the tympanic membrane
➤ To determine mobility of the tympanic membrane
➤ To evaluate persistent middle ear effusions
➤ To evaluate patency of pressure-equalization tubes
➤ To assess middle ear function when patient is unable to cooperate with audiometry
➤ To verify middle ear abnormalities

## CONTRAINDICATIONS

### Absolute
➤ Canal totally obstructed by cerumen
➤ External otitis media

### Relative
➤ Age younger than 7 months

## EQUIPMENT

Tympanometer tool with 220 to 226 Hz probe tone and air pressure range of –400 decaPascals (daPa) to +200 daPa ◆ otoscope ◆ various size ear tips

## ESSENTIAL STEPS

➤ Explain the procedure to the patient or parent and describe how the patient should indicate hearing the tone. Answer any questions.
➤ Seat the patient in a comfortable, upright position or allow the patient to sit independently or in a parent's lap.
➤ Using an otoscope, inspect the ear canal for cerumen obstruction or evidence of infection. If the patient is a child, allow him to hold the tympanometer.
➤ Select the proper ear tip that provides a tight seal of the ear canal, insert it snugly, and activate the tympanometer.
➤ Gently apply traction to the pinna, pulling up and back on an older child and adult or pulling back on an infant or child under age 3, to produce a good seal.
➤ When an appropriate seal is achieved, the tympanometer will automatically transmit the sound, measure the air pressures, record readings, and print out results.
➤ Interpret the results of tympanometer reading. Low compliance measurements indicate a stiff or obstructed middle ear, while high compliance measurements indicate flaccid or highly mobile tympanic membrane.
➤ Review results with the patient or parents.

## PATIENT TEACHING

➤ Explain the results and, if a problem is identified, explain the epidemiology.
➤ Discuss choices for therapeutic interventions and expected resolution timetable.
➤ Discuss any environmental factors, such as allergies, smoking, and loud noises, that

may be contributing to the problem and appropriate avoidance measures.

➤ Instruct the patient or parent of the need for follow-up care and evaluation and specify the date for each.

➤ Provide instructions verbally and in written form. Any referrals should include the provider's name, address, and phone number.

➤ Instruct the patient or parents to call you if the symptoms continue after 72 hours or if they worsen in any way.

## COMPLICATIONS

None known

## SPECIAL CONSIDERATIONS

➤ If problems are indicated, consult with an ear, nose, and throat specialist and consider immediate referral.

➤ If external otitis media is present and the ear canal is occluded with purulent material, consult with a physician about treatment options.

➤ If the tympanic membrane is occluded with cerumen, order cerumen softener and have patient return in 48 to 72 hours for cerumen removal and tympanogram.

 **CULTURAL TIP** Some cultural groups, such as Hispanics and Mexicans, may use an alternative therapy for an earache such as willow and garlic ear oil. The oil is warmed to slightly higher than body temperature, placed in the ears, and covered with cotton. It is possible that your Mexican patients may be particularly reluctant to mention the use of such alternative therapies out of respect for your belief in Western medicine.

## DOCUMENTATION

➤ Note the reason for tympanometry.

➤ Document the number, type, and frequency of problems.

➤ Record previous treatment modalities.

➤ Include a copy of the tympanogram on the chart and list findings and plan of care.

# Cerumen impaction removal

**CPT CODE**
*69210    Removal of impacted cerumen (one or both ears)*

## DESCRIPTION

The goal of cerumen impaction removal is to mobilize and evacuate cerumen from the external ear canal. Although cerumen is an ear canal lubricant and protector, it may become dried and hardened. If ceruminolytic ear drops are ineffective in removing cerumen, manual disimpaction is most commonly done by irrigation. Irrigating the ear involves washing the external auditory canal with a stream of solution to clean the canal of discharges, to soften and remove impacted cerumen, or to dislodge a foreign body. Sometimes, irrigation aims to relieve localized inflammation and discomfort. The procedure must be performed carefully to avoid causing patient discomfort or vertigo and to avoid increasing the risk of otitis externa. Because irrigation may contaminate the middle ear if the tympanic membrane is ruptured, an otoscopic examination always precedes ear irrigation.

## INDICATIONS

➤ To remove symptomatic cerumen impaction that is causing pain, dizziness, and hearing loss

➤ To improve impaired visualization of the tympanic membrane due to cerumen buildup

## CONTRAINDICATIONS

### Absolute
➤ Suspected tympanic membrane perforation
➤ Infectious process present

### Relative
➤ Recent ear or head trauma
➤ Large foreign body present
➤ Tympanic membrane or ear canal deformities present

## EQUIPMENT

Otoscope with aural speculum ◆ tuning fork ◆ prepackaged or sterile ear curette ◆ ear irrigation syringe ◆ emesis basin and irrigation reservoir setup ◆ towel or absorbent drape ◆ cotton-tipped applicators ◆ gloves ◆ warm water (body temperature), mineral oil, or ceruminolytic agent such as triethanolamine polypeptide oleate-condensate (Cerumenex)

## PREPARATION OF EQUIPMENT

➤ Select the appropriate syringe, and obtain the prescribed irrigant.
➤ Put the container of irrigant into the large basin filled with hot water to warm the solution to body temperature: 98.6° F (37° C). Avoid extreme temperature changes because they can affect inner ear fluids, causing nausea and dizziness.
➤ Test the temperature of the solution by sprinkling a few drops on your inner wrist.
➤ Inspect equipment (syringe or catheter tips) for breaks or cracks; inspect all metal tips for roughness. Ensure adequate lighting is available.

## ESSENTIAL STEPS

➤ Explain the procedure and equipment to the patient. Place him in a sitting position. Cover the patient with an absorbent towel or drape.
➤ Wash hands and put on gloves.
➤ With the patient seated, assess the external ear canal with the otoscope. (Remember to pull the pinna up and back on an older child and adult; pull the pinna back on an infant or child under age 3.) Look for consistency, amount, and color of ear canal matter, as well as the surrounding ear canal wall tissue. Using the tuning fork, perform Weber and Rinne tests for hearing status.
➤ Fill the ear irrigation syringe with body-temperature warm water.
➤ Tilt the patient's head to the side. Have him participate by instructing him to hold the reservoir or emesis basin to the ear being irrigated. (See *How to irrigate the ear canal*.)
➤ Remove equipment from the ear and dry external area.
➤ Assess external ear canal with an otoscope.
➤ If necessary, use an ear curette to remove existing cerumen.
➤ If cerumen remains hardened, instill a commercial preparation or mineral oil to soften it. Wait approximately 5 to 10 minutes for preparation to soften cerumen.
➤ Reassess the external ear with the otoscope.
➤ Gently flush the ear canal again with body-temperature water. Observe and assess debris eliminated. Do not use more than 500 ml of irrigating solution during this procedure.
➤ Repeat ear curette usage if necessary.
➤ Reassess the ear canal with the otoscope. Inspect ear canal walls for redness, bleeding, and irritation. Assess the tympanic membrane for infections, perforations, and landmarks. Perform postprocedure Weber and Rinne hearing tests.
➤ If cerumen remains hardened, it may be necessary to instill products into the ear canal to soften over a period of time

(1 to 2 days), then instruct the patient to return for proper irrigation.
➤ Dry the pinna and outer ear canal area with cotton-tipped applicators.
➤ Properly dispose of debris material and solutions.
➤ Wash hands.

## PATIENT TEACHING

➤ Tell the patient that he should notice immediate relief from any ear pressure or fullness and restoration of hearing after complete evacuation of impacted cerumen.
➤ Instruct the patient to contact you if any abnormal discharge, pain, vertigo, or hearing problems ensue. Instruct him to follow up with you in 1 to 2 days to evaluate hearing and check for infection.
➤ Instruct the patient in proper ear care to prevent future cerumen impaction. This may include the use of over-the-counter earwax preparations at regular intervals, avoidance of self-irrigation, and preventing insertion of foreign objects into ears for self-evacuation.

## COMPLICATIONS

➤ *Trauma to mucous membranes* is minimized by gentle handling and careful aiming of the stream of fluid into the ear. *Bleeding* is handled with pressure to the site.
➤ *Infection* is treated on a case-by-case basis and may result from the foreign body or the extraction. Options include local or systemic antibiotics or consultation with collaborating physician or an ear, nose, and throat (ENT) specialist.
➤ *Inability to remove the impacted cerumen* requires consultation or referral to a physician, ENT specialist, or an acute care facility.
➤ *Nausea and vomiting* typically resolve within a few hours.
➤ *Tinnitus* may result from stimulation of the vestibular system with cold water. This can be minimized by using tepid wa-

### HOW TO IRRIGATE THE EAR CANAL

Follow these guidelines for irrigating the ear canal.
➤ Gently pull the pinna up and back to straighten the ear canal. (For a child, pull the pinna back.)
➤ Have the patient hold an emesis basin beneath the ear to catch returning irrigant. Position the tip of the irrigating syringe at the meatus of the auditory canal. Don't block the meatus because you'll impede backflow and raise pressure in the canal.

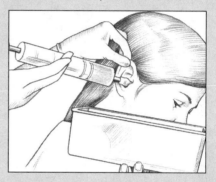

➤ Tilt the patient's head toward you, and point the syringe tip upward and toward the posterior ear canal. This angle prevents damage to the tympanic membrane and guards against pushing debris further into the canal.

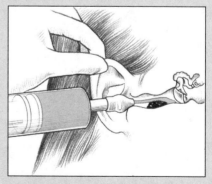

➤ Direct a steady stream of irrigant against the upper wall of the ear canal, and inspect return fluid for cloudiness, cerumen, blood, or foreign matter.

ter but will resolve spontaneously without treatment.

## SPECIAL CONSIDERATIONS

➤ If the canal begins to become irritated, swollen, or bleed, stop the procedure to avoid an outer ear infection. The procedure should also be stopped if the patient complains of increasing discomfort because this may indicate tympanic membrane rupture.

➤ If signs of infection are present, irrigation may cause the infection to spread inward. In this case, remove cerumen plugs with a cerumen spoon.

➤ Avoid dropping or squirting irrigant on the tympanic membrane. This may startle the patient and cause discomfort. If you're using an irrigating catheter instead of a syringe, adjust the flow of solution to a steady, comfortable rate with a flow clamp. Don't raise the container more than 6″ (15.2 cm) above the ear. If the container is higher, the resulting pressure could damage the tympanic membrane.

➤ If you place a cotton pledget in the ear canal to retain some of the solution, pack the cotton loosely. Instruct the patient not to remove it.

➤ If irrigation doesn't dislodge impacted cerumen, instruct the patient to instill several drops of glycerin, carbamide peroxide (Debrox), or a similar preparation two to three times daily for 2 to 3 days, and then have the ear irrigated again.

## DOCUMENTATION

➤ As indicated, document the reason for not performing disimpaction and if the patient was referred to an ENT specialist for further evaluation.

➤ Record preprocedure and postprocedure hearing (including Weber and Rinne testing) results and otoscope assessment.

➤ Document the type of procedure performed and irrigant used.

➤ Record the patient's response to the procedure and assessments, such as hearing status changes and comfort level, as well as the type and amount of ear canal debris removed.

➤ Document instructions given to the patient and his understanding.

# Foreign body removal from the ear

## CPT CODES

*69200   Removal of foreign body from external auditory canal without general anesthesia*
*69210   Removal of impacted cerumen (one or both ears)*

## DESCRIPTION

Removal of foreign bodies from the ear involves manually removing an object from the ear. Cerumen is the most common foreign body in most adults. However, in children and mentally incapacitated persons, other objects also become lodged in the external ear, such as parts of toys, beans, peas, nuts, coins, cotton-tipped applicators, and insects. It's important to get a firm grip on the foreign body to avoid pushing it deeper into the ear canal.

## INDICATIONS

➤ To remove foreign body in the outer two-thirds of external ear canal

## CONTRAINDICATIONS

### Absolute

➤ Visibility obscured due to trauma
➤ Tympanic membrane perforation or infection suspected
➤ Object likely to swell with moisture (such as a pea or bean)

## Relative

➤ Noncompliant patient
➤ Object not easily accessible or visible

## EQUIPMENT

Otoscope ◆ ear speculum ◆ gloves ◆ ear curette, loop, or hook (plastic or wire) curette with soft tubing, bulb syringe ◆ alligator forceps ◆ small magnet ◆ alcohol or peroxide ◆ cotton-tipped applicator ◆ protective cover ◆ towel ◆ 4″ × 4″ gauze pad ◆ viscous lidocaine, topical anesthetics, or mineral oil (optional) ◆ otic antibiotic or corticosteroid such as Cortisporin (optional) ◆ adjustable light such as a gooseneck lamp

## ESSENTIAL STEPS

➤ Explain the procedure in detail to the patient and parents and answer any questions they have. Explain that there will be some discomfort.
➤ Wash your hands and put on gloves.
➤ Inspect the external ear for signs of infection or injury. Refer patients with trauma to the ear canal to an ear, nose, and throat (ENT) specialist or the emergency department.
➤ Using the otoscope, inspect the external ear canal for edema and erythema, and determine the presence and type of foreign body. Determine the appropriate extraction tool. For vegetation and fabric, choose alligator forceps. For smooth objects, such as beads, popcorn kernels, or nuts, choose the loop. Harder objects such as batteries may be retrieved with a 1-mm right-angle hook. Metal items may be retrieved with a small magnet. Insects need to be immobilized or killed before removal is attempted; instill viscous lidocaine, mineral oil, or topical anesthetic into the ear canal and allow 5 minutes for these agents to work.
➤ Grasping the pinna of the ear, straighten the external ear canal by pulling the ear up and back (on an adult) and back (on a child).
➤ Hold the patient's head in place with your nondominant hand. Rest your dominant hand on the patient's head to steady it and to move with the patient if he moves suddenly.
➤ Insert the ear speculum, then introduce the retrieval instrument through the speculum. Grasp the object firmly with the forceps, or place the loop or hook behind the object. Withdraw the instrument and speculum with a slow, steady motion.
➤ If these steps are ineffective, try flushing out the object. However, if the object may swell (such as might occur with an organic foreign body), don't instill fluid into the ear canal. If removal is successful, but small particles or debris remain, irrigate the ear.
➤ Inspect the external ear canal for patency after extraction; repeat the procedure as needed until the canal is clear.
➤ Dry the external ear canal to remove any blood and swab with an alcohol or peroxide saturated cotton-tipped applicator to reduce the risk of otitis externa.
➤ Instill a topical antibiotic or corticosteroid (such as Cortisporin) to control external edema, erythema, and infection.

## PATIENT TEACHING

➤ Tell the patient not to clean the external ear with a cotton-tipped applicator and not to place any small objects into the ear canal.

## COMPLICATIONS

➤ *Risk of tympanic membrane rupture and laceration of the external ear canal* are minimized with gentle handling but may be unavoidable. Depending on the extent of injury, consider consulting with your collaborating physician or an ENT specialist.
➤ *Middle ear effusion* is more common with ear irrigation if the tympanic mem-

brane is perforated. This infection and otitis externa may be treated with local antibiotics such as chloramphenicol.

## SPECIAL CONSIDERATIONS

➤ If the object is a live insect, try placing the patient in a dark room and shining a penlight into the ear canal. Many times the insect will move towards the light, easing extraction.

➤ Don't push the foreign body toward the tympanic membrane during extraction; doing so could cause injury.

➤ Stop trying to extract the object if the patient experiences pain, severe vertigo, or nausea.

➤ Battery parts can leak acid and irrigation would spread caustic material throughout the canal.

➤ Patients, particularly small children, may require sedation before attempting removal.

➤ Refer the patient to the collaborating physician or otolaryngologist if the extraction effort wasn't successful or if the patient has a perforated tympanic membrane, myringotomy tubes, or chronic otitis media.

➤ If the patient has impacted cerumen, consider instilling carbamide peroxide or mineral oil three times a day for 3 to 5 days to soften it before attempting removal.

## DOCUMENTATION

➤ Document which ear was affected, and identify the suspected foreign body, if possible.

➤ Note the date and time of extraction, including the instruments used for manual extraction and if irrigation was necessary.

➤ Record your assessment of the appearance of the ear canal, noting any signs of infection and any change in hearing ability both before and after the procedure. Note how the patient tolerated the procedure and any concerns he had, particularly related to his hearing acuity.

➤ Document patient teaching and that patient was instructed to notify you for any signs or symptoms of infection such as increasing pain, drainage, swelling, or fever.

# Auricular hematoma evacuation

## CPT CODES

69000    *Draining external ear, abscess or hematoma, simple*
69005    *Draining external ear, abscess or hematoma, complicated*

## DESCRIPTION

Auricular hematoma evacuation is the drainage of a blood collection in the pinna followed by compression to prevent further bleeding. An auricular hematoma may result from direct or indirect trauma to the external ear. Early intervention prevents further damage to the ear tissue, infection process, and preventable permanent ear deformities. If the hematoma site is too large, a referral to a plastic surgeon may be considered.

## INDICATIONS

➤ To alleviate local pressure or discomfort

➤ To assess vascular compromise causing a blue tint and swelling of the auricle

## CONTRAINDICATIONS

### Absolute

➤ Laceration or complex injury

## EQUIPMENT

1% lidocaine ◆ #15 scalpel blade with handle ◆ 18G or 20G needle and 3-ml syringe ◆ 30G needle and 3-ml syringe ◆ curved hemostat ◆ sterile towels or drape ◆ povidone-iodine topical antiseptic ◆ sterile gloves ◆ 4" × 4" gauze ◆ 2" gauze roll ◆ nonadherent gauze ◆ antibiotic ointment (such as Neosporin) ◆ goggles ◆ gloves ◆ tape ◆ 4-0 or 5-0 nylon sutures with a straight suture needle (optional)

## ESSENTIAL STEPS

➤ Explain the procedure to the patient, obtain informed consent, and answer any questions he has. Advise the patient there will be some discomfort but it's crucial to stay still.
➤ Position the patient in the supine position with injured ear accessible.
➤ Drape the patient's head to expose the injured ear only.
➤ Assess the ear and hematoma site for size, consistency, tenderness, drainage, and color.
➤ Put on gloves and goggles.
➤ Clean the ear site using gauze and antiseptic solution.
➤ Dispose of gloves and put on sterile gloves.
➤ Inject the hematoma site anteriorly, posteriorly, and directly with 1% lidocaine anesthetic using a 30G needle and a 3-ml syringe.
➤ Insert an 18G or 20G needle attached to a 3-ml syringe into the hematoma and aspirate.
➤ If unable to aspirate with the syringe and needle, make a 4- to 5-mm incision into the hematoma site with #15 scalpel with handle. The more time that has passed since the trauma, the greater the likelihood of needing multiple incisions for evacuation.

➤ Use a curved hemostat and manual pressure to probe, release, and expel remaining fluid and clots.
➤ When the area is fully evacuated, cover the incision site with antibiotic ointment, then a nonadherent gauze, and apply a dry sterile auricular pressure dressing (with 2" gauze and roll to ½" thickness).
➤ Prescribe analgesics and antibiotics as indicated, such as cephalexin or cefadroxil for 5 to 7 days.
➤ Keep pressure dressing in place for 48 to 72 hours postprocedure.
➤ Reevaluate the hematoma site in 48 to 72 hours.

## PATIENT TEACHING

➤ Tell the patient that some bleeding can be expected for 24 hours and full recovery from this procedure may take up to 2 weeks.
➤ Instruct the patient to follow up with you in 48 hours for reevaluation of the site, and further postprocedure instructions.
➤ Tell the patient to contact you immediately if he experiences bleeding or drainage from site, a foul odor, fever, or an increase in pain or discomfort.
➤ Tell the patient to use cool compresses or ice on the surrounding area for comfort.
➤ Inform the patient that Tylenol with codeine may be taken if necessary for the first day. After that, regular acetaminophen should be adequate. If pain persists, he should call you.
➤ Provide dressing instructions to the patient and emphasize that pressure must be maintained to prevent bleeding and scarring.

## COMPLICATIONS

➤ *Cosmetic scarring or auricular deformity* may occur, depending on the size of the hematoma, procedure difficulties, or inadequate or lack of postprocedure site care.

## APPLYING AN AURICULAR PRESSURE DRESSING

If you're unable to apply a pressure dressing with tape alone, consider suturing it in place. To do this, first apply the antibiotic ointment to the incision. Form two rolls, using 2" gauze, each rolled to ½" thickness. Then take a straight suture needle and 4-0 or 5-0 nylon suture material and pass it through the anterior roll and then through the ear (close to the incision) in an anterior-to-posterior direction. Pass the needle back and forth through the posterior roll twice before piercing the ear in the posterior-to-anterior direction. After again passing through the anterior roll, ensure that both rolls are snug against the ear and tie the suture in place to form a pressure dressing on the anterior and posterior surfaces of the auricular hematoma site.

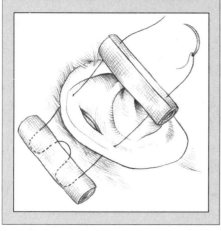

➤ *Infection* risk is minimized by aseptic technique and prophylactic antibiotics as needed.

## SPECIAL CONSIDERATIONS

➤ If you are unable to apply a pressure dressing with tape, place 4-0 or 5-0 nylon sutures through the dressing and the pinna and tie to hold the pressure dressing in place. (See *Applying an auricular pressure dressing*.)

## DOCUMENTATION

➤ Document the indications for the procedure and if informed consent was obtained.
➤ Record an assessment of the ear preprocedure and postprocedure, including changes in function or appearance.
➤ Document the type of procedure used and postprocedure patient status (site evaluation, pain tolerance, temperature).
➤ List any instructions given to the patient and any medications prescribed.
➤ Document the patient's understanding of postprocedure instructions (such as dressing change procedure and when to schedule an appointment).

# Ear piercing

CPT CODE
*69090    Ear piercing*

## DESCRIPTION

Ear piercing is generally a voluntary procedure that is requested by patients of all ages, usually for cosmetic reasons. The procedure involves inserting a needle or piercer through the earlobe, then inserting a hypoallergenic earring in the hole. Informed consent may be necessary before the procedure.

## INDICATIONS

➤ To perform an elective procedure

## CONTRAINDICATIONS

### Relative
➤ Immunocompromised patient
➤ Predisposed to keloid formation
➤ Coagulopathy
➤ Skin disorder at the site

## EQUIPMENT

Commercial ear-piercing tool ◆ topical antiseptic skin cleanser such as alcohol swabs ◆ surgical marking pen ◆ ice pack ◆ gloves ◆ sterile earrings (use 14-karat gold or surgical steel posts)

## ESSENTIAL STEPS

➤ Explain the procedure, answer questions, and obtain informed consent, if necessary.
➤ Assess external ear for shape, symmetry, defects, and other ear puncture sites.
➤ Position the patient either sitting in high Fowler's position or lying on her side. Wash hands well.
➤ Ask the patient to point to the area where she wants the piercing to take place. Mark the site with a surgical marking pen, anteriorly. Have the patient verify placement selection.
➤ Apply an ice pack to the front and back of the earlobe for 2 minutes.
➤ Put on gloves.
➤ Clean the piercing site with topical antiseptic cleanser, such as alcohol.
➤ Position the earlobe between the front and rear portions of the piercing tool with the nose of the device over the placement box. (See *Piercing the earlobe*.)
➤ Clean around the earring and new puncture site with an alcohol swab.
➤ Repeat procedure to the opposite earlobe, if desired.

## PATIENT TEACHING

➤ Tell the patient that minimal and temporary pain is anticipated with this procedure and that cool compresses may be applied to the earlobes for comfort. Tell her to contact with you if any colored discharge, swelling, redness, or ongoing pain is noted.
➤ Teach the patient to clean new piercing site daily with soap and water or alcohol.

### PIERCING THE EARLOBE

After marking the site and inserting the earring post and back into the ear-piercing tool, insert the earlobe and depress the handle. To release the earring back, stop applying pressure and ease the earlobe forward.

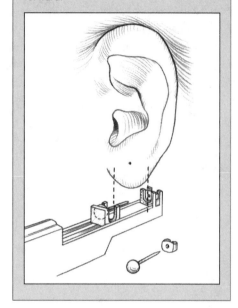

➤ Teach the patient to turn earrings while remaining inside the ear two to four times daily for the first few weeks.
➤ Tell the patient to call you if the earlobe becomes tender, red, and crusty.

## COMPLICATIONS

➤ *Infection* may occur at puncture site if appropriate postprocedure care isn't initiated and maintained.
➤ *Keloid formation* is reduced by minimizing trauma during insertion but keloids may be permanent.
➤ *Ear deformity* due to the earring pulling through the earlobe can be avoided by inserting more than ¼" (0.5 cm) from the edge of the lobe.

➤ *Auricular hematoma* is treated with pressure and drainage as needed.
➤ *Nickel dermatitis* is avoided by using 14-karat gold or surgical steel earrings.
➤ *Embedded earring post or backing* risk is minimized by turning the earring in the hole several times daily.

## SPECIAL CONSIDERATIONS

➤ For the first ear piercing, mark the site at the center of each earlobe. For second piercings, existing earring must be removed and the second mark should be place approximately ⅜″ (1 cm) up from the first hole along the natural line of the earlobe.
➤ Earrings must remain in place for 6 weeks before being removed or replaced with different earrings so that complete healing and epithelialization of the earlobe sinus tract can occur.

## DOCUMENTATION

➤ Document if informed consent was received, if necessary.
➤ Record the preprocedure and postprocedure assessment of ear.
➤ Document procedure, method of puncture, and location.
➤ Note the patient's understanding of instructions, such as site care, pain control, and when to contact you.

# NOSE PROCEDURES

## Epistaxis control

CPT CODES
*30901    Control nasal hemorrhage, anterior, simple (limited cautery or packing), any method*

*30903    Control nasal hemorrhage, anterior, complex (extensive cautery or packing), any method*
*30905    Control nasal hemorrhage, posterior, with posterior nasal packs or cautery, initial*
*30906    Control nasal hemorrhage, posterior, with posterior nasal packs or cautery, subsequent*

## DESCRIPTION

Epistaxis is spontaneous, usually self-limited bleeding from the nasal cavity or nasopharynx. One in 10 persons experience at least one significant episode in their lifetime. However, recurrent or persistent episodes may signal an underlying disorder.

There are two main types of nosebleeds. The first type is *anterior epistaxis*, where moderate, continuous bleeding typically occurs in one nostril. Almost all cases of nosebleeds in children and adults are of this type. The blood typically has a venous source, although elderly people are more prone to arterial bleeding because of vascular and mucosal atrophy. Episodes typically last from a few minutes to half an hour. The second type is *posterior epistaxis*, which occurs in about 10% of nosebleeds where bleeding is heavier and the blood may run from both nostrils if the patient is leaning forward. The blood may also flow into the pharynx, causing profound nausea and possibly coffee-ground emesis. Bleeding is brisk and intermittent, and the source of blood is typically arterial. This type of epistaxis occurs most frequently in elderly people. It's often difficult to treat because the rupture is usually slightly superior or inferior to the posterior tip of the inferior turbinate.

There are several causes of epistaxis including trauma such as direct trauma to the nose or nose-picking, which is a primary cause of disruption to nasal mucosa. Other causes include allergies, a dry environment that may cause excessive heat to dry and crack the nasal mucosa, and infections, especially upper respiratory tract infections and influenza. A spontaneous rupture of a blood vessel (typical in children and elderly people, usually in the anterior septum) and cocaine use (which induces vasospasm and can lead to tissue necrosis) can also trigger epistaxis. If an X-ray of the patient's sinuses appears opaque and he has a sinus infection that doesn't respond to conservative therapy, the epistaxis may indicate the presence of a neoplasm.

## INDICATIONS

➤ To control nasal hemorrhage

## CONTRAINDICATIONS

### Relative
➤ Nasal trauma that might involve internal structure injury
➤ Coagulopathy
➤ Potential cerebrospinal fluid leak

## EQUIPMENT

### For anterior and posterior packing
Gowns ◆ goggles ◆ masks ◆ sterile gloves ◆ emesis basin ◆ facial tissues ◆ patient drape (towels, incontinence pads, or gown) ◆ nasal speculum ◆ tongue depressors (may be in preassembled head and neck examination kit) ◆ directed illumination source (such as headlamp or strong flashlight) or fiber-optic nasal endoscope ◆ suction apparatus with sterile suction-connecting tubing and sterile nasal aspirator tip ◆ sterile bowl ◆ sterile saline solution for flushing out suction apparatus ◆ sterile tray or sterile towels ◆ sterile cotton-tipped applicators ◆ local anesthetic spray (topical 4% lidocaine) or vial of local anesthetic solution (such as 2% lidocaine or 1% to 2% lidocaine with epi-

nephrine 1:100,000) ◆ sterile cotton balls or cotton pledgets ◆ 10-ml syringe with 22G 1½″ needle ◆ silver nitrate sticks ◆ small-tip topical nasal vasoconstrictor (such as 1.5% to 2% phenylephrine or 4% cocaine) ◆ absorbable hemostatic (such as Gelfoam, Avitene, Surgicel, or thrombin) ◆ sterile normal saline solution (1-g container and 60-ml syringe with luer-lock tip, or 5-ml bullets for moistening nasal tampons) ◆ hypoallergenic tape ◆ antibiotic ointment ◆ equipment for measuring vital signs ◆ equipment for drawing blood

### For anterior packing
Two packages 1½″ (4-cm) petroleum strip gauze (3′ to 4′ [0.9 to 1.2 m]) ◆ bayonet forceps or two nasal tampons

### For posterior packing
Two #14 or #16 French catheters with 30-cc balloon or two single- or double-chamber nasal balloon catheters ◆ marking pen ◆ 4″ × 4″ gauze ◆ suture material

## PREPARATION OF EQUIPMENT

➤ Wash your hands.
➤ Assemble all equipment. Make sure the headlamp or flashlight works.
➤ Create a sterile field. (Use the sterile towels or the sterile tray). Using aseptic technique, place all sterile equipment on the sterile field. Thoroughly lubricate the anterior or posterior packing with antibiotic ointment.

## ESSENTIAL STEPS

➤ Put on protective equipment, including gown, gloves, goggles, and mask.
➤ Check vital signs and observe for hypotension with postural changes. Also monitor airway patency.
➤ Explain the procedure, offer reassurance, and answer any questions the patient has.

➤ To prevent blood from going down the nasopharynx and to reduce venous pressure, position the patient sitting up and leaning forward.
➤ To inspect the naval cavity, use a nasal speculum and an external light source or a fiber-optic nasal endoscope. To remove collected blood and help visualize the bleeding vessel, use cotton-tipped applicators and wick away the blood. Consider applying a topical vasoconstrictor such as phenylephrine to slow bleeding and aid visualization.
➤ Apply continuous external pinching pressure with the thumb and forefinger to the anterior nasal septum for 15 minutes without stopping if bleeding is located anteriorly.
➤ If blood still hasn't clotted, insert a cotton pledget of vasoconstricting nasal drops or epinephrine into the nasal passage. Apply pressure for an additional 10 minutes.
➤ Remove the pledget to observe for rebleeding.
➤ If these measures fail, anesthetize the mucous membrane with a cotton pledget of 4% lidocaine.
➤ If you can see the bleeding site and it's accessible, apply a silver nitrate stick to the site and any prominent vessels.
➤ If bleeding recurs after a short time, repeat the previous two steps immediately and then pack the nasal passage with a petroleum gauze strip or oxidized regenerated cellulose for 24 hours.

## For anterior nasal packing
➤ Apply topical vasoconstricting agents to control bleeding or use chemical cautery with silver nitrate sticks. To enhance the vasoconstrictor's action, apply continuous external pinching pressure with the thumb and forefinger to the anterior nasal septum for 15 minutes without stopping.
➤ If bleeding persists, insert an absorbable hemostatic nasal pack directly on the bleeding site. The pack swells to form an artificial clot. If these methods fail, insert an-

terior nasal packing. Even if only one side is bleeding, both sides may require packing to control bleeding. (See *Types of nasal packing*.)
➤ While the anterior pack is in place, instruct the patient or parent to use cotton-tipped applicators to apply petroleum jelly to the patient's lips and nostrils to prevent drying and cracking.
➤ Alternatively, nasal balloon catheters may be used to control epistaxis. (See *Nasal balloon catheters*, page 310.)

## For posterior nasal packing
➤ Wash your hands and put on sterile gloves.
➤ Roll 4″ × 4″ gauze and tie with suture material, leaving ends long enough to tie to the catheters.
➤ If the bleeding source is in the posterior nasal cavity, lubricate the soft catheters to ease insertion. Instruct the patient to open his mouth and to breathe normally through his mouth during catheter insertion to minimize gagging as the catheters pass through the nostril.
➤ Advance one or two soft catheters into the patient's nostrils. As they appear in the nasopharynx, grasp them with a clamp and pull them out through the mouth. Tie the two end sutures to the catheter and gently pull the catheter back out from the nose until the rolled gauze passes the uvula and is snug against the nasal passage.
➤ Help the patient assume a comfortable position with his head elevated 45 to 90 degrees.
➤ Assess him for airway obstruction or any respiratory changes.

## PATIENT TEACHING
➤ Instruct the patient to contact you for recurrent bleeding within 1 hour or for a second episode within 1 week.
➤ Tell the patient to schedule an appointment for removal of the nasal packing, usually in 2 to 5 days. After an anterior pack

## TYPES OF NASAL PACKING

Your patient's nosebleed may be controlled with anterior or posterior nasal packing.

### Anterior nasal packing
You may treat an anterior nosebleed by packing the anterior nasal cavity with a 3' to 4' (0.9- to 1.2-m) strip of antibiotic-impregnated petroleum gauze or with a nasal tampon.

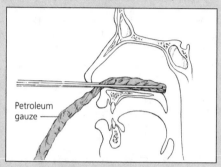

Petroleum gauze

A nasal tampon is made of tightly compressed absorbent material with or without a central breathing tube. Insert a lubricated tampon along the floor of the nose (shown above) and, with the patient's head tilted backward, instill 5 to 10 ml of antibiotic or normal saline solution. The tampon expands as a result, stopping the bleeding. Instruct the patient to moisten the tampon periodically.

In a child or a patient with blood dyscrasia, you may fashion an absorbable pack by moistening a gauzelike, regenerated cellulose material with a vasoconstrictor. Applied to a visible bleeding point, this substance will swell to form a clot. The packing is absorbable and doesn't need removal.

### Posterior nasal packing
Posterior packing consists of a gauze roll shaped and secured by three sutures (one suture at each end and one in the middle). To insert the packing, advance a soft catheter or catheters into the patient's nostrils. When the catheter tips appear in the nasopharynx, grasp them with a Kelly clamp or bayonet forceps

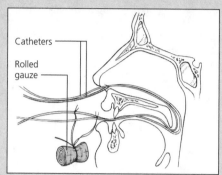

Catheters

Rolled gauze

and pull them forward through the mouth. Secure the two end sutures on the nasal packing to the catheter tip and draw the catheters back through the nostrils (shown above). This step brings the packing into place with the end sutures hanging from the patient's nostril. (The middle suture emerges from the patient's mouth to free the packing, when needed.)

You may weight the nose sutures with a clamp. Then pull the packing securely into place behind the soft palate and against the posterior end of the septum (nasal choana).

After you examine the patient's throat (to ensure that the uvula hasn't been forced under the packing), insert anterior packing and secure the whole apparatus by tying the posterior packing sutures around rolled gauze or a dental roll at the nostrils (shown below).

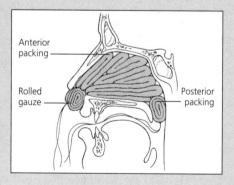

Anterior packing

Rolled gauze

Posterior packing

is removed, instruct the patient to avoid rubbing or picking his nose, inserting any object into his nose, and blowing his nose forcefully for 48 hours.

➤ Tell the patient to expect reduced smell and taste ability. Make sure he has a working smoke detector at home.

## NASAL BALLOON CATHETERS

To control epistaxis, you may use a balloon catheter instead of nasal packing. Self-retaining and disposable, the catheter may have a single balloon or a double balloon to apply pressure to bleeding nasal tissues.

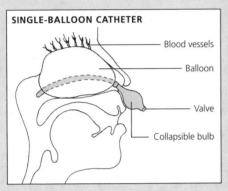

**SINGLE-BALLOON CATHETER**

Blood vessels
Balloon
Valve
Collapsible bulb

Once inserted and inflated, the single-balloon catheter (shown above) used for anterior bleeding compresses the blood vessels while a soft, collapsible external bulb prevents the catheter from dislodging posteriorly.

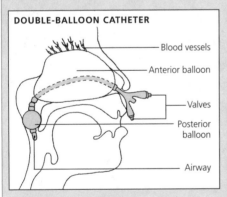

**DOUBLE-BALLOON CATHETER**

Blood vessels
Anterior balloon
Valves
Posterior balloon
Airway

The double-balloon catheter (shown above) is used for simultaneous anterior and posterior nasal packing. It compresses the posterior vessels serving the nose and the posterior bleeding vessels; the anterior balloon compresses bleeding intranasal vessels. This catheter contains a central airway for breathing comfort.

### Insertion

To insert a single- or double-balloon catheter, prepare the patient as you would for nasal packing. Be sure to discuss the procedure thoroughly to alleviate the patient's anxiety and promote his cooperation.

Explain that the catheter tip will be lubricated with an antibiotic or a water-soluble lubricant to ease passage and to prevent infection. The tip of the single-balloon catheter will be inserted in the nostrils until it reaches the posterior pharynx. Then the balloon will be inflated with normal saline solution, pulled gently into the posterior nasopharynx, and secured at the nostrils with the collapsible bulb. With a double-balloon catheter, the posterior balloon is inflated with normal saline solution; then the anterior balloon is inflated.

### Routine care

To prevent damage to nasal tissue, order the balloon deflated for 10 minutes every 24 hours. If bleeding recurs or remains uncontrolled, reinflate the balloon immediately.

### Recognizing complications

The patient may report difficulty breathing, swallowing, or eating, and the nasal mucosa may sustain damage from pressure. Balloon deflation may dislodge clots and nasal debris into the oropharynx, which could prompt coughing, gagging, or vomiting. If these occur, remove the catheter. Under these circumstances, arterial ligation, cryotherapy, or arterial embolization should be considered.

➤ Advise him to eat soft foods because his eating and swallowing abilities will be impaired. Instruct him to drink fluids often or to use artificial saliva to cope with dry mouth.

➤ Teach him measures to prevent nosebleeds, and instruct him to seek medical help if these measures fail to stop bleeding.

➤ Suggest rubbing a lubricant (such as A&D ointment or bacitracin) over the nasal septum twice a day for 3 to 5 days to promote healing and hydration. Suggest using a humidifier or pot of water on the ra-

## HOW TO STOP AND PREVENT A NOSEBLEED

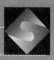

DEAR PATIENT:

Even a minor bump can start a nosebleed. To keep from panicking, learn how to stop the bleeding. Even a child can learn to control nosebleeds with a bit of guidance from an adult. Here are some steps to follow.

### Apply pressure

When your nose bleeds, pinch the lower half of it tightly shut between your thumb and fingers. Breathe through your mouth while you hold your nose like this for 10 minutes continuously.

If your hand or fingers tire, switch hands by placing the thumb and fingers of your rested hand above the fingers of your tired hand. Start pinching with the rested hand as you let go with your tired hand. Then slide your fingers down your nose until they're pinching the lower half of your nose as before.

Practice this technique. This way you'll learn how much pressure to apply and you'll know how your fingers feel when they're in the right position.

Be sure you compress the entire lower half of your nose, not just the tip.

### Other tips

➤ Learn to sit down (quietly and calmly) whenever your nose starts to bleed.
➤ Tilt your head slightly forward so that you don't swallow or choke on your blood.
➤ Don't tilt your head backward, lie down, or stuff a tissue in your nose.
➤ Spit out any blood that gets in your mouth or throat. Spit into a container if possible. This will allow you to estimate blood loss.

➤ You can resume activity when the bleeding stops. Restrict vigorous activity to keep the bleeding from starting again.
➤ Don't pick or blow your nose after a nosebleed because the bleeding may recur.

### Get help

Contact your practitioner if a nosebleed won't stop after two sets of compression lasting 10 minutes each or if bleeding starts again. Stay calm and walk (not run) to find help if it's needed. Hold your head straight or bent slightly downward and keep applying pressure on your nose until you find help.

### Preventing recurrent nosebleeds

➤ Because nosebleeds can result from dry mucous membranes, use a cool mist vaporizer or humidifier, as needed, especially in dry environments.
➤ If you get a nosebleed despite these precautions, keep your head higher than your heart and, using your thumb and forefinger, press the soft portion of the nostrils together and against the facial bones. (Don't use direct pressure if you have a facial injury or nasal fracture.) Maintain pressure for 10 minutes continuously, and then reassess bleeding. If it's uncontrolled, reapply pressure for another 10 minutes with ice between the thumb and forefinger.
➤ After a nosebleed, avoid rubbing or picking your nose, putting a handkerchief or tissue in your nose, or blowing your nose forcefully for at least 48 hours. After this time, you may blow your nose gently and use salt-water nasal spray to clear nasal clots.

diator to increase humidity in the home, especially in sleeping areas and during the winter.

➤ If the patient is a child, tell parents to keep their child's fingernails trimmed.

➤ Provide the patient with a handout on epistaxis management. (See *How to stop and prevent a nosebleed*, page 311.)

## COMPLICATIONS

➤ *Blood loss and infection* are treated on a case-by-case basis.

➤ *Hypoxemia* is treated with oxygen by mask and monitored closely.

➤ *Airway obstruction* is relieved by adjusting or removing the packing.

➤ *Pressure necrosis* risk is minimized by not pulling the packing too tight and removing it as soon as possible.

➤ *Hypotension* is treated with fluid replacement, rest, and blood transfusion (if needed).

## SPECIAL CONSIDERATIONS

➤ Refer the patient to an otolaryngologist or emergency medical facility for massive bleeding, persistent and continuous epistaxis, an inaccessible or poorly visualized bleeding site, or posterior epistaxis.

➤ Patients with posterior packing may be hospitalized for monitoring.

➤ Once the packing is in place, compile assessment data carefully to help detect the underlying cause of nosebleeds. Mechanical factors include a deviated septum, injury, and a foreign body. Environmental factors include drying and erosion of the nasal mucosa. Other possible causes are upper respiratory tract infection, anticoagulant or salicylate therapy, blood dyscrasia, cardiovascular or hepatic disorders, tumors of the nasal cavity or paranasal sinuses, chronic nephritis, and familial hemorrhagic telangiectasia.

➤ If significant blood loss occurs or if the underlying cause remains unknown, order a complete blood count and coagulation profile as soon as possible. As indicated, order an arterial blood gas analysis to detect any pulmonary complications, and arterial oxygen saturation monitoring to assess for hypoxemia. If necessary, administer supplemental humidified oxygen with a face mask. Prescribe antibiotics, decongestants, and analgesics without aspirin or ibuprofen, as indicated.

➤ If needed, obtain hemoglobin and hematocrit studies (if the patient has a history of significant bleeding); type and crossmatch (if the patient may need a transfusion); prothrombin time, partial thromboplastin time, and international normalized ratio (if the patient tends to bleed easily from external stimuli); or sinus X-rays (if you suspect a neoplasm).

## DOCUMENTATION

➤ List a detailed history, including frequency and duration of nosebleeds, associated trauma or history, and coagulopathies.

➤ Document any measures for hemostasis utilized and outcomes. Record the type of packing and when it should be removed. Note the patient's vital signs, any laboratory studies performed, and the results. Record any complications and measures taken.

➤ Record patient instructions and verification of comprehension.

# Foreign body removal from the nose

CPT CODE
*30300 Removal of foreign body, intranasal without anesthetic*

## DESCRIPTION

The primary goal of foreign body removal from the nose is to remove the object without trauma to the nasal cavity and without aspiration of the object. For extremely anxious or noncompliant patients, sedation may help the practitioner perform a safe and effective removal.

Children and mentally incapacitated patients are among the high-risk groups for placing foreign bodies in the nose (and ears). Small toy parts and beans are among the most common intruders, but a wide variety of objects have been reported. Children may inform parents that they have inserted objects into their noses. However, sometimes the history is not as clear, and the child may present with a purulent nasal discharge from the obstructed nostril. A visual examination may reveal the object, or it may show a grossly inflamed area with purulent discharge. Once the diagnosis is made, every attempt should be made to remove the foreign body noninvasively and with direct visualization of the object.

Noninvasive steps should be taken first to reduce the incidence of trauma to the patient or the nose. Noninvasive methods include blowing the nose forcefully, mouth-to-mouth technique, and bag-valve mask positive pressure. Invasive methods include the hooked probe (bayonet or alligator forceps), suction, and balloon technique with Foley or Fogarty catheters.

## INDICATIONS

➤ To remove known foreign body

## CONTRAINDICATIONS

### Relative
➤ Combative or uncooperative patient
➤ Large amount of swelling around the object (Patients with edema around the object that inhibits removal may require general anesthesia and referral to an ear, nose, and throat [ENT] specialist.)

## EQUIPMENT

Phenylephrine spray ◆ topical lidocaine epinephrine solution ◆ suction machine ◆ #3 or #5 curved suction catheter ◆ #4 Fogarty catheter ◆ alligator forceps ◆ bayonet forceps ◆ bright portable light source ◆ gloves ◆ drape or towel ◆ suction tips ◆ nasal speculum ◆ tissues ◆ bag-valve mask (optional)

## ESSENTIAL STEPS

➤ Explain the procedure in detail to the patient and parents. Explain that there will be some discomfort and that aspiration deeper into the nasal cavity or posterior nasopharynx is possible. Answer any questions and obtain written consent from parent or guardian for minors or mentally incapacitated patients.

➤ Place the patient in a supine position. This allows for increased patient comfort and facilitates the procedure for the practitioner.

➤ Stress the importance of the patient remaining completely still for the procedure.

➤ Put on gloves and drape the patient to protect clothing.

➤ Using a nasal speculum and a bright light source, inspect the nostril and try to visualize the object. Extending the head may aid visualization.

➤ Suction any pus or debris that may occlude visualization of the object.

➤ Administer phenylephrine and lidocaine into affected nostril to reduce intranasal inflammation and provide topical anesthesia. Sedate if necessary.

 **ALERT** Some children may need to be physically restrained to perform the procedure. If difficulty continues, stop and refer the patient to an ENT specialist due to the risk of forcing the object further inside.

## Noninvasive procedures

➤ If the patient is cooperative and able, tell him to forcefully blow his nose into a tissue while occluding the unaffected nostril. This should help dislodge the object.

➤ Another noninvasive technique is the mouth-to-mouth technique. Instruct the parent to blow a sharp breath into the child's mouth while occluding the opposite nostril. The positive pressure from behind the object should help dislodge it. This technique allows for parental involvement, which may help to calm the child and is especially useful with infants.

➤ The bag-valve mask works similarly to the mouth-to-mouth technique, providing a positive pressure force behind the object. Again, the unaffected nostril is occluded while delivering positive pressure into the mouth of the patient using a bag-valve mask.

## Invasive procedures

➤ If noninvasive methods are unsuccessful and you're able to visualize the object, choose an extraction tool based on the type of object. Use alligator forceps to withdraw soft objects, such as paper, cotton, and cloth. Harder objects can be removed with bayonet forceps.

➤ Insert the chosen tool gently into the nose with the patient lying completely still. If you meet resistance or the patient is combative, refer the patient to an ENT specialist.

➤ Open the clamps as you approach the object. Grasp it and withdraw slowly.

➤ Use a suction catheter for smooth, round objects that are difficult to grasp with the above tools. Place the suction catheter gently against the object and then turn on the suction while removing the catheter. Be careful not to push the object further into the nasal passage.

➤ A Foley or Fogarty (balloon technique) catheter can also be used. Pass the catheter carefully past the object, inflate the balloon with approximately 1 cc of air, and withdraw slowly pulling the object out of the nose.

## PATIENT TEACHING

➤ Although the risk of infection is small, instruct the patient and parents to observe for signs and symptoms. These include increased pain within 24 hours of the procedure, increased temperature, yellow or green drainage from nose, and foul odor. If any of these symptoms appear, the patient should return to the office as soon as possible. Otherwise, he should follow-up with you 1 to 2 days after the procedure. Following removal of nasal foreign bodies, the patient should irrigate with normal saline solution two to three times per day for 2 to 3 days.

➤ Educate parents that there is a significant risk in aspiration of these objects in small children, especially those under the age of 5. Parents should also be educated about objects often found lodged in the nose and ears, such as marbles and beads. Advise them that young children shouldn't be allowed to play with small objects.

## COMPLICATIONS

➤ *Trauma to mucous membranes* increases the possibility of postprocedure bleeding or infection and may require application of a topical hemostatic agent.

➤ *Injury to nasal passages* can be life-threatening. To prevent this, refer combative patients to an ENT specialist.

➤ *Aspiration or deeper progression of the object* resulting in the inability to remove the object requires referral to an acute care facility or an ENT specialist.

## SPECIAL CONSIDERATIONS

➤ The nasal mucosa may be premedicated with 0.5% phenylephrine (Neo-Synephrine) and aerosolized lidocaine or tetracaine to reduce any mucosal edema and to provide local anesthesia. However, some practitioners prefer using nebulized epinephrine instead. Parents can hold the nebulizer mask close to the child's face. The inhaled medication helps reduce nasal inflammation and makes removing the object easier. Children generally tolerate this better than nasal inhalers and removal with instrumentation may be avoided.

➤ Patients with edema around the object that inhibits removal may require general anesthesia and referral to an ENT specialist.

➤ Usually instillation of lidocaine into the nose provides sufficient anesthesia. However, with the combative child, it may be necessary to administer I.V. sedation.

➤ In all procedures, using any instrument that is to be placed into the nasal canal should be done with a steady hand resting on the patient's head in case of sudden movement, which can be an involuntary response to pain.

➤ After the foreign body is removed, inspect the nasal cavity again for additional foreign bodies or bleeding.

➤ Any bleeding can be stopped by inserting cotton into the nostril temporarily.

➤ Some practitioners recommend always using a topical anesthetic (for comfort) and a vasoconstrictive agent (to decrease edema in surrounding tissues) before attempting to remove a nasal foreign body.

➤ It's important to rule out a foreign body as the source of any unilateral nasal discharge.

 **ALERT** Always use care when performing these procedures. Aspiration of foreign bodies has resulted in death in some children under age 5.

## DOCUMENTATION

➤ Document the patient's condition on arrival, history and duration of symptoms, any behavioral changes, and if the object was visualized.

➤ Note the actual procedure, instruments used (if any), technique, and how the patient tolerated it.

➤ List any and all medications given to the patient and if any restraints were used.

➤ Document any instructions given to patient and parents postprocedure, including preventive measures to avoid a recurrence.

# Gynecologic Procedures

## 7

Women are more likely than men to seek information; as they become better informed, they look to find quality gynecologic care. Advances in technology and treatments of gynecologic disorders reflect a growing interest in improving women's health care. Today, practitioners must be more able to assess, counsel, teach, treat, and refer these patients, while considering such relevant factors as the desire to have children, problems of sexual adjustment, and self-image.

In no part of the body do so many interrelated physiologic functions occur in such proximity as in the area of the female reproductive tract. Frequently, the situation is complicated further by the fact that multiple gynecologic and obstetric abnormalities often occur simultaneously. For example, a patient with dysmenorrhea may also have trichomonal vaginitis, dysuria, and unsuspected infertility. Her condition may be further complicated by associated urologic disorders, due to the proximity of the urinary and reproductive systems. This tendency for patients to have multiple and complex disorders requires a thorough understanding of normal and abnormal anatomy and physiology before initiating any gynecologic procedure.

In addition, it is important that you apply sensitivity and thought when approaching a woman with gynecologic issues. Due to the intimate nature of contact during gynecologic procedures, a patient may be more likely to remember or relate past abuse, trauma, or other concerns. To provide the best response, facilitating health and a strong practitioner-patient relationship, you must consider the possibilities and appropriate responses *before* the situation occurs.

 **CULTURAL TIP** Many cultural groups have modesty issues about the pelvic region that require extra care in providing privacy and draping. Gypsies, Arabians, Central Americans, and Vietnamese may be more uncomfortable if any part of their lower body (including their legs) is exposed. In some cases, such as with the Samoan culture, women may be more concerned with exposing their thighs than their breasts.

Puerto Rican women may prefer to meet with you before changing into a gown and prefer not to use the word sex *(sexo);* the preferred term is "to have intimate relations" *(tener relaciones).*

In addition, West Indian women may display extreme modesty. Embarrassment, which the patient may refer to as "shame," is increased if you are of the opposite gender or you are younger than the patient. Draping the patient well and providing a secure environment will minimize this discomfort.

Female circumcision (clitoridectomy) or infibulation (removal of labia minora, clitoris, and sewing of labia majora, leaving just a small hole for micturition and menstruation) are procedures practiced by some Arabic cultural groups, African tribes, and Muslims. These practices are also known as female genital mutilation (FGM). Some parents may arrange to have school-age or adolescent girls return to their homeland to have the procedure done, or arrange to have it done here in the United States (despite that it's illegal in this country). Patients who have undergone this procedure are unlikely to volunteer this information, particularly if they are monolingual or have an interpreter with a bias about this cultural practice. Patients may not relate their symptoms to FGM or be aware of normal anatomy and physiology, as these procedures are frequently done at a young age. The most valuable tools if you are in contact with these patients are a compassionate, nonjudgmental attitude (as FGM is done in the belief that it's in the girl's best interest) and information. For additional information, access the Rising Daughters Aware Web site *www.fgm.org;* contact Forward USA Against FGM, 2040 Forest Ave., Suite 2, San Jose, CA 95128; or call (408) 298-3798.

# DIAGNOSTIC TESTING

## Papanicolaou test

### CPT CODES
*88142 Cytopathology, cervical or vaginal, collected in preservative fluid, automated thin layer preparation; manual screening under physician supervision*
*88144 Cytopathology, cervical or vaginal, collected in preservative fluid, automated thin layer preparation; with manual screening and computer-assisted rescreening under physician supervision*
*88147 Cytopathology, cervical or vaginal; screening by automated system under physician supervision*

*88150 Cytopathology, cervical or vaginal; manual screening under physician supervision*

## DESCRIPTION

Also known as the Pap test or Pap smear, this cytologic test was developed in the 1920s by George N. Papanicolaou and allows early detection of cervical cancer. The test involves scraping secretions from the cervix. The cells are then spread on a slide and immediately coated with fixative spray or solution to preserve specimen cells for nuclear staining. Alternatively, the collection device is rinsed in a vial of preservative solution and sent to the laboratory. Cytologic evaluation then outlines cell maturity, morphology, and metabolic activity. Although cervical scrapings are the most common test specimen, the Pap test also permits cytologic evaluation of the vaginal pool, prostatic secretions, urine, gastric secretions, cavity fluids, bronchial aspirations, and sputum.

## INDICATIONS

➤ To perform annual screening
➤ To evaluate abnormal vaginal bleeding or discharge
➤ To assess lower abdominal pain
➤ To identify cervical lesions that are visible or palpable
➤ To rule out cervical dysplasia or malignancy noted on previous Pap test
➤ To evaluate history of sexually transmitted diseases or multiple sexual partners

## CONTRAINDICATIONS
### Relative
➤ Current menses, acute infection, or inflammation
➤ Douching or intercourse within previous 72 hours

## EQUIPMENT

Bivalve vaginal speculum ◆ gloves ◆ cervical sampling device (wooden spatula, Cervexbrush, or Cytobrush) ◆ long cotton-tipped applicator ◆ glass microscope slides or vial of preservative (such as ThinPrep) ◆ fixative for slide (a commercial spray or 95% ethyl alcohol solution) ◆ adjustable lamp ◆ drape ◆ laboratory request forms

## PREPARATION OF EQUIPMENT

➤ Select a speculum of the appropriate size, and gather the equipment in the examining room. If preparing smear specimens, label the frosted end of the glass slides with the patient's name and "E" and "C" to differentiate endocervical and cervical. If the patient has had a hysterectomy, label one slide "V" to differentiate a vaginal specimen. If using Thinprep, obtain the vial of preservative and open it.

## ESSENTIAL STEPS

➤ Explain the procedure to the patient and answer any questions she has.
➤ Instruct the patient to void. This will relax the perineal muscles and facilitate bimanual examination of the uterus, which will be performed after the Pap test.
➤ Provide privacy, and instruct the patient to undress below the waist but to wear her shoes, if desired, to cushion her feet against the stirrups. Then instruct her to sit on the examining table and to drape her genital region.
➤ Wash your hands.
➤ Place the patient in the lithotomy position, with her feet in the stirrups and her buttocks extended slightly beyond the edge of the table. Adjust the drape.
➤ Adjust the lamp so that it fully illuminates the genital area. Then fold back the corner of the drape to expose the perineum.

➤ Put on gloves. Examine the vulva, including Bartholin's and Skene's glands. Note the pattern of hair growth for Tanner scale evaluation, any discharge, and any abnormal anatomy.
➤ Take the speculum in your dominant hand and moisten it with warm water to ease insertion. Avoid using water-soluble lubricants, which can interfere with accurate laboratory testing.
➤ Warn the patient that you're about to touch her to avoid startling her. Then, gently separate the labia with the thumb and forefinger of your nondominant hand.
➤ Instruct the patient to take several deep breaths. Insert the speculum into the vagina, applying gentle pressure posteriorly as you advance it. Make sure you can see the entire cervix as you open the speculum. If you can't, remove the speculum, insert your index finger into the vagina, and locate the cervix; then reinsert the speculum. Once it's in place, slowly open the blades to expose the cervix; lock the blades in place.
➤ Note any signs of inflammation, infection, dysplasia, or structural abnormalities. Identify the transformation zone. Note the appearance of any cervical mucus and gently blot mucus or discharge to permit a full view.
➤ Being careful not to traumatize the cervix, insert a cotton-tipped applicator or sampling device through the speculum ⅕" (5 mm) into the cervical os. Rotate the applicator 360 degrees to obtain an endocervical specimen. Then remove the sampling device and, if using slides, gently roll it in a circle across the slide marked "E." Refrain from rubbing the applicator on the slide to prevent cell destruction. Immediately place the slide in a fixative solution or spray it with a fixative to prevent drying of the cells.
➤ Insert the small curved end of the Pap stick or sampling device through the speculum and place it directly over the cervical os. Rotate the stick gently but firmly to scrape cells loose from the ectocervix. Re-

move the sampling device, spread the specimen across the slide marked "C," and fix it immediately, as before. It's important to obtain cells from both the endocervix and the transformational zone. (See *Obtaining an adequate Pap test specimen*)

➤ Alternatively, a plastic sampling device and a Thinprep vial may be used. Obtain specimens as above and rinse the sampling device in the preservative solution in the Thinprep vial.

➤ If the patient has had a hysterectomy, insert the opposite end of the Pap stick or a cotton-tipped applicator through the speculum, and scrape the posterior fornix or vaginal pool, an area that collects cells from the endometrium, vagina, and cervix. Remove the stick or applicator, spread the specimen across the slide marked "V," and fix it immediately, as before. If any abnormalities are seen in this area, another specimen should be obtained and sent as a separate specimen.

➤ Unlock the speculum to ease removal and avoid accidentally pinching the vaginal wall. Then examine the vaginal walls as you slowly withdraw the speculum.

➤ Remove the glove from your nondominant hand and lubricate the glove on your dominant hand. Perform the bimanual examination, which usually follows the Pap test. Note the mobility of the uterus as well as any palpated abnormalities or tenderness as you assess the introitus, vagina, fornices, cervix, Skene's glands (on the external vulva) and Bartholin's glands (at the base of the vaginal opening).

➤ Instruct the patient to bear down and then cough as you assess for urinary leakage and prolapse of the uterus or cervix. Insert a lubricated gloved finger rectally to check for masses and to obtain a specimen for fecal occult blood testing if any stool is obtained from the rectal vault.

➤ Remove your other glove and discard both gloves. Gently remove the patient's feet from the stirrups and assist her to a sitting position. Provide privacy for her to

## OBTAINING AN ADEQUATE PAP TEST SPECIMEN

It's important to obtain cells from the endocervix and the transformational zone in order to have an adequate Pap test specimen. First, take the sampling device and lightly scrape around the ectocervix.

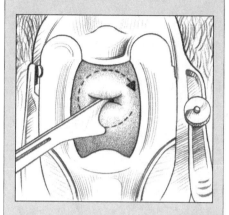

Then insert the sampling device into the endocervix, turning it 360 degrees. If you obtain a great deal of mucus, wipe it away without swabbing the endocervix.

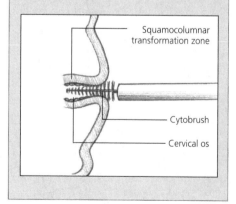

Squamocolumnar transformation zone

Cytobrush

Cervical os

dress. Fill out the appropriate laboratory request forms, including the date of the patient's last menses, any clinical findings and risk factors.

*(Text continues on page 323.)*

PATIENT-TEACHING AID

## HOW TO PREPARE FOR A PELVIC EXAM

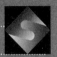

DEAR PATIENT,

If just thinking about a pelvic exam makes you feel uncomfortable, remember this: The exam won't hurt, and it could save your life. How? During the exam, you'll have a Pap test, which is a simple, painless, cervical smear that can detect cancer cells.

The pelvic exam can also help your practitioner verify that your reproductive organs are healthy and detect sexually transmitted diseases and other infections while they're treatable. Another plus — the exam takes only about 5 minutes.

### Before the exam
First, the practitioner will ask about your health history, take your blood pressure, and request a urine specimen.

Next, you'll enter an examination room, remove your clothes, and put on a front-opening examination gown. Then you'll sit on an examining table, and the assistant will give you a sheet to drape across your legs.

### A brief physical
The practitioner may check your throat, neck, heart, lungs, and breasts. (Ask how to perform a breast self-examination if you don't already know how.)

### Positioning
Then you'll need to position yourself so that your buttocks are at the table's edge and your heels are in the table's stirrups. Once a sheet is draped over your legs, you'll be instructed to spread your knees apart.

### Inspection
The practitioner will inspect your external genitals (called the perineum) for irritation or other abnormalities.

Next, she'll insert a speculum into your vagina. This instrument enables her to inspect your vagina and cervix. It may feel cool, but usually it will be warmed and lubricated so that it slides easily and causes little sensation.

If you resist the speculum, however, you may feel uncomfortable. So take a deep breath and relax.

### Obtaining cell samples
Using a thin wooden or plastic spatula, tiny brush, and cotton-tipped swab, the practitioner will obtain cell samples for tests, such as a Pap smear — most women don't feel this at all. Once that is done, she will remove the speculum.

### Checking internal organs
Next, the practitioner will perform a two-handed (bimanual) exam to feel your internal organs. She'll insert two gloved and lubricated fingers into your vagina up to the cervix. Then, with her other hand on your abdomen, she'll feel the size, shape, and location of your uterus, ovaries, and fallopian tubes and check for tenderness, masses, and other abnormalities. If you tense up, take a deep breath to relax.

### After the exam
When the examination is over, remember to ask any questions you have. Then wipe the lubricant from your perineum with a tissue and get dressed in private.

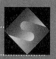

# HOW TO EXAMINE YOUR BREASTS

**DEAR PATIENT:**

Because women themselves discover about 90% of breast cancers, it's important to learn and practice breast self-examination techniques. You should examine your breasts once a month. If you haven't reached menopause, the best examination time is immediately after your menstrual period. If you're past menopause, choose any convenient, easy-to-remember day each month — the first of the month, for example. Here is how to proceed.

**1** Undress to the waist, and stand or sit in front of the mirror with your arms at your sides. Observe your breasts for any change in their shape or size. Look for any puckering or dimpling of the skin.

**2** Raise your arms and press your hands together behind your head. Observe your breasts as before.

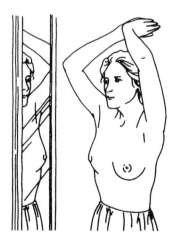

**3** Press your palms firmly on your hips and observe your breasts again.

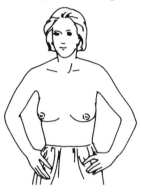

**4** Now, lie flat on your back. This position flattens and spreads your breasts more evenly over the chest wall. Place a small pillow under your left shoulder, and put your left hand behind your head.

**5** Examine your left breast with your right hand, using a circular motion and progressing clockwise, until you've examined every portion. You'll notice a ridge of firm tissue in the lower curve of your breast; this is normal.

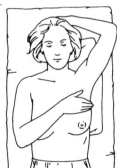

*(continued)*

**6** Check the area under your arm with your elbow slightly bent. If you feel a small lump that moves freely under your armpit, don't be alarmed. This area contains your lymph glands, which may become swollen when you're sick. Check the lump daily. Call the practitioner if it doesn't go away in a few days or if it gets larger.

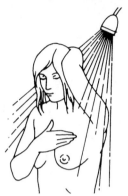

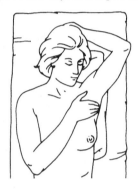

**7** Gently squeeze your nipple between your thumb and forefinger, and note any discharge. Repeat steps 4 through 7 on your right breast, using your left hand.

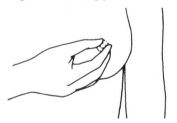

**8** Finally, examine your breasts while you're in the shower or bath, lubricating your breasts with soap and water. Using the same circular, clockwise motion, gently inspect both breasts with your fin-

gertips. After you've toweled dry, squeeze each nipple gently, and note any discharge.

**9** If you feel a lump, don't panic — most lumps aren't cancerous. First, note whether you can easily lift the skin covering it and whether the lump moves when you do so.

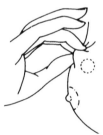

Next, notify your practitioner. Be prepared to describe how the lump feels (hard or soft) and whether it moves easily under the skin. Chances are, your practitioner will want to examine the lump. Then she can advise you about what treatment (if any) you need. Although self-examination is important, it isn't a substitute for examination by your practitioner. Be sure to see her annually or semiannually (if you're considered a risk).

## PATIENT TEACHING

➤ Advise the patient to abstain from intercourse, douching, or using any vaginal medications, spermicidal foams, creams, or gels for 2 days prior to the appointment. These activities may wash away cells or alter test results (see *How to prepare for a pelvic exam,* page 320).

➤ Tell the patient that minor bleeding after the procedure is common.

➤ Advise the patient that further testing may be necessary.

➤ Inform the patient that results should be available within 10 days of the procedure. If she isn't contacted within that time, she should call the office.

➤ Review self-breast examination technique (see *How to examine your breasts,* pages 321 and 322).

## COMPLICATIONS

➤ *Discomfort, bleeding, and flashbacks of trauma or abuse* require supportive care and cessation of the procedure if the adverse reaction is severe.

## SPECIAL CONSIDERATIONS

➤ False negative results are minimized by ensuring an adequate specimen and routine follow-up testing.

➤ Annual or semiannual breast examination is typically completed at the same time as the pelvic examination and the Pap test.

➤ Look for lesions on the cervix and in the vaginal area and include cells from this area on the Pap smear, making a note of it on the slip that is sent to the laboratory. Also note on the slip if any bleeding occurred and note "contact bleeding" in the patient's chart.

➤ Any lesions that are seen or palpated may require colposcopy, which may be performed at the time of the Pap smear.

➤ If using a broom collection device, such as the Cytobrush or Cervexbrush, rotate it

360 degrees on the cervix five times to obtain specimens from the endocervix and ectocervix at the same time.

➤ If the patient appears anxious or upset during the pelvic examination, stop at once, make eye contact, and ask if she wants you to stop. If she does, stop the examination but discuss the importance of having a pelvic examination and Pap test at the next visit or with another provider. When the patient has dressed, discuss your observations (for example, hands balled into fists, pallor, tears, and changes in breathing pattern) and ask if she wants to discuss anything. Think about your response in advance; you don't want to respond with hesitancy or silence if the patient discloses trauma or abuse.

## DOCUMENTATION

➤ Document indications for and details of the procedure, including a detailed description of any abnormalities noted.

➤ Note specimens sent, the patient's reaction to the procedure, medications ordered, time frame for follow-up evaluation, and instructions given to the patient.

# Colposcopy and cervical biopsy

### CPT CODES
*57452  Colposcopy (separate procedure)*
*57454  Colposcopy with biopsy of cervix or endocervical curettage*
*57500  Biopsy, single or multiple, or local excision of lesion*
*57505  Endocervical curettage (separate procedure)*

## DESCRIPTION

Colposcopy is an integral part of cervical cancer detection and treatment programs.

## UNDERSTANDING HOW A COLPOSCOPE WORKS

The colposcope is a binocular microscope on a stand. It incorporates a light source, usually tungsten or halogen bulbs; some use a fiber-optic light source. The colposcope used in gynecologic examinations must be supplied with a green or blue filter that can be used to amplify findings. The filter absorbs red light reflected from blood vessels on the surface of the cervix, making them appear black against the surrounding tissue and enhancing their evaluation.

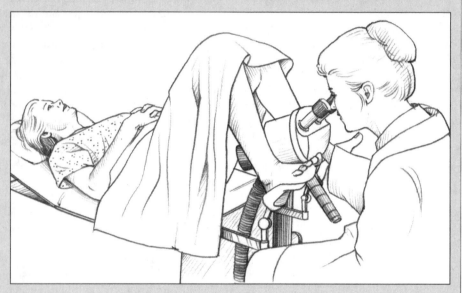

Colposcopy more closely examines the cervix with the assistance of a special mounted microscope. It may be used to keep track of precancerous abnormalities and look for recurrent abnormalities after treatment. (See *Understanding how a colposcope works*.)

### INDICATIONS

➤ To evaluate abnormal Pap smear result indicating cervical pathology
➤ To treat suspicious lesions visualized or palpated during pelvic examination
➤ To rule out suspected human papilloma virus
➤ To assess history of high-risk of dysplasia

### CONTRAINDICATIONS

#### Relative

➤ Current menses, inflammation, or infection

### EQUIPMENT

Colposcope ◆ gloves ◆ speculums ◆ biopsy forceps ◆ curettes ◆ endocervical speculum (optional) ◆ 3% to 5% acetic acid ◆ normal saline solution ◆ Lugol's iodine solution ◆ Monsel's solution ◆ sponge forceps ◆ cotton-tipped and gynecologic applicator such as a Scopette ◆ sanitary napkins ◆ 4″ × 4″ sponges ◆ glass slide and preservative or vial with preservative

## PREPARATION OF EQUIPMENT

➤ Gather equipment and warm the room.

## ESSENTIAL STEPS

### For colposcopy

➤ Prepare the woman for the examination by describing the procedure. Obtain consent, especially if a biopsy (either endocervical or cervical) may be taken. Sensations that may be experienced and should be discussed include stinging, which may accompany the application of acetic acid solution; biopsy of the cervix is experienced as a "pinch"; and cramping that may accompany the endocervical curettage. Verify through history and testing, if indicated, that she isn't pregnant. Evaluate the patient's comfort level and pursue areas of concern as appropriate.

➤ Wash your hands.

➤ After she has removed her undergarments, voided, and is appropriately draped, assist her to the lithotomy position. Adjust the colposcope's height to the examining table, chair, and yourself.

➤ Put on gloves. Examine the external genitalia visually.

➤ Using one gloved finger lubricated with water only, palpate the vaginal walls gently to detect subepithelial nodules or masses.

➤ Also ascertain the plane of the cervix so that insertion of the speculum will be atraumatic.

➤ Insert a warmed and clean, water-lubricated speculum of the appropriate size and open it to expose the cervix. (*Note:* To help the patient relax the pelvic musculature and ease the discomfort, encourage her to try to "push out" the speculum as you insert it.)

➤ Obtain a Pap test specimen and cultures at this time, if needed.

➤ Gently move the cervix with a cotton-tipped or gynecological applicator to clearly visualize the vaginal fornices.

➤ Using a gynecologic applicator or a 4″ × 4″ sponge held by a forceps, apply normal saline or acetic acid solution and clean the cervix of secretions. If acetic acid is used, it's necessary to wait several minutes before examining the cervix with the colposcope to allow aceto-whitening to fade.

➤ Move the colposcope into position and focus for the most clear cervical appearance. Examine the cervix under magnification. (See *Abnormal findings*, page 326.)

➤ Next, repeat the examination under blue or green light. This action makes abnormal surface blood vessels visible as black structures on the cervix.

➤ After a complete and thorough examination, reapply 3% to 5% acetic acid to the cervix.

➤ Allow at least 15 seconds for aceto-whitening to occur and reexamine the cervix with the colposcope without the light filter and then with the light filter. If aceto-whitening fades during the examination, additional acetic acid can be applied without danger to the patient.

### For cervical biopsy

➤ Repeat your examination for abnormal findings of the cervix.

➤ Alternatively, some practitioners use Lugol's solution to paint the cervix for examination (Schiller's test). Lugol's is taken up by normal, mature, glycogenated squamous epithelium, causing the tissue to attain a rich, mahogany color. Abnormal or neoplastic epithelium doesn't contain glycogen and won't stain, but looks a dirty yellow. Schiller's test is helpful in identifying the margins of lesions.

➤ At this time, biopsy specimens of abnormal appearing cervical tissues are taken with the biopsy forceps. Always warn the patient before obtaining the biopsy that she will feel a pinch. When identifying areas to biopsy, look for an area that will af-

## ABNORMAL FINDINGS

During the examination, you're observing the appearance of the original squamous epithelium, the transformation zone (the area between the original squamous epithelium and columnar epithelium), and the columnar epithelium. Abnormal findings should be described in detail, such as whether the lesion is flat, micropapillary, or microconvoluted. Iodine-negative epithelium results in a yellow color, as opposed to the normal iodine reaction, which is a dark mahogany color. The presence of atypical vessels in any lesion suggests more severe dysplasia. Leukoplakia is evidenced by white, thickened patches that can't be rubbed off and that sometimes show a tendency to fissure. Other abnormal findings that indicate the need for biopsy include the following:

➤ Aceto-white epithelium (Note if it's mildly or intensely aceto-white.)

➤ Punctation with no blood vessel pattern and a pitted appearance

➤ Mosaic with no blood vessel pattern and a geographic appearance

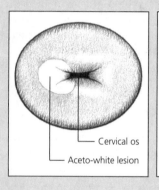

Cervical os
Aceto-white lesion

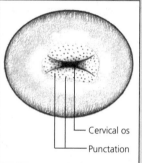

Cervical os
Punctation

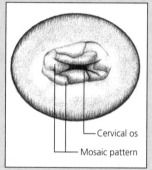

Cervical os
Mosaic pattern

ford the pathologist with a border of normal and abnormal tissue, although it isn't required. (See *Obtaining a cervical biopsy*.)

 **ALERT** Biopsy abnormal areas on the posterior cervix before obtaining specimens from the anterior cervix. If anterior lesions are biopsied first, the area will bleed, obscuring the view of the posterior cervix and its lesions.

➤ Place the specimens immediately in preservative for transport to pathology.

➤ Next, inform the patient that you'll be scraping cells from the canal of the cervix. Insert the curette ¾" to 1¼" (2 to 3 cm) into the cervical canal and scrape toward the external os. Repeat this procedure until you have scraped the canal two or three times in each quadrant (two or three times between 9 o'clock and 12 o'clock).

➤ Place the endocervical specimen in preservative for transport to pathology.

➤ Using an applicator, apply Monsel's solution to the biopsy areas to obtain hemostasis. Pressure may also be applied by a Scopette to control bleeding.

➤ Remove the speculum, dispose of soiled equipment and supplies, then assist the patient to a seated position. Instruct her that she may rest for a few minutes and then dress. Provide her with a sanitary pad.

## PATIENT TEACHING

➤ Tell the patient that bleeding may continue like a light period for several days and that cramping may continue for the next few hours. Advise her that ibuprofen

will relieve the cramps. Tell her to use sanitary napkins or panty liners for bleeding.
➤ Instruct the patient to schedule follow-up in the office when results of biopsies are received to discuss further therapy and plan of care.
➤ Explain to the patient that the Monsel's solution will drain out over the next day or so and will look like coffee grounds.
➤ Tell the patient not to use tampons or vaginal preparations, not to douche unless instructed otherwise, and to abstain from intercourse for 1 week.
➤ Inform the patient to contact you if heavier bleeding, temperature higher than 100.4° F (38° C), discharge with foul odor or burning or itching, and other symptoms that cause concern occur.
➤ Discuss lifestyle changes with the patient to reduce the risk of cervical cancer, including using condoms, stopping smoking, and avoiding exposure to sexually transmitted diseases by limiting the number of sexual partners.

## COMPLICATIONS

➤ *Excessive bleeding* is treated with a second application of Monsel's solution.
➤ *Infection* requires evaluation, testing, and treatment.

## SPECIAL CONSIDERATIONS

➤ Ideally, the time to perform the colposcopy in premenopausal women is at midcycle.
➤ When scheduling a colposcopy, instruct the woman to avoid having intercourse or using vaginal medication, contraceptives, or douching for 48 hours before the examination.
➤ Refer to algorithms available for diagnostic decision making related to abnormal Pap smears and the performance of colposcopy (for example, at the National Testing Laboratories Worldwide Web site,

### OBTAINING A CERVICAL BIOPSY

Biopsy forceps are used to obtain a specimen of abnormal-appearing cervical tissues. The specimen should include the border of the lesion so the pathologist can compare normal and abnormal tissue.

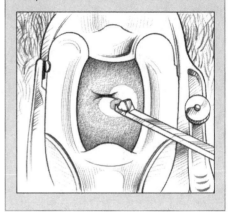

*http://www.cervicography.com/evaluating.html*).
➤ There are a variety of colposcopy instruments available. Models with magnifications between 10X and 16X are practical for most diagnostic situations.
➤ Graves metal bivalve specula are preferred. Specula with matte finishes may be used to overcome reflection problems.
➤ The Kevorkian curette is used in a cervix with a wide os to obtain a specimen. The Novak curette is more suitable for the narrow cervical os. A skin hook (optional) may be applied to the anterior cervical lip to stabilize the cervix if the curette does not slip easily into the os.
➤ Cervicography is an adjunctive cervical screening procedure, intended to increase the sensitivity of the Pap smear in screening for cervical abnormalities. After a routine Pap test is obtained, the cervix is swabbed with an acetic acid solution and the outside of the cervix is photographed

with a special camera, such as a cerviscope. The photos are then sent out for evaluation by an expert. The slide is projected on a screen 10' (3 m) or greater in width and observed at a distance of 3' (1 m). This process approximates a colposcopic examination, and the information obtained can be used to allow the specialist to triage patients and see those with more severe dysplasia quickly. This is not a substitute for colposcopy, but rather is performed as a prelude to colposcopy in areas where colposcopists are not routinely available.

➤ When performing cervicography, examine the cervix carefully and remove any hair, discharge, or other obstruction to visualization without rubbing or traumatizing tissue. Obstruction is the most common reason for a "technically defective" cervicography result.

## DOCUMENTATION

➤ Chart the indications for and the patient's response to the procedure. An efficient way to document colposcopic findings is by drawing the cervix with areas of aceto-whitened epithelium (AWE), abnormal vessels (AV), mosaic (MO), punctation (PU), or leukoplakia (LEU) drawn in and labeled as visualized. Areas biopsied (BX) should be marked by o'clock locations. It's important to draw lesions to scale to avoid misunderstanding about the size by professionals or laypersons who may review the chart in the future.

➤ Classify the colposcopy as satisfactory (entire squamocolumnar junction visualized) or unsatisfactory (unable to inspect complete squamocolumnar junction).

➤ Document teaching, instructions for follow-up care, and the need for further treatment or referral.

# Gram stain, wet mount, and potassium hydroxide

## CPT CODES
*87205    Smear, primary source, with interpretation; routine stain for bacteria, fungi, or cell types*
*87210    Smear, primary source, with interpretation; wet mount with simple stain, for bacteria, fungi, ova, and parasites*
*87220    Tissue examination for fungi*

## DESCRIPTION

Specimen collection involves obtaining a fluid sample from the vagina for testing. As a procedure in gynecology, a Gram stain is used to assist in the diagnosis of sexually transmitted diseases (STDs), particularly *Neisseria gonorrhoeae*. The Gram stain enhances detection of bacteria and polymorphonuclear (PMN) leukocytes. A thin smear of cervical secretions is dried, then Gram-stained. Under oil emersion microscopy (100X), gram-negative *N. gonorrhoeae* can be visualized as pink diplococci within PMN cells of the specimen.

The wet mount is another technique used to assist in the diagnosis of vaginal disorders. Specimens of vaginal discharge are taken from several sites on the vaginal walls and fornices with a clean applicator. The specimen is then mixed with normal saline or 10% to 20% potassium hydroxide (KOH) on a glass slide. The slide is viewed microscopically at 10X and 40X, and any of the following may be identified: *Candida albicans* (and other *Candida* species), *Trichomonas vaginalis*, and the clue cells of bacterial vaginosis. The presence of candidiasis and trichomoniasis may be confirmed by wet mount. Diagnosis of bacterial vaginosis is further confirmed by a vaginal pH of more than 4.7 measured by litmus tape, and a fishy odor (caused by release of amines) when KOH is mixed with the vaginal secretions.

## INDICATIONS

➤ To identify suspected STD
➤ To assess vaginal discharge, itching, burning, or irritation

## CONTRAINDICATIONS

➤ Current menses
➤ Recent intercourse, douching, or intravaginal medication

## EQUIPMENT

Gloves ◆ cotton-tipped applicators ◆ glass slide ◆ coverslips ◆ dropper bottle of normal saline ◆ dropper bottle of 10% to 20% KOH ◆ small test tubes (optional) ◆ microscope ◆ vaginal speculum ◆ litmus paper ◆ drape

## ESSENTIAL STEPS

➤ Explain the procedure to the patient. Evaluate the patient's comfort level and pursue areas of concern as appropriate.
➤ Have the patient disrobe from the waist down and put on a gown or drape. Assist her into the lithotomy position.
➤ Wash your hands.
➤ Put on gloves, examine the external genitalia and mons, and insert a warmed speculum that has been moistened with water.
➤ Visualize the cervix and collect a Pap smear if appropriate.
➤ Collect the specimen for Gram stain from the cervical os using a cotton-tipped applicator. Roll a thin specimen of the secretions onto a glass slide and set aside to air dry before Gram-staining.
➤ Discard the applicator.

➤ Collect a specimen for the wet mount from several areas along the vaginal walls and fornices on another cotton-tipped applicator.
➤ Touch the applicator to a sample of litmus paper and note the pH.
➤ *Option 1 (slide):* Set this applicator on a glass slide while you complete the speculum examination.
➤ *Option 2 (test tube):* Place the applicator in a glass test tube with 0.5 to 1.0 ml of normal saline. Repeat this step, placing the second applicator in 0.5 to 1.0 ml KOH.
➤ Remove the speculum.
➤ Perform a bimanual examination and evaluate carefully for tenderness in the uterus or adnexa.
➤ Remove soiled gloves, and wash your hands; explain your findings to the patient and assist her to a seated position.
➤ Instruct her to dress while you complete the laboratory studies.
➤ Put on a clean pair of gloves. Take the applicator you placed on the clean slide or the test tube to the microscope.
➤ *Option 1:*
– Apply a thin sample of discharge directly to a glass slide from the cotton-tipped applicator.
– Allow a drop of normal saline to fall on the specimen and use the wooden applicator end to mix.
➤ *Option 2:*
– Gently agitate the cotton-tipped applicator in the normal saline. Transfer a drop of the saline solution to a glass slide.
➤ Cover the slide with a coverslip.
➤ Prepare the KOH slide similarly.
➤ Alternatively, use two slides, placing both the normal saline and KOH specimens on a single slide at opposite ends. Standardize your technique by always placing normal saline at one end of the slide and KOH at the other end of the slide.
➤ Place a slide under the microscope. Allow the other to air dry.
➤ Examine the normal saline slide first under 10X and then 40X power. Examine

## IDENTIFYING MICROSCOPIC FINDINGS

To identify microscopic findings, first examine the specimen with saline. Potential findings are trichomonads, leukocytes, and clue cells.

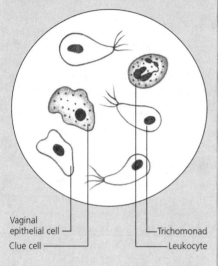

Vaginal
epithelial cell
Clue cell
Trichomonad
Leukocyte

Next, examine the specimen with potassium hydroxide. Potential findings are pseudohyphae, spores, and leukocytes.

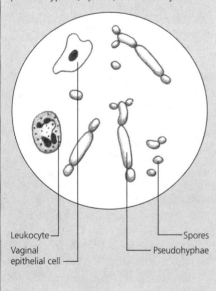

Leukocyte
Vaginal
epithelial cell
Spores
Pseudohyphae

the KOH slide the same way. Examine at least five different microscopic fields. (See *Identifying microscopic findings*.)

➤ Retrieve the first slide that air-dried. Apply Gram stain and see if it adheres to the specimen. If it "stains" the sample, the result is gram-positive. If it doesn't adhere to the sample, it's gram-negative.

➤ Correlate laboratory findings with clinical information and diagnose the cause of the complaint. (See *Differential diagnosis of vaginal discharge*.)

## PATIENT TEACHING

➤ Tell the patient that the appropriate therapy for the identified vaginal malady will generally resolve the abnormal discharge and that no complications are common with this procedure.

➤ Instruct the patient to complete the course of drug therapy and schedule a follow-up appointment after drug therapy is completed. As appropriate, teach the patient how to administer vaginal medication (see *How to administer a vaginal medication*, pages 332 and 333).

➤ Review proper use of condoms as indicated. (See *How to use a condom*, pages 334 and 335).

➤ Advise the patient to contact you if symptoms aren't resolved by completion of the medication, if symptoms escalate or don't improve, or if additional symptoms develop.

 **ALERT** Warn the patient that vaginal preparations suspended in petrolatum will weaken latex condoms and diaphragms. Advise her to use an alternate form of birth control while treatment for vaginal infection continues.

Behaviors to control vaginal infections include wearing cotton underwear; avoiding tight-fitting jeans, nylons, and slacks; wiping from front to back after going to the bathroom; using mild soap; and avoiding douching.

*(Text continues on page 336.)*

# DIFFERENTIAL DIAGNOSIS OF VAGINAL DISCHARGE

Although individual presentations vary, there are some common findings that help differentiate the causes of vaginal discharge. To review these findings, check below.

| DISORDER AND CAUSATIVE ORGANISM | CHARACTERISTICS OF DISCHARGE | VULVOVAGINAL FINDINGS | DIAGNOSTIC TESTS |
|---|---|---|---|
| **Candidal vaginitis** | | | |
| *Candida albicans, C. glabrata, C. tropicalis* | Mild more than profuse; thin more than thick; white, curdlike discharge; adherent to vaginal walls | Possible erythema, excoriation, edema | ➤ pH 4.0 to 4.7<br>➤ KOH: positive for hyphae or spores<br>➤ Saline: White blood cells (WBCs)<br>➤ Gram stain: positive for budding *Candida* |
| **Trichomonal vaginitis** | | | |
| *Trichomonas vaginalis* | Yellow to gray to green odorous discharge; varying consistency; may have bubbles | Possible erythema, and edema; may have "strawberry" patches | ➤ pH greater than 6.0<br>➤ KOH: amine odor<br>➤ Saline: motile trichomonads, elevated WBCs, decreased lactobacilli present on Pap smear |
| **Bacterial vaginosis** | | | |
| Polybacterial *Mobiluncus, Bacteroides, Peptococcus, Peptostreptococcus, Eubacterium, Fusobacterium, Mycoplasma hominis* | White to gray or yellow to green; thin, homogenous, malodorous discharge; adherent to walls and at introitus; may have erythema | Discharge at introitus; may have erythema | ➤ pH 5.5 to 7.0<br>➤ Saline: increased parabasal cells; decreased lactobacilli<br>➤ Gram stain: *G. vaginalis, Mobiluncus* |
| **Cytolytic vaginitis** | | | |
| None; exfoliative vaginitis and greater turnover of squamous epithelial cells secondary to overproduction of lactobacilli | Thick, white discharge | Within normal limits; may see thick vaginal discharge | ➤ pH 4.0 to 4.5<br>➤ Saline: increased epithelial cells, increased lactobacilli, elevated or decreased WBCs<br>➤ Gram stain: lactobacilli, gram-positive rods |

PATIENT-TEACHING AID

## HOW TO ADMINISTER A VAGINAL MEDICATION

DEAR PATIENT:

Your practitioner has prescribed a vaginal medication for you. To insert the medication, follow these instructions.

**1** Plan to insert the vaginal medication after bathing and just before bedtime to ensure that it will stay in the vagina for an appropriate amount of time.
Collect the equipment you'll need: the prescribed medication (suppository, cream, ointment, tablet, or jelly), an applicator, water-soluble lubricating jelly (such as K-Y jelly), a towel, a hand mirror, paper towels, and a sanitary pad.

**2** Next, empty your bladder, wash your hands, and place the towel on the bed. Sit on the towel, and open the medication wrapper or container.

**3** Using the hand mirror, carefully inspect your perineum. If you see signs of increased irritation, don't insert the medication. Notify the practitioner. She may change your medication.

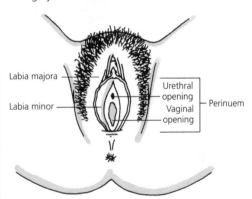

**4** Place a vaginal suppository or tablet in the applicator or fill the applicator with cream, ointment, or jelly.

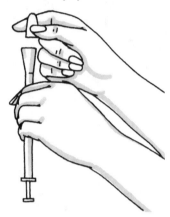

**5** To make insertion easier, lubricate the suppository or applicator tip with water or water-soluble lubricating jelly.

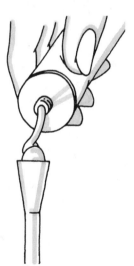

## HOW TO ADMINISTER A VAGINAL MEDICATION *(continued)*

Now lie down on the bed with your knees flexed and legs spread apart.

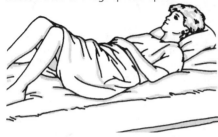

Spread apart your labia with one hand, and insert the applicator with the other hand. Advance the applicator about 2 inches (5 cm), angling it slightly toward your tailbone.

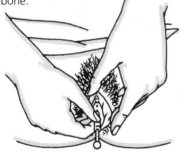

**6** Push the plunger to insert the medication. Be aware that the medication may feel cold.

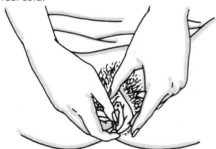

**7** Remove the applicator and discard it, if it's disposable. If it's reusable, thoroughly wash it with soap and water, dry it with a paper towel, and return it to its container.

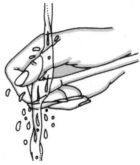

**8** If your practitioner prescribes it, apply a thin layer of cream, ointment, or jelly to the vulva (the area including the vagina, labia majora, and labia minora).

**9** Remain lying down for about 30 minutes so the medicine won't run out of your vagina. Apply the sanitary pad to avoid staining your clothes or bed linens. Then check your vagina for signs of an allergic reaction. If the area seems unusually red or swollen, contact your practitioner.

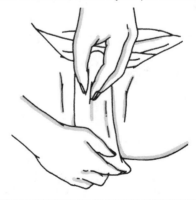

PATIENT-TEACHING AID

# HOW TO USE A CONDOM

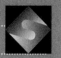

## DEAR PATIENT

Sexual abstinence is the only sure way to prevent sexual transmission of diseases. But if you use a new condom every time you have sex — and use it correctly — this will help protect you and your partner from infection. The suggestions below will help you choose, store, and use condoms.

### Buying condoms

Buy only latex condoms. They give better protection. If you are allergic to latex, use condoms made of polyurethane.

Be sure the condom has a reservoir tip (or receptacle end). Notice that the package has a manufacturer's date — and an expiration date if the product contains spermicide.

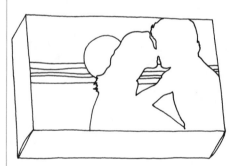

### Storing condoms

Store unused condoms in a cool, dry place. Don't keep them in a warm place, such as your hip pocket or the glove compartment of your car. Heat can damage the latex.

### Using condoms

Follow these steps to apply and remove a condom.

**1** Open the wrapper carefully because a jagged fingernail can tear the condom. Hold the rolled condom by the reservoir tip to squeeze out the air and make room for the semen when you ejaculate.

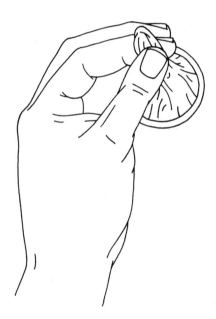

**2** If the condom isn't lubricated inside, apply a water-based lubricant or plain water to your penis to increase sensation.

Once you have an erection, pull back the foreskin if you're uncircumcised.

Next, place the rolled condom on the end of your penis.

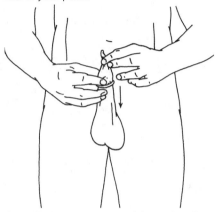

**3** Hold the reservoir tip with one hand, and unroll the condom onto your erect penis with the other hand. Unroll it until it touches your pubic hair. If the condom doesn't have a reservoir tip, keep ½ inch free at the end to collect semen.

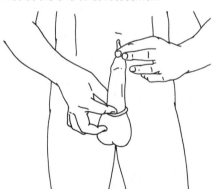

**4** If you need extra lubrication, rub it on the outside of the condom after applying it. Use a spermicidal lubricant containing nonoxynol 9 (which kills HIV, the AIDS virus) for vaginal intercourse and a water-based lubricant for anal intercourse. Don't use petroleum jelly or oil — they can weaken the latex.

If the condom breaks or tears during intercourse, have your partner insert contraceptive foam, cream, or jelly containing nonoxynol 9 into the vagina or rectum immediately.

**5** To remove the condom, pinch the tip with one hand to keep the semen from spilling, and roll the condom off your penis with the other hand.

**6** Flush the condom down the toilet immediately, or discard it in a closed, rigid plastic or metal container such as a coffee can. Never use a condom twice.

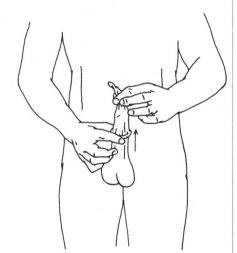

**7** Wash your penis and hands with soap and water.

## COMPLICATIONS

None known

## SPECIAL CONSIDERATIONS

➤ With the availability of over-the-counter (OTC) vaginal medications, the patient may come for diagnosis after overtreating. Her disorder isn't caused by fungal, protozoal, or bacterial elements. Cytolytic vaginitis is a reaction that occurs from treatment or overtreatment of vaginal infections. An overgrowth of lactobacilli produces excess acid that results in cytolysis of epithelial cells. The discharge of cytolytic vaginitis contains no pathogens. Treatment is alkaline douche (1 tsp baking soda in 1 pint of warm water) once or twice as necessary.

➤ Consider postponing specimen collection until the next day if the patient has douched, used intravaginal medication, or had intercourse within the previous 24 hours.

➤ Consider testing all patients with vaginal complaints, especially if the symptoms don't resolve with treatment.

➤ The specimen for Gram stain may be sent out for analysis, at which time the laboratory technician will also review the slide for diplococci.

➤ Discuss the presence of natural vaginal lubrication. Advise the patient against excessive treatment of simple vaginal discharge (one unaccompanied by itching, irritation, or malodor) with over-the-counter preparations.

## DOCUMENTATION

➤ Record subjective data, such as complaints, symptoms, duration, exacerbating or ameliorating factors, remedies tried, and effects of remedies.

➤ Document findings of examination of external genitalia and pelvic examination and findings on wet mount, normal saline, and KOH slides. Documentation of wet mount is in the form of what is present on the slide (for example, normal saline: no hyphae, positive for motile trichomonads, no clue cells; KOH: positive for whiff).

➤ List the prescribed treatment for diagnosed vaginal malady and follow-up care as appropriate.

➤ Document any patient teaching and patient's understanding.

# Postcoital test

CPT CODE
*89300    Semen analysis; presence and motility of sperm including Huhner test (postcoital)*

## DESCRIPTION

The postcoital test (PCT) involves obtaining a specimen that is used to evaluate the cervical mucus following intercourse. Often used early in the infertility workup, the PCT determines the following:

➤ if the ejaculate is delivered appropriately during intercourse

➤ the quantity and quality of preovulatory cervical mucus

➤ the character of the cervical os

➤ the sperms' ability to survive in the cervical mucus

➤ the adequacy of the number of sperm

➤ the presence of an immunologic incompatibility.

A PCT is performed during the late follicular phase (before ovulation, which occurs in the proliferative phase of the menstrual cycle), when cervical mucus is most receptive to sperm. It is performed a minimum of 3 hours but no more than 12 hours following intercourse.

## INDICATIONS

➤ To evaluate the interaction between sperm and cervical mucus

## CONTRAINDICATIONS

### Relative

➤ Any condition that would preclude un-protected sexual intercourse
➤ Bacterial cervicitis or vaginitis

## EQUIPMENT

Glass slides and coverslips (two) ◆ tuber-culin syringe without needle or endome-trial biopsy device such as a Pipelle ◆ speculum ◆ gloves ◆ drape ◆ 4″ × 4″ gauze ◆ microscope

## ESSENTIAL STEPS

➤ Explain the procedure to the patient and answer questions.
➤ Have the patient undress from the waist down and apply drape.
➤ Assist the patient into a dorsal lithoto-my position.
➤ Wash your hands and put on gloves.
➤ Insert a vaginal speculum lubricated with warm water.
➤ Gently swab the vagina with a 4″ × 4″ gauze.
➤ Assess the cervical os (it should be open and hyperemic) and the cervical mucus quality and quantity (it should be watery, clear, abundant and stretchy; also known as spinnbarkeit).
➤ Insert a tuberculin syringe without a needle or a Pipelle 2 to 3 mm into the cervix.
➤ Pull back on the suction applicator and withdraw about 2 ml of cervical mucus and cap the syringe or Pipelle.
➤ On the first slide, place a drop of cervi-cal mucus; immediately cover with a cov-erslip to view under a microscope.

➤ Evaluate the mucus for clarity and vol-ume. Perform the spinnbarkeit test to de-termine how far the mucus will stretch without breaking. This may be done with forceps as they are withdrawn from the vaginal opening or by placing mucus be-tween the gloved index finger and thumb.
➤ Spinnbarkeit greater than 10 cm indi-cates a high level of estrogen and mucus conducive to ovulation. Spinnbarkeit less than 3 cm isn't conducive to ovulation as sperm are unlikely to be capable of pene-trating the mucus.
➤ On the second slide, spread remaining mucus on the pipette tip uniformly across the slide and allow to air-dry to evaluate the ferning pattern (present with high es-trogen levels).
➤ View the first slide and evaluate sperm, cell characteristics, and pH:
– A finding of 20 or more sperm is gener-ally associated with a sperm count above 20 million/ml.
– A finding of 5 to 15 motile sperm with good linear progression is interpreted as a good PCT.
– The presence of white blood cells, clue cells, or trichomonads may indicate an in-fection.
➤ View the second slide for a ferning pat-tern; if present, it indicates adequate es-trogen production.

## PATIENT TEACHING

➤ Before the PCT is scheduled, explain the purpose, procedure, and timing of the test (see *Understanding the menstrual cy-cle*, page 338):
– Carefully review the ovulation determi-nation technique she will use, and instruct her to schedule the postcoital test 1 to 2 days before the expected ovulation.
– Advise her to have intercourse 4 to 12 hours before the appointment and not to use lubricants, douche, or take a tub bath after intercourse.
– She may shower before the appointment.

# UNDERSTANDING THE MENSTRUAL CYCLE

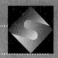

DEAR PATIENT:

Your menstrual cycle has three distinct phases: menstrual, proliferative, and secretory.

## Menstrual phase

Starting on the first day of menstruation, your body's levels of the hormones estrogen and progesterone fall if an ovum (or egg) has not been fertilized and implanted in the lining of your uterus (called the endometrium). As a result, the tissues of the endometrium's superficial layer break down and flow through the vaginal opening and out of the body. This outflow, called the menses or menstrual period, consists of blood, mucus, and unneeded tissue.

## Proliferative phase

During this phase, estrogen levels rise, causing the endometrium to thicken. At the same time, follicles (containing eggs) in your ovary are maturing in preparation for possible pregnancy.

## Secretory phase

During this phase, the endometrium continues to thicken by the following process: At ovulation, around day 14, one of the developing follicle cells ruptures, releasing an egg from the ovary. The ruptured follicle cells develop into the corpus luteum, which starts secreting progesterone as well as estrogen. These hormones prepare the endometrium for implantation and nourishment of the embryo should fertilization occur. Without fertilization, the top layer of the endometrium breaks down, and the cycle begins again.

The menstrual cycle repeats itself about every 28 days.

### HOW YOUR ENDOMETRIUM CHANGES DURING YOUR MENSTRUAL CYCLE

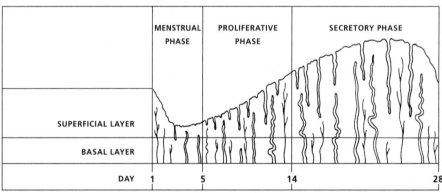

➤ The PCT involves the insertion of a speculum and the removal of cervical mucus and takes approximately 15 minutes.
➤ Tell the patient that no complications are commonly associated with this procedure and it shouldn't be painful.
➤ Inform the patient that test results are known immediately and can be used to guide the next step in the infertility evaluation.

## COMPLICATIONS

None known

## SPECIAL CONSIDERATIONS

➤ A pH below 7 may be treated with a precoital baking soda douche.
➤ Some couples may find the PCT to be intrusive and interfering with the privacy of their sexual relationship. Also, some women may feel self-conscious and uncomfortable seeing a practitioner so soon after intercourse.

## DOCUMENTATION

➤ Before scheduling the PCT, document that patient education and counseling have taken place, and that the patient verbalizes an understanding of ovulation determination technique and importance of proper timing for the PCT.
➤ On the day of the PCT, document the cycle day and when intercourse occurred. Document the appearance of the cervical os, the quality and quantity of cervical mucus, and the presence and quality of spinnbarkeit and ferning. Document the number and motility of the sperm. Document the patient counseling that was provided after the procedure and the plan for further evaluation.

# TREATMENTS

## Bartholin's gland abscess incision and drainage

CPT CODE
*56420   Incision and drainage of Bartholin's gland abscess*

## DESCRIPTION

A Bartholin's cyst forms when the gland duct is occluded. The cause of ductal occlusion is unknown, but sources suggest that congenital stenosis or atresia, thickened mucus, or trauma may contribute to accumulated secretions. Small, asymptomatic cysts require no therapy. However, the dilated gland may become infected. Common organisms cultured from infected cysts include *Escherichia coli*, *Bacteriodes*, *Proteus*, *Peptostreptococcus*, and *Chlamydia trachomatis*; however, 10% are caused by *Neisseria gonorrhoeae*. Because a sexually transmitted disease (STD) may be the source of the Bartholin's gland abscess, tests for *Chlamydia* and gonorrhea should be performed before treatment is initiated.

Conservative therapy for an acute Bartholin's gland abscess may be sitz baths for 72 hours, although the patient must be informed that spontaneous rupture is often accompanied by recurrence. Broad-spectrum antibiotics may be used in early bartholinitis; however, this therapy may delay ripening of the abscess.

After incising and draining a Bartholin's gland abscess, Word catheter insertion is commonly done. The purpose of using the Word catheter is to create a temporary fistulous tract from the Bartholin's gland to the vaginal vestibule to facilitate drainage of the abscess.

## INDICATIONS

➤ To treat acute, symptomatic Bartholin's gland or abscess
➤ To assess tenderness, pain and throbbing of labia, dyspareunia, and pain when walking or sitting

## CONTRAINDICATIONS

### Relative
➤ Pregnancy (refer to a gynecologist)

## EQUIPMENT

Disposable scalpel with pointed knife blade ◆ Word catheter ◆ syringe with 2 to 4 ml sterile water ◆ lidocaine 1% and 10-ml syringe ◆ povidone-iodine solution or a dilute Hibiclens solution ◆ 4″ × 4″ gauze sponges ◆ drape ◆ curved hemostat ◆ 25G needle ◆ sterile gloves ◆ optional equipment: irrigant (peroxide and normal saline mixed 1:1), #16 angiocatheter with inserter needle removed, 5-ml syringe ◆ cotton-tipped applicator with transport medium

## PREPARATION OF EQUIPMENT

➤ Set up a sterile field with gauze, scalpel, needle, and syringes.
➤ Using the 10-ml syringe and 25G needle, draw up 5 to 10 ml of lidocaine.
➤ Inflate the Word catheter with 2 to 4 ml of sterile water to ensure that the catheter bulb functions. Deflate the catheter and leave the syringe attached to the catheter port to lessen manipulation after the catheter is placed.

## ESSENTIAL STEPS

➤ Explain the procedure and alternatives to the patient, show her the Word catheter, and answer any questions. Obtain informed consent.
➤ Instruct the patient to empty her bladder. Have her undress from the waist down.
➤ Assist the patient to the lithotomy position and drape the perineum appropriately.
➤ Wash your hands and put on gloves; maintain strict asepsis throughout the procedure.
➤ Verify that the patient is not allergic to iodine and clean the skin near the Bartholin's gland abscess and vaginal introitus with povidone-iodine and 4″ × 4″ gauze in a circular manner from the site outward.
➤ Anesthetize with lidocaine along a vertical line at the medial aspect of the abscess by inserting the needle and then slowly infusing as the needle is withdrawn.
➤ Stab the scalpel tip into the abscess near the ductal opening (usually between the hymenal ring and labia majora at 4 o'clock or 8 o'clock, near the fourchette). Successful incision will result in the spontaneous release of purulent drainage and be just large enough to allow catheter insertion.
➤ Obtain a specimen for culture at this time, if indicated, using the cotton-tipped applicator. Place it in a plastic transport tube and crush the tip to release the culture medium.
➤ Insert a gloved finger into the vaginal opening, positioning your finger medial to the abscess and applying gentle pressure to express all material possible.
➤ Gently insert curved hemostat to aid inspection and to break any septa leading to fluid-filled cavities. Grasp the cyst wall with the hemostat to stabilize the tract opening.
➤ Irrigate the cyst cavity with a 1:1 solution of normal saline and peroxide, using

the 5-ml syringe with a needleless angio-catheter to perform the irrigation, if necessary.

➤ Insert the tip of the Word catheter into the cyst and inflate the retention balloon with sufficient water (from 2 to 4 ml) to retain catheter tip inside the cyst. Remove the syringe from Word catheter's self-sealing port.

 **ALERT** Be certain to maintain pressure on the syringe while verifying that the catheter is inflated enough to stay in place. Without adequate pressure, the catheter will eject fluid into the syringe and slip out of place.

➤ Tuck catheter tip into the vagina.

## PATIENT TEACHING

➤ Advise the patient that although the procedure may be uncomfortable, pain relief often accompanies initial evacuation of purulent fluid.

➤ Inform the patient that the Word catheter remains in place for 4 to 6 weeks while the cavity heals and that the expected outcome is drainage from the site for up to 6 weeks until complete resolution of the abscess and infection occurs.

➤ Instruct the patient to return in 1 week for Word catheter and abscess examination.

➤ Advise the patient to take over-the-counter pain medications, such as ibuprofen (Advil) and acetaminophen (Tylenol), every 4 to 6 hours as necessary to relieve pain. Sitz baths also provide pain relief. Three or four sitz baths a day promote healing as well as clean the area.

➤ Tell the patient that sexual intercourse may be resumed when tenderness subsides.

➤ Discuss the etiology and nature of acute abscess with her. Advise the patient that there is an association between abscesses and sexually transmitted diseases (STDs). Review the necessity for safer-sex practices. Suggest that the patient's partner be examined for STDs before resuming in-

tercourse. Inform the patient of confidential testing options such as public health clinics and self-testing, as appropriate. (See *Performing a home HIV test*, pages 342 and 343.)

➤ Instruct the patient to contact the office if pain increases, if discharge increases or changes in color, if fever is greater than 100.4° F (38° C), or if bleeding from cavity or catheter occurs.

## COMPLICATIONS

➤ *Overinflation of the Word catheter bulb* may cause pressure necrosis of the cyst wall with formation of a chronic defect and requires referral to a gynecologist.

➤ *Recurrence of Bartholin's gland cyst or abscess* is an indication for referral to a gynecologist.

## SPECIAL CONSIDERATIONS

➤ Use gentle pressure only, when expressing material from the cyst.

➤ Deflate catheter bulb only if drainage has stopped or if the bulb is causing discomfort. Reinsertion is difficult once the catheter becomes dislodged.

➤ For cyst incision and drainage (without inserting a Word catheter), pack the site with iodoform gauze, making sure to leave at least ¼″ (0.6 cm) of iodoform gauze protruding from the cavity to allow for removal easy removal of the gauze later. Half the gauze is generally removed at 24 hours, and half at 48 hours.

➤ Primary Bartholin's cyst in a woman over 40 years of age may indicate a neoplastic process and should be referred to a gynecologist for treatment.

## DOCUMENTATION

➤ Record any subjective indications for the procedure including unilateral swelling of the labia, tenderness, pain, dyspareu-

*(Text continues on page 344.)*

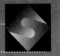

# PERFORMING A HOME HIV TEST

## DEAR PATIENT:

Human immunodeficiency virus (HIV) is a virus that attacks your immune system and causes acquired immunodeficiency syndrome (AIDS). By testing your blood, you can determine if you've been infected with HIV. Remember that even if you've been exposed to HIV, it may not become evident in your blood for 6 months. If you have any questions about your test results or the risk factors associated with HIV, always consult your practitioner. Follow these steps to learn how to obtain a blood sample and how to perform the test.

### Getting ready

**1** Begin by assembling the necessary equipment included in the packet: a lancet, a test card with your personal identification number (to receive the confidential and anonymous test results), and the envelope in which to send the test card to the laboratory.

**2** Read the instructions thoroughly before you stick your finger. Instructions appear in English and Spanish. Remove the personal identification card from the bottom of the test card and place it in a safe place.

### Obtaining blood

**1** Wash your hands thoroughly and dry them. Choose a site on the end or side of any fingertip. To enhance blood flow, hold your finger under warm water for a minute or two.

**2** Hold your hand below your heart, and milk the blood toward the fingertip you plan to pierce. Squeeze that fingertip with the thumb of the same hand. Place your fingertip, with your thumb still pressed against it, on a firm surface such as a table.

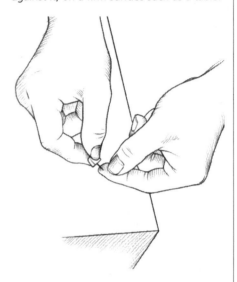

**3** Twist off the lancet's protective cap. Then grasp the lancet and quickly pierce your fingertip just to the side of the finger pad, where you have more blood vessels and fewer nerve endings.

**4** Remove your thumb from your fingertip to permit blood flow. Then milk your finger gently until you get a large, hanging drop of blood.

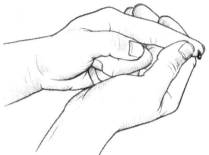

**5** Point your finger down directly over the three circles on the test card. Completely fill each circle with blood.

**6** Place any used lancets in the containers attached to the mailing card. Slip the test card in the postage-paid mailer, seal the mailer, and send it to the address printed on the front. Save the part of the card that lists the toll-free phone number to call for results.

### Obtaining the results
In about 1 week, call the toll-free number on the identification card. Give the person who answers your identification number and wait for the results. If your test is positive for HIV, a specially trained counselor will advise you what to do next and will tell you about nationwide HIV and AIDS organizations. If your test results are negative for HIV, the trained counselor will advise

you how to maintain your negative HIV status.

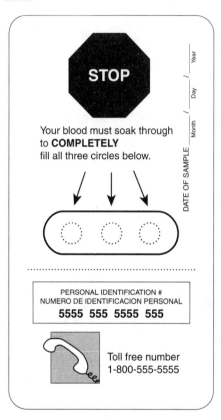

Remember, a negative test result doesn't necessarily mean you're free from HIV infection. It may simply mean that the antibodies are not yet present in your blood. To be certain, repeat the test in 6 months.

nia; pain when walking or sitting; and a previous history of Bartholin's cyst or abscess.

➤ Note all objective findings, such as erythema, acute tenderness, edema, a fluctuant mass located lateral to the vestibule, purulent drainage, and tender and enlarged inguinal nodes.

➤ Document all physical findings that indicate Bartholin's gland cyst or abscess, carcinoma of Bartholin's gland, STDs, inclusion cyst, sebaceous cyst, lipoma, or fibroma.

➤ Chart the procedure as performed, medications used (amount of lidocaine injected), and how the procedure was tolerated. Record plan for subsequent follow-up or referral including the provider's name, address, phone number, and a specific time frame for follow-up.

➤ Document any patient teaching and patient's understanding.

## Condyloma acuminatum treatment

### CPT CODES
*56501 Destruction of lesion(s), vulva; simple, any method*
*56515 Destruction of lesion(s), vulva; extensive, any method*

## DESCRIPTION

Human papillomavirus (HPV) is a slow-growing deoxyribonucleic acid virus that causes intradermal papilloma and is a sexually transmitted disease (STD). HPV infection creates the lesions commonly called genital warts. HPV may be external or internal. External HPV lesions may be removed by self-applied medications (Condylox or Podofilox), 80% to 90% trichloroacetic acid (TCA), or 10% to 25%

podophyllin. Cryotherapy with liquid nitrogen, vaporization with a carbon dioxide laser, electrodiathermy loop excision procedure, surgical excision, and interferon or 5-fluorouracil are methods used by physicians to treat internal lesions. The methods most commonly used by nurse practitioners (TCA and podophyllin) are discussed here. Both of these methods are relatively inexpensive but can cause skin irritation. When choosing between them, remember that podophyllin and Podofilox have a low systemic absorption rate, and TCA penetration is difficult to control. Practitioners who specialize in dermatology or STD clinics or those who perform colposcopy may use additional therapies.

The purpose of therapy is to remove genital warts and prevent progression of neoplasias. Because HPV is a virus and resides in human tissues even when dormant, is isn't possible to eradicate the infection and recurrence of lesions is common.

## INDICATIONS

➤ To treat external genital or vaginal condylomata
➤ To remove symptomatic condylomata

## CONTRAINDICATIONS

### Relative
➤ Pregnancy
➤ Internal HPV treatment
➤ Suspected malignancy

## EQUIPMENT

80% to 90% TCA or 10% to 25% podophyllin ◆ cotton-tipped applicators ◆ petroleum jelly ◆ light source ◆ gloves ◆ paper cup ◆ 3% to 5% acetic acid ◆ 4″ × 4″ gauze pads ◆ antiseptic such as povidone-iodine ◆ fenestrated drape (optional) ◆ tuberculin syringes (optional) ◆ interferon (optional) ◆ 27G or 30G needle (optional)

## ESSENTIAL STEPS

➤ Explain the procedure to the patient, obtain informed consent, and answer any questions she may have.
➤ Wash your hands.
➤ Provide privacy, and instruct the patient to undress below the waist but to wear her shoes, if desired, to cushion her feet against the stirrups. Then instruct her to sit on the examining table and to drape her genital region. Place the patient in the lithotomy position, with her feet in the stirrups and her buttocks extended slightly beyond the edge of the table.
➤ Adjust the lamp so that it fully illuminates the genital area. Then fold back the corner of the drape to expose the perineum.
➤ Put on gloves. Warn the patient that you're about to touch her to avoid startling her.
➤ Using cotton-tipped applicators or gauze soaked with acetic acid, swab the area. Areas with HPV-DNA will turn white (called aceto-whitening).

### Topical application

➤ Apply a fenestrated drape, making sure all lesions are easily accessible.
➤ Using gloved fingers, coat the healthy skin adjacent to the lesions with petroleum jelly.
➤ Remove 0.5 ml of podophyllin from the container and place in a paper cup or open the TCA container. Dip a cotton-tipped applicator into the podophyllin or TCA.
➤ Warn the patient that the medicine may sting within minutes of application but usually resolves in about 5 minutes. Apply the podophyllin or TCA to lesions, taking care to avoid touching the chemicals to healthy tissue. With TCA, the lesions will turn white.
➤ Dispose of each applicator after it touches tissues and use additional applicators until all lesions are treated.
➤ Tell the patient to wash the podophyllin off in 2 to 4 hours.

### Lesion injection

➤ Taking 4″ × 4″ gauze pads and an antiseptic such as povidone-iodine, clean the area in a circular motion from the site of the lesions outward.
➤ Apply the fenestrated drape, ensuring that all lesions are easily accessible.
➤ Using a separate tuberculin syringe for each lesion with a maximum of five lesions treated at one visit, fill each syringe with 0.05 ml of interferon.
➤ Insert the needle into the base of the lesion and form a wheal with the interferon. Repeat for each lesion.
➤ Repeat procedure twice weekly for 1 to 2 months for each lesion, depending on response to treatment.

## PATIENT TEACHING

➤ Inform the patient that the area treated will be tender but should improve in a few hours. Tissues may be red, and leukorrhea may develop. These symptoms resolve in 2 to 3 days. Lesions will become smaller and finally disappear if therapy is successful.
➤ Advise the patient to take sitz baths of warm water to relieve perineal discomfort.
➤ If lesions are too sore to touch with a towel, tell the patient to use a hair dryer on low setting.
➤ Tell the patient that over-the-counter (OTC) pain relievers (acetaminophen or ibuprofen) may be used. Topical anesthetics may provide relief, but may also irritate.
➤ Teach the signs and symptoms of podophyllin toxicity (nausea, vomiting, lethargy, coma, or paralysis), as indicated.
➤ Instruct the patient to contact you if symptoms are not managed by sitz baths and OTC medications. Persistent tissue redness or leukorrhea may indicate infection.
➤ Teach the patient and the patient's partners, if necessary, that although the first outbreak occurs after a 1- to 6-month in-

cubation period, it isn't always sympto-matic. Recurrent outbreaks can occur years later. Thus, diagnosing a patient with condyloma acuminata for the first time is not "proof" of having intercourse with an infected person within the recent past.

➤ Instruct the patient to use condoms to decrease the risk of transmitting the infection.

## COMPLICATIONS

➤ *Tissues may be red, swollen, and tender* within a few hours after treatment with TCA or podophyllin. Sloughing of treated tissue may occur and referral to a gynecologist is indicated.

➤ *Anaphylactic reactions to podophyllin* require emergency treatment.

## SPECIAL CONSIDERATIONS

➤ Use podophyllin and TCA on external HPV *only*. Use no more than 0.5 ml of podophyllin per treatment and treat less than 10 cm² per session.

➤ Inject only five lesions per visit if using intralesional interferon.

➤ Podophyllin preparations aren't used during pregnancy.

➤ If there is no apparent improvement, an alternative therapy will be used or the patient may be referred for surgical or electrocautery removal.

 **CULTURAL TIP** It's important to be aware of who the decision-maker is in the patient's relationship with their partner. If it isn't the patient, it's important to provide the option of being present when the patient discusses the diagnosis with her partner to avoid untoward repercussions. Cultural groups in which the male is likely to have more decision-making power than the female include Arabic, Chinese, Colombian, Cuban, Hmong, Iranian, Japanese, Mexican, South Asian, Vietnamese, and West Indian.

## DOCUMENTATION

➤ Document the onset, duration, symptoms, remedies tried, and outcomes.

➤ Describe the lesions and their number, size, location, and distribution.

➤ Note the differential diagnoses, which may include condyloma lata, molluscum contagiosum, carcinoma, and other STDs, such as syphilis, gonorrhea, and chlamydia.

➤ Record the number and approximate area of lesions treated and protection of adjacent skin with petrolatum if topical agents used.

➤ Report the immediate reaction of the patient to therapy.

➤ Record follow-up instructions and educational materials given as appropriate and patient's understanding of instructions and materials.

## Cryocautery of cervix

CPT CODE
*57511    Cryocautery of cervix, initial or repeat*

## DESCRIPTION

Used to treat cervical intraepithelial neoplasia (CIN), cryocautery uses freezing temperatures to destroy the outermost layers of cervical cells. Temperatures of –4° F (–20° C) or lower for about 1 minute kill the infected or cancerous cervical cells. To perform the procedure, a probe that uses a refrigerant, such as nitrous oxide, to reach temperatures as low as –103° F (–75° C) is placed on the tissue and forms an ice ball (also called a cryolesion). Repeated cycles of freezing and thawing produce more tissue destruction than one freezing treatment that lasts an equal amount of time, provided that each freezing cycle produces the maximum effect. Smaller lesions may require only one treatment, but larger lesions may require multiple freeze cycles; persistent disease may require retreatment.

Three basic scenarios exist, only the first of which is an indication for cryocautery:
– The lesion is covered by the 20- or 25-mm probe.
– The lesion extends beyond the probe, and the ice ball can only extend to the lesion periphery but not uniformly beyond 4 mm of the extent of the lesion.
– The lesion extends onto the vaginal fornices.

## INDICATIONS

➤ To remove CIN grade I or II lesion, precancerous cervical lesions, or carcinoma in situ

## CONTRAINDICATIONS

### Absolute
➤ History of hypersensitivity or adverse reaction to cryotherapy
➤ Invasive cancer or dysplasia more than grade II
➤ Positive endocervical curettage
➤ Pregnancy
➤ Lack of correlation between a Pap test or colposcopic impression and biopsies
➤ Inability to see entire lesion or lesion is greater than 2 cm in diameter
➤ Lesion extends beyond the reach of the probe or lesion is greater than 2 cm in diameter
➤ Current sexually transmitted disease besides human papillomavirus
➤ Expected onset of menses within the next week

### Relative
➤ Collagen disorders or immunoproliferative disorders
➤ Ulcerative colitis
➤ Glomerulonephritis

➤ High cryoglobulin levels (abnormal proteins that dissolve at body temperature but precipitate when cooled)
➤ History of endocarditis, syphilis, Epstein-Barr virus infection, high-dose steroid use, cytomegalovirus infection, or chronic hepatitis B (because high-dose corticosteroid use can result in exaggerated tissue damage)

## EQUIPMENT

Cryogun with nitrous oxide tank and 20- and 25-mm flat and slightly conical cryoprobes ◆ warm water ◆ normal saline solution ◆ water-soluble lubricant ◆ timer or watch with a second hand ◆ vaginal speculum ◆ vaginal side-wall retractors or glove to place over the speculum ◆ drape

## ESSENTIAL STEPS

➤ Have the patient premedicate with a nonsteroidal anti-inflammatory drug, such as ibuprofen 800 mg, 1 hour before the procedure to decrease associated cramping and discomfort.
➤ Explain the procedure to the patient, address any concerns, answer any questions she might have, and obtain informed consent.
➤ Wash your hands.
➤ Provide privacy, and have the patient undress from the waist down except for shoes and socks and cover herself with a drape. Assist the patient into the lithotomy position and position the drape so the perineal area is visible.
➤ If the vaginal walls are at risk for contact with the cryoprobe (such as for an obese patient), use vaginal retractors. If one isn't available, you can cut the finger off a glove and snip the fingertip off as well. Slip this over the speculum before inserting it. When the speculum opens, the vaginal walls will be splinted.
➤ Dip the speculum in warm water. Instruct the patient to take several deep

breaths while you insert the speculum into the vagina. Once it's in place, slowly open the blades to expose the lesion. Then lock the blades in place.

➤ Select a cryoprobe tip that will cover the lesion plus 5 mm beyond the lesion's borders.

➤ Select a flat or slightly conical tip. This will minimize the depth of freezing beyond diseased tissues. Dip the cryoprobe in warm water or saline solution and apply a thin layer of water-soluble lubricant to maintain good contact between the probe tip and the cervix.

➤ Turn on the nitrous oxide tank and check the pressure. Insufficient pressure increases the time it takes the tissue to freeze.

➤ Apply the cryoprobe and activate the freezing mechanism. Start timing the freeze, and tell the patient you've started the procedure. When adherence occurs (after 5 seconds), apply gentle outward traction to center the probe in the cervix. Your goal is to prevent the healthy tissue from being affected without tearing the cryoprobe free.

➤ For benign cervicitis, freeze for one 3-minute period. For dysplastic CIN, freeze long enough to form an ice ball that extends at least 5 mm beyond the lesion (approximately 3 minutes). After freezing is stopped, allow the cryoprobe to defrost enough to fall away by itself. Most units automatically defrost the probe when freezing ceases. After the tissue thaws completely (5 to 10 minutes), repeat the process (called the freeze-thaw-refreeze cycle). Keep in mind that the timing isn't as important as formation of an adequate ice ball.

➤ Between freeze cycles, place the tip in warm water to increase efficacy.

## PATIENT TEACHING

➤ Tell the patient that mild cramping noted at the time of the procedure resolves within an hour in most cases.

➤ Instruct her to return to the office in 4 weeks for a postoperative examination, and tell her to follow up with a Pap test in 4 months; send her a reminder notice at that time.

➤ Tell the patient that cryosurgery will treat her cervical abnormality in the least invasive effective manner, preventing progression or worsening of the abnormality.

➤ Explain that a heavy, watery discharge for at least 3 weeks — occasionally up to 8 weeks — can be normal; the discharge may be blood-tinged for a few days but should change to darker red to brown and lessen over time. Suggest that she wear a sanitary pad and change it at least every 4 hours. After 3 weeks she may douche with 1 tbs of vinegar in 1 cup of water or use a povidone-iodine vaginal suppository if odor becomes a problem.

➤ Tell her that she can resume normal activities but must refrain from sexual intercourse and from putting anything in the vagina, including tampons, for 2 weeks.

 **ALERT** Tell the patient to call you for severe cramping, bleeding, temperature above 100° F (38° C), or discharge that lasts longer than 3 weeks.

## COMPLICATIONS

➤ *Cramping and flushing* commonly occur during the procedure but resolve spontaneously. The squamocolumnar junction may be deeper in the os after the procedure, making subsequent examinations more difficult.

➤ *Cervical stenosis* may occur if a long tip is used.

➤ *Infertility, bleeding, menstrual irregularities for up to 3 months, and infection* are rare, but are indications for referral to a gynecologist.

## SPECIAL CONSIDERATIONS

➤ To produce an adequate cryolesion, make sure that the temperature at the periphery of the lesion and at 5-mm depth in the cervix reaches at least –4° F (–20° C) and is maintained for at least 1 minute. Adequate cryonecrosis at a depth of 5 mm requires a freeze-thaw-refreeze cycle of 5 minutes for each part of the cycle.

➤ For larger lesions, consider using a 25-mm probe, which may produce better results than a 20-mm probe.

➤ Be aware that many cryosurgical units have a defrost function that causes the cryoprobe to detach less than 15 seconds after freezing stops but the gas must remain on to activate this defrost function.

➤ Keep in mind the following factors that increase freeze time: increased size of the ice ball needed, low tank pressure, increased vascularity, extra keratin covering on the cervix (remove or moisten the keratin to decrease freeze time), and poor physical contact between the cryoprobe and lesion. The type of system used also affects freeze time.

➤ Most patients receive treatment in the office setting and don't need an anesthetic.

## DOCUMENTATION

➤ Document a detailed description of the site pre- and postprocedure, the patient's reaction to the procedure, medications ordered, time frame for follow-up evaluation, and instructions given to the patient.

## Pessary insertion

CPT CODE
*57160    Fitting and insertion of pessary or other intravaginal support device*

## DESCRIPTION

A pessary is a device that is worn internally, such as a diaphragm, and supports the uterus, bladder, or rectum. Vaginal supportive pessaries are helpful in managing uterine prolapse, uterine retrodisplacement, and stress urinary incontinence, as well as pathology associated with these conditions.

## INDICATIONS

➤ To alleviate uterine prolapse, cystocele, genital hernias, dysmenorrhea, dyspareunia, retroverted incompetent cervix (the pessary tilts the cervix, promoting fertility)

➤ To treat bladder incontinence

➤ To be used when surgery is contraindicated for the patient

➤ To be used as an intermediate measure while awaiting surgery

## CONTRAINDICATIONS

### Absolute

➤ Genital infection
➤ Atrophic vaginitis
➤ Adherent uterus

## EQUIPMENT

Sterile pessary (Gehrung for cystocele; ring, ball, inflatable, or other option for cystocele or rectocele; Gelhorn, Hodge, Cube, or Napier for uterine prolapse) ◆ drape ◆ sterile gloves ◆ antiseptic such as povidone-iodine ◆ sterile basin ◆ sterile ring forceps or claw forceps ◆ water-soluble lubricant such as K-Y jelly ◆ mirror

## ESSENTIAL STEPS

➤ Explain the procedure and answer any questions the patient may have.

➤ Have the patient void and undress from the waist down except shoes and socks.

➤ Assist the patient into the lithotomy position.

## PESSARY INSERTION

To insert a pessary, apply gentle pressure to the patient's pelvic opening with your nondominant hand to enlarge the introitus. Grasp the pessary with the forceps and squeeze them to minimize the pessary. Insert the pessary toward the back of the vagina behind the suprapubic bone, stopping when you feel resistance. Release the pessary and close and remove the forceps. Assess fit — there should be a fingerswidth on all sides and the pessary shouldn't be visible at the introitus.

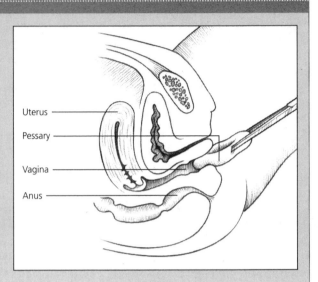

Uterus

Pessary

Vagina

Anus

➤ Drape the patient, wash your hands and put on gloves.

➤ Measure the internal dimensions to determine the size of the pessary. For length, measure from the introitus to the top of the posterior vaginal vault and then subtract ⅓″ (1 cm) from this measurement. For the width, insert the ring forceps into the vagina to the level of the cervix, open them until they touch the walls, and note the distance between the handles of the forceps. Remove the forceps, open them to the same distance between the handles, and measure the distance between the tips. Average these two measurements to determine the pessary diameter.

➤ Soak the pessary in a basin of povidone-iodine.

➤ Lubricate the pessary with water-soluble gel.

➤ Apply gentle pressure to the pelvic opening with your nondominant hand to enlarge the introitus. (See Pessary insertion.)

➤ Instruct the patient to urinate, walk, and squat to evaluate placement. Adjust

the pessary if the patient reports discomfort or if the pessary becomes displaced.

➤ Using a mirror, teach the patient how to insert and remove the pessary herself.

➤ Instruct her to schedule an appointment for 2 weeks after to evaluate for proper fit, infection, irritation, and technique for inserting and removing it.

## PATIENT TEACHING

➤ Teach the patient about the specific type of pessary inserted, including its purpose (for instance, to maintain the position of the uterus or bladder). (See How a pessary functions.)

➤ Explain that she should remove the pessary daily or monthly as appropriate for that type of pessary, and clean it with soap and water. If any vaginal infection is detected, the patient should soak the pessary in alcohol for 20 minutes, then dry and insert.

➤ Never use powder or perfume on the pessary.

➤ Tell the patient she can douche using a 1:1 solution of vinegar and water to lower the risk of infection and decrease odor. Tell her to follow up as appropriate but not to wait more than 3 months. She should bring the pessary to her routine gynecologic examinations so fit can be reevaluated and it can be replaced annually.

 **ALERT** Tell the patient to call you for urinary retention, frequency, and urgency; dysuria; foul odor; and unusual vaginal discharge.

## COMPLICATIONS

➤ *Vaginal and urinary tract infections* are treated with cessation of pessary use, which may be reinstituted after completion of antimicrobial treatment.
➤ *Vaginal burning and itching, dysuria, and urinary retention, frequency, and urgency* are indications for cessation of pessary use, and may be indications for referral.

## SPECIAL CONSIDERATIONS

➤ The patient may find a pessary that doesn't exert pressure on the bowel or bladder (such as the Cube) more comfortable, but because suction holds such a pessary in place, the patient needs to remove it daily to prevent erosion of vaginal mucosa. The Gelhorn and ring-type pessaries exert pressure on the bowel or bladder, but may be left in for up to 3 months at a time.
➤ Strongly consider using estrogen vaginal cream with the pessary.
➤ Provide routine follow-up, focusing on inspecting for lacerations and ulcerations.

## DOCUMENTATION

➤ Document indications for and details of the procedure, including the patient's reaction to the procedure and ability to demonstrate proper technique, time frame for follow-up evaluation, and patient instructions given.

### HOW A PESSARY FUNCTIONS

A pessary may be used to support the posterior vaginal fornix and push the cervix slightly backward and upward into the pelvis. It's purpose is to maintain the position of the uterus or bladder.

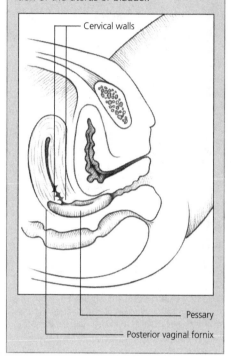

# CONTRACEPTION

## Cervical cap fitting

**CPT CODE**
*57170  Diaphragm or cervical cap fitting with instructions*

## DESCRIPTION

The cervical cap is a barrier method of contraception with an efficacy rate of about 80%. It is similar to the diaphragm but smaller in size — a thimble-shaped soft rubber cup that the patient places over the cervix. The cervical cap may be worn by women who are not suited for the diaphragm. The cap requires less spermicide, is less likely to become dislodged during coitus, and does not require refitting with a change in weight. For parous women, the cap is less effective than the diaphragm or the female condom. For nulliparous women, the cap and diaphragm provide similar contraceptive efficacy during typical use. Failure of the cervical cap is commonly due to neglect to use the device or inappropriate use of the device.

## INDICATIONS

➤ To provide contraceptive protection during sexual intercourse

## CONTRAINDICATIONS

➤ Perpendicular cervical angle
➤ Unusually long or short cervix
➤ Allergy to latex or spermicides
➤ Vaginal stenosis or pelvic abnormalities
➤ Personal factors that interfere with insertion and removal
➤ History of toxic shock syndrome, cervical warts, or polyps

## EQUIPMENT

Cervical cap fitting set ◆ gloves ◆ goggles

## ESSENTIAL STEPS

➤ Check the patient's history for allergies, especially to latex.

➤ Following appropriate education and counseling, escort the patient into the examining room. Instruct her to undress below the waist and assist her into a dorsal lithotomy position.
➤ Wash hands and put on gloves. Perform a bimanual pelvic examination and Pap testing as indicated.
➤ During the bimanual examination, assess the degree of vaginal tone and estimate the length, diameter, and symmetry of the cervix:
–The length of the cervix must be at least ½" (1.5 cm), and the width of the cervix must be ⅓" to 1" (1 to 2.5 cm).
– The cervix must be fairly symmetrical, without extensive laceration or scarring that may interfere with proper fit.
– The cervix should be in the same angle as the vagina, and fairly distal to the introitus.
– Vaginal tone should be good, and vaginal length should be adequate to minimize dislodgment of the cap and partner complaints.
➤ Determine the appropriate cap size:
– Caps come in four sizes: 22, 25, 28, and 31 mm.
– The cap diameter is measured across the cap rim.
– The cap depth increases with the diameter.
– The internal ring creates a "suction" seal on the cervix.
➤ Insert the best estimated cap size (try at least two):
– With cap rim dry, hold cap in the middle and squeeze fingers together, separate labia, and insert cap.
– Once inside the vagina, reposition fingers to either side of the cap rim.
– Move cap opening toward the cervix and cover cervix completely.
➤ Assess the fit. (See *Fitting a cervical cap*.)
➤ Trace the entire upper rim of the cap to determine that the cervical base is fully covered.

## FITTING A CERVICAL CAP

With the proper fit, the "gap" or space between the base of the cervix and the inside of the cap ring, should be 1 to 2 mm (to reduce the possibility of dislodgment), and the rim should fill the cervicovaginal fornix. Leave the cap in place for a minute or two. Then, with the cervical cap in place, pinch the dome until there is a dimple.

A dimple that takes about 30 seconds to resume a domed appearance indicates good suction and a good fit. If the cap is too small, the rim leaves a gap where the cervix remains exposed. If the cap is too large, it isn't snug against the cervix and is more easily dislodged.

| CORRECT FIT | CAP TOO SMALL | CAP TOO BIG |
| --- | --- | --- |
| 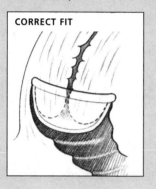 | 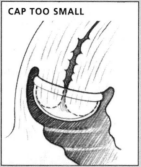 | 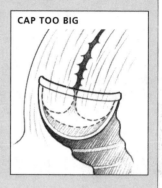 |

➤ Ensure that the cap rim fits completely against the vaginal fornices. The dome of the cap should be deep enough so that it does not rest on the cervical os.

➤ After a minute or two, assess the cap's suction.

➤ Assess the ability of the cap to relocate itself to the cervix when dislodged — an indicator of good fit.

➤ Involve the patient before and during the fitting:

– Allow her to view her cervix (plastic speculum offers the best unobstructed view).

– Instruct her to check the cap's placement by tracing the entire upper rim (360 degrees) around her cervix.

➤ Remove the cap:

– Insert fingers and push cap rim to one side to dislodge.

– Remove the cap sideways with one or two fingers.

➤ Facilitate the patient's comfort level with cap insertion and removal:

– Ask the patient to feel her cervix and note where the cap was.

– Review cap placement and removal techniques.

– Ask her to insert the cap in a squatting position with her back upright. Check for proper fit; and give feedback.

– Ask her to remove the cap by pushing the rim to one side to dislodge and removing it with one or two fingers.

➤ Put on goggles and demonstrate how to properly clean the cap with warm soapy water and pay special attention to the groove on the inside rim.

## PATIENT TEACHING

➤ Tell the patient to return in 3 months to reassess fit, and her skill and comfort level with the cap.

➤ Emphasize the importance of using the cap every time she and her partner have intercourse. Reinforce that this doesn't prevent infection.

➤ Before each insertion, instruct the patient to fill the cap one third full with a spermicidal cream or jelly. Overfilling the cap may interfere with its suction.

➤ Before inserting the cap, instruct her to be sure her fingers and the rim of the cap are dry.

➤ Advise her to grasp the cap in the middle of the rim, folding it together. Once inside the vagina, the open part of the cap is pushed toward the cervix.

➤ Teach the patient how to check for proper placement. She should trace the entire upper cap rim. If it's correctly positioned, she won't feel her cervix (it's inside the cap and feels similar to a nose).

➤ Instruct the patient about the following:

– Slightly turning the cap by a quarter to a half-turn may improve its suction and fit. This is done by pushing the rim up and to the side.

– If the cap is dislodged during intercourse, it should not be moved or removed. Instead, the patient should insert an applicator full of spermicide into her vagina and remain in a reclining position for at least 30 minutes.

– The cap must remain in place at least 8 hours following intercourse and it may safely remain in place up to 48 hours at one time.

– The cap must not be worn during menses because menstrual flow will interfere with the fit.

– The cap may be inserted up to 1 day before intercourse.

– With repeated intercourse, additional spermicide is not necessary.

– The cap should not be reinserted for at least 8 hours after removal.

➤ Teach the patient how to properly care for the cervical cap. After removal, wash the cap with warm, soapy water and be careful to clean the groove on the inside rim. Allow it to air dry completely and store the cap in its plastic container in a cool,

dry place. Never apply powder, oil-based lubricants, or medications to the cap. Inspect the cap at least once a month for any holes or damage to the latex.

➤ Tell the patient that the cap should be replaced every two 2 years, and may require refitting following any delivery or cervical surgery.

➤ Advise the patient that cap use should be temporarily discontinued and you should be notified if the patient suspects she has a vaginal, urinary, or pelvic infection; if pain is associated with use of the cap; if the cap repeatedly dislodges; if she suspects she is pregnant; if she has abnormal Pap test results; if she suspects she has toxic shock syndrome; or if she has continued problems associated with the cap.

## COMPLICATIONS

➤ *Pregnancy, leukoplakia, endometriosis, urinary tract infection (risk is less than with a diaphragm), toxic shock syndrome (a theoretical risk), and cervical dysplasia* are all indications for referral to a gynecologist.

## SPECIAL CONSIDERATIONS

➤ Standard precautions must be observed during fitting, cleaning, and disinfecting cervical caps. Eye splash protection and gloves must be worn during cleaning. Because caps come into contact with intact mucous membrane, fitting caps are classified as semicritical devices that require processing with a high-level disinfectant according to Occupational Safety and Health Administration guidelines. Following disinfection, allow the caps to air dry, and then store them in a disinfected container.

## DOCUMENTATION

➤ Preprocedure, document that patient education and counseling has taken place. Note that history and physical examination have been performed and reflect no absolute or relative contraindications to the patient using the cervical cap.

➤ Postprocedure, record the size of the cervical cap fitted and the patient's demonstrated ability to properly insert and remove the cervical cap properly. Note the patient was instructed to schedule a return visit for 3 months postprocedure.

# Diaphragm fitting

## CPT CODE
*57170    Diaphragm or cervical cap fitting with instructions*

## DESCRIPTION

The diaphragm is a barrier contraception method that mechanically blocks sperm from entering the cervix. A diaphragm consists of a soft latex rubber dome that is supported by a round metal spring on the outside. Diaphragms are available in various sizes and must be fitted to the individual. When used with spermicidal jelly, its effectiveness ranges from 80% to 93% for new users and increases to 97% for long-term users.

## INDICATIONS

➤ To be used in patients who prefer or require reversible contraception

## CONTRAINDICATIONS

### Absolute
➤ History of toxic shock syndrome or repeated urinary tract infections (UTIs)
➤ Vaginal stenosis
➤ Pelvic abnormalities
➤ Allergy to spermicidal jellies or rubber
➤ Less than 6 weeks postpartum

➤ Inability or unwillingness to learn proper techniques for care and insertion of the diaphragm

### Relative
➤ Uterine prolapse or retroversion
➤ Large cystocele or rectocele

## EQUIPMENT

Diaphragm fitting rings or set of fitting diaphragms ◆ diaphragm ◆ water-soluble lubricant ◆ diaphragm introducer (optional) ◆ gloves ◆ goggles

## ESSENTIAL STEPS

➤ Check the patient's history for allergies, especially to latex.
➤ After explaining the procedure to the patient, instruct her to undress below the waist and assist her into the lithotomy position.
➤ Wash hands and put on gloves.
➤ If not done recently, perform a pelvic examination and Pap test.
➤ Insert your index and middle fingers as if performing a pelvic examination.
➤ Measure from the symphysis bone to the posterior of the cervix by touching the posterior fornix with your middle finger and raising your hand until the index finger touches the pubic arch.
➤ Use your thumb tip of the inserted hand, to mark where the pubic bone touches the middle finger.
➤ While maintaining your thumb position, withdraw your hand from the patient.
➤ Place one end of the diaphragm rim or fitting ring on the tip of the middle finger with the opposite side lying just in front of the thumb. This action will give you the approximate diameter of the diaphragm. Diaphragms are manufactured in sizes of 60 to 90 mm, with the average being 75 to 80 mm. (See *Proper diaphragm measurement*, page 356.)

## PROPER DIAPHRAGM MEASUREMENT

To ascertain the correct size of the diaphragm, hold your index and middle fingers extended together and insert them into the patient's vagina. With the middle finger touching the posterior fornix, raise your hand until your index finger touches the pubic arch. Press your thumb against your hand directly under the pubic bone.

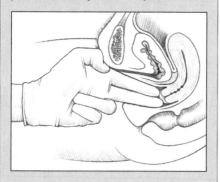

Keep your hand in that position and smoothly withdraw it. The correctly sized diaphragm is the one that fits with one end of the diaphragm rim on the tip of the middle finger and the opposite side of the rim lying just in front of the thumb tip. Common diaphragm sizes are 75 to 80 mm.

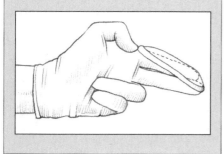

➤ Select the appropriate sized diaphragm and lubricate the rim or dome. (See *Inserting the diaphragm.*)
➤ Check the diaphragm to ensure that it fits snugly against the vaginal walls. Follow the edges of the diaphragm ring, feeling for gaps. It may be necessary to insert and remove several diaphragms until the proper size is found.
➤ To remove the diaphragm, insert your index finger under the symphysis pubis and hook the diaphragm under the proximal rim. Gently pull the diaphragm down and out. Alternatively, slide one finger under the rim until the suction is released.
➤ Teach the patient how to insert and remove the diaphragm. Then leave the patient with the diaphragm in place so that she can practice inserting and removing it in private, leaving it in when she has finished.
➤ Examine her to see if she inserted the diaphragm correctly. With the diaphragm inserted, have the patient squat and move around to ensure proper fit.
➤ Put on goggles and demonstrate how to properly clean the diaphragm with warm, soapy water.

## PATIENT TEACHING

➤ Tell the patient that minimal discomfort during the procedure typically resolves by the end of the procedure.
➤ Emphasize that she's to call you for symptoms of toxic shock syndrome that include fever greater than 101° F; nausea, vomiting, diarrhea, sore throat, body aches, a rash, or feeling dizzy, faint, or weak.
➤ If the patient is new to diaphragm use and misses a menstrual cycle, she should consider a pregnancy test; contraceptive failure is more common in new users.
➤ Instruct the patient to return for follow up for any complications or concerns. Proper fit should be verified annually after weight change of more than 15 lb (6.8 kg); after giving birth; after pelvic surgery or an abortion; or for symptoms such as dyspareunia, cramping, and bladder or rectal pain. Diaphragms are replaced every 2 years even if they still fit well.
➤ Emphasize to the patient the importance of using the diaphragm with sper-

## INSERTING THE DIAPHRAGM

Instruct the patient as you insert the diaphragm, identifying structures and associated feelings to prepare her for inserting it herself.
  Lubricate the rim or dome of the fitting ring or diaphragm to lessen the discomfort of insertion.

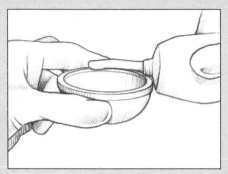

Slide the folded diaphragm into the vagina and toward the posterior cervicovaginal fornix.

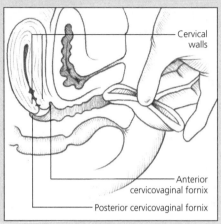

Cervical walls

Anterior cervicovaginal fornix

Posterior cervicovaginal fornix

Hold the vulva open with your other hand. Fold the diaphragm in half with one hand by pressing the opposite sides together.

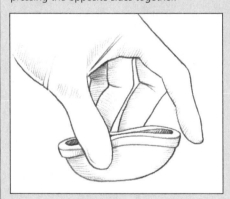

It should fit from below the symphysis and cover the cervix. The proximal rim should fit behind the pubic arch with minimal pressure. Note that the cervix is palpable behind the diaphragm. The cervix feels like a "nose."

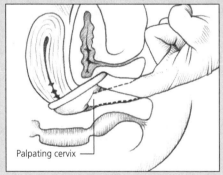

Palpating cervix

micidal jelly every time she has intercourse. Explain that she should apply about a teaspoon of spermicidal jelly (such as nonoxynol 9) to the concave surface and a thin layer around the rim. Never use oil-based products as they will cause the diaphragm to deteriorate.
➤ Teach her to insert one rim behind the pubic bone and the opposite rim behind the cervix and to confirm placement by feeling the cervix behind the dome.
➤ Tell her that for subsequent intercourse, she should leave the diaphragm in place and insert more spermicidal jelly into the vagina; she shouldn't douche.
➤ Tell her to leave the diaphragm in place at least 6 hours after the last session of intercourse (but less than 24 hours).

➤ Instruct the patient to wash the diaphragm with mild soap and dry it after each use, and inspect it at least once a month for holes and wear of the latex.
➤ To ease insertion, advise the woman to try inserting the diaphragm while squatting, laying on her back with both knees bent, or by standing and putting one foot on a stool.

## COMPLICATIONS

➤ *Pregnancy* from not using spermicidal jelly or from improperly placing the diaphragm (the result of poor technique or body changes, such as weight gain or loss of more than 15 lb [6.8 kg] and surgery); *teratogenic effects* from the spermicidal jelly (if the patient becomes pregnant) can occur.
➤ *Recurrent UTIs, discomfort, or ulceration from an improper fit* are indications for removal.

## SPECIAL CONSIDERATIONS

➤ Although you shouldn't use spermicidal jelly for the demonstration, explain to the patient that she'll use it whenever she uses the diaphragm.
➤ You can obtain diaphragm fitting rings free from such companies as Ortho Pharmaceuticals in sizes that increase in 5-mm increments.
➤ Several types of diaphragms exist.
– The arching spring is the most common in the United States and has a firm rim, needs no introducer, and is helpful to patients who have less pelvic support, cystocele, rectocele, or a retroverted uterus. It tends to be easier to insert.
– The coil spring has a flexible rim and needs no introducer, but requires good internal support and the cervix in the midplane or anterior position. The flat spring has flat-plane flexibility and may need an introducer. It's recommended for smaller women, those with a narrow pelvic shelf,

and women who have never been pregnant.
➤ Alternatively a diaphragm introducer may be used to insert the diaphragm.

## DOCUMENTATION

➤ Document details of the procedure, including the patient's reaction to the procedure, the diaphragm size, ability to demonstrate proper technique, time frame for follow-up evaluation, and instructions given to the patient.

# Intrauterine device insertion and removal

CPT CODES
58300   *Insertion of intrauterine device (IUD)*
58301   *Removal of IUD*

## DESCRIPTION

The intrauterine device (IUD) is a plastic contraceptive device inserted into the uterus through the cervical canal. The IUD is inserted into and removed from the uterus most easily during the menses, when the cervical canal is slightly dilated. It also reduces the likelihood of inserting an IUD into a pregnant uterus.

Two types of IUDs are available in the United States: the Paragard-T and the Progestasert System. A third device containing the hormone levonorgestrel may be approved in the near future. The Paragard is a T-shaped, polyethylene device with copper wrapped around the vertical stem. A knotted monofilament retrieval string is attached through a hole in the stem. The Progestasert IUD is a T-shaped device made of an ethylene vinyl acetate copolymer. The Progestasert device may relieve excessive menstrual blood loss and dysmenorrhea.

Progesterone is stored in the hollow vertical stem, suspended in an oil base. A knotted monofilament retrieval string is attached through a hole in the vertical stem.

After consultation with the physician, a properly trained and experienced practitioner may insert an IUD. An IUD is effective for 8 years.

## INDICATIONS

➤ To be used in women who have contraindications to hormonal contraceptives
➤ To be used in women who desire reversible contraception

## CONTRAINDICATIONS

### Absolute

➤ Active, recent, or recurrent pelvic inflammatory disease (PID)
➤ Infection or inflammation of the genital tract
➤ Sexually transmitted disease (STD)
➤ Diseases that suppress immune function, including human immunodeficiency virus
➤ Unexplained cervical or vaginal bleeding or malignancy
➤ Previous problems with an IUD
➤ History of ectopic pregnancy, severe vasovagal reactivity, difficulty obtaining emergency care, valvular heart disease, anatomic uterine deformities, anemia, or nulliparity

### Relative

➤ Small uterus
➤ Wilson's disease

## EQUIPMENT

### Insertion

Sterile single-toothed tenaculum ◆ sterile uterine sound ◆ sterile scissors ◆ speculum ◆ light source ◆ cotton-tipped applicator ◆ antiseptic cleansing agent such as povidone-iodine solution or Hibiclens

◆ 4″ × 4″ gauze pads ◆ sterile gloves ◆ urine pregnancy test ◆ drape ◆ gloves ◆ IUD and insertion tube

### Removal

Sponge forceps ◆ sterile gloves ◆ drape ◆ speculum ◆ tenaculum (optional)

## PREPARATION OF EQUIPMENT

➤ Review the product documents and instructions for IUD insertion and ensure that the proper equipment is available before the insertion is scheduled.
➤ Place the contents of the IUD pack on a sterile field close to the lithotomy table.
➤ Slide the IUD into the insertion tube. Make sure the arms are bent and within the tube just enough to ensure they remain in the tube during insertion. Place the inserter rod into the barrel of the tube and advance it until it touches the IUD.

## ESSENTIAL STEPS

### Insertion of the IUD

➤ Explain the procedure to the patient, answer questions, and obtain informed consent.
➤ Obtain urine for a pregnancy test. If negative, offer ibuprofen to reduce postinsertion cramping.
➤ After she has removed her undergarments, assist her onto the examining table and drape the area.
➤ Assist the woman into the lithotomy position. Place light in position.
➤ Wash hands, put on gloves. Warn the patient that you're about to touch her to avoid startling her.
➤ Perform a bimanual examination to ascertain uterine position, size, and shape. Evaluate for tenderness suggestive of PID.
➤ Insert a warmed, moistened speculum and visualize the cervix.
➤ Verify the patient isn't allergic to iodine and clean the cervix in concentric circles

from the os outward with povidone-iodine or Hibiclens soaked 4″ × 4″gauze. Tell the woman she may notice a cold sensation in the vagina as you complete the preparation. Explain to the woman that you'll be applying an instrument to the cervix.

➤ Pinch and grasp the anterior lip of the cervix at 12 o'clock with the single-toothed tenaculum. Close the clamp slowly, avoiding jerking motions.

➤ Holding the tenaculum in the non-dominant hand and the uterine sound in the dominant hand, insert the sound slowly and gently through the cervical canal and into the uterus. Gentle traction on the tenaculum may aid insertion. Tell the woman she may experience cramping during the uterine sounding. When the fundus of the uterus is reached, resistance will be felt.

➤ Place a clean, cotton-tipped applicator beside the uterine sound, touching the cervix.

➤ Remove the sound and applicator simultaneously. The distance between the tip of the sound and the tip of the swab gives an approximate measure of the depth of the fundus.

➤ Note the distance in centimeters. Remove the soiled gloves and put on sterile gloves.

➤ Set the movable flange on the inserter barrel to the depth the uterus sounded. Ensure that the flange and the arms of the T are aligned in the same plane. (See *IUD insertion*.)

➤ If needed, use the single-toothed tenaculum to secure the cervix. Introduce the loaded inserter tube through the cervical canal and into the uterus until the flange reaches the cervical opening.

➤ Insert the IUD by retracting the inserter as you hold the inserting rod in place.

➤ Gently advance the inserter and plunger until resistance is felt.

➤ Withdraw the solid rod while holding the insertion barrel stationary and then withdraw the insertion barrel and rod from the cervix.

➤ Clip the IUD strings about 1″ to 2″ (3 to 5 cm) from the cervical os with sterile scissors.

➤ Remove the speculum and assist the woman to a seated position. When she feels comfortable, show her how to check for the IUD string.

**Removal of the IUD**

➤ Explain the procedure for removing the IUD to the patient. Tell her she will need another method of birth control after removal of the IUD unless she intends to become pregnant.

➤ After she undresses from the waist down and drapes herself, assist the woman into the lithotomy position.

➤ Wash hands and put on gloves.

➤ Insert a speculum for adequate exposure of the cervix.

➤ Identify the IUD strings on the surface of the cervix. If the strings are missing, consult a physician.

➤ Grasp the IUD strings in the sponge forceps and apply gentle traction. The IUD should gradually appear at the cervical os. If resistance is experienced, a tenaculum may be used to apply gentle traction on the cervix as traction on the string is applied. This action may straighten an anteflexion or retroflexion that is hampering removal.

➤ If the IUD cannot easily be removed, consult a physician.

➤ Remove and discard soiled supplies. Assist the woman to a sitting position.

**PATIENT TEACHING**

➤ Tell the patient that she can expect her period to be heavier after an IUD insertion. Cramping may accompany insertion, and continue for a time after insertion. Cramping should lessen gradually over the next few days.

## IUD INSERTION

Set the movable flange on the inserter barrel to the depth the uterus sounded in centimeters. Introduce the loaded inserter tube through the cervical canal and into the uterus while applying gentle, steady traction on the tenaculum. Advance the inserter tube to the flange.

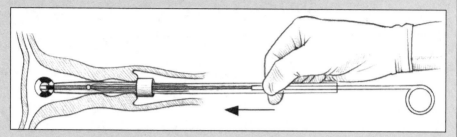

Insert the intrauterine device (IUD) by retracting the inserter slowly about ½″ (1.3 cm) over the plunger, holding the plunger still. This allows the arms to open.

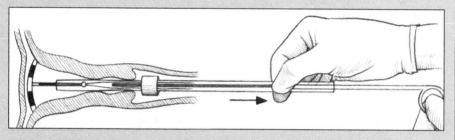

Now gently advance the inserter and plunger until resistance is felt. This action ensures high fundal placement of the IUD and may reduce the potential for expulsion.

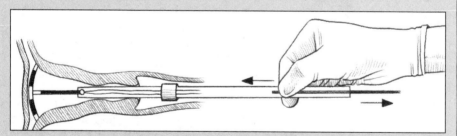

Withdraw the solid rod while holding the insertion barrel stationary. Withdraw the insertion barrel from the cervix. Clip the IUD strings about 1″ to 2″ (3 to 5 cm) from the cervical os. This action leaves sufficient string for the woman to check and for removal of the IUD.

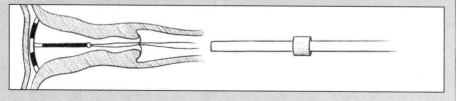

➤ Instruct the patient to schedule a return visit after the next menses for an IUD check.

➤ Tell her that if she experiences pain, the best analgesic is a prostaglandin inhibitor such as ibuprofen.

➤ Inform the patient that the contraceptive action of the IUD is immediate. Foam and condoms may be used as backup contraception during the first month until retention of the IUD is more certain.

➤ Advise the patient that the IUD offers *no* protection from STDs.

➤ Tell the patient to check the strings at least weekly the first month. This action increases confidence in the IUD's presence. Also, tell her to check the strings each month after her menses.

➤ Instruct the patient to watch for signs of infection, such as fever, pelvic pain, tenderness, severe cramping, and unusual vaginal bleeding or discharge. Tell her to call you or the office immediately to report infection symptoms. Emphasize to her that untreated infections can progress to PID, which may necessitate a hysterectomy.

➤ Emphasize the symptoms of PID:
– fever of 101° F (38.3° C) or greater
– purulent vaginal discharge
– abdominal or pelvic pain
– dyspareunia
– cervicitis
– suprapubic tenderness or guarding
– pain with cervical motion
– tenderness on bimanual examination
– adnexal tenderness or mass.

➤ Tell the patient to chart her menses. If a period is late, tell her to call you immediately.

➤ Tell the patient to report severe cramping or bleeding; if the IUD causes increased menstrual pain and bleeding, it can be removed.

➤ Instruct the patient not to attempt to remove the IUD herself or allow her partner to attempt to remove it.

➤ Give the patient the mnemonic, PAINS, to recall the signs of IUD complications:

– P: period late, abnormal bleeding, or spotting
– A: abdominal pain, pain with intercourse
– I: infection, exposure to an STD, abnormal discharge
– N: not feeling well, fever, chills
– S: string missing, shorter or longer.

## COMPLICATIONS

➤ *Uterine perforation* signs include pain, loss of strings, or the plastic of the device is felt or visible in the cervix. Ultrasound can help to confirm perforation. If perforation is suspected, refer the patient to a physician or gynecologist.

➤ *Vasovagal syncopal episodes* may accompany IUD insertion. Symptoms are dizziness, flushing, tachycardia, and hypotension. Treatment is immediate removal of the IUD.

➤ *Anemia* secondary to spotting or bleeding requires monitoring. Remove the IUD if the hemoglobin is less than 9 g.

➤ *Pain and cramping* relieved with nonsteroidal anti-inflammatory drugs after uterine perforation, cervical or pelvic infection, and pregnancy (intrauterine or ectopic) are ruled out.

➤ *Pregnancy* may occur after insertion. There is an increased risk of septic abortion if pregnancy occurs. If menses is are delayed, evaluate for pregnancy and infection and remove the IUD if either occurs.

➤ *PID* risk increases. Most cases of PID occur during the first 3 months after insertion. After 3 months, the chance of PID is lower unless preinsertion screening failed to identify a person at risk for STDs.

## SPECIAL CONSIDERATIONS

➤ The Paragard IUD can't be used by women with Wilson's disease because of their inability to metabolize copper properly.

➤ Remove the IUD during the menstrual period if possible, or during midcycle when the cervix is softer, to minimize trauma to the cervical os.
➤ Ectopic pregnancy rates are higher among Progestasert users. With the Progesetasert IUD in place:
– 50% will experience spontaneous abortion.
– 25% will abort if the IUD is removed.
– 5% will have an ectopic pregnancy.
– severe pelvic infection and death can occur.

## DOCUMENTATION

➤ Document the patient's desire for this method of birth control and that a thorough discussion of options, advantages, and disadvantages took place.
➤ Record findings of the pelvic examination and pregnancy test. Detail the procedure for insertion of the IUD, including the depth of the uterus (sounded) and the depth the IUD was inserted. Include the length of strings protruding from the cervical os after trimming.
➤ Note the patient's tolerance of the procedure; any adverse reactions, such as a vasovagal reaction; and actions taken.
➤ Record your instructions related to how to check the string, symptoms to observe for, and when to return for a follow-up examination.

## Norplant insertion

### CPT CODES

*11975   Insertion of implantable contraceptive capsules*
*11977   Removal of implantable contraceptive capsules with reinsertion of implantable contraceptive capsules*

## DESCRIPTION

The Norplant System (levonorgestrel implants) of birth control consists of six thin, flexible capsules of soft silastic tubing sealed at each end with silicone. Each capsule contains 36 mg of dry crystalline levonorgestrel and is 34 mm long and 2.4 mm in diameter. The capsules are very stable; levonorgestrel is released over a period of 5 years. During the first year, 80 mcg/day is released. Gradually, the release of levonorgestrel decreases to 30 to 40 mcg/day.

The Norplant System is the first and only sustained-release subdermal contraceptive delivery system. It provides effective contraception for up to 5 years. Norplant is a progestin-only contraceptive and differs from the progestin-only mini-pill by maintaining a constant level of levonorgestrel. It has two possible mechanisms of action: (1) ovulation is suppressed in most of the menstrual cycles because Norplant maintains a consistent low level of progestin; or (2) cervical mucus is thickened, providing a hostile passage for sperm and preventing sperm penetration into the lining of the uterus.

The placement of the Norplant System involves a counseling visit, followed by the office procedure in which the capsules are inserted.

## INDICATIONS

➤ To be used in patients desiring long-term reversible contraception
➤ To be used in patients who are considering sterilization
➤ To be used in patients who have difficulty remembering to take daily birth control pills
➤ To be used in patients who cannot tolerate other forms of contraception, such as birth control pills, and coitus-dependent techniques, such as condoms and diaphragms

➤ To be used in patients who cannot tolerate estrogen administration

➤ To be used in patients who have contraindications to intrauterine device use (nulliparous, history of ectopic pregnancy, pelvic inflammatory disease, nonmonogamous relationships)

## CONTRAINDICATIONS

### Absolute

➤ Active thrombophlebitis or thromboembolic disease

➤ Undiagnosed abnormal genital bleeding

➤ Possible pregnancy

➤ Acute liver disease

➤ Benign or malignant liver tumors

➤ Known or suspected carcinoma of the breast

➤ Lack of informed consent

➤ Unwillingness to accept amenorrhea or metrorrhagia for at least 6 to 9 months

➤ Excessive concern over the minimal scar that will occur at the site of placement

➤ Patient who is less than 6 weeks postpartum

➤ Foreign body carcinogenesis

### Relative

➤ Cigarette smokers under age 35

## EQUIPMENT

Norplant System (set of six Norplant System capsules, Norplant System obturator and trocar, #11 scalpel, 5-ml syringe, two 25G needles, package of skin closures, package of three gauze sponges, stretch bandage, two sterile drapes, fenestrated surgical drape) ◆ urine pregnancy test ◆ butterfly adhesive strip ◆ 5 ml of 1% or 2% lidocaine without epinephrine ◆ sterile and clean gloves ◆ antiseptic solution such as povidone-iodine solution ◆ sterile drape ◆ normal saline solution ◆ ice pack ◆ Elastoplast (optional) ◆ template

to mark the locations for insertion (optional)

## ESSENTIAL STEPS

➤ Review the method of insertion with the patient and answer any questions. If there are no contraindications and the patient indicates that she would like to use the Norplant System, obtain an informed consent. (*Note:* The company provides a model arm; you can show the display, sample capsules, and the site of the insertion to the patient.)

➤ Obtain a pregnancy test.

### Insertion of the Norplant System

➤ Instruct the patient to lie down on her back on the examination table with her left arm (if the patient is left-handed, the right arm) flexed, the elbow externally rotated so that her hand is lying by her head.

➤ Wash your hands and put on gloves. Verify that the patient isn't allergic to iodine and clean the patient's upper arm with antiseptic solution. Cover the arm above and below the insertion area with a sterile drape.

➤ Open the sterile Norplant System package carefully by pulling apart the sheets of the pouch, allowing the capsules to fall onto a sterile cloth. Count the six capsules.

➤ Fill a 5-ml syringe with local anesthetic.

➤ Anesthetize the insertion area by first inserting the needle under the skin at a 45-degree angle and injecting a small amount of the anesthetic as you withdraw the needle. Then anesthetize six areas about 1½″ to 1¾″ (4 to 4.5 cm) long, to mimic the fanlike position of the implanted capsules.

 **ALERT** Use only lidocaine without epinephrine because epinephrine can cause cutaneous ulceration.

➤ Put on sterile gloves.

➤ Use the scalpel to make a small, shallow incision (about 2 mm) through the skin. The optimal insertion area is in the inside of the upper arm about 3" to 4" (8 to 10 cm) above the elbow crease.

➤ Insert the tip of the trocar subdermally through a small 2-mm incision beneath the skin at a shallow angle. Once the trocar is inserted, it should be oriented with the bevel up toward the skin to keep the capsules in a superficial plane. Correct subdermal placement of the capsules facilitates removal.

➤ Advance the trocar gently under the skin to the first mark near the hub of the trocar. The tip of the trocar is now at a distance of about 1½" to 1¾" (4 to 4.5 cm) from the incision. Do not force the trocar; if resistance is felt, try another direction.

➤ The skin should be visibly tented at all times as the trocar is advanced. Keep the trocar superficial even though this typically requires more force than subcutaneous insertion.

➤ When the trocar has been inserted the appropriate distance, remove the obturator and load the first capsule into the trocar using the thumb and forefinger.

➤ Gently advance the capsule with the obturator toward the tip of the trocar until you feel resistance. Never force the obturator.

➤ Hold the obturator steady and retract the trocar until it touches the handle of the obturator.

➤ As the trocar is withdrawn, hold the distal tip of the capsule in place through the skin. Proximally, as the trocar is withdrawn to the mark near the tip, you should be able to feel the capsule fall from the tip. Place your index finger over this newly inserted capsule to prevent the trocar from catching on it. If the trocar catches the capsule, it could damage it or force it back under the skin where it will lie in a bent position.

➤ Don't remove the trocar from the incision until all capsules have been inserted.

## CHECKING CAPSULE PLACEMENT

After insertion, once again identify the six subdermal implants. If the capsules are dropped or if the patients expels a capsule, it can be returned to the company and replaced without cost to the patient or you.

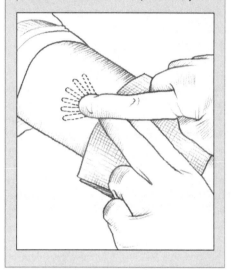

The trocar is withdrawn only to the mark close to its tip. Each succeeding capsule is inserted next to the previous capsule with the forefinger and middle finger of the free hand.

➤ Advance the trocar along the tips of the fingers. This action will ensure a suitable distance of about 15 degrees between capsules and keep the trocar from puncturing previously inserted capsules. Leave a distance of about 5 mm between the incision and the tips of the capsules. This action will help to prevent spontaneous expulsions. Ensure the correct position of the capsules by feeling them after the insertion has been completed. (See *Checking capsule placement*.)

➤ Press the edges of the incision together, and close the incision with a butterfly adhesive strip.

366 ◆ Gynecologic procedures

➤ Cover the insertion area with gauze sponges, and wrap the stretch bandage around the arm to ensure hemostasis. Observe the patient for a few minutes for signs of syncope or bleeding from the incision before she is discharged.

➤ Apply an ice pack to the site. Instruct the patient to remove the dressing in 1 day and to keep the area clean and dry for 3 days.

## PATIENT TEACHING

➤ Emphasize that Norplant doesn't provide protection from diseases. As appropriate, review barrier methods such as a female dam or partner's use of a condom.

➤ Review the history of effectiveness of the Norplant System with the patient. Inform the patient that this method is not absolutely foolproof, but that it is one of the best contraceptive devices available, with a failure rate of less than 1%.

➤ Discuss the advantages of the Norplant System, including the absence of estrogen, the long duration of use, the effectiveness, the reversibility, and the fact that nothing needs to be remembered and it's independent of coitus. The capsules don't interfere with activity in any way. It's effective within 24 hours of insertion if inserted within 7 days of the onset of menses.

➤ Review the possible adverse effects of the Norplant System, including arm pain, weight gain, headaches, bloating, nausea, depression, dizziness, sore breasts, and acne.

➤ Tell the patient that irregular bleeding occurs in 60% of women; the patient can expect to experience an alteration of menstrual patterns during the first year. The menstrual cycle usually becomes more regular within 9 to 12 months.

➤ Inform the patient that there is a low incidence of thromboembolic phenomena. However, the patient subjected to prolonged immobilization due to surgery or other illness should have the capsules removed before surgery for thrombophlebitis prophylaxis.

➤ The effect on cholesterol and blood sugar is minimal.

➤ Tell the patient that she may have arm pain and a large ecchymotic area may develop at the insertion site. She can expect this symptom to resolve in approximately 2 weeks.

➤ Instruct the patient to ice the area immediately after insertion to decrease bruising.

➤ Tell the patient to take acetaminophen (Tylenol) or ibuprofen (Motrin) every 4 to 6 hours as needed for pain.

➤ Tell the patient that the gauze may be removed after 1 day; the butterfly bandage, as soon as the incision has healed (normally in 3 days).

➤ Advise the patient to keep the insertion area dry for 2 to 3 days.

## COMPLICATIONS

➤ *Infection near the site of insertion* is very uncommon (0.7%); however, if the site becomes infected, the capsules must be removed and the area must be allowed to heal. The practitioner will decide if all capsules need to be removed.

➤ *Expulsion of a capsule* can occur. This is more common if the placement is too shallow or if infection occurs at the time of insertion. A new, sterile capsule must be placed because fewer than six capsules may provide inadequate contraception.

➤ *Ulceration over the area* is possible and may possibly be more common when the local anesthetic contains epinephrine. Removal of capsules to allow healing is required.

## SPECIAL CONSIDERATIONS

➤ It's important to let women know of the more common adverse effects, which include irregular menses, weight gain, some hair loss, headaches, and hyperpigmentation at the site. Depression and premenstrual symptoms may either improve or become worse.

➤ Removal of the implants can be difficult because of scar tissue that forms around the implants.

➤ You should stress the necessity of annual Pap smears to the patient using long-term contraceptive systems — even though she doesn't need a new prescription.

➤ Studies on the Norplant System focused on women ages 18 to 40; however, many practitioners don't impose a lower or upper age limit.

➤ Modification of the Norplant System (Norplant II) is currently undergoing trials and will consist of only two subdermal capsules.

## DOCUMENTATION

➤ Always document that the patient has read over the patient education handouts and that you have discussed the risks, benefits, possible complications, and alternatives.

➤ Include indications for the procedure, the number of capsules placed, the insertion site, the patient's response to the procedure, site appearance postprocedure, instructions given, and any patient concerns.

## Norplant removal

CPT CODES
*11976 Removal of implantable contraceptive capsules*
*11977 Removal of implantable contraceptive capsules with reinsertion of implantable contraceptive capsules*

## DESCRIPTION

Removal of the Norplant System involves incising the area and withdrawing the capsules with forceps, taking about 20 minutes to perform. It requires more skill and patience than does insertion. Removal can be complicated by an initial irregular placement or by a fracture of the silastic capsules.

The modified U technique requires half the time for removal but requires a modified #11 scalpel vasectomy clamp. Local anesthesia is used only at the site of removal.

## EQUIPMENT

Sterile fenestrated drape ◆ sterile gloves ◆ antiseptic solution ◆ local anesthetic with 30G needle ◆ 3-ml syringe ◆ #11 scalpel ◆ forceps (straight and curved mosquito) ◆ butterfly adhesive strips such as Steri-Strips ◆ 4″×4″ sterile gauze ◆ Elastoplast or a stretch bandage ◆ sterile skin marker (optional)

## ESSENTIAL STEPS

➤ Wash hands and put on gloves. Draw anesthetic into 3-ml syringe with 30G needle. Clean the area with gauze and antiseptic in a circular motion from the site outward. Apply the fenestrated drape to the insertion area.

➤ Locate the implanted capsules by palpation, marking the position with a sterile skin marker if desired. Apply a small amount of local anesthetic under the capsule ends nearest the original incision site by inserting the needle at a 45-degree angle and injecting. This action will serve to raise the ends of the capsules. Anesthetics injected over the capsules will obscure them and make removal more difficult. Additional small amounts of anesthetic can

## REMOVING CONTRACEPTIVE CAPSULES

Push each capsule gently toward the incision with your fingers. When the tip is visible or near to the incision, grasp it with a mosquito forceps.

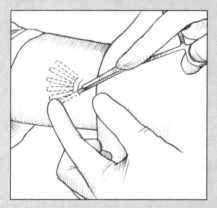

Very gently, use the scalpel to open the tissue sheath that has formed around the capsule. Remove the capsule from the incision with the straight forceps.

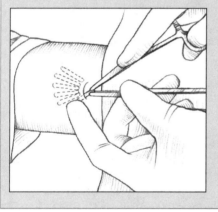

be used for removing each of the capsules, if required.

➤ Make a 4-mm incision with the scalpel close to the ends of the capsules. Don't make a large incision.

➤ Push each capsule gently towards the incision with the fingers, then grasp it with a mosquito forceps. (See *Removing contraceptive capsules*.)

➤ After the procedure is completed, close the incision with a butterfly adhesive strip and bandage as with insertion.

## PATIENT TEACHING

➤ Tell the patient that following removal, a return to the previous level of fertility is usually prompt, and pregnancy may occur at any time.

➤ Instruct the patient to keep the upper arm dry for 3 days.

## COMPLICATIONS

➤ *Infection* requires evaluation and possible culture and sensitivity study; it is treated with a broad-spectrum antibiotic until laboratory results allow refined treatment. If capsules remain under the skin, refer the patient to a gynecologist.

➤ *Ulceration* is avoided by ensuring there is no epinephrine in the anesthetic agent.

## SPECIAL CONSIDERATIONS

➤ If the patient wishes to continue using the method, a new set of Norplant System capsules can be inserted through the same incision in the same or opposite direction.

➤ Patients who meet eligibility requirements may receive the Norplant System at no cost by the Norplant Foundation. They may be reached at (703) 706-5933.

➤ If the Norplant capsules have been in for a while, there will be a fibrous structure encapsulating them.

➤ Capsules can sometimes be nicked during removal. However, the incidence of overall difficulties, including damage to capsules, has been 13.2% percent; less than half of the difficulties occurring during removal have caused inconvenience to the patient.

➤ If the removal of some of the capsules proves difficult, schedule the patient to return for a second visit. The remaining capsules will be easier to remove after the area has healed. If contraception is still desired, a barrier method should be advised until all capsules are removed.

## DOCUMENTATION

➤ Record the indications for the procedure, patient education, the patient's response to the procedure, how many capsules removed, wound appearance, and follow-up plan.

Because of its profound emotional implications for mother and child, maternal care requires expertise that goes beyond clinical skills and must combine clinical competence, sensitivity, and good judgment. Maternal care must consider the patient's sexuality and self-image and recognize changing social attitudes and values — especially those concerning conventional and alternative methods of conception and childbirth.

More than 4 million infants are born in the United States each year. Many of them are born with considerably less medical intervention than was customary in previous decades, and many of them were conceived with considerably more intervention. As a result, you must be prepared to implement or assist with a wide range of procedures.

When working with a pregnant patient, you'll need to use your teaching skills. For instance, you may be called on to organize and direct natural childbirth classes or to teach a pregnant patient how to breathe and control pain during childbirth. Or you may also teach fathers and other support persons to participate in childbirth by providing comfort and direction.

You may also be asked about childbirth options. Although most births still occur in a hospital, many patients inquire about delivery in a birth center. Usually located in the maternity unit of a hospital or sponsored by a childbirth association, a birth center combines the advantages of a home-like setting with the emergency medical and nursing interventions available in a hospital. A practitioner may staff or direct the birth center.

Today, a women's health or obstetric practitioner brings advanced technical skills and certification to diverse communities — urban center to rural community — working in collaboration with a single obstetrician or a group.

**CULTURAL TIP** Being aware of cultural beliefs can prepare you for unusual behaviors and increase your ability to help a patient make informed choices. For example, some Hispanics may believe that wearing proper clothing, or protective objects, will ensure a safe birth. Other cultural groups, such as Southeast Asian, believe in following a specific diet and behaving in a certain fashion during pregnancy. These beliefs may cause a patient not to seek early and regular prenatal care.

Counseling sessions must emphasize confidentiality and help patients when issues related to sexuality, including birth control, may be unacceptable in the community. This may be more crucial in some cultural groups than in others. In the Amish society, family life is important and families tend to be large, with many children. It is also common for several generations to live together. Family members are available to provide support and assistance after childbirth. However, the Amish society is patriarchal — women are not considered equal in authority and are expected to be submissive. Members of Hispanic and Asian cultural groups may also hold these beliefs.

In the case of spontaneous abortion, a patient from a cultural group such as Native American may request the products of conception for proper burial.

Women from certain cultural groups, including Muslim, Hindu, and Hispanic, may be resistant to examination by males, as their culture dictates that a woman's reputation depends on demonstrated modesty. The patient may seek her husband's permission before allowing a procedure to be performed.

In some cultural groups, including native African and Muslim, infibulation is common. You must be prepared for how the genitals will look, how to minimize the significantly increased pain associated with childbirth, and how to present the patient with information she can use to make an informed decision about the options available to her.

# FETAL ASSESSMENT

## Fetal heart rate monitoring

CPT CODE
No specific code has been assigned.

### DESCRIPTION

A major clue to fetal well-being during gestation and labor, the fetal heart rate (FHR) may be assessed by auscultating with a fetoscope or a Doppler ultrasound stethoscope placed on the maternal abdomen. This ultrasound device emits low-energy, high-frequency sound waves that rebound from the fetal heart to a transducer, which transmits the impulses to a monitor strip for recording.

### FINDING FETAL HEART TONES

When explaining the procedure to the patient, reassure her that you may reposition the listening instrument frequently to hear the loudest fetal heart tones. If you are unable to detect the fetus with the fetoscope, use a Doppler stethoscope to locate the heartbeat first, then place the fetoscope in the same spot. It is a good idea to develop a systematic approach to locating fetal heart tones so that you don't miss or unnecessarily repeat areas.

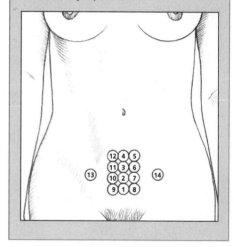

Because FHR normally ranges from 110 to 160 beats/minute, auscultation yields only an average rate at best. However, because auscultation can detect gross (but often late) fetal distress signs (tachycardia and bradycardia), the technique remains useful in an uncomplicated, low-risk pregnancy. In a high-risk pregnancy, indirect external or direct internal electronic fetal monitoring gives more accurate information on fetal status.

### INDICATIONS

➤ To screen for fetal distress

## INSTRUMENTS FOR HEARING FETAL HEART TONES

The fetoscope and the Doppler stethoscope are basic instruments for auscultating fetal heart tones and assessing fetal heart rate.

### Fetoscope

This instrument can be used to help determine gestational age. If you can hear fetal heart tones (FHTs) with a fetoscope between 18 and 20 weeks' gestation, it can either confirm or lend support to the estimated due date. The FHTs are best heard when the tubing of the fetoscope is not longer than 10". The fetoscope must be placed with the metal against your forehead. Metal against bone facilitates the conduction of sound. Use of a fetoscope later in pregnancy may not require the use of your forehead, because the uterus is thinner. When listening for early FHTs with the fetoscope, you may need to turn off air conditioners and have the patient empty her bladder.

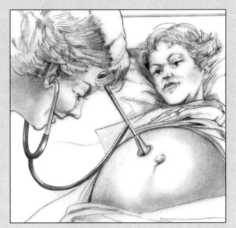

### Doppler stethoscope

This instrument can detect fetal heartbeats as early as the 10th gestational week. Useful throughout labor, the Doppler stethoscope has greater sensitivity than the fetoscope.

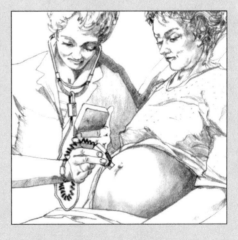

## CONTRAINDICATIONS

None known

## EQUIPMENT

Fetoscope or Doppler stethoscope ◆ water-soluble lubricant (for ultrasound instrument) ◆ watch with second hand ◆ drape

## ESSENTIAL STEPS

➤ Explain the procedure to the patient, wash your hands, and provide privacy. Reassure the patient that you may reposition the listening instrument frequently to hear the loudest fetal heart tones. (See *Finding fetal heart tones,* page 371.)

➤ Assist the patient to a supine position, and drape her appropriately to minimize exposure. If you're using a Doppler stethoscope, apply the water-soluble lubricant to the patient's abdomen. (See *Instruments for hearing fetal heart tones*.) This gel or paste creates an airtight seal between the skin and the instrument and promotes optimal ultrasound wave conduction and reception.

## Calculating FHR during gestation

➤ To assess FHR in a fetus age 20 weeks or older, place the earpieces in your ears and position the bell of the fetoscope or Doppler stethoscope on the abdominal midline above the pubic hairline of the patient.

➤ After 20 weeks' gestation, when you can palpate fetal position, use Leopold's maneuvers to locate the back of the fetal thorax. Then position the listening instrument over the fetal back. (See *Performing Leopold's maneuvers*, page 374.) Because the presentation and position of the fetus may change, most practitioners don't perform Leopold's maneuvers until 32 to 34 weeks' gestation.

➤ Using a Doppler stethoscope, place the earpieces in your ears and press the bell gently on the patient's abdomen. Start listening at the midline, midway between the umbilicus and the symphysis pubis. If using a fetoscope, place the earpieces in your ears with the fetoscope positioned centrally on your forehead. Gently press the bell about ½″ (1.3 cm) into the patient's abdomen. Remove your hands from the fetoscope to avoid extraneous noise.

➤ Move the bell of either instrument slightly from side to side, as necessary, to locate the loudest heart tones. After locating these tones, palpate the maternal pulse.

➤ While monitoring the maternal pulse rate (to avoid confusing maternal heart tones with fetal heart tones), count the fetal heartbeats for at least 15 seconds. If the maternal radial pulse and FHR are the same, try to locate the fetal thorax by us-

ing Leopold's maneuvers; then reassess FHR. Usually, the fetal heart beats faster than the maternal heart does. Record FHR.

## Counting FHR during labor

➤ Position the fetoscope or Doppler stethoscope on the abdomen — midway between the umbilicus and symphysis pubis for cephalic presentation or at the umbilicus or above for breech presentation. Locate the loudest heartbeats, and simultaneously palpate the maternal pulse to ensure that you're monitoring fetal rather than maternal pulse.

➤ Monitor maternal pulse rate and count fetal heartbeats for 60 seconds during the relaxation period between contractions to determine baseline FHR. In a low-risk labor, assess FHR every 60 minutes during the latent phase, every 30 minutes during the active phase, and every 15 minutes during the second stage of labor. In a high-risk labor, assess FHR every 30 minutes during the latent phase, every 15 minutes during the active phase, and every 5 minutes during the second stage of labor.

➤ Auscultate FHR during a contraction and for 30 seconds after the contraction to identify fetal response to the contraction.

➤ Notify the collaborating physician immediately if you observe marked changes in FHR from baseline values (especially during or immediately after a contraction when signs of fetal distress typically occur). If fetal distress develops, begin indirect or direct electronic fetal monitoring.

➤ Repeat the procedure as indicated.

➤ Also auscultate before administration of medications, before ambulation, and before artificial rupture of membranes.

➤ Auscultate after rupture of membranes, after any changes in the characteristics of the contractions, after vaginal examinations, and after administration of medications.

## PERFORMING LEOPOLD'S MANEUVERS

You can determine fetal position, presentation, and attitude by performing Leopold's maneuvers. Ask the patient to empty her bladder, assist her to a supine position, and expose her abdomen. Then perform the four maneuvers in order.

### First maneuver
Face the patient, and warm your hands. Place them on the patient's abdomen to determine fetal position in the uterine fundus. Curl your fingers around the fundus. With the fetus in vertex position, the buttocks feel irregularly shaped and firm. With the fetus in breech position, the head feels hard, round, and movable.

### Second maneuver
Move your hands down the sides of the abdomen, and apply gentle pressure. If the fetus lies in vertex position, you'll feel a smooth, hard surface on one side — the fetal back. Opposite, you'll feel lumps and knobs — the knees, hands, feet, and elbows. If the fetus lies in breech position, you may not feel the back at all.

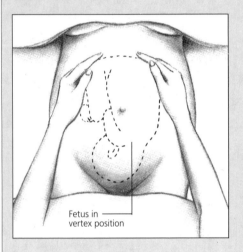

Fetus in vertex position

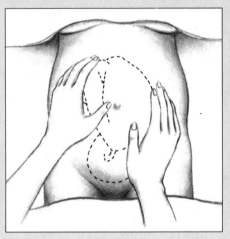

## PATIENT TEACHING

➤ Tell the patient that the FHR will be assessed periodically to evaluate the status of the fetus.
➤ If using a Doppler stethoscope, tell the patient that the lubricant will feel cold and wet.

## COMPLICATIONS

None known

## SPECIAL CONSIDERATIONS

➤ Allow the patient and her support person to listen to the fetal heart if they wish. This helps to make the fetus a greater reality for them. Record their participation.
➤ Auscultating the FHR is a noninvasive method that screens for fetal distress while leaving the patient mobile and unencumbered. However, this method may not be adequate and an external or internal monitor may become necessary as labor progresses.
➤ If you're auscultating FHR with a Doppler stethoscope, be aware that obe-

### Third maneuver

Spread apart the thumb and fingers of one hand. Place them just above the patient's symphysis pubis. Bring your fingers together. If the fetus lies in vertex position and hasn't descended, you'll feel the head. If the fetus lies in vertex position and has descended, you'll feel a less distinct mass.

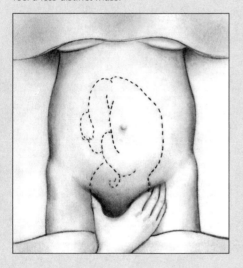

### Fourth maneuver

Use this maneuver in late pregnancy. The purpose of the fourth maneuver is to determine flexion or extension of the fetal head and neck. Place your hands on both sides of the lower abdomen. Apply gentle pressure with your fingers as you slide your hands downward, toward the symphysis pubis. If the head presents, one hand's descent will be stopped by the cephalic prominence. The other hand will be unobstructed.

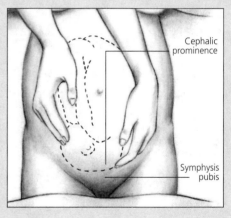

Cephalic prominence

Symphysis pubis

sity and hydramnios can interfere with sound-wave transmission, making accurate results more difficult to obtain. For continuous FHR monitoring, apply the ultrasound transducer (also called a tocotransducer) to the patient's abdomen. The monitor will provide a printed record of FHR.

➤ The tocotransducer may also be applied to monitor the contractile pattern.

## DOCUMENTATION

➤ Record both FHR and maternal pulse rate on the flowchart.

➤ Document each auscultation and indications for monitoring.
➤ Note the patient's and her support person's participation of counting FHR during labor.

## External fetal monitoring

CPT CODE
No specific code has been assigned.

## DRAWBACKS OF EXTERNAL FETAL MONITORING

Use of external fetal monitoring is uncomfortable for a laboring woman. It restricts her movement and changes of position due to possible dislodgment of the transducers. The transducers and straps need frequent adjustments. The transducers pick up maternal activity, anything that brushes the surface of the transducer (such as hands or sheets), as well as the patient's internal noises (bowel sounds), creating static noise. These extra sounds interfere with obtaining a clear recording of either the fetal heart rate or uterine activity. Support and comfort measures are limited for women with an external fetal monitor.

The need for a supine position may interfere with placental blood flow, thus causing supine hypotensive syndrome (caused by the weight of the uterus and its contents on the maternal inferior vena cava).

There is a direct correlation between the use of continuous external fetal monitoring and an increase in the number of cesarean sections.

## DESCRIPTION

An indirect, noninvasive procedure, external fetal monitoring uses two devices strapped to the patient's abdomen to evaluate fetal well-being during labor. The use of the external fetal monitor has a number of drawbacks. (See *Drawbacks of external fetal monitoring*.)

One device used for fetal monitoring, an ultrasound transducer, transmits high-frequency sound waves through soft body tissues to the fetal heart. The waves rebound from the heart, and the transducer relays them to a monitor. Another device used for fetal monitoring, a pressure-sensitive tocotransducer, responds to the pressure exerted by uterine contractions and simultaneously records their duration and

frequency. (See *Applying external fetal monitoring devices*.) The monitoring apparatus traces fetal heart rate and uterine contraction data onto the same printout paper.

## INDICATIONS

➤ To monitor fetal status in high-risk pregnancy
➤ To monitor fetal status in oxytocin-induced labor
➤ To monitor fetal status during antepartal nonstress and contraction stress test

## CONTRAINDICATIONS

None known

## EQUIPMENT

Electronic fetal monitor ◆ ultrasound transducer and cable ◆ tocotransducer and cable ◆ conduction gel ◆ transducer straps ◆ damp cloth ◆ printout paper

## PREPARATION OF EQUIPMENT

➤ Because fetal monitor features and complexity vary, review the operator's manual before proceeding. If the monitor has two paper speeds, select the slower speed (typically 3 cm/minute) to ensure an easy-to-read tracing. At higher speeds (for example, 1 cm/minute), the printed tracings are difficult to decipher and interpret accurately. Plug the tocotransducer cable into the uterine activity jack and the ultrasound transducer cable into the phono-ultrasound jack. Attach the straps to the tocotransducer and the ultrasound transducer. Label the printout paper with the patient's identification number or birth date and name, the date, maternal vital signs and position, the paper speed, and the number of the strip paper to maintain accurate, consecutive monitoring records.

## APPLYING EXTERNAL FETAL MONITORING DEVICES

To ensure clear tracings that define fetal status and labor progress, be sure to precisely position external monitoring devices, such as an ultrasound transducer and a tocotransducer.

### Fetal heart monitor
Palpate the uterus to locate the fetus's back. If possible, place the ultrasound transducer over this site where the fetal heartbeat sounds the loudest. Then tighten the belt. Use the fetal heart tracing on the monitor strip to confirm the transducer's position.

### Labor monitor
A tocotransducer records uterine motion during contractions. Place the tocotransducer over the uterine fundus where it contracts, either midline or slightly to one side. Place your hand on the fundus, and palpate a contraction to verify proper placement. Secure the tocotransducer's belt; then adjust the pen set so that the baseline values read between 5 and 15 mm Hg on the monitor strip.

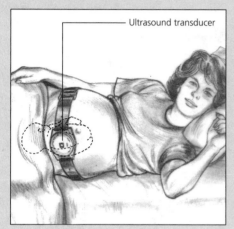

Ultrasound transducer

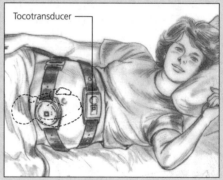

Tocotransducer

## ESSENTIAL STEPS

➤ Explain the procedure to the patient and obtain informed consent. Answer any questions she or her support person may have.
➤ Wash your hands and provide privacy.

### Beginning the procedure
➤ Assist the patient to the semi-Fowler or left-lateral position with her abdomen exposed. Don't let her lie supine because pressure from the gravid uterus on the maternal inferior vena cava may cause maternal hypotension and decreased uterine perfusion and may induce fetal hypoxia.
➤ Palpate the patient's abdomen to locate the fundus — the area of greatest muscle density in the uterus. Then, using transducer straps, secure the tocotransducer over the fundus.
➤ Adjust the pen set tracer controls so that the baseline values read between 5 and 15 mm Hg on the monitor strip. This prevents triggering the alarm that indicates the tracer has dropped below the paper's margins. The proper setting varies among tocotransducers.
➤ Apply conduction gel to the ultrasound transducer crystals to promote an airtight seal and optimal sound-wave transmission.
➤ Use Leopold's maneuvers to palpate the fetal back, through which fetal heart tones resound most audibly.

➤ Start the monitor. Then apply the ultrasound transducer directly over the site having the strongest heart tones.

➤ Activate the control that begins the printout. On the printout paper, note any coughing, position changes, drug administration, vaginal examinations, and blood pressure readings that may affect interpretation of the tracings.

### Monitoring the patient

➤ Observe the tracings to identify the frequency and duration of uterine contractions, but palpate the uterus to determine intensity of contractions.

➤ Mentally note the baseline fetal heart rate (FHR) — the rate between contractions — to compare with suspicious-looking deviations. FHR normally ranges from 110 to 160 beats/minute.

➤ Assess periodic accelerations or decelerations from the baseline FHR. Compare the FHR patterns with those of the uterine contractions. Note the time relationship between the onset of an FHR deceleration and the onset of a uterine contraction, the time relationship of the lowest level of an FHR deceleration to the peak of a uterine contraction, and the range of FHR deceleration. These data help distinguish fetal distress from benign head compression.

➤ Move the tocotransducer and the ultrasound transducer to accommodate changes in maternal or fetal position. Readjust both transducers every hour, and assess the patient's skin for reddened areas caused by the strap pressure. Document skin condition.

➤ Clean the ultrasound transducer periodically with a damp cloth to remove dried conduction gel, which can interfere with ultrasound transmission. Apply fresh gel as necessary. After using the ultrasound transducer, place the cover over it.

## PATIENT TEACHING

➤ Inform the patient and her support person that "external fetal monitoring" is the term used for measuring the FHR as it reacts to her uterine contractions during labor. The FHR and the pattern of the patient's contractions are displayed as a graph on the monitor. This helps you know how the fetus is handling the stress of labor.

➤ Inform the patient and her support person that the monitor may make noise if the pen set tracer moves above or below the printed paper. Reassure them that this doesn't indicate fetal distress. As appropriate, explain other aspects of the monitor to help reduce maternal anxiety about fetal well-being.

➤ Explain to the patient and her support person how to time and anticipate contractions with the monitor. Inform them that the distance from one dark vertical line to the next on the printout grid represents 1 minute. The support person can use this information to prepare the patient for the onset of a contraction and to guide and slow her breathing as the contraction subsides.

➤ Advise the patient and her support person that external fetal monitoring may be done for about 20 minutes at the start of labor, then for a few minutes each hour. The monitor may be left on for continuous monitoring as well. The monitor allows you to see signs of fetal distress early and take steps to help the fetus.

➤ Explain to the patient that the external fetal monitors are held in place by straps around her abdomen. A pressure gauge measures the pressure of the contractions and an ultrasonic device detects fetal heart rate. The monitors don't cause any pain and don't stop the patient from changing positions; however movement can temporarily interfere with monitoring information.

➤ Advise the patient that either the nurse or you are able to disconnect the monitor temporarily to allow her to walk around or go to the bathroom.

## COMPLICATIONS

None known

## SPECIAL CONSIDERATIONS

➤ If the monitor fails to record uterine activity, palpate for contractions. Check for equipment problems as the manufacturer directs, and readjust the tocotransducer.

➤ If the patient reports discomfort in the position that provides the clearest signal, try to obtain a satisfactory 5- or 10-minute tracing with the patient in this position before assisting her to a more comfortable position. As the patient progresses through labor and abdominal pressure increases, the pen set tracer may exceed the alarm boundaries.

➤ Monitoring devices, such as phonotransducers and abdominal electrocardiogram transducers, are available. However, facilities use these devices less frequently than they use the ultrasound transducer.

➤ The Association of Women's Health, Obstetric, and Neonatal Nurses (AWHONN) maintains that intermittent auscultation of the fetal heart with a 1:1 nurse-patient ratio is equivalent to continuous external fetal monitoring. For low-risk patients, the suggested auscultation frequency is 30-minute intervals in active first-stage labor and 15-minute intervals in second-stage labor. For high-risk patients, the suggested auscultation frequency is 15-minute intervals in active first-stage labor and 5-minute intervals in second-stage labor.

## DOCUMENTATION

➤ Make sure you've numbered each monitor strip in sequence and labeled each printout sheet with the patient's identification number or birth date and name, the date, the time, maternal vital signs and position, the paper speed, and the number of the strip paper.

➤ Record the time of any vaginal examinations, membrane rupture, drug administration, and maternal or fetal movements.

➤ Record maternal vital signs and the intensity of uterine contractions.

➤ Document each time that you moved or readjusted the tocotransducer and ultrasound transducer, and summarize this information in your notes.

## Internal fetal monitoring

CPT CODE
No specific code has been assigned.

## DESCRIPTION

Also called direct fetal monitoring, this sterile, invasive procedure uses a spiral electrode and an intrauterine catheter to evaluate fetal status during labor. By providing an electrocardiogram (ECG) of the fetal heart rate (FHR), internal electronic fetal monitoring assesses fetal response to uterine contractions more accurately than does external fetal monitoring. It precisely measures intrauterine pressure, tracks labor progress, and allows evaluation of short- and long-term FHR variability.

Internal fetal monitoring is indicated whenever direct, beat-to-beat FHR monitoring is required. However, internal monitoring is performed only if the amniotic sac has ruptured, the cervix is dilated at

## CRITERIA FOR AND RISKS OF INTERNAL FETAL MONITORING

Use of the internal fetal monitor requires that the membranes be ruptured because the fetal electrode is attached directly to the fetus and the intrauterine pressure catheter (IUPC) is placed in the uterine cavity. Criteria for the insertion of either the internal fetal monitor or IUPC are:
➤ 2 cm of cervical dilation
➤ presenting part of fetus needs to be down to at least −1 station.

Rupture of the fetal membranes carries potential hazards to the fetus because amniotic fluid, within the membranes, protects the fetal head and the umbilical cord from undue and uneven pressure. Some changes common when amniotic fluid is missing are more extensive molding of the head, which may exhibit itself by periodic heart rate pattern changes, identifiable as early decelerations resulting from head compression, as well as more extensive formation of caput succedaneum.

Studies have shown that uneven head compression, which may occur without the protective membranes, causes abnormal changes in fetal electroencephalogram findings and may cause brain damage due to trauma. Without the protection of the fetal membranes containing the amniotic fluid, the umbilical cord may be compressed between the uterus and the fetus during contractions, particularly if the cord has looped itself around the trunk or neck or the fetus. Spontaneous rupture of membranes normally occurs at the end of the first stage of labor; membranes that remain intact up to that point protect the fetus from uneven and undue pressure during the process of dilation.

least 2 cm, and the presenting part of the fetus is at least at the −1 station.

## INDICATIONS

➤ To monitor fetal status in maternal diabetes or hypertension
➤ To monitor fetal status in fetal postmaturity
➤ To monitor fetal status when intrauterine growth retardation is suspected
➤ To monitor fetal status if amniotic fluid is meconium-stained
➤ To detect possible distress as indicated by external fetal monitoring

## CONTRAINDICATIONS

### Absolute
➤ Maternal human immunodeficiency virus
➤ Maternal blood dyscrasias
➤ Virus infection
➤ Other high-risk factors for fetal infection
➤ Suspected fetal immune deficiency, herpes simplex virus, and hepatitis B virus
➤ Placenta previa

### Relative
➤ Face presentation or uncertainty about presenting part (although an internal fetal monitor electrode can also be placed on the fetal sacrum in the case of a breech presentation). (See *Criteria for and risks of internal fetal monitoring*.)

## EQUIPMENT

Electronic fetal monitor ◆ spiral electrode and a drive tube ◆ disposable leg plate pad or reusable leg plate with Velcro belt ◆ conduction gel ◆ antiseptic solution ◆ hypoallergenic tape ◆ gown ◆ goggles ◆ mask ◆ two pairs of sterile gloves ◆ sterile drape ◆ intrauterine pressure catheter (IUPC) and connection cable ◆ printout paper ◆ operator's manual

## PREPARATION OF EQUIPMENT

➤ Be sure to review the operator's manual before using the equipment. If the monitor has two paper speeds, set the speed at 3 cm/minute to ensure a readable tracing.

A tracing at 1 cm/minute is more condensed and harder to interpret accurately. Connect the IUPC cable to the uterine activity outlet on the monitor. Wash your hands, and open the sterile equipment, maintaining aseptic technique.

## ESSENTIAL STEPS

➤ Describe the procedure to the patient and her support person, if present, and explain how the equipment works. Tell the patient that you will first perform a vaginal examination to identify the position of the fetus.

➤ After explaining the procedure and answering all questions, obtain a signed consent form.

➤ Label the printout paper with the patient's identification number or name and birth date, the date, the paper speed, and the number of the monitor strip.

### Monitoring contractions

➤ Assist the patient into the lithotomy position for a vaginal examination.

➤ Attach the connection cable to the appropriate outlet on the monitor marked UA (uterine activity). Connect the cable to the IUPC. Next, zero the IUPC with a gauge provided on the distal end of the catheter. This will help determine the resting tone of the uterus, usually 5 to 15 mm Hg.

➤ Put on gown, goggles, mask, and sterile gloves.

➤ Cover the patient's perineum with a sterile drape. Then clean the perineum with antiseptic solution, according to facility policy. Using aseptic technique, insert the IUPC into the uterine cavity while performing a vaginal examination. The IUPC is advanced to the black line on the catheter and secured with hypoallergenic tape along the patient's inner thigh.

➤ Observe the monitoring strip to verify proper placement of the IUPC and to ensure a clear tracing. Periodically evaluate

the monitoring strip to determine the exact amount of pressure exerted with each contraction. Note all such data on the monitoring strip and on the patient's medical record.

➤ The IUPC is usually removed during the second stage of labor. Dispose of the catheter, and clean and store the cable according to facility policy. (See *Applying an internal electronic fetal monitor*, page 382.)

### Monitoring FHR

➤ Apply conduction gel to the leg plate. Then secure the leg plate to the patient's inner thigh with Velcro straps or 2″ tape. Connect the leg plate cable to the ECG outlet on the monitor.

➤ Put on sterile gloves.

➤ Perform a vaginal examination to identify the fetal presenting part (which is usually the scalp or buttocks), to determine the level of fetal descent, and to apply the electrode. Place the spiral electrode in a drive tube and advance through the vagina to the fetal presenting part. To secure the electrode, mild pressure will be applied and the drive tube will be turned clockwise 360 degrees.

➤ After the electrode is in place and the drive tube has been removed, connect the color-coded electrode wires to the corresponding color-coded leg plate posts.

➤ Turn on the recorder, and note the time on the printout paper.

➤ Assist the patient to a comfortable position, and evaluate the strip to verify proper placement and a clear FHR tracing.

### Monitoring the patient

➤ Begin by noting the frequency, duration, and intensity of uterine contractions. Normal intrauterine pressure ranges from 8 to 12 mm Hg. (See *Reading a fetal monitor strip*, page 383.)

➤ Next, check the baseline FHR. Assess periodic accelerations or decelerations from the baseline FHR.

## APPLYING AN INTERNAL ELECTRONIC FETAL MONITOR

During internal electronic fetal monitoring, a spiral electrode monitors the fetal heart rate (FHR) and an internal pressure catheter monitors uterine contractions.

### Monitoring FHR

The spiral electrode is inserted after a vaginal examination that determines the position of the fetus. As shown at right, the electrode is attached to the presenting fetal part, usually the scalp or buttocks.

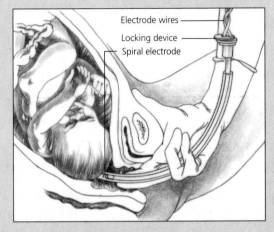

Electrode wires
Locking device
Spiral electrode

### Monitoring uterine contractions

The intrauterine pressure catheter is inserted up to a premarked level on the tubing and then connected to a monitor that interprets uterine contraction pressures.

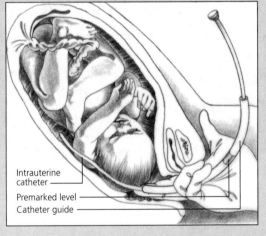

Intrauterine catheter
Premarked level
Catheter guide

➤ Compare the FHR pattern with the uterine contraction pattern. Note the interval between the onset of an FHR deceleration and the onset of a uterine contraction, the interval between the lowest level of an FHR deceleration and the peak of a uterine contraction, and the range of FHR deceleration.

➤ Determine the baseline FHR within 10 beats/minute; then assess the degree of baseline variability. Note the presence or absence of short-term or long-term variability. Identify periodic FHR changes such as decelerations (early, late, variable, or mixed) and nonperiodic changes such as a sinusoidal pattern.

## READING A FETAL MONITOR STRIP

Presented in two parallel recordings, the fetal monitor strip records the fetal heart rate (FHR) in beats/minute in the top recording and uterine activity (UA) in mm Hg in the bottom recording. You can obtain information on fetal status and labor progress by reading the strips horizontally and vertically.

Reading horizontally on the FHR or the UA strip, each small block represents 10 seconds. Six consecutive small blocks, separated by a dark vertical line, represent 1 minute.

Reading vertically on the FHR strip, each block represents an amplitude of 10 beats/minute. Reading vertically on the UA strip, each block represents 5 mm Hg of pressure.

Assess the baseline FHR — the "resting" heart rate — between uterine contractions when fetal movement diminishes. This baseline FHR (normal range: 110 to 160 beats/minute) pattern serves as a reference for subsequent FHR tracings produced during contractions.

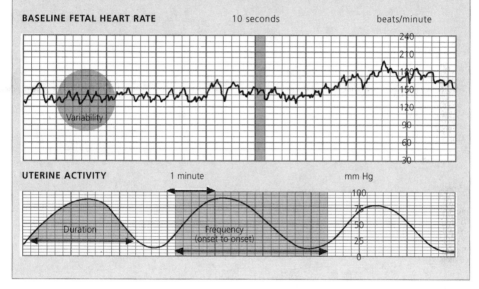

**BASELINE FETAL HEART RATE**  10 seconds  beats/minute

**UTERINE ACTIVITY**  1 minute  mm Hg

## PATIENT TEACHING

➤ Advise the patient and her support person that the information from an external monitor isn't always adequate. An internal monitor, a tiny wire placed on the baby's scalp provides more information. You and a nurse will evaluate the results from the monitor along with other factors to determine how well the fetus is doing.
➤ Tell the patient and her support person that the monitor will show if the fetus is distressed. A heart rate that is too fast or

slow, or doesn't change with contractions may mean that the fetus isn't getting enough oxygen. This information allows you to take steps to help a fetus in distress early.
➤ Inform the patient and her support person that a vaginal examination is done first to ensure that the electrode isn't attached to in an area that would cause the fetus harm such as the suture lines, fontanels, face, or genitalia.

*(Text continues on page 388.)*

## IDENTIFYING BASELINE FHR IRREGULARITIES

Fetal heart rate (FHR) variability is an indication of fetal oxygen reserve as well as of neurologic integrity and stability. It is important to identify FHR irregularities quickly and accurately in order to be able to manage them appropriately. For a quick review, consult the chart below.

| IRREGULARITY | CLINICAL SIGNIFICANCE |
|---|---|

### BASELINE TACHYCARDIA

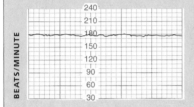

Fetal tachycardia alone is not usually associated with poor outcome in the term fetus. In the preterm fetus (whose organ systems are immature) and the postterm fetus (when the placenta has begun aging), tachycardia is an indication for closer observation. Fetal tachycardia plus either late decelerations or prolonged variable decelerations (even without meconium), and absent variability, is indicative of fetal distress.

### BASELINE BRADYCARDIA

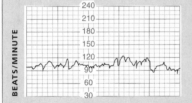

Bradycardia is a baseline FHR level in the range of 100 to 110 beats/minute. Marked bradycardia is a baseline below 100 beats/minute that lasts for more than 10 minutes. Bradycardia with average variability generally is not clinically significant as an indicator of fetal distress. If fetal bradycardia occurs, however, you should assess for signs and symptoms of fetal distress (presence of prolapsed cord, duration of bradycardia, variability, late or prolonged variable decelerations, and the expected time until delivery).

| POSSIBLE CAUSES | INTERVENTIONS |
| --- | --- |
| ➤ Extreme prematurity<br>➤ Maternal dehydration<br>➤ Fetal anemia related to Rh sensitization, nonimmune hydrops, fetal-maternal hemorrhage, or placental abruption<br>➤ Maternal ingestion of high doses of caffeine<br>➤ Early fetal hypoxia<br>➤ Maternal fever<br>➤ Parasympathetic agents, such as atropine and scopolamine<br>➤ Beta-adrenergic blocking agents, such as ritodrine and terbutaline<br>➤ Amnionitis (inflammation of inner layer of fetal membrane, or amnion)<br>➤ Maternal hyperthyroidism<br>➤ Fetal anemia<br>➤ Fetal heart failure<br>➤ Fetal arrhythmias | ➤ Intervene to correct the cause of fetal distress. Administer supplemental oxygen as needed. Also administer I.V. fluids.<br>➤ Discontinue oxytocin infusion to reduce uterine activity.<br>➤ Turn the patient onto her left side and elevate her legs.<br>➤ Continue to observe FHR.<br>➤ Document interventions and outcomes.<br>➤ Notify your collaborating physician; further medical intervention may be necessary. |
| ➤ Late fetal hypoxia<br>➤ Beta-adrenergic blocking agents, such as propranolol, and anesthetics<br>➤ Maternal hypotension<br>➤ Prolonged umbilical cord compression<br>➤ Maternal hypothermia<br>➤ Prolapsed umbilical cord: occult, complete, or intermittent cord compression<br>➤ Fetal hypoxemia or asphyxia (acute or chronic) usually preceded by non-reassuring fetal heart patterns and absent or decreased variability<br>➤ Vagal stimulation due to maternal pushing efforts, vaginal examination, rapid descent, posterior or transverse position of the fetal head in vertex presentation<br>➤ Fetal cardiac anomalies<br>➤ Fetal congenital heart block (possibly related to maternal autoimmune diseases such as lupus erythematosus) | ➤ Intervene to alleviate the cause of fetal distress. Administer supplemental oxygen, as needed. Also administer I.V. fluids.<br>➤ Discontinue oxytocin infusion to reduce uterine activity.<br>➤ Turn the patient onto her left side and elevate her legs.<br>➤ Continue to observe the FHR.<br>➤ Document interventions and outcomes.<br>➤ Notify your collaborating physician; further medical intervention may be necessary. |

*(continued)*

## IDENTIFYING BASELINE FHR IRREGULARITIES *(continued)*

| IRREGULARITY | CLINICAL SIGNIFICANCE |
|---|---|

### EARLY DECELERATIONS

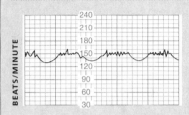

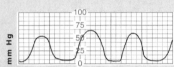

Early decelerations are benign, indicating fetal head compression at dilation of 4 to 7 cm. Early decelerations descend gradually from the onset to nadir (in 30 seconds or more) and last less than 2 minutes in duration. Early decelerations occur repetitively, and the onset and the recovery coincide with the beginning, the peak, and the end of the contraction. They are usually benign if there is prompt recovery of the fetal heart to baseline after the end of the contraction. This is usually an indication of fetal head compression at 4 to 7 cm and during second-stage pushing.

### LATE DECELERATIONS

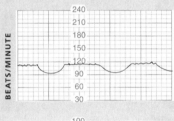

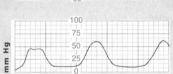

Uncorrected late decelerations may be life-threatening. The severity of the fetal distress cannot be measured by the depth of the deceleration. A shallow deceleration is most dangerous because it is easy to miss and is just as serious as a deep deceleration.

| POSSIBLE CAUSES | INTERVENTIONS |
|---|---|
| ➤ Fetal head compression | ➤ Reassure the patient that the fetus isn't at risk.<br>➤ Observe the FHR.<br>➤ Document the frequency of decelerations. |
| ➤ Uteroplacental circulatory insufficiency (placental hypoperfusion) caused by decreased intervillous blood flow during contractions or a structural placental defect, such as abruptio placentae<br>➤ Uterine hyperactivity caused by excessive oxytocin infusion<br>➤ Maternal hypotension<br>➤ Maternal supine hypotension<br>➤ Uteroplacental insufficiency, which may be caused by:<br>– Fetal anemia associated with Rh sensitization, nonimmune hydrops, or fetal-maternal hemorrhage<br>– Maternal sickle cell crisis<br>– Abnormal placentation (placenta previa, infarction of one of the lobes of the placenta, poorly controlled diabetes)<br>– Abruption associated with hypertension, cocaine use, overdistention of the uterus<br>– Hypertensive disorders (pregnancy-induced hypertension, chronic hypertension, or both), positioning, conduction anesthesia, severe dehydration, or septic shock<br>– Hypertonic uterine contractions such as those caused by administration of oxytocin or prostaglandin $E_2$<br>– Postmaturity | ➤ Turn the patient onto her left side and elevate her legs but not her body (don't place in Trendelenburg's position).<br>➤ Discontinue oxytocin infusion to reduce uterine activity.<br>➤ Increase or start administration of I.V. fluids; don't use a solution that contains glucose.<br>➤ Administer oxygen by mask at 6 to 8 L/minute, as indicated.<br>➤ If late decelerations are related to epidural administration, check the patient's blood pressure; correct hypotension with hydration or ephedrine administration.<br>➤ If late decelerations are due to excessive uterine activity, tocolytic therapy (drugs that halt contractions) may be prescribed. |

*(continued)*

| IRREGULARITY | CLINICAL SIGNIFICANCE |
|---|---|

**VARIABLE DECELERATIONS**

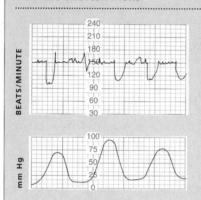

Variable decelerations are the most common deceleration pattern in labor because of contractions and fetal movement. The seriousness of variable decelerations depends on their frequency, depth, rate of recovery, effect on baseline fetal heart rate, and variability. Variable decelerations that return to baseline quickly and have average variability aren't associated with hypoxemia and acidosis. However, variable decelerations that return to baseline slowly (regardless of depth of fall), plus an increased baseline rate (tachycardia) or absence of variability, may indicate serious fetal compromise.

## COMPLICATIONS

➤ *Uterine perforation* and *intrauterine infection* are maternal complications that can result from internal fetal monitoring and require evaluation by a specialist such as an obstetrician.

➤ *Abscess, hematoma,* and *infection* are fetal complications that can result from internal fetal monitoring and require evaluation by a specialist such as a neonatalogist.

## SPECIAL CONSIDERATIONS

➤ Keep in mind that acute fetal distress can result from any change in the baseline FHR that causes fetal compromise. If necessary, take steps to counteract FHR changes. (See *Identifying baseline FHR irregularities*, pages 384 to 389, and *Evaluating and managing abnormal tracings*, page 390.)

➤ A spiral electrode is the most commonly used device for internal fetal monitoring. Shaped like a corkscrew, the electrode is attached to the presenting fetal part (usually the scalp). It detects the fetal heartbeat and then transmits it to the monitor, which converts the signals to a fetal ECG waveform.

➤ Measurements of intrauterine pressure or amniotic fluid pressure are made possible by inserting an IUPC. IUPCs are used for two different purposes:
– Internal monitoring of the contractions for evaluation of the fetal heart.
– Amnioinfusion, the transcervical infusion of sterile, balanced salt solutions during labor. Amnioinfusion is used to ameliorate variable decelerations of the fetal heart rate tracing that are suspected to be due to umbilical cord compression. It is

| POSSIBLE CAUSES | INTERVENTIONS |
|---|---|
| ➤ Umbilical cord compression causing decreased fetal oxygen perfusion | ➤ Help the patient change position. No other intervention is necessary unless you detect fetal distress. <br> ➤ Assure the patient that the fetus tolerates cord compression well. Explain that cord compression affects the fetus the same way that breath-holding affects her. <br> ➤ Assess the deceleration pattern for reassuring signs: a baseline FHR that isn't increasing, short-term variability that isn't decreasing, abruptly beginning and ending decelerations, and decelerations lasting less than 50 seconds. If assessment doesn't reveal reassuring signs, consult with your collaborating physician. <br> ➤ Start I.V. fluids and administer oxygen by mask at 10 to 12 L/minute, as indicated. <br> ➤ Discontinue oxytocin infusion to reduce uterine activity. <br> ➤ Document interventions and outcomes. |

additionally used to dilute thick meconium.

➤ The use of an IUPC requires the same criteria as the internal fetal monitor: at least 2 cm of cervical dilation and at least a –1 station of the presenting part of the fetus is required.

## DOCUMENTATION

➤ Document date and time of initiation of procedure including placement of the spiral electrode.

➤ Document all activity related to monitoring. (A fetal monitoring strip becomes part of the patient's permanent record, and is considered a legal document.) Be sure to record the type of monitoring your patient received as well as all interventions.

➤ Identify the monitoring strip with the patient's name, your name, and the date

and time. Also document the paper speed and electrode placement.

➤ Record the patient's vital signs at regular intervals. Note her pushing efforts, and record any change in her position.

➤ Document any I.V. line insertion and any changes in the I.V. solution or infusion rate. Note the use of oxytocin, regional anesthetics, or other medications.

➤ After a vaginal examination, document cervical dilation and effacement as well as fetal station, presentation, and position.

➤ Also document membrane rupture, including the time it occurred and whether it was spontaneous or artificial. Note the amount, color, and odor of the fluid. (See *Terms for documentation of fetal monitoring*, page 391.

(Text continues on page 392.)

## EVALUATING AND MANAGING ABNORMAL TRACINGS

Although you must evaluate each patient individually, the following algorithm outlines general treatment protocols for evaluating and managing abnormal tracings.

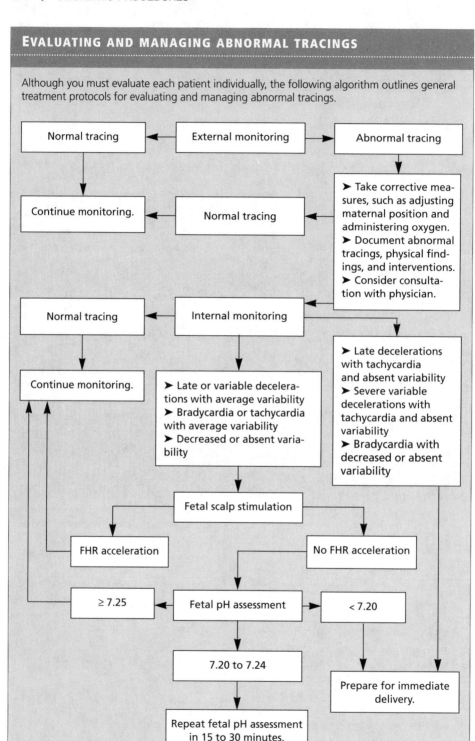

# TERMS FOR DOCUMENTATION OF FETAL MONITORING

Many terms have changed in obstetric care, and it's important that practitioners define them uniformly to ensure clear communication. Listed below are common terms for the documentation of fetal monitoring.

The new normal fetal heart rate (FHR) range is 110 to 160 beats/minute. Bradycardia is a baseline of less than 110 beats/minute, and tachycardia is a baseline of greater than160 beats/minute. Patterns are categorized as either baseline, periodic, or episodic.

➤ *Baseline:* The approximate FHR during a 10-minute segment excluding periodic or episodic changes or marked FHR variability or segments of the baseline that differ by greater than 25 beats/minute. The baseline must be at least 2 minutes in length, or it's documented as indeterminate.

➤ *Periodic* changes are associated *with* uterine contractions. Periodic patterns are described on the basis of waveform, "abrupt" versus "gradual" onset.

➤ *Episodic* changes are those *not* associated with contractions.

*Variability* is the irregular fluctuation of the FHR baseline that occurs as a result of changes between each computed heartbeat. Variability is a function of the baseline.

➤ Variability is based on the amplitude of the complexes, with the exclusion of the sinusoidal pattern.

➤ Variability is quantified as the amplitude of the peak-to-trough in beats/minute:
– Amplitude range undetectable: *absent* FHR variability
– Amplitude range of less than 5 beats/minute: *minimal* FHR variability
– Amplitude range of 6 to 25 beats/minute: *moderate* FHR variability
– Amplitude range of more than 25 beats/minute: *marked* FHR variability (usually due to cord compression).

*Acceleration* is greater than or equal to 15 beats/minute *above most recent baseline* lasting for 15 seconds or more and less than 2 minutes. Because gestational age affects the characteristics of FHR patterns, it must be considered in the full description of the pattern. Expectations for a fetus at less than 32 weeks' gestation (with no proven ability to initiate 15 beats/minute × 15-second accelerations) are 10 beats/minute × 10-second accelerations.

➤ *Prolonged acceleration* lasts 2 minutes or more but less than 10 minutes in duration.

➤ Acceleration of 10 minutes or more must be considered a baseline change.

*Decelerations* are periodic FHR changes that are associated with uterine contractions.

➤ *Late decelerations* descend *gradually* from onset of decrease to the return to baseline in association with the contractions. Usually the onset of the decelerations occurs near the nadir (or the bottom most point of the decelerations) and the recovery occurs after the end of the contraction.

➤ *Early decelerations* descend gradually from onset to nadir (in 30 seconds or more) and last less than 2 minutes in duration. Early decelerations occur repetitively. Timing of the onset and recovery coincide with the beginning and end of the contraction.

➤ *Prolonged deceleration* is a decrease in the FHR that lasts 2 minutes but no longer than 10 minutes.

➤ *Variable deceleration* is a decrease in FHR that usually falls significantly below the baseline (by 15 beats/minute or more), descends abruptly from the baseline to nadir (in less than 30 seconds), and lasts at least 15 seconds but no more than 2 minutes in duration.

## QUICK GUIDE TO STAGES OF LABOR

Normal labor advances through the four stages summarized below. Offer your patient encouragement and progress reports throughout the stages.

### First stage
Regular contractions, which repeat at 15- to 20-minute intervals and last between 10 and 30 seconds, signal the onset of labor's first stage. This stage has three phases: latent, active, and transitional. In primiparous patients, the first stage of labor may range from 3.3 to 19.7 hours; in multiparous patients, it may range from 0.1 to 14.3 hours.

In the *latent phase* (characterized by irregular, brief, and mild contractions), the cervix dilates to 3 or 4 cm. Other signs and symptoms include abdominal cramping and backache. The patient may expel the mucus plug during this phase. This phase averages 8.6 hours in primiparous patients and 5.3 hours in multiparous patients.

During the *active phase,* cervical dilation increases to between 5 and 7 cm. Contractions occur every 3 to 5 minutes, last 30 to 45 seconds, and become moderately intense. In primiparous patients, this phase averages 5.8 hours; in multiparous patients, this phase averages 2.5 hours.

In the *transitional phase,* the cervix dilates completely (8 to 10 cm). Uterine contractions grow intense, last between 45 and 60 seconds, and repeat at least every 2 minutes. The patient may thrash about, lose control of breathing techniques, and experience nausea and vomiting. This phase typically lasts less than 3 hours in primiparous patients and less than 1 hour in multiparous patients.

### Second stage
In the second stage of labor, contractions occur every 1½ to 2 minutes and last up to 90 seconds. This stage commonly ends within 1 hour for a primiparous patient and possibly 15 minutes for a multiparous patient.

Signs and symptoms signaling onset of the second stage include increased bloody show, rupture of membranes (if they're still intact), severe rectal pressure and flaring, and reflexive bearing down with each contraction. The fetal head approaches the perineal floor and emerges at the vaginal opening. The second labor stage concludes with birth.

### Third stage
Strong but less painful contractions expel the placenta, which normally emerges within 30 minutes after the neonate emerges. Signs indicating normal separation of the placenta from the uterine wall include lengthening of the umbilical cord, a sudden gush of dark blood from the vagina, and a palpable change in uterine shape from disclike to globular.

### Fourth stage
This stage begins with placental expulsion and extends through the next 4 hours, while the patient's body rests and begins adjusting to the postpartum state.

# LABOR AND DELIVERY

## Uterine contraction palpation

### CPT CODE
No specific code has been assigned.

## DESCRIPTION

Periodic, involuntary uterine contractions characterize normal labor and cause progressive cervical effacement and dilation, impelling the fetus to descend. Uterine palpation can tell you the frequency, duration, and intensity of contractions and the relaxation time between them. The character of contractions varies with the stage of labor and the body's response to labor-inducing drugs, if administered. As labor advances, contractions become more intense, occur more often, and last longer. (See *Quick guide to stages of labor*.)

## INDICATIONS

➤ To assess labor and patient's response to interventions

## CONTRAINDICATIONS

None known

## EQUIPMENT

Watch with a second hand ◆ sheet (for draping)

## ESSENTIAL STEPS

➤ Review the patient's admission history to determine the onset, frequency, duration, and intensity of contractions. Also, note where contractions feel strongest or exert the most pressure.
➤ Wash your hands and provide privacy.
➤ Describe the palpation procedure to the patient and answer any questions she may have. Because she may be ticklish or sensitive to touch, forewarn her that you'll palpate her abdominal area over the uterus.
➤ Assist the patient to a comfortable side-lying position to relieve pressure on the inferior vena cava and promote uteroplacental circulation. This position also relieves direct pressure on the sacral area from the fetal head and eases backache.
➤ Drape the patient with a sheet.
➤ Plant the palmar surface of your fingers on the uterine fundus, and palpate lightly to assess contractions. Note the uterine tightening and abdominal lifting that occur with contractions. Each contraction has three phases: increment (rising), acme (peak), and decrement (letting down or ebbing).
➤ Palpate several contractions. Simultaneously use the second hand on your watch to assess and measure such contraction qualities as frequency, duration, and intensity.
➤ To assess frequency of the contraction, time the interval between the beginning of one contraction and the beginning of the next. In normal labor, contractions begin slowly and gradually occur more frequently with briefer relaxation intervals.
➤ To assess duration of the contraction, time the period from when the uterus begins tightening until it begins relaxing. As labor progresses, contractions usually last longer.
➤ To assess intensity of the contraction, press your fingertips into the uterine fundus when the uterus tightens. During mild contractions, the fundus indents easily and feels like a chin. During moderate contractions, the fundus indents less easily and feels like a nose; during strong contractions, the fundus resists indenting and feels like a forehead.
➤ Determine how the patient copes with discomfort by assessing her breathing and relaxation techniques, if any. This may help guide your intervention choices. Naturally, you'll provide ongoing emotional support in any event.
➤ Observe the patient's response to contractions to evaluate whether she needs an analgesic, anesthetic, or other appropriate measure, such as repositioning and back massage.
➤ Assess contractions at least hourly during the latent phase of first-stage labor and every 30 minutes throughout the active phase. During second-stage labor, assess contractions every 15 minutes.

## PATIENT TEACHING

➤ Tell the patient that her uterine contractions will be assessed periodically to determine their interval, character, and duration. This information is helpful in the assessment of how labor is progressing and permits early intervention if there isn't an adequate interval between contractions. The interval between contractions is important, not only to allow her respite, but also to permit a return of full blood flow to the fetus.

➤ Advise the patient that uterine contraction palpation involves placing fingertips lightly on the edge of the uterus farthest from the vaginal opening, and feeling the changes in muscle tension that occur with contractions. Normal uterine contractions are like waves, with the muscle hardness slowly building to a peak, (also called an acme), and then subsiding.

## COMPLICATIONS

None known

## SPECIAL CONSIDERATIONS

➤ Because the patient may become irritable or anxious during the transitional phase of first-stage labor — when the cervix dilates fully — and because abdominal palpation may aggravate her distress, assess contractions only as necessary. If appropriate, teach her support person to palpate and record contractions.

➤ If any contraction lasts longer than 90 seconds and isn't followed by uterine muscle relaxation, further evaluate maternal and fetal well-being. Also evaluate further a brief relaxation period between contractions because inadequate relaxation intervals increase the risk of fetal hypoxia and exhaust the patient.

➤ Be aware that false labor (or Braxton Hicks) contractions occur at irregular intervals and vary in intensity. They're felt over the abdomen and are often relieved by walking. During false labor, membranes remain intact, and there is no show of blood or progressive cervical dilation or effacement.

## DOCUMENTATION

➤ Record the frequency, duration, and intensity of contractions.

➤ Keep track of the relaxation time between contractions, and describe the patient's response to contractions.

# Vaginal examination

CPT CODE
No specific code has been assigned.

## DESCRIPTION

Vaginal examination is performed during first-stage labor to assess cervical dilation, effacement, membrane status, and fetal presentation, position, and engagement.

Important considerations during the examination include respecting the patient's privacy, providing simple explanations for her and her support person, maintaining eye contact when possible, and using aseptic technique. This enables the examination to proceed precisely and efficiently.

## INDICATIONS

➤ To check for cervical changes before ruling out labor
➤ To perform routine assessment during labor
➤ To check for rupture of membranes (ROM)
➤ To exclude the presence of cord prolapse following spontaneous ROM
➤ To evaluate cervical changes prior to the administration of analgesics

## CONTRAINDICATIONS

### Relative
➤ Premature labor (prior to the completion of 37 weeks' gestation)
➤ Premature ROM (prior to the completion of 37 weeks' gestation)
➤ Active genital herpes

➤ Known placenta previa
➤ Less than 4 hours since the last vaginal examination
➤ Excessive vaginal bleeding, which may signal placenta previa or placental abruption

## EQUIPMENT

Sterile gloves ◆ sterile water-soluble lubricant or sterile water ◆ linen-saver pads ◆ sterile gauze

## ESSENTIAL STEPS

➤ Explain the procedure to the patient and answer any questions she may have. Give her an opportunity to empty her bladder because a distended bladder may interfere with accurate examination findings.
➤ Use Leopold's maneuvers to identify the fetal presenting part and position. Then help the patient into a lithotomy position for the vaginal examination.
➤ Wash your hands. Place a linen-saver pad under the patient's buttocks, and put on sterile gloves.
➤ Inform the patient when you are about to touch her to avoid startling her.
➤ Apply sterile lubricating gel to your index and middle finger.
➤ Spread the labia with the thumb and ring finger of your examining hand.
➤ Ask the patient to relax by taking several deep breaths and slowly releasing the air. Then insert your lubricated fingers (palmar surface down) into the vagina. Keep your uninserted fingers flexed to avoid the rectum. Be mindful of where your thumb is. Your thumb should be in a tucked position. (Flexing the thumb or even resting it against the clitoris can cause the patient undue discomfort.) (See *Step-by-step vaginal examination,* page 396.)
➤ Palpate the cervix, keeping in mind that it may assume a posterior position in early labor and be difficult to locate. Once you find the cervix, note its consistency. The

cervix gradually softens throughout pregnancy, reaching a buttery consistency before labor begins. (See *Cervical effacement and dilation,* page 397.)
➤ After identifying the presenting fetal part and position, evaluating dilation and effacement, assessing fetal engagement and station, and verifying membrane status, gently withdraw your fingers. Let the patient clean her perineum herself with sterile gauze if she can walk to the bathroom. If she's confined to bed, you can clean her perineum and change the linen-saver pad.
➤ To encourage the patient and help reduce her anxiety, describe how labor is progressing, and define the stage and phase if appropriate.

## PATIENT TEACHING

➤ Notify the patient of the degree of dilation. Be certain to emphasize that the cervix opens very slowly until it's about halfway dilated, then it opens fully very quickly.

## SPECIAL CONSIDERATIONS

➤ Patients with immunoglobulin A deficiency are at increased risk of an anaphylactic reaction.
➤ In early labor, perform the vaginal examination between contractions, focusing primarily on the extent of cervical dilation and effacement. At the end of first-stage labor, perform the examination during a contraction, when the uterine muscle pushes the fetus downward. This examination will focus on assessing fetal descent.
➤ If the amniotic membrane ruptures during the examination, record the fetal heart rate. Then note the time, and describe the color, odor, and approximate amount of fluid. Determine fetal station, and check for umbilical cord prolapse. After the membranes rupture, perform the vaginal examination only when labor changes sig-

## STEP-BY-STEP VAGINAL EXAMINATION

Begin the vaginal examination — usually in early labor — by inserting your gloved index and middle fingers palm side down into the vagina. Use your nondominant hand to gently but firmly press on the uterus to steady the fetal presenting part against the cervix for examination.

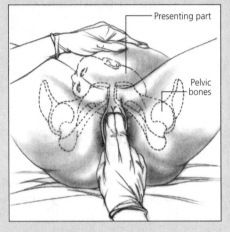

### Confirm the presenting part and position

Rotate your fingers to palpate and confirm the fetal presenting part (a fetal head feels firm, the buttocks soft) and position (left, right, anterior, posterior, or transverse), identified by using Leopold's maneuvers.

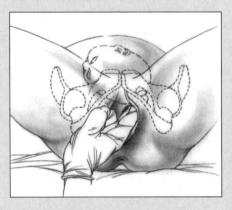

### Assess cervical effacement and dilation

Estimate cervical dilation by palpating the internal os. Each fingerbreadth of dilation averages 1.5 to 2 cm, depending on the width of the examiner's finger.

Next, determine the percentage of effacement by palpating the ridge of tissue around the cervix. Assign a low percentage of effacement to defined and thick cervical tissue. Indistinct, wafer-thin cervical tissue scores 100%.

### Assess fetal engagement and station

Estimate the extent of fetal engagement (descent of the fetal presenting part into the pelvis). Then palpate the presenting part and grade the fetal station (where the presenting part lies in relation to the ischial spines of the maternal pelvis). A zero grade indicates that the presenting part lies level with the ischial spines.

Station grades range from –3 (3 cm above the maternal ischial spines) to +4 (4 cm below the maternal ischial spines, causing the perineum to bulge).

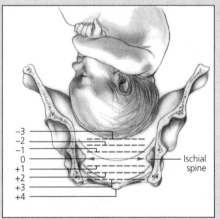

### Evaluate membrane status

If appropriate, also check amniotic membrane status. If you feel a bulging, slick surface over the presenting fetal part, you know the membranes remain intact.

## CERVICAL EFFACEMENT AND DILATION

As labor advances, so do cervical effacement and dilation, thereby facilitating birth. During effacement, the cervix shortens and its walls become thin, progressing from 0% effacement (palpable and thick) to 100% effacement (fully indistinct — or effaced — and paper thin). Full effacement obliterates the constrictive uterine neck to create a smooth, unobstructed passage for the fetus.

At the same time, dilation occurs. This progressive widening of the cervical canal — from the upper internal cervical os to the lower external cervical os — advances from 0 to 10 cm. As the cervical canal opens, resistance decreases. This further eases fetal descent.

**NO EFFACEMENT OR DILATION**

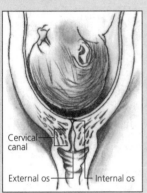

**EARLY EFFACEMENT AND DILATION**

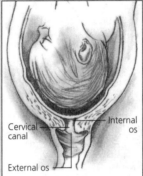

**FULL EFFACEMENT AND DILATION**

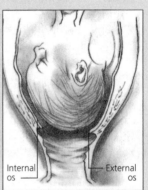

nificantly to minimize the risk of introducing intrauterine infection.

## DOCUMENTATION

➤ After each examination, record the percentage of effacement, dilation, the station of the presenting fetal part, amniotic membrane status, and the patient's tolerance of the procedure.

## Cervical ripening

**CPT CODE**
*59200 Insertion of cervical dilator
(such as prostaglandin)*

## DESCRIPTION

Elective induction for the patient's or practitioner's convenience is never justified. Methods of induction and augmentation of labor are used only when the benefits to either the patient or the fetus outweigh the benefits of continuing the pregnancy. Labor is induced most commonly for postdates, which occur in more than 13% of deliveries in the United States. In the event that induction or augmentation of labor becomes necessary, nonpharmacological advances (such as sexual intercourse and stripping the membranes) and recent pharmacological advances may facilitate a vaginal birth.

Cervical ripening with prostaglandin $E_2$ ($PGE_2$) or dinoprostone (such as Cervidil or Prepidil) is the most common pharmacological method of induction or augmentation of labor. PGE$_2$ may prove beneficial if the cervix is unfavorable for induction. The application of PGE$_2$ gel into the endocervical canal has the effect of ripening (or softening) the cervix and provides an oxytoxic effect. This method of action directly stimulates the collagenase of the cervix, breaking down the collagen network and softening it for induction. The gel can be applied via an intracervical route with greater efficacy. Alternatively, a 10 mg vaginal insert (Cervidil) is available and provides a lower rate of release of medication than the gel and is single dose only, removed upon onset of active labor or 12 hours after insertion. Should hyperstimulation occur, Cervidil also has the added advantage of easy removal.

Likewise, Prepidil (up to three doses) may be applied at 6-hour intervals for a maximum cumulative dose of 1.5 mg (0.5 mg of gel in three applications). Following the placement of PGE$_2$ and the recommended waiting time after the last dose (12 hours), administration of I.V. oxytocin can be initiated.

Recently, misoprostol, a prostaglandin E$_1$ analog, has been used for preinduction cervical ripening and labor induction. Although the U.S. Food and Drug Administration has not approved its use for these indications, it is being used more frequently. Misoprostol is less expensive and is stable at room temperature. Uterine hyperstimulation has not been a problem when a dosage of 25 mcg is used every 4 hours (for a maximum of six doses in a 24-hour time period). Be sure to follow your facility's protocol for use of misoprostol.

## INDICATIONS

➤ To induce a patient with premature rupture of membranes if maternal temperature is rising, if the patient is at term with a positive cervical culture for group B beta hemolytic streptococci, or if the management plan is to impose a limited number of hours before delivery

➤ To induce a patient with chorioamnionitis, severe pregnancy-induced hypertension, maternal diabetes mellitus, polyhydramnios (the accumulation of an excessive amount of amniotic fluid), oligohydramnios (too little amniotic fluid), or Rh incompatibility (fetus is being sensitized due to blood type incompatibility between the mother and fetus)
➤ To induce a patient who is postterm with gestational age past 42 weeks
➤ To induce a patient in which fetal demise has occurred
➤ To induce labor when the biophysical profile score is less than eight (See *Understanding the biophysical profile score.*)

## CONTRAINDICATIONS

### Absolute
➤ Patients with low-lying or marginal placentas or with any vaginal bleeding
➤ Patients in whom oxytocic drugs are contraindicated or where prolonged contractions of the uterus are considered inappropriate
➤ History of cesarean section or major uterine surgery
➤ A clinical suspicion or definite evidence of fetal compromise where delivery is not imminent
➤ Known hypersensitivity to prostaglandins
➤ Evidence of cephalopelvic disproportion
➤ A history of six or more term pregnancies
➤ Active herpes genitalis
➤ Patients receiving oxytoxic drugs
➤ Nonvertex presentations
➤ History of difficult labor or traumatic delivery

### Relative
➤ Fetal demise after 28 weeks' gestation
➤ With fetal demise, PGE$_2$ is contraindicated in the case of maternal cyanotic or ischemic cardiac disease, or severe asthma

► Use of PGE$_2$ with a history of asthma, glaucoma, or increased intraocular pressure, renal, or hepatic dysfunction

## EQUIPMENT

PGE$_2$ administered with a 20-mm endocervical catheter if the cervix is not effaced or a 10-mm endocervical catheter if the cervix is 50% effaced ◆ sterile speculum ◆ sterile gloves ◆ external electronic fetal monitor ◆ linen-saver pads

## ESSENTIAL STEPS

► Explain the procedure to the patient and its risks and benefits.
► Answer any questions the patient may have and obtain consent for the procedure.
► Have the patient empty her bladder prior to the examination.
► Identify and record the fetal heart rate (FHR) with an external fetal monitor. Continue to monitor FHR throughout the procedure and after the procedure following your facility's protocol.
► Help the patient into the lithotomy position with slight elevation, placing the patient's feet in stirrups with her buttocks near the end of the table as for a vaginal examination.
► Place a linen-saver pad under the buttocks.
► Wash your hands and put on sterile gloves. Using a sterile speculum, locate the cervix.
► Apply the PGE$_2$ preparation or misoprostol.
► After the procedure, return the patient to a supine or semi-Trendelenburg position for 15 to 30 minutes to minimize leakage. Then return patient to a more comfortable position while monitoring the FHR and contractions following your facility's protocol. At a minimum, the FHR should be monitored by external fetal monitor for at least 30 minutes and for up to 2 hours

## UNDERSTANDING THE BIOPHYSICAL PROFILE SCORE

A biophysical profile is a real-time ultrasound performed for a maximum of 30 minutes. In conjunction with a nonstress test (NST), a biophysical score is able to identify a healthy or compromised fetus and helps in the development of rational management schemes. Frequency of biophysical profiling should be based on the clinical circumstances for each individual case.

Parameters included in the biophysical profile are:
► fetal tone (fisted hand, fat folds in neck, flexion of extremities)
► fetal movement
► fetal breathing
► amniotic fluid volume
► fetal heart rate activity (28 to 32 weeks' gestation) usually performed by NST.

Each parameter is given either two points or zero, with a healthy score being ten points. Amniotic fluid volume is the most profound criteria. It is measured in quadrants of the uterus. An amniotic fluid volume of less than 5 ml indicates oligohydraminos, and induction should be considered (this finding would receive a score of zero in the biophysical profile). A volume of more than 23 ml indicates polyhydraminos and requires careful observation, as it may lead to preterm labor.

In understanding the management with relation to the biophysical profile, the risk of asphyxia is extremely rare in scores of:
► 10 out of 10
► 8 out of 10 (normal fluid)
► 8 out of 8 (NST not done).

**Alert**
If the test result is 8 out of 10 (with abnormal fluid), this is a strong indication for intervention. There is probable chronic fetal compromise.

after the PGE$_2$ is placed in the endocervical canal.

## PATIENT TEACHING

➤ Tell the patient that the dosage can be repeated in 6 hours for a maximum of three doses.
➤ Tell the patient that labor will usually ensue within 12 hours.

## COMPLICATIONS

➤ If *uterine hyperstimulation* occurs, the woman should be placed on her left side and oxygen should be administered. If uterine hyperstimulation persists, a tocolytic agent may be used to reverse the action of the prostaglandin.
➤ *Hypertonus* or *maternal fluid overload* can occur, and the patient should be vigilantly observed.

## SPECIAL CONSIDERATIONS

➤ Oxytocin may be started 12 hours after the last dose of prostaglandin.
➤ If $PGE_2$ gel is to be used in the case of fetal demise after 28 weeks' gestation, use caution due to risk of uterine rupture.
➤ An interval of 6 hours before repeating the dose or 12 hours before starting I.V. oxytocin or a maximum cumulative dose of 1.5 mg (0.5 mg of gel in three applications) in 24 hours is recommended to avoid hyperstimulation.
➤ Gel should not be placed above the internal cervical os; this may lead to hyperstimulation.

## DOCUMENTATION

➤ Document the indication for the procedure, along with the date and time and how the patient tolerated it.
➤ Record FHR and establish a baseline prior to the administration of prostaglandin. Record maternal vital signs and fetal response to the administration of the medication. Document the contraction pattern

hourly or more frequently, as conditions warrant.

# Oxytocin administration

CPT CODE
No specific code has been assigned.

## DESCRIPTION

The hormone oxytocin stimulates the uterus to contract, thereby facilitating cervical dilation. Oxytocin (Pitocin or Syntocinon) may be indicated to induce or augment labor or to control bleeding and enhance uterine contraction after the placenta is delivered. Usually, you'll administer oxytocin I.V. To regulate dosage and to help prevent uterine hyperstimulation, always use an infusion pump. Additional responsibilities include managing the infusion and monitoring maternal and fetal responses.

## INDICATIONS

➤ To induce a patient with pregnancy-induced hypertension, prolonged gestation, maternal diabetes, Rh sensitization, premature or prolonged rupture of membranes, incomplete or inevitable abortion, or fetal distress after 31 weeks' gestation

## CONTRAINDICATIONS

### Absolute
➤ Placenta previa
➤ Diagnosed cephalopelvic disproportion
➤ Fetal distress
➤ Prior classic uterine incision or uterine surgery
➤ Active genital herpes

## Relative

➤ Overdistended uterus or a history of cervical surgery, uterine surgery, or grand multiparity

## EQUIPMENT

Administration set for primary I.V. line ◆ infusion pump and tubing ◆ I.V. solution ◆ external or internal fetal monitoring equipment ◆ oxytocin ◆ 20G 1″ needle ◆ label ◆ venipuncture equipment ◆ autosyringe (optional) ◆ 20G angiocath

## PREPARATION OF EQUIPMENT

➤ Prepare the oxytocin solution. Rotate the I.V. bag to disperse the drug throughout the solution. Label the I.V. container with the name of the medication. Then attach the infusion pump tubing to the I.V. container, and connect the tubing to the pump.

➤ Because infusion pump features vary, review the operator's manual before proceeding. Attach the 20G 1″ needle to the tubing to piggyback it to the primary I.V. line, or use an autosyringe connected to the primary I.V. line. Then set up the equipment for internal or external fetal monitoring.

## ESSENTIAL STEPS

➤ Explain the procedure to the patient and provide privacy. Wash your hands. Describe the equipment, and forewarn the patient that she may feel a pinch from the venipuncture.

### Administering oxytocin during labor and delivery

➤ Help the patient to a lateral-tilt position, and support her hip with a pillow. Don't let her lie supine. In the supine position, the gravid uterus presses on the maternal great

vessels, producing maternal hypotension and reduced uterine perfusion.

➤ Identify and record the fetal heart rate (FHR), and assess uterine contractions occurring in a 20-minute span to establish baseline fetal status and evaluate spontaneous maternal uterine activity.

➤ Start the primary I.V. line using at least a 20G angiocath. Use this line to deliver not only oxytocin but also fluids, blood, or other medications as needed.

➤ Piggyback the oxytocin solution (metered by the infusion pump) to the primary I.V. Using the Y injection site nearest the venipuncture ensures that the primary line holds the lowest concentration of oxytocin if you must stop the infusion.

➤ Begin the oxytocin infusion. The typical recommended labor-starting dose ranges between 0.5 and 1.0 mU/minute. (The maximum dose is 20 mU/minute.)

➤ Because oxytocin begins acting immediately, be prepared to start monitoring uterine contractions.

➤ Increase the oxytocin dosage as indicated. As a rule, each increase should range no more than 1 to 2 mU/minute infused once every 30 to 60 minutes. When induced labor simulates normal labor (contractions occurring every 2 to 3 minutes and lasting 40 to 60 seconds) and cervical dilation progresses at least 1 cm/hour in first-stage, active-phase labor, you can stop increases. However, continue the infusion at the dosage and rate that maintain the activity closest to normal labor.

➤ Before each increase, be sure to time the frequency and duration of contractions, palpate the uterus to identify contraction intensity, and assess maternal vital signs and fetal heart rhythm and rate to ensure safety and to anticipate possible complications. If you're using an external fetal monitor, the uterine activity strip or grid should show contractions occurring every 2 to 3 minutes. The contractions should last for about 60 seconds and be followed by uterine relaxation. If you're using an internal fetal monitor, look for an optimal baseline value ranging from 5 to 15 mm Hg. Your aim is to verify uterine relaxation between contractions.

➤ Assist with comfort measures, such as repositioning the patient on her other side, as needed.

➤ Continue assessing maternal and fetal responses to the oxytocin. For example, every 10 to 15 minutes, evaluate FHR, maternal response to increased contraction activity and subsequent discomfort, and maternal pulse rate and pattern, blood pressure, respiration rate and quality, and uterine contractions. Also, review the infusion rate to prevent uterine hyperstimulation. Signs of hyperstimulation include contractions less than 2 minutes apart and lasting 90 seconds or longer, uterine pressure that doesn't return to baseline between contractions, and intrauterine pressure that rises over 75 mm Hg.

➤ To reduce uterine irritability, try to increase uterine blood flow. Do this by changing the patient's position and increasing the infusion rate of the primary I.V. line. Avoid exceeding the maximum total infusion of 20 mU/minute.

➤ To manage hyperstimulation, discontinue the infusion and administer oxygen.

➤ After hyperstimulation resolves, resume the oxytocin infusion. Depending on maternal and fetal conditions, select one of the following methods: resume the infusion beginning with oxytocin 0.5 mU/minute, increase the dosage to 1 mU/minute every 15 minutes, and increase the rate, as before; resume the infusion at one-half of the last dosage given and increase the rate as before; or resume the infusion at the dosage given before hyperstimulation signs occurred. Check your facility's policy for the appropriate method.

➤ Monitor and record intake and output. Output should be at least 30 ml/hour. Oxytocin has an antidiuretic effect at rates of 16 mU/minute and more, so you may need to administer an electrolyte-containing I.V. solution to maintain electrolyte balance.

## Administering oxytocin after delivery

➤ After delivery, administer 10 to 40 units of oxytocin added to 1,000 ml of physiologic electrolyte solution. Infuse at a rate titrated to decrease postpartum bleeding or uterine atony after placental delivery. As an alternative, administer 10 units of oxytocin I.M. until you can establish an I.V. line.

## PATIENT TEACHING

➤ Talk to the patient and her support person as you proceed, letting them know what you're doing and that the procedure is producing the expected results.

## COMPLICATIONS

➤ *Uterine hyperstimulation* can be caused by oxytocin and may progress to tetanic contractions, which last longer than 2 minutes. Other potential complications include *fetal distress, abruptio placentae,* and *uterine rupture.* All indicate a need for collaboration or referral to a specialist.

➤ *Maternal seizures* or *coma* from water intoxication can result from oxytocin. Watch for signs of oxytocin hypersensitivity, such as *elevated blood pressure.* This requires immediate cessation of oxytocin and contact with your collaborating physician.

## SPECIAL CONSIDERATIONS

➤ Most facilities require use of an infusion pump to ensure accurate dosage and titration.

➤ Without an infusion pump, administer oxytocin through a minidrop system (60 drops/ml) or an autosyringe, and observe the patient closely. Without an electronic fetal monitor, frequently palpate and assess contractions. Auscultate FHR every 5 to 15 minutes.

## DOCUMENTATION

➤ Record maternal response to contractions, blood pressure, pulse rate and pattern, and respiratory rate and quality on the labor progression chart.
➤ Document FHR, oxytocin infusion rate, and intake and output amounts.
➤ Describe uterine activity.

# Amniotomy

CPT CODE
No specific code has been assigned.

## DESCRIPTION

In amniotomy, you'll use a sterile amniohook to rupture the amniotic membranes. This controversial but common procedure prompts amniotic fluid drainage, which enhances the intensity, frequency, and duration of uterine contractions by reducing uterine volume.

Amniotomy is performed to induce or augment labor when the membranes fail to rupture spontaneously. This procedure helps to expedite labor after dilation begins and helps to facilitate the insertion of an intrauterine catheter and a spiral electrode for direct fetal monitoring.

Oxytocin infusion may precede amniotomy or follow it by 6 to 8 hours if labor fails to progress. If birth doesn't occur within 24 hours after amniotomy, the physician may decide to perform a cesarean section to reduce the risk of infection.

When deciding whether to perform amniotomy, you should consider such factors as fetal presentation, position, and station; the degree of cervical dilation and effacement; contraction frequency and intensity; the fetus's gestational age; existing complications; and maternal and fetal vital signs.

## INDICATIONS

➤ To promote labor failing to progress

## CONTRAINDICATIONS

### Absolute
➤ The presenting fetal part is unengaged (because of the risk of transverse lie and umbilical cord prolapse)

### Relative
➤ High-risk pregnancies, unless more accurate fetal assessment using internal fetal monitoring is necessary

## EQUIPMENT

Povidone-iodine solution ◆ linen-saver pads ◆ bedpan ◆ soap and water ◆ 4″× 4″ gauze pads ◆ external electronic fetal monitoring equipment or a fetoscope or Doppler stethoscope ◆ two pairs of sterile gloves ◆ sterile amniohook

## ESSENTIAL STEPS

➤ Explain the procedure, answer the patient's questions, and obtain informed consent.
➤ Wash your hands and put on sterile gloves.
➤ Clean the perineum with soap and water or 4″× 4″ gauze pads moistened with povidone-iodine solution.
➤ Position the patient and the bedpan so that the bedpan receives the amniotic fluid. Then elevate the head of the bed about 25 degrees. Alternatively, place linen-saver pads under the patient if the bedpan is too

## UNDERSTANDING AMNIOINFUSION

Amnioinfusion is the intrapartal administration of warmed saline solution into the uterus via a hollow intrauterine pressure catheter. This procedure increases the fluid around the fetus and cushions the umbilical cord.

Amnioinfusion is used to relieve severe or prolonged variable decelerations caused by umbilical cord compression, particularly in patients with oligohydramnios or premature rupture of the membranes. It's also used to dilute and lavage meconium from the uterus and, occasionally, to administer antibiotics.

### Assembling the equipment
Gather the following items:
➤ 1,000 ml of normal saline solution, pre-warmed to 98.6° F (37° C)
➤ intrauterine pressure catheter
➤ infusion pump
➤ tubing.

### Administering the infusion
➤ Attach the infusion tubing to an infusion pump.
➤ Insert the intrauterine catheter.
➤ Next, attach the tubing to the catheter.

➤ As ordered, administer a loading volume — usually 10 ml/minute (600 ml/hour) — for 1 hour. Continue to administer the infusion at the ordered rate — usually 60 to 120 ml/hour.

### Special considerations
➤ Be aware that the duration of the infusion and the total amount of saline solution infused will depend on the patient's condition and the nature of her problem.
➤ Make sure that continuous fetal and maternal monitoring are maintained.
➤ Measure and record intrauterine pressures every 15 to 30 minutes.
➤ Measure the amount of fluid leaking from the vagina to help prevent polyhydramnios.
➤ Change the patient's underpads frequently because of the constant fluid leakage.
➤ If variable decelerations persist, consult with your collaborating physician immediately.

### Minimizing complications
Possible complications of amnioinfusion include uterine overdistention and an increase in the uterine resting tone. Releasing some of the fluid can help relieve these problems.

uncomfortable, and then permit the amniotic fluid to drain on the linen-saver pads.
➤ Note the baseline fetal heart rate (FHR). Use external fetal monitoring throughout the procedure. Alternatively, use the fetoscope or Doppler stethoscope before and after the procedure.
➤ Using aseptic technique, open the amniohook package. Change into a second pair of sterile gloves, remove the amniohook from the package.
➤ If indicated, have an assistant apply pressure to the uterine fundus as you insert the amniohook vaginally to the cervical os. This helps to keep the fetal presenting part engaged and reduces the risk of cord prolapse. Then, carefully avoiding contact with the fetal presenting part, rupture the amniotic membrane at the internal os.
➤ If not using external electronic fetal monitoring equipment, use a fetoscope or Doppler stethoscope to evaluate FHR for at least 60 seconds after the membrane ruptures to detect bradycardia. Otherwise, check the monitor tracing for large, variable decelerations in FHR that suggest cord compression. If these FHR changes occur, perform a vaginal examination to check for cord prolapse. For cord compression, consider performing amnioinfusion. (See *Understanding amnioinfusion.*)
➤ Clean and dry the perineal area, and remove the bedpan. When necessary, replace the linen-saver pad.

➤ Inspect the amniotic fluid for meconium, blood, or foul odor. Note the color and measure the amount of fluid.

➤ Monitor the patient's temperature every 2 hours to detect possible infection. If her temperature rises to 100° F (37.8° C), begin hourly checks. Continue to monitor uterine contractions and labor progress.

## PATIENT TEACHING

➤ Tell the patient that amniotomy is done for one of three reasons: to induce or speed labor, to check for meconium, or to place the internal fetal monitor on the neonate's scalp.

➤ Talk to the patient and her support person as you proceed, letting them know what you're doing and that the procedure is producing the expected results.

➤ Reassure the patient that while some patient's find this painful, most notice hardly any discomfort when amniotomy is performed.

➤ Inform the patient that while amniotomy increases some risks such as the possibility of a cord prolapse, these may be minimized by bedrest until delivery.

## COMPLICATIONS

➤ *Umbilical cord prolapse* — a life-threatening potential complication of amniotomy — is an emergency requiring immediate cesarean delivery to prevent fetal death. It occurs when amniotic fluid, gushing from the ruptured sac, sweeps the cord down through the cervix. The risk of prolapse is higher if the fetal head is not engaged in the pelvis before the rupture occurs.

➤ *Intrauterine infection* can result from failure to use aseptic technique for amniotomy or from prolonged labor after amniotomy.

## SPECIAL CONSIDERATIONS

➤ During a vaginal examination after amniotomy, maintain strict aseptic technique to prevent uterine infection. For the same reason, minimize the number of vaginal examinations.

## DOCUMENTATION

➤ Document the date and time of the procedure.

➤ Record FHR before, and at frequent intervals immediately after, amniotomy (every 5 minutes for 20 minutes and then every 30 minutes).

➤ Note the appearance of the amniotic fluid, particularly the presence of any meconium or blood.

➤ Measure the amount of fluid, and note whether the fluid has an odor.

## Emergency delivery

CPT CODES
59409   *Vaginal delivery only (with or without forceps or episiotomy)*
59410   *Vaginal delivery only (with or without forceps or episiotomy) plus postpartum care*

## DESCRIPTION

Emergency delivery, the unplanned birth of a neonate outside of a health care facility, may occur when labor progresses very quickly or when circumstances prevent the patient from entering a facility. Whether assisting at an emergency delivery or instructing the person who is, your objectives include establishing a clean, safe, and private birth area; promoting a controlled delivery; and preventing injury, infection, and hemorrhage.

# EQUIPMENT

Unopened newspaper or large, clean cloth (such as a tablecloth, towel, or curtain) ◆ bath towel, blanket, or coat (to cushion and support the patient's buttocks) ◆ gloves ◆ at least two small, clean cloths ◆ clean, sharp object for cutting (such as a pair of scissors, new razor blade, knife, or nail file) ◆ ligating material (such as string, yarn, ribbon, or new shoelaces) ◆ clean blanket or towel (to cover the neonate) ◆ boiling water

# PREPARATION OF EQUIPMENT

➤ Boil the ligating and cutting materials for at least 5 minutes, if possible.

# ESSENTIAL STEPS

➤ Offer support and reassurance to help relieve the patient's anxiety. Encourage the patient to pant during contractions to promote a controlled delivery. To the extent possible, provide privacy, wash your hands, and put on gloves.
➤ Position the patient comfortably on a bed, a couch, or the ground. Open the newspaper or the large, clean cloth and place it under the patient's buttocks to provide a clean delivery area. Elevate the buttocks slightly with the bath towel, blanket, or coat to provide additional room for delivery.
➤ Check for any combination or all of these signs of imminent delivery — bulging perineum, an increase in bloody show, urgency to push, or crowning of the presenting part.
➤ As the fetal head reaches and begins to pass the perineum, instruct the patient to pant or blow through the contractions because bearing down forcefully could cause extensive maternal lacerations. Place one hand gently on the perineum to cover the fetal head, control birth speed, and prevent sudden expulsion.

➤ Avoid forcibly restraining fetal descent because undue pressure can cause cephalohematoma or scalp lacerations, head trauma, and vagal stimulation. Undue pressure may also occlude the umbilical cord, which may cause fetal bradycardia, circulatory depression, and hypoxia.
➤ As the fetal head emerges, immediately break the amniotic sac if it's intact. Support the head as it emerges. Instruct the patient to continue blowing and panting.
➤ Locate the umbilical cord. Insert one or two fingers along the back of the emerging head to be sure the cord isn't wrapped around the neck. If the cord is wrapped loosely around the neck, slip it over the head to prevent strangulation during delivery. If it's wrapped tightly around the neck, ligate the cord in two places. Then carefully cut between the ligatures, using a clean, sharp object or, if possible, a sterile one.
➤ Carefully support the head with both hands as it rotates to one side (external rotation). Gently wipe mucus and amniotic fluid from the nose and mouth in a downward motion with a clean, small cloth to prevent aspiration.
➤ Instruct the patient to bear down with the next contraction to aid delivery of the shoulders. Position your hands on either side of the neonate's head, and support the neck. Exert gentle downward pressure to deliver the upper shoulder. Then exert gentle upward pressure to deliver the lower shoulder. Don't force the shoulder — this could damage the neonate's spinal cord. Instead, wait for the patient to bear down again. (See *Delivering the neonate's shoulders*.)

 **ALERT** Remember that amniotic fluid and vernix are slippery, so take care to support the neonate's body securely after freeing the shoulders. Cup one hand around the head and grasp the buttocks or feet as they emerge.

## DELIVERING THE NEONATE'S SHOULDERS

Depending on the neonate's size, delivering the shoulders may be rapid or slow. You should deliver the shoulders with the contraction following that which frees the head. Tell the patient to breathe quickly four times, exhaling as if she's blowing out a candle, then to push hard.

Place a hand on either side of the neonate's head for support. As the contraction begins, gently guide the neonate's head downwards to deliver the upper shoulder, as shown.

Then, at the next contraction, guide the neonate's head upward to help deliver the lower shoulder, as shown.

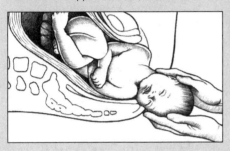
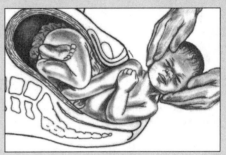

➤ Keep the neonate in a slightly head-down position to encourage mucus to drain from the respiratory tract. Wipe excess mucus from his face. If the neonate doesn't breathe spontaneously, gently pat the soles of his feet or stroke his back. Never suspend a neonate by his feet.
➤ Note the time of delivery.
➤ Dry and cover the neonate quickly with the blanket or towel. Ensure that his head is well covered to minimize exposure and heat loss.

 **ALERT** Cradle the neonate at the level of the maternal uterus until the umbilical cord stops pulsating. This prevents the neonatal blood from flowing to or from the placenta and leading to hypovolemia or hypervolemia, respectively. Hypovolemia can lead to circulatory collapse and neonatal death; hypervolemia can cause hyperbilirubinemia.
➤ Place the neonate on the mother's abdomen in a slightly head-down position. Encourage the mother to start breast-feeding right away if she wants to. Skin-to-skin

contact will warm the neonate. Cover the patient and neonate with a warm blanket, but leave the patient's legs uncovered so you can deliver the placenta.
➤ Ligate the umbilical cord at two points, 1″ to 2″ (2.5 to 5 cm) apart. Place the first ligature 4″ to 6″ (10 to 15 cm) from the neonate. Ligation prevents autotransfusion, which may cause hemolysis and hyperbilirubinemia.
➤ Cut the umbilical cord between the two ligatures, using sterile equipment if available.
➤ Watch for signs of placental separation, such as a slight gush of dark blood from the vagina, cord lengthening, and a firm uterine fundus rising within the abdominal area. Usually, the placenta separates from the uterus within 5 minutes after delivery (though it may take as long as 30 minutes). When you see these signs, encourage the patient to bear down to expel the placenta. As she does, apply gentle downward pressure on her abdomen to aid placental delivery. Never tug on the

umbilical cord to initiate or aid placental delivery because this may invert the uterus or sever the cord from the placenta.

➤ Examine the expelled placenta for intactness. Retained placental fragments may cause hemorrhage or lead to intrauterine infection.

➤ Place the cord and the placenta inside the towel or blanket covering the neonate to provide extra warmth and also to ensure that the cord and placenta will be transported to the hospital for closer examination.

➤ Palpate the maternal uterus to make sure it's firm. Gently massage the atonic uterus to encourage contraction and prevent hemorrhage. Encourage breast-feeding, if appropriate, to stimulate uterine contraction.

➤ Check the patient for excessive bleeding from perineal lacerations. Apply a perineal pad, if available, and instruct the patient to press her thighs together. Provide comfort and reassurance, and offer fluids if available. Have someone summon an emergency medical service or arrange transportation to the hospital for the patient and neonate. Make sure that the patient and neonate are warm and dry while they await transport.

## PATIENT TEACHING

➤ Provide information to patient and her support person as appropriate. (See *How to handle your baby* and *How to breast-feed your baby*, pages 410 and 411.)

➤ As you perform each step, calmly explain what you're doing to the patient. If a support person is present, encourage him to help the patient focus on her breathing. Initially, she'll need to take small panting breaths. As the baby emerges she needs to breathe quickly four times, exhaling as if she's blowing out a candle, then taking a deep breath as she bears down.

## SPECIAL CONSIDERATIONS

➤ Maintain a warm environment and close all doors and windows to prevent heat loss from the neonate.

➤ Never introduce any object into the vagina to facilitate delivery. This increases the risk of intrauterine infection as well as injury to the cervix, uterus, fetus, cord, or placenta.

➤ In a breech presentation, make every effort to transport the patient to a nearby hospital. If the patient begins to deliver, carefully support the fetal buttocks with both hands. Gently lift the body to deliver the posterior shoulder. Then lower the neonate slightly to deliver the anterior shoulder. Flexion of the head usually follows. Never apply traction to the body to avoid lodging the head in the cervix. Allow the neonate to rotate and emerge spontaneously.

➤ If the umbilical cord emerges first, elevate the presenting part throughout delivery to prevent occluding the cord and causing fetal hypoxia. This obstetric emergency usually necessitates a cesarean section.

➤ If the neonate fails to breathe spontaneously after birth, begin to breathe for him. Place your open mouth over his nose and mouth. Using air collected in your cheeks, deliver four short puffs. Next, check the umbilical cord for pulsation. If you find no pulse, begin cardiopulmonary resuscitation (CPR). Place your index and middle fingers over the lower third of the neonate's sternum. The other hand supports the back with the fingers encircling the torso. Administer a breath of air; then use your fingers gently but firmly to pump the heart making sure the chest wall returns to its relaxed position between compressions. Pump five times for each breath of air delivered for a rate of 100 beats/minute. Continue performing CPR until the neonate breathes and his heart beats.

➤ Some patients prefer to squat or sit at the edge of a chair, letting gravity aid the

*(Text continues on page 412.)*

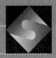

DEAR PATIENT:

New parents often worry about handling fragile-looking newborns or active older babies. The following tips will help you lift and hold your baby safely.

**Lifting your baby**

1 If your baby is lying on his stomach, turn him onto his back by supporting his head and neck with your palm while keeping your arm alongside his body. Put your other hand under his body and roll him onto his back, taking care not to pin his arm under him.

2 To lift him, support his head, neck, and shoulders with your lower hand and arm, keeping your thumb over his shoulder and your fingers under his arms. Reach under his legs and grasp his thighs and buttocks with your other hand, creating two points of contact. Now lift.
    *Never* lift him by his arms.

**Cradle hold**

Cradle the baby's head in the bend of your elbow, with your forearm around the outside of his body and your fingers holding his outer leg. Support his back and buttocks with your opposite hand and forearm.

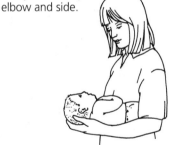

**Shoulder hold (burping position)**

Hold the baby against your chest and shoulder with one hand supporting his buttocks and the other hand supporting his head and back. Once he has some head control, support just his back with your second hand.

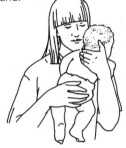

**Football hold**

Support the baby's head and neck in your palm, and support his upper body with your forearm. Hold the rest of his body firmly between your elbow and side.

Never toss a baby into the air or shake him by the shoulders or arms — it can cause brain damage or even death. And never hold a baby on you lap in a car — always put him in a safety seat.

## HOW TO BREAST-FEED YOUR BABY

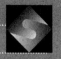

**DEAR MOTHER:**

For most babies, breast milk is the ideal food for the first 6 months of life. But breast-feeding can be awkward and frustrating at first. These pointers will help you get the knack.

**Relax and get comfortable**
After washing your hands, sit with your back straight or bent slightly forward. Support your back with a pillow if you want. Or put a pillow on your lap to raise your baby to breast level. If you've had a cesarean section, you may lie on your side to relieve pressure on your suture line. That way, you can support your baby with your lower arm.

**Feeding your baby**
**1** If you are sitting, rest your baby's head in the crook of your elbow and support his back with your hand as shown. Turn his body — not just his head — to face you. Then cup your breast, fingers under, thumb above.

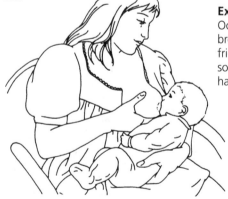

**2** Touch your baby's cheek nearest you to make him turn his head. Then touch your nipple to his mouth to stimulate his rooting and sucking reflexes. He'll open his mouth.

**3** Pull him toward you so your nipple and areola (dark area around the nipple) are in his mouth and the tip of his nose touches the top of your breast. Be sure the entire areola is in his mouth; otherwise, his sucking will be ineffective for him and painful for you.

**4** To remove your baby from your breast, gently pull his chin down or insert a finger into the corner of his mouth to break the suction. Never just pull — it can cause sore nipples.

**5** Let your baby feed from both breasts at each feeding — from 2 to 5 minutes for each breast at first, then 10 to 15 minutes regularly. Remember to burp your baby after he finishes feeding from each breast.

**Expressing breast milk**
Occasionally, you may need to express your breast milk to relieve engorgement or to refrigerate or freeze for later use. Here are some guidelines for expressing your milk by hand or by breast pump.

### Expressing milk by hand

**1** Wash and dry your hands. Apply lotion to them to prevent friction and breast irritation. (But don't rub lotion on the nipple area.) Have a sterilized baby bottle or other container ready.

**2** Massage your breasts to stimulate the milk flow. Place your thumb above the areola and your fingers below it. Then press in toward your chest gently but firmly.

   Squeeze your thumb and fingers together rhythmically, pressing toward the nipple (but not squeezing the nipple itself) until the milk flows into the container. Repeat these actions, rotating your fingers around the areola to empty all milk ducts (20 to 30 minutes for each breast).

### Expressing milk by pump

**1** Using hot, soapy water and a non-scratching brush, clean the pump parts initially and after each use. Rinse them well.

   Read the manufacturer's directions. Then put together the pump.

**2** Wash your hands. Then massage one breast until milk begins to flow, as described above.

**3** Now moisten the inside of the pump's breast cup with warm water, and place your nipple and areola in the cup. Then gently press toward your breast, centering your nipple in the cup, as shown at the top of the next column.

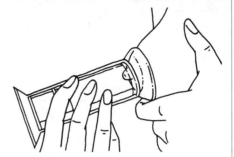

**4** Slowly pump the outside cylinder to keep the milk flowing. Alternate breasts to prevent soreness.

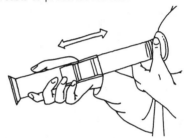

**5** When milk flow decreases, remove the pump and empty the milk into a storage container. Either repeat the procedure on your other breast, or massage the same breast again, and continue pumping until the flow decreases to drops.

   At first, limit pumping to 5 to 10 minutes per breast. Work up to 15 minutes per breast.

### Aftercare

After either breast-feeding or expressing milk, air-dry your nipples. Wear a comfortable, supportive bra. If your breasts leak milk, wear nursing pads or a soft cloth in your bra.

delivery. If that is the case, be prepared to catch the neonate so it won't hit the floor.
➤ Never try to delay the birth or tell the patient to wait. Also, don't deny that the birth is about to take place.

 **ALERT** Never try to deliver a neonate whose foot, arm, or shoulder appears first. The neonate and the mother could die in this situation. Instead, make every effort to get the patient in contact with a more experienced practitioner.

➤ Some neonates emerge quickly and all neonates are very slippery at birth, so cup one hand around the head and grasp the buttocks or feet as they emerge.

## DOCUMENTATION

➤ Give the medical care team the following information, if possible: the time of delivery; the presentation and position of the fetus; any delivery complications, such as the cord wrapped around the neonate's neck; the color, character, and amount of amniotic fluid; and the patient's blood type and Rh factor if known.
➤ Note the time of placental expulsion, the placental appearance and intactness, the amount of postpartum bleeding, the status of uterine firmness (tone) and contractions, and the patient's response.
➤ Document the sex of the neonate, his estimated Apgar score, and any resuscitative measures used.
➤ Record whether the patient began breast-feeding the neonate.
➤ Identify and quantify any fluids given to the patient.

## Episiotomy

CPT CODE
*59300    Episiotomy or vaginal repair, by other than attending physician*

## DESCRIPTION

An episiotomy is an incision into the perineum to enlarge the vaginal opening in preparation for fetal delivery. It is performed in 60% of vaginal deliveries. The American College of Obstetrics and Gynecology no longer recommends routine episiotomy. Instead, efforts should be made to assist the natural thinning of the perineum. Episiotomies are performed during the second stage of labor. The decision to perform an episiotomy is usually made after the fetal cranium has distended the introitus.

There are two types of episiotomy incisions, midline and mediolateral. (See *Episiotomy options*.) After delivery of the placenta, the episiotomy is repaired.

## INDICATIONS

➤ To relieve fetal or maternal distress
➤ To facilitate delivery in patients with significant cardiac disease such as mitral stenosis
➤ To facilitate delivery in patients with a prolonged second stage of labor
➤ To reduce the risk of significant perineal trauma

### Fetal
➤ To aid in delivery of prematurity or breech presentation
➤ To facilitate delivery of a fetus in significant distress during second stage of labor

## CONTRAINDICATIONS

➤ Patient refusal
➤ Severe scarring or peritoneal malformation
➤ Extensive condyloma

## EQUIPMENT

Sterile blunt, sharp scissors ◆ syringe (size dependent on care provider preference)

◆ two pair sterile gloves ◆ local anesthetic ◆ absorbable sutures (such as 2-0 or 3-0 chromic or vicryl absorbable sutures)

## ESSENTIAL STEPS

### To perform an episiotomy

➤ Tell the patient you are about to perform the episiotomy.
➤ Insert the index and middle finger of your gloved, nondominant hand between the fetal scalp and the maternal perineum and gently push the perineum towards the anus. (See *Performing an episiotomy,* page 414.)
➤ Place your thumb on the exterior perineum to define the bottom of the episiotomy.
➤ Administer a local anesthetic if the area is not already sufficiently anesthetized.
➤ Insert the open sterile scissors with one edge under the perineum and cut an incision parallel and between your fingers taking care to protect the fetus and to avoid damaging the external sphincter of the anus.
➤ Extend the incision 2 cm to 4 cm up the vaginal mucosa to prevent tearing.
➤ Continue with delivery.

### To repair an episiotomy

➤ Inspect for tears beyond the initial episiotomy and palpate 6 cm of the rectal mucosa to identify damage to anal sphincter or rectal mucosa.
➤ Put on a new pair of sterile gloves.
➤ Examine the remainder of lower urogenital tract for lacerations not related to the episiotomy.
➤ Examine the episiotomy to make sure that the edges will close evenly.
➤ Suture the vaginal incision starting at the apex on the vaginal incision and run down in locked sutures to the introitus taking care to not enter the rectum.
➤ Approximate the bulbocavernosus at the base of the introitus and insert a crown stitch.

---

### EPISIOTOMY OPTIONS

An episiotomy may be performed using the midline or mediolateral approach, as indicated below.

Infant's head — Midline episiotomy / Mediolateral episiotomy

---

➤ Close the deep perineum with a running stitch down toward the sphincter.
➤ Close the skin of the perineum with a subcuticular stitch.
➤ Alternatively, the deep perineal tissues can be reapproximated with buried interrupted stitches and then closed with a second layer of interrupted sutures before placing the subcuticulars.
➤ Perform a final rectal-to-vaginal examination to verify that rectal mucosa is intact.

## PATIENT TEACHING

➤ Instruct the patient to observe strict perineal cleanliness and spray the area with a peri bottle after each void and defecation. This helps to aid the healing process.
➤ Inform the patient to wash her hands before and after giving herself perineal care.
➤ Tell the patient not to touch stitch area with fingers.

## PERFORMING AN EPISIOTOMY

To minimize bleeding after the episiotomy, wait until a 3- to 4-cm diameter of fetal scalp is visible and delivery is expected within the next three contractions. Using your nondominant hand, insert your index and middle finger between the perineum and the fetal scalp. Your fingers will form a protective barrier between the fetus and the scissors and will be able to feel the anal sphincter. Where the tip of your thumb touches the exterior perineum is the maximum incision length, to minimize the risk of forming a recto-vaginal fistula.

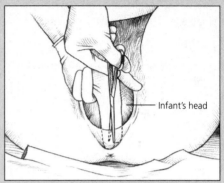

Infant's head

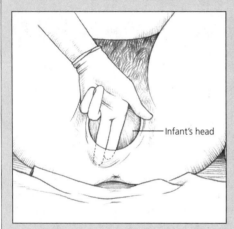

Infant's head

Insert the scissors between your fingers with the cutting edge parallel to your fingers and directed toward the anus. When you are able to fully visualize the area to be cut, make an incision with one stroke from 2 to 4 cm in length.

For routine episiotomy repair, it's crucial to approximate the wound edges well. Using 3-0 polyglycolic thread, place a buried stitch above the apex of the incision line in the vaginal mucosa and tie it. Without cutting the thread, form a continuous buried perineal suture line. Then form a superficial suture line to close off the episiotomy. In the illustration below, the buried suture line is completed and the first superficial suture is being placed.

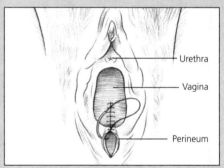

Urethra

Vagina

Perineum

➤ Have the patient fill the entire peri bottle with warm water and empty the entire bottle each time.

➤ Inform the patient to pat or wipe dry from front to back and discard wipe. Repeat with a new wipe if necessary.

➤ Instruct the patient to be careful not to touch the side of sanitary pad that is to be worn next to the perineum.

➤ Have the patient apply the sanitary pad from front to back and snug enough so it won't slide back and forth with movements but not so snug as to be uncomfortable.

➤ Tell the patient to change pads frequently or with each void or defecation.

➤ Have the patient hold a sanitary wipe or sterile 4″ × 4″ pad on the perineum during the first bowel movement to give extra support and to allay fears that the episiotomy repair may split open during defecation.

## HOW TO TAKE A SITZ BATH

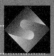

DEAR PATIENT:

Taking a warm-water sitz bath can decrease pain and swelling in the perineal and anal area. What is more, a sitz bath can soothe discomfort and promote healing after surgery or childbirth. Take two or three sitz baths a day, especially after bowel movements and before bedtime. Continue the baths until your symptoms subside and your pain is relieved.

The hospital may give you a sitz bath kit before discharge. Otherwise, you can buy one at a drugstore. The kit contains a plastic pan and a plastic bag with attached tubing. To take a sitz bath, follow these steps:

**1** Raise the toilet seat, and fit the plastic pan over the toilet bowl. Be sure the drainage holes are in back and the single slot is in front.

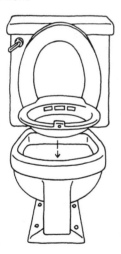

**2** Close the clamp on the plastic bag's tubing, and fill the bag with warm water. If the practitioner ordered medication for your sitz bathwater, add it to the bag now.

**3** Insert the free end of the tubing into the slot at the front of the pan. Then hang the bag on a doorknob or towel bar. Just remember to keep the bag higher than the toilet.

**4** Now, sit in the pan, and open the clamp on the tubing. The warm water will flow from the bag and fill the pan. The excess water will flow out the drainage holes; continue to sit in the pan until the water begins to cool.

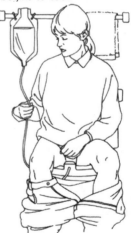

Afterward, dry yourself completely. Apply an ointment or dressing if the practitioner orders it.

➤ Advise the patient to soak in a warm sitz bath for 10 to 20 minutes two or three times per day after the first 24 hours. The warmth of the water increases circulation and promotes healing. (See *How to take a sitz bath*.)

➤ Tell the patient that most patients are nervous or fearful about the first defecation after delivery. This is a common reaction and knowing that they are not the only ones that experience this reaction is helpful to patients. Laxatives are commonly prescribed for patients with an episiotomy or laceration repair.

➤ Have the patient apply witch hazel compresses for 20 to 30 minutes as needed. Witch hazel both reduces edema and has analgesic effects. Compresses can be made by pouring witch hazel on a 4″ × 4″ gauze pad or using a commercial preparation such as Tucks.

➤ Have the patient contact you for signs of infection, severely painful or lumpy breasts, or calf pain or heat that occurs with or without leg edema.

## COMPLICATIONS

➤ *Blood volume loss* — observe the patient carefully and treat with fluid replacement.

➤ *Hematoma formation* may require consultation with your collaborating physician. The hematoma should be opened and drained.

➤ *Infection* is treated with systemic antibiotics.

➤ *Dehiscence* requires collaboration with a physician after immediate application of a nonadherent dressing.

➤ *Extensions (tears)* may require collaboration with a physician for repair.

➤ *Fistulas* may be caused by direct trauma or from infection or necrosis associated with suturing. Referral to a physician may be necessary.

## SPECIAL CONSIDERATIONS

➤ A single cut should be made, not repeated snipping (leaving jagged edges).

➤ The cut should be large enough to meet the purpose for deciding to cut.

➤ The incision should be timed appropriately.

➤ Avoid cutting too early to decrease unnecessary blood loss.

➤ Cut when the perineum is bulging.

➤ Cut when the vaginal orifice is distended and approximately 3 cm of the presenting part is visible between contractions.

➤ Cut when the birth is expected between the next one to three contractions.

➤ Signs and symptoms of infected episiotomies or lacerations include:
– localized or abdominal pain
– dysuria
– low-grade temperature — seldom above 101° F (38.3° C)
– pulse usually below 100 beats per minute
– acute sudden chill and spike in temperature 104° F (40° C)
– edema
– red and inflamed repair edges
– wound separation or dehiscence (bursting open)
– foul or odorous vaginal discharge.

➤ Once perineal pain is determined to be normal, the following measures may help in alleviating it:
– Ice packs or bags should be wrapped in a sterile peri-chux for protection against ice burn. Optimal benefit is achieved if the ice packs are applied for 30 minutes three times per day for the first 24 hours.
– Topical anesthetics such as Dermoplast or Nupercaine may provide relief.

## DOCUMENTATION

➤ Document the indications for episiotomy.

➤ Document that procedure, options, and risks were discussed at length with the patient and the patient wanted an episiotomy performed.

➤ Document any complications, what action was taken, and the outcome. Note whether collaboration or referral takes place, the outcome, and your follow-up evaluation.

# Postpartum fundal assessment

## CPT CODE
*59430 Postpartum care only*

## DESCRIPTION

After delivery, the uterus gradually shrinks and descends into its prepregnancy position in the pelvis — a process known as involution. You'll evaluate normal involutional progress by palpating and massaging the uterus to identify uterine size, firmness, and descent. (See *Hand placement for fundal palpation and massage.*)

Involution normally begins immediately after delivery, when the firmly contracted uterus lies midway between the umbilicus and the symphysis pubis. (See *Fundal height measurement,* page 418.)

When the uterus fails to contract or remain firm during involution, uterine bleeding or hemorrhage can result because placental separation after delivery exposes large uterine blood vessels, which uterine contractions close off (like a tourniquet). Fundal massage, synthetic oxytocic delivery, or natural oxytocic substances released during breast-feeding help to maintain or stimulate contractions.

Typically, fundal palpation and massage are performed while you are caring for the perineum and evaluating healing. (See *Postpartum perineal care,* page 419.)

## INDICATIONS

➤ To evaluate the position of the uterus in the postpartal period

## CONTRAINDICATIONS

None known

## HAND PLACEMENT FOR FUNDAL PALPATION AND MASSAGE

A full-term pregnancy stretches the ligaments supporting the uterus, placing the uterus at risk for inversion during palpation and massage. To guard against this, use your hands to support and fix the uterus in a safe position.

Place one hand against the patient's abdomen at the symphysis pubis level. This steadies the fundus and prevents downward displacement.

Place the other hand at the top of the fundus, cupping it.

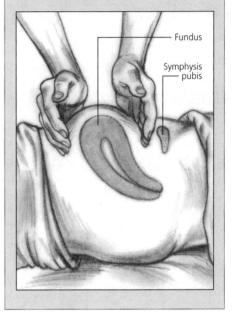

Fundus

Symphysis pubis

## EQUIPMENT

Gloves ◆ analgesics ◆ perineal pad ◆ urinary catheter (optional)

## ESSENTIAL STEPS

➤ Explain the procedure to the patient and answer any questions she may have. Provide privacy. Wash your hands and put on gloves.

## FUNDAL HEIGHT MEASUREMENT

Involution normally begins immediately after delivery, when the firmly contracted uterus lies midway between the umbilicus and the symphysis pubis. Soon the uterus rises to the umbilicus; after the first postpartum day, it begins returning to the pelvis. The average descent rate is 1 cm or fingerbreadth daily — slightly slower if the patient had a cesarean section. By the 10th postpartum day the now unpalpable uterus lies deep in the pelvis, at or below the symphysis pubis.

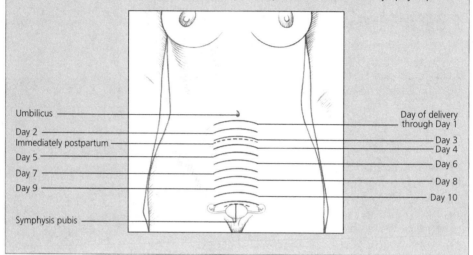

Umbilicus ———
Day 2 ———
Immediately postpartum ———
Day 5 ———
Day 7 ———
Day 9 ———
Symphysis pubis ———

Day of delivery through Day 1
Day 3
Day 4
Day 6
Day 8
Day 10

➤ Generally, schedule fundal assessments every 15 minutes for the 1st hour after delivery, every 30 minutes for the next 2 to 3 hours, every hour for the next 4 hours, every 4 hours for the rest of the first postpartum day, and every 8 hours until the patient's discharge. Offer analgesics before fundal checks if indicated.

➤ Encourage the patient's efforts to urinate because bladder distention impairs uterine contraction by pushing the uterus up and aside. You may need to catheterize the patient if she can't urinate or if the uterus becomes displaced with increased bleeding.

➤ Lower the head of the bed until the patient lies supine. If this position causes discomfort — especially if she has had cesarean surgery — keep the head of the bed slightly elevated.

➤ Expose the abdomen for palpation and the perineum for observation. Watch for bleeding, clots, and tissue expulsion while massaging the fundus.

➤ Gently compress the uterus between both hands to evaluate uterine firmness. Note the level of the fundus above or below the umbilicus in fingerbreadths or centimeters.

➤ If the uterus seems soft and boggy, gently massage the fundus with a circular motion until it becomes firm. Simply cupping the uterus between your hands may also stimulate contraction. Alternatively, massage the fundus with the side of the hand above the fundus. Without digging into the abdomen, gently compress and release, always supporting the lower uterine segment with the other hand. Observe for lochia flow during massage.

➤ Massage long enough to produce firmness. The sensitive fundus needs only gentle pressure. This should produce the desired results without causing excessive discomfort.

➤ Notify the collaborating physician immediately if the uterus fails to contract and if heavy bleeding occurs. If the fundus becomes firm after massage, keep one hand on the lower uterus, and press gently toward the pubis to expel clots.

➤ Clean the perineum, and apply a clean perineal pad. Help the patient into a comfortable position.

## PATIENT TEACHING

➤ Tell the patient that you are measuring the height of the fundus to make sure it is dropping towards a prepregnancy level. Fundal massage will help the uterus contract and decrease bleeding and is done if the fundus is above the umbilicus in the first hour after delivery or feels soft and boggy.

➤ Demonstrate fundal massage so the patient can perform it herself. She supports the lower aspect of the uterus with one hand while gently massaging the top, sides, and front of the fundus by moving the loose abdominal tissues over the fundus.

➤ Teach the patient about the amount, color, and consistency of lochial flow she can expect during the postpartal period.

➤ Advise the patient of the importance of emptying her bladder at regular intervals to prevent urinary retention and promote uterus contraction.

➤ Teach the patient relaxation techniques (such as deep breathing) to help her cope with the discomfort associated with fundal palpation and massage. Advise the patient who has had a cesarean section that there is some discomfort because you are touching near the incision but that this resolves quickly.

## POSTPARTUM PERINEAL CARE

Vaginal birth (which stretches and sometimes tears the perineal tissues) and episiotomy (which may minimize tissue injury) usually leave the patient with perineal edema and tenderness. Postpartum perineal care aims to relieve this discomfort, promote healing, and prevent infection.

Performed after the patient eliminates, perineal hygiene involves cleaning and drying the perineum and assessing the wound area and the lochia (blood and debris sloughed from the placental site and the decidua). Red immediately after delivery, the lochia turns pinkish brown in 4 to 7 days and appears white during the 2nd and 3rd weeks after delivery. This discharge decreases gradually but may continue for up to 6 weeks.

### Cleaning the perineum

Teach the patient to use a water-jet irrigation system or a peri bottle to clean the perineum. Here are the basic steps:

➤ If using a water-jet irrigation system, insert the prefilled cartridge containing antiseptic or medicated solution into the handle, and push the disposable nozzle into the handle until it audibly clicks into place. While sitting on the commode, place the nozzle parallel to the perineum and turn on the unit. Rinse the perineum for at least 2 minutes from front to back. Then turn off the unit, remove the nozzle, and discard the cartridge. Dry the nozzle, and store it appropriately for later use.

➤ If using a peri bottle, fill it with cleaning solution, and pour it over the perineal area.

➤ Stand up before you flush the commode to avoid spraying the perineum with contaminated water.

➤ Apply a new perineal pad before returning to bed. Apply the pad front to back to avoid infection.

➤ Be alert for such signs of infection as unusual swelling, pain, and foul-smelling drainage.

## COMPLICATIONS

➤ *Pain* is the most common complication of fundal palpation and massage because the uterus and its supporting ligaments are usually tender after delivery. Avoid excessive massage which can stimulate premature uterine contractions, causing undue muscle fatigue and leading to uterine atony or inversion.

## SPECIAL CONSIDERATIONS

➤ Because incisional pain makes fundal palpation uncomfortable for the patient who has had a cesarean section, provide pain medication beforehand as ordered. If the lochia flow diminishes after 4 hours, consider performing fewer fundal checks than usual, especially if the patient is receiving oxytocin.
➤ If the patient has had a vertical abdominal incision for a cesarean section, palpate the uterus from the sides to determine tone.
➤ Beware if no lochia appears. This may signal a clot blocking the cervical os. Subsequent heavy bleeding may result if a position change dislodges the clot. Take vital signs to assess for hypovolemic shock. If vital signs are stable, massage with slightly increased pressure to help expel any clots and to help the uterus contract further.

## DOCUMENTATION

➤ Record vital signs, fundal height in centimeters or fingerbreadths, and position (midline or off-center) and tone (firm, or soft and boggy) of the uterus.
➤ Document massage and note the passage of any clots.
➤ Note how the patient tolerated the procedure.
➤ Record excessive bleeding or other complications, your actions, and the outcome.

# NEONATAL PROCEDURES

## DeLee suctioning

CPT CODE
*99440    Newborn resuscitation*

## DESCRIPTION

The objective of DeLee suctioning is to minimize meconium aspiration and to decrease respiratory distress when the possibility of aspiration is high, such as in neonates who are gasping at the time of delivery. This procedure is used to clear secretions from the upper airways and the stomach before delivery of the shoulders occurs.

## INDICATIONS

➤ To remove secretions present in the nose and mouth
➤ To decompress the stomach to decrease the potential for further aspiration of meconium or amniotic fluid prior to the first breath

## CONTRAINDICATIONS

### Absolute
➤ Suspected choanal atresia
➤ Thick, sticky meconium

## EQUIPMENT

DeLee suction device or a #8 or #10 French suction catheter ◆ wall or mechanical portable suction machine that does not exceed –100 mm of mercury (Hg) ◆ small bulb syringe ◆ oxygen apparatus and tubing ◆ 3 or 3.5 mm endotracheal tube ◆ mask ◆ protective eye cover ◆ sterile gloves

## ESSENTIAL STEPS

➤ Wash and prepare as though for a surgical procedure, and apply a mask and protective eye cover. Scrub and glove in the approved manner for your facility.
➤ Check the package for sterility and the suction apparatus for proper functioning suction.
➤ Open the package and unfold the collection trap; attach the suction end of the device to the suction system.
➤ When the patient bears down and the neonate's head presents at the perineum, prior to the delivery of the shoulders, take the bulb syringe and clear out the initial mucus and secretions from the mouth and then the nose.
➤ Keeping the catheter as sterile as possible, insert one finger of your gloved hand with the catheter into the neonate's mouth. Using your gloved finger continue to guide the catheter down the back of the throat until it enters the esophagus and only 5 to 10 cm of the catheter is visible outside the mouth. The catheter should be in the neonate's esophagus.

 **ALERT** You will know that the catheter is in the esophagus if the neonate has not become *more* distressed during this insertion; for example, becoming cyanotic, struggling, or gasping deeply.
➤ Alternatively, you can use a #8 or # 10 French suction catheter instead of the DeLee device. Be sure to crimp the tubing prior to inserting it in the neonate's mouth, and don't uncrimp the tubing until you are ready to apply suction.
➤ Attach the suction end of the DeLee device to the source of suction, and occlude the opening on the device with your thumb. Check the suction reading to ensure that it does not exceed 110 mm of suction. Ap-

ply suction for a few seconds to empty the stomach contents, and then gently but steadily pull back on the catheter to remove it, suctioning as you go.
➤ If time allows, suction secretions from the nares, using the same technique. The actual suctioning should take no more than 10 to 15 seconds.

 **ALERT** Assess for any respiratory distress during this procedure, and, if noted, reposition the neonate's head so that his neck is only slightly hyperextended and more neutral in its position relative to his chest.

## PATIENT TEACHING

➤ Mention to the patient and her support person that the neonate will appear blue and this is to be expected during the first few minutes of life.
➤ Be sure to talk to the patient and her support person as you proceed, telling her what you are doing and that the procedure is producing the results expected.
➤ Await the complete delivery of the neonate prior to reassuring the patient and her support person that all is well. Reassure them that the procedure went well and that the neonate is breathing as expected. Mention that you do not expect the neonate to have any after effects from the procedure.

## COMPLICATIONS

 **ALERT** *Vagal nerve response,* which could cause a transient apnea, bradycardia, and distress may occur any time you insert a tube into a neonate's throat (esophagus or trachea). Remove the catheter immediately and reposition the neonate for optimal airway management. Be sure to have a supply of oxygen at hand and a 3 or 3.5 mm endotracheal tube handy.

➤ *Tissue damage* of the mouth, nose, esophagus, and stomach can occur if suctioning is performed too vigorously or is done with too much suction.

➤ *Apnea* or *respiratory distress* may result from applying suction to the catheter for extended periods of time. Limit suctioning to no more that 10 to 15 seconds at one time.

## SPECIAL CONSIDERATIONS

➤ If the neonate has a tracheoesophageal fistula that is large and of the "H" type, there is a danger that the DeLee catheter could enter the trachea instead of the esophagus. This could result in respiratory distress. Simply removing the catheter should open up the airway again.

➤ Thick, sticky meconium cannot be adequately removed with a DeLee suctioning device. In this instance, you would use the bulb syringe to clear the oral cavity and proceed with the endotracheal tube. If dark, thick meconium is present after the neonate is delivered completely, an endotracheal tube should be inserted into the trachea and deep suctioning performed.

## DOCUMENTATION

➤ Document the time and date of the delivery of the neonate's head, the amount of time the spent suctioning, the maximal amount of suction pressure used, and the results or appearance of the aspirate. Note the approximate quantity of the aspirate and the degree of tenacity or difficulty in removing it from the neonate.

➤ Note that the suctioning was only performed once prior to delivery of the neonate's torso.

➤ Note any respiratory distress and any measures taken to relieve the distress.

➤ Note any instructions for further follow-up of the neonate that were given either to the patient and her support person or to the health care team.

## Apgar scoring

CPT CODE
No specific code has been assigned.

## DESCRIPTION

Named after its developer, Virginia Apgar, the Apgar score quantifies the neonatal heart rate, respiratory effort, muscle tone, reflexes, and color. Each category is assessed 1 minute after birth and again 5 minutes later. Scores in each category range from 0 to 2. The highest Apgar score is 10 — the greatest possible sum of the five categories.

The evaluation at 1 minute indicates the neonate's initial adaptation to extrauterine life. The evaluation at 5 minutes gives a clearer picture of overall status. If the neonate doesn't breathe or his heart rate is less than 100 beats/minute, call for help and begin resuscitation at once without waiting for a 1-minute Apgar test score.

## INDICATIONS

➤ To evaluate the neonate's adaptation to extrauterine life

## CONTRAINDICATIONS

None known

## EQUIPMENT

Apgar score sheet or neonatal assessment sheet ◆ stethoscope ◆ clock with second hand or Apgar timers ◆ gloves

## PREPARATION OF EQUIPMENT

➤ If you use Apgar timers, make sure both timers are on at the instant of birth.

## ESSENTIAL STEPS

➤ Note the exact time of delivery. Wear gloves for protection from blood and body fluids. Dry the neonate to prevent heat loss.
➤ Place the neonate in a 15-degree Trendelenburg position to promote mucus drainage. Then position his head with the nose slightly tilted upward to straighten the airway.
➤ Assess the neonate's respiratory efforts. If necessary, supply stimulation by rubbing his back or gently flicking his foot.

 **ALERT** If the neonate exhibits abnormal respiratory responses, begin neonatal resuscitation according to the guidelines of the American Heart Association and the American Academy of Pediatrics. Then use the Apgar score to judge the progress and success of resuscitation efforts. Should resuscitation efforts prove futile, you'll need to be prepared to meet the patient and her support person's needs, even if they seem unusual or inappropriate to you.

 **CULTURAL TIP** In the Gypsy culture, if the neonate dies, the parents must avoid it and so may leave suddenly. Grandparents may avoid a dead neonate as well to avoid bad luck.

Some Koreans believe that any problems that occur with the neonate may be attributed to what they believe is the mother's incorrect behavior. Although this is obviously not the case, it is important to reassure her and all concerned that no one is to blame.
➤ If the neonate exhibits normal responses, assign the Apgar score at 1 minute after birth.
➤ Repeat the evaluation and record the score at 5 minutes after birth.

## Assessing neonatal heart rate

➤ Using a stethoscope, listen to the heartbeat for 30 seconds, and record the rate. To obtain beats per minute, double the rate. Alternatively, palpate the umbilical cord where it joins the abdomen, monitor pulsations for 6 seconds, and multiply by 10. Assign a 0 for no heart rate, a 1 for a rate under 100 beats/minute, and a 2 for a rate greater than 100 beats/minute.

## Assessing respiratory effort

➤ Count unassisted respirations for 60 seconds, noting quality and regularity (a normal rate is 30 to 50 respirations/minute). Assign a 0 for no respirations; a 1 for slow, irregular, shallow, or gasping respirations; and a 2 for regular respirations and vigorous crying.

## Assessing muscle tone

➤ Observe the extremities for flexion and resistance to extension. This can be done by extending the limbs and observing their rapid return to flexion — the neonate's normal state. Assign a 0 for flaccid muscle tone, a 1 for some flexion and resistance to extension, and a 2 for normal flexion of elbows, knees, and hips, with good resistance to extension.

## Assessing reflex irritability

➤ Observe the neonate's response to nasal suctioning or to flicking the sole of his foot. Assign a 0 for no response, a 1 for a grimace or weak cry, and a 2 for a vigorous cry.

## Assessing color

➤ Observe skin color, especially at the extremities. Assign a 0 for complete pallor and cyanosis, a 1 for a pink body with blue extremities (acrocyanosis), and a 2 for a completely pink body. To assess color in a dark-skinned neonate, inspect the oral mucous membranes and conjunctiva, the lips, the palms, and the soles.

## PATIENT TEACHING

➤ If the patient and her support person don't know about the Apgar score, discuss it with them during early labor, when they will be more receptive to new knowledge. To prevent confusion or misunderstanding at delivery, explain to them what will occur and why. Add that this is a routine procedure.

## COMPLICATIONS

None known

## SPECIAL CONSIDERATIONS

➤ If the neonate requires emergency care, make sure that a member of the delivery team offers appropriate support to the patient.
➤ Closely observe the neonate whose mother receives heavy sedation just before delivery. Despite a high Apgar score at birth, he may show secondary effects of sedation in the nursery. Be alert for depression or unresponsiveness.

## DOCUMENTATION

➤ Record the Apgar score on the Apgar score sheet or the neonatal assessment sheet required by your facility. Be sure to indicate the total score and the signs for which points were deducted to guide postnatal care.

## Eye prophylaxis (Credé's treatment)

CPT CODE
No specific code has been assigned.

## DESCRIPTION

Named for its developer, Credé's treatment prevents damage and blindness from conjunctivitis due to *Neisseria gonorrhoeae*, which is transmitted to the neonate during birth if the mother has gonorrhea. It's also used to treat chlamydial conjunctivitis transmitted during birth.

Required by law in the United States, Credé's treatment consists of instilling 1% silver nitrate solution into the neonate's eyes. Most states permit alternative treatment with 1% tetracycline ointment or 0.5% erythromycin ophthalmic ointment. By this method, the neonate may avoid chemical irritation from silver nitrate yet benefit from the antimicrobial effects of broad-spectrum antibiotics.

You'll instill the solution or ointment in the conjunctival sac (from the eye's inner canthus to its outer canthus). The treatment, which may cause conjunctival swelling, may also disturb the typically quiet but alert neonate at birth. So, although silver nitrate treatment is usually given at delivery, it can be delayed for up to 1 hour to allow initial parent-child bonding.

## INDICATIONS

➤ To prevent *Neisseria gonorrhoeae* infection in all neonates

## CONTRAINDICATIONS

None known

## EQUIPMENT

Silver nitrate ampule or ophthalmic antibiotic ointment ◆ sterile needle or pin supplied by silver nitrate manufacturer (as needed) ◆ gloves

## PREPARATION OF EQUIPMENT

➤ Puncture one end of the wax silver nitrate ampule with the needle or pin. If you're administering ophthalmic antibiotic ointment (such as tetracycline or erythromycin), remove the cap from the ointment container. A single-dose ointment tube should be used to prevent contamination and spread of infection.

## ESSENTIAL STEPS

➤ Wash your hands and put on gloves. To ensure comfort and effectiveness, shield the neonate's eyes from direct light, tilt his head slightly to the side of the intended treatment, and instill the medication. (See *How to instill medication for Credé's treatment.*)
➤ Close and manipulate the eyelids to spread the medication over the eye.

## PATIENT TEACHING

➤ If the patient and her support person are present for the procedure, explain that state law mandates Credé's treatment. Forewarn them that the neonate may cry and that the treatment may irritate his eyes. Reassure them that these are temporary effects.

## COMPLICATIONS

➤ *Chemical conjunctivitis* may cause redness, swelling, and drainage especially after silver nitrate instillation.

## SPECIAL CONSIDERATIONS

➤ Instill another drop if the silver nitrate solution touches only the eyelid or eyelid margins to ensure complete prophylaxis.

### HOW TO INSTILL MEDICATION FOR CREDÉ'S TREATMENT

Using your nondominant hand, gently raise the neonate's upper eyelid with your index finger and pull down the lower eyelid with your thumb. Using your dominant hand, apply the ophthalmic antibiotic ointment, such as tetracycline or erythromycin, in a line along the lower conjunctival sac (as shown). Repeat the procedure for the other eye.

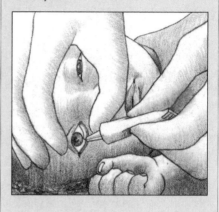

➤ If chemical conjunctivitis occurs or if the skin around the neonate's eyes discolors, reassure the patient that these temporary effects will subside within a few days.

## DOCUMENTATION

➤ If you perform Credé's treatment in the delivery room, record the treatment on the delivery room form.
➤ If you perform the treatment in the nursery, document it in your notes.

# Maternal Procedures

## RhoGAM administration

CPT CODES
*90384    Rh_o(D) immune globulin (RhIG), human (with principal code 90782)*
*90782    Therapeutic injection, intramuscular (specify medication injected)*

## Description

$Rh_o(D)$ human immune globulin (RhoGAM) is a concentrated solution of immune globulin containing $Rh_o(D)$ antibodies. Intramuscular injection of RhoGAM keeps the Rh-negative mother from producing active antibody responses and forming anti-$Rh_o(D)$ to Rh-positive fetal blood cells and endangering future Rh-positive infants. It should be given within 72 hours of precipitating event to prevent future maternal sensitization. Maternal immunization to the Rh antigen commonly results from transplacental hemorrhage during gestation or delivery. If unchecked during gestation, incompatible fetal and maternal blood can lead to hemolytic disease in the neonate. RhoGAM is indicated for the Rh-negative mother with a neonate having $Rh_o(D)$-positive or $D^u$ positive blood and Coombs'-negative cord blood.

## Indications

➤ To treat an Rh-negative patient with low Rh-positive antibody titers
➤ To protect the fetus of an Rh-negative mother

➤ To treat Rh-positive exposure (full-term pregnancy or termination of pregnancy)
➤ To treat Rh-positive exposure resulting from amniocentesis, threatened abortion, abruptio placentae, or abdominal trauma during pregnancy
➤ To treat blood transfusion exposure

## Contraindications

### Absolute
➤ Rh (D)-positive
➤ Previously immunized to Rh (D) blood factor
➤ History of hypersensitive response to human globulin

### Relative
➤ Immunoglobulin A deficiency
➤ More than 72 hours has passed since indication for RhoGAM occurred

## Equipment

3-ml syringe ◆ 22G 1½" needle ◆ RhoGAM vial ◆ alcohol sponges ◆ triplicate form and patient identification (from the blood bank or laboratory)

## Essential Steps

➤ Identify the patient. Explain RhoGAM administration to the patient, and answer her questions.
➤ Obtain a history of allergies and reaction to immunizations.
➤ Two nurses must check the vial's identification numbers and sign the triplicate form that comes with the RhoGAM. Complete the form as indicated. Attach the top copy to the patient's chart. Send the remaining two copies, along with the empty RhoGAM vial, to the laboratory or blood bank.
➤ Withdraw the RhoGAM from the vial with the needle and syringe. Clean the

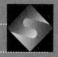

# RECEIVING RHOGAM

DEAR PATIENT,

Your practitioner has recommended that you receive RhoGAM. This sheet reviews why this injection is so important.

## The Rh factor

Rh factor refers to the D antigen that is found on the red blood cells (RBCs) of most people. It is called Rh because it was first discovered in Rhesus monkeys.

People who have the D antigen on their RBCs are called Rh-positive. People without it are called Rh-negative. About 15% of people in the United States are Rh-negative.

## Antibodies

A woman can become sensitized to Rh factor in a number of ways. Contact with small amounts of Rh-positive blood can occur in several ways, including the baby's blood that enter the mother's bloodstream during the course of the pregnancy, during amniocentesis, or abdominal trauma. A transfusion containing the Rh factor can also sensitize the mother. This minute exposure can cause the mother's body to mount a defense against this foreign substance, forming antibodies to the Rh factor. These antibodies seek out any Rh factor and try to eliminate it.

## Rh and pregnancy

These antibodies to Rh factor go throughout the mother's body, and the unborn baby's body. Although the mother may not feel any change, the antibodies may be targeting RBCs in the baby. This destruction of RBCs can cause anemia, high bilirubin levels, and even heart failure in the baby.

With each pregnancy, the Rh-negative mother should undergo screening to determine if she has Rh antibodies.

## How RhoGAM helps

RhoGAM is an injection that contains Rh antibodies. It is given to the Rh-negative mother during pregnancy (around the 28th week) and soon after delivery if the baby is Rh-positive. These antibodies neutralize any Rh-positive RBCs in the mother's blood. This stops the mother's body from developing her own Rh antibodies.

## Adverse effects of RhoGAM

RhoGAM may cause some discomfort at the injection site and a slight chance of a mildly elevated temperature.

## When to receive RhoGAM

RhoGAM is recommended around the 28th week of pregnancy. If the baby is Rh-positive, the mother should receive RhoGAM within 72 hours after delivery.

RhoGAM is recommended after an amniocentesis, ectopic pregnancy, tubal pregnancy, dilatation and curettage (also called a D & C), or any fetal death.

For any additional questions or concerns, speak with your practitioner.

ADDITIONAL INSTRUCTIONS:

.............................................................................

.............................................................................

.............................................................................

.............................................................................

gluteal injection site, and administer the RhoGAM I.M.

➤ Give the patient a card that identifies her Rh-negative status, and instruct her to carry it with her or keep it in a convenient location.

## PATIENT TEACHING

➤ Advise the patient on the importance RhoGAM administration. (See *Receiving RhoGAM*, page 427.)

## COMPLICATIONS

➤ *Fever, myalgia, lethargy, discomfort, splenomegaly,* or *hyperbilirubinemia* may occur after multiple injections (such as given after Rh mismatch). Complications rarely occur after a single RhoGAM injection; when they do, they're mild and confined to the injection site.

## SPECIAL CONSIDERATIONS

➤ After the procedure, watch for redness and soreness at the injection site.

➤ Provide an opportunity for the patient to voice any guilt or anxiety she may feel if she perceives her body as acting against the fetus.

➤ Administration of RhoGAM at approximately 28 weeks' gestation can also protect the fetus of the Rh-negative mother. The dose is determined according to the fetal packed red blood cell (RBC) volume that enters the mother's blood. A volume under 15 ml usually calls for one vial of RhoGAM; a significant fetal-maternal hemorrhage calls for more than one vial if the fetal packed RBC volume is greater than 15 ml.

## DOCUMENTATION

➤ Record the date, the time, and the site of the RhoGAM injection.

➤ If applicable, note the patient's refusal to accept a RhoGAM injection and a summary of the risks that were explained to the patient inherent in that refusal.

➤ Document patient teaching about RhoGAM.

➤ Note that the patient received a card identifying her Rh-negative status.

# NEONATAL AND PEDIATRIC PROCEDURES  9

Caring for neonatal and pediatric patients demands specialized knowledge and skills. Because infants and children lack the physiologic maturity of adults, their response to both illness and treatment increases, and their small size narrows the margin for error in treatment. Additionally, although children tend to recover more rapidly from an illness than adults, they have a higher risk for serious complications.

The neonatal period extends from birth to 28 days. During this time the neonate must adjust to extrauterine life. You need to recognize the neonate's normal physiologic status and be alert for possible problems.

When you treat a child, you need to consider his level of growth and development. For example, a young child has only rudimentary motor skills, limited comprehension, and limited ability to comply with a practitioner's instructions. This makes him especially prone to injury and, for this reason, you need to remain alert to potentially dangerous situations and take steps to ensure the child's safety.

Remember also to include the parents or caregivers in all aspects of their child's care. Encourage them to maintain their roles as caregivers and to continue including the child as a member of the family — especially those with long-term disorders. Doing so will help to achieve one of the overall goals of care — to create a positive environment that promotes the physical and emotional health of the child and his family. Conversely, if a parent or caregiver declines to participate, explore the reasons and try to find an acceptable way for them to be involved. Many parents or caregivers do not want their child to associate them with the painful or traumatizing memory of the procedure. The parents or caregivers may also have feelings of guilt about not being able to prevent pain or discomfort and from not being with their child during the procedure. Your acceptance and support can ease the burden for the parents or caregivers and help develop a strong working relationship with them.

 **CULTURAL TIP** In many cultural groups, problems with a child are not automatically presented to the mother. For instance, when caring for a pediatric patient in Colombian, Cuban, Ethiopian, Filipino, Japanese, Vietnamese, or West Indian cultural groups, discuss how to present medical information to the mother with the father, maternal grandmother, or other family members. In the Iranian culture, it is correct to contact the father to give information and to consult for decisions. In other cultural groups, such as the Hmong and Samoan, the mother and adult female relatives normally deal with the infant's needs. Likewise, Puerto Rican and Russian mothers typically want immediate notification of problems with the infant.

In terms of caring for a child, some Russians believe that it is necessary to keep the baby warm at all times to allow normal bone development and to prevent illness. Covering the baby's head when exposed to environmental changes is a normal practice.

In the Gypsy cultural group, babies are often tightly swaddled and are considered vulnerable to the evil eye, which may evidence itself in fussiness or colic. To undo the evil eye, the person responsible must make a cross with spittle on the baby's forehead. If asked to do this, it is usually best to comply — no blame is assigned if you give the evil eye as it is believed a person can't help it. People with thick eyebrows or lots of body hair are often thought to have the evil eye. Some Gypsies believe that if a baby dies the parents must avoid it and so may leave the situation suddenly. As well, the grandparents may avoid a dead baby to avoid bad luck.

Additionally, some Koreans believe that any problems that occur with the infant may be attributed to what they believe is incorrect behavior on the part of the mother. It is important to reassure the mother and all concerned that no one is to blame.

Other cultural beliefs that may be encountered include Samoan mothers not standing in front of windows with a new baby at night, Southeast Asian mothers and their newborns remaining homebound for the first 40 days; and Muslims shaving their newborn's head.

# TREATMENTS

## Oxygen administration

CPT CODES
*94656   Ventilation assist and management, initiation of pressure or volume*

*preset ventilators for assisted or controlled breathing; first day*
*94657   Ventilation assist and management; subsequent days*
*94660   Continuous positive airway pressure ventilation (CPAP), initiation and management*
*99440   Newborn resuscitation*

## DESCRIPTION

The infant with signs and symptoms of respiratory distress will probably need oxygen. Because of his small size and respiratory requirements, he'll need special equipment and administration techniques.

In an emergency, a handheld resuscitation bag and a small oxygen mask may be sufficient until more permanent measures can be initiated. The oxygen can be delivered by means of an oxygen hood or nasal prongs when the infant requires additional oxygen above the ambient concentration. He may receive oxygen through a nasopharyngeal or an endotracheal (ET) tube if he needs continuous positive airway pressure (CPAP) to prevent alveolar collapse at the end of a breath (as in respiratory distress syndrome). Oxygenation typically improves with CPAP and any pulmonary shunting tends to decrease. If the infant can't breathe on his own or needs to conserve his energy, he may receive oxygen through a ventilator.

Oxygen administration is potentially hazardous to the infant no matter which system delivers the oxygen. The gas must be warmed and humidified to prevent hypothermia and dehydration. Oxygen in high concentrations over prolonged periods can cause retrolental fibroplasia (which results in blindness). If the oxygen concentration is too low, hypoxia and central nervous system damage may occur. Additionally, oxygen can contribute to bronchopulmonary dysplasia, depending on how it's delivered.

In some cases, extracorporeal membrane oxygenation, an alternative to oxygen administration, may help infants who have severe hypoxia. This technique also relies on a supplemental oxygen source.

## INDICATIONS

➤ To treat signs and symptoms of respiratory distress, such as cyanosis, pallor, tachypnea, nasal flaring, bradycardia, hypothermia, retractions, hypotonia, hyporeflexia, expiratory grunting
➤ To treat arterial blood gas (ABG) levels indicating hypoxia

## CONTRAINDICATIONS

No contraindications exist when indications are present.

## EQUIPMENT

Oxygen source (wall, cylinder, or liquid unit) ◆ compressed air source ◆ flowmeters ◆ nasal prongs ◆ blender or Y-connector ◆ large- and small-bore oxygen tubing (sterile) ◆ warming-humidifying device ◆ sterile water ◆ blood gas analyzer ◆ thermometer ◆ stethoscope ◆ nasogastric (NG) tube

### For handheld resuscitation bag and mask delivery
Specially sized mask with manual resuscitation bag ◆ manometer with connectors (the resuscitation bag must have a pressure-release valve)

### For oxygen hood delivery
Appropriate-sized oxygen hood ◆ oxygen analyzer

### For CPAP delivery
Manometer with connectors ◆ nasopharyngeal or ET tube ◆ hypoallergenic tape ◆ water-soluble lubricant

### For delivery with a ventilator
Ventilator unit with manometer and in-line thermometer ◆ specimen tubes for ABG analyses ◆ pulse oximeter or transcutaneous oxygen monitor (optional)

## PREPARATION OF EQUIPMENT

➤ Wash your hands. Gather the necessary equipment and assemble it conveniently.

### To calibrate the oxygen analyzer
➤ Turn the analyzer on, and read the results. Room air should be about 21% oxygen.
➤ Check the analyzer power or battery level.
➤ Expose the analyzer probe to 100% oxygen and adjust sensitivity as necessary. Then recheck the amount of oxygen in room air.

### To set up a manual resuscitation bag and mask
➤ Place the resuscitation bag and mask in the crib.
➤ Connect the large-bore oxygen tubing to the mask outlet. Then use connectors and small-bore tubing to connect a manometer to the bag.
➤ Next, connect the free end of the oxygen tubing to the warming-humidifying device, and fill the device with sterile water.
➤ Turn on the device when ready to use it, or prepare the device according to the manufacturer's instructions.
➤ Connect another piece of small-bore tubing to the inlet of the warming-humidifying device.
➤ Attach a Y-connector to the opposite end of this tubing.
➤ Place a piece of small-bore tubing on each end of the Y-connector, and connect the pieces of tubing to the flowmeters.

➤ Place an in-line thermometer as close as possible to the delivery end of the apparatus.

### To set up an oxygen hood
➤ Bring a clean oxygen hood (and tubing, if needed) to the infant's bedside.
➤ If the infant was receiving oxygen via bag and mask, remove them from the connecting tubing.
➤ Attach the oxygen hood to this tubing.
➤ Place an in-line thermometer as close to the infant as possible whenever using warmed oxygen.

## ESSENTIAL STEPS

➤ Explain the procedure to the parents or caregivers to reduce their anxiety and to ensure cooperation.

### Using a handheld resuscitation bag and mask
➤ Turn on the oxygen and compressed air flowmeters to the prescribed flow rates.
➤ Place the mask on the infant's face. Don't cover the infant's eyes. Check pressure settings and mask size to ensure that air doesn't leak from the mask's edges.
➤ Provide 40 to 60 breaths/minute. Use enough pressure to cause a visible rise and fall of the infant's chest. Provide enough oxygen to maintain pink nail beds and mucous membranes. Deliver the oxygen percentage defined by your facility's protocol.
➤ Continuously watch the infant's chest movements, and listen to breath sounds. Avoid overventilation, which will blow off too much carbon dioxide and cause apnea. If the infant's heart rate falls below 100 beats/ minute and doesn't rise, continue to use the handheld resuscitation bag until the heart rate rises to 100 beats/minute or higher.
➤ Insert an NG tube to vent air from the infant's stomach.

### Using an oxygen hood
➤ Remove the connecting tubing from the face mask, and connect it to the oxygen hood. Activate oxygen and a compressed air source, if needed, at ordered flow rates.
➤ Place the oxygen hood over the infant's head.
➤ Measure the amount of oxygen the infant is receiving with the oxygen analyzer. Be sure to place the analyzer probe close to the infant's nose and set the oxygen rate.

### Using nasal prongs
➤ Match the prong size to the infant's nose. Apply a small amount of water-soluble lubricant to the outside of the prongs. Turn on the oxygen and compressed air, if necessary. Connect the prongs to the oxygen tubing. Insert the prongs into the nose and steady them.

### Using CPAP
➤ Position the infant on his back with a rolled towel under his neck to keep the airway open without hyperextending the neck.
➤ Obtain the correct size tube if you're administering oxygen through a nasopharyngeal or an ET tube. Turn on the oxygen and compressed air source. Insert the ET tube, attach the oxygen delivery system (as set up for mask and bag delivery), and tape the tube in place. Next, insert an NG tube, and leave it in place to keep the stomach decompressed, if indicated. Leave it open unless the infant is receiving gavage feedings. Write orders for suctioning of the nasal passages and oropharynx every 2 hours or as needed to maintain an open airway.

### Using a ventilator
➤ Turn on the ventilator, and adjust the controls.
➤ Insert the ET tube.
➤ Connect the ET tube to the ventilator, and tape the tube securely.

➤ As with any delivery system, carefully watch the manometer to maintain pressure at the prescribed level. Also monitor the in-line thermometer for correct temperature.

➤ Monitor ABG levels every 15 to 20 minutes — or as indicated — after any changes in oxygen concentration or pressure. Draw blood samples for ABG analysis from an umbilical artery catheter, radial artery catheter, or radial artery puncture. If desired, obtain capillary blood by warmed heel stick — this gives accurate levels of pH and carbon dioxide but not oxygen. If indicated, monitor oxygen perfusion with transcutaneous oxygen monitoring, pulse oximetry, or mixed venous oxygen saturation monitoring.

➤ Monitor ABG levels so you can make appropriate changes in oxygen concentration. Usually, partial pressure of oxygen is maintained between 60 and 90 mm Hg for an arterial sample and between 40 and 60 mm Hg for a capillary sample.

➤ Auscultate the lungs for crackles, rhonchi, and bilateral breath sounds.

## PATIENT TEACHING

➤ As soon as possible, explain the situation and the procedures to the parents or caregivers. Review safety precautions to avoid fire or explosion. Explain measures to keep the infant warm because hypothermia impedes respiration.

➤ If the infant will receive oxygen over a lengthy time span, prepare his parents or caregivers to administer oxygen at home. (See *Comparing home oxygen delivery systems*.)

## COMPLICATIONS

➤ *Infection* or *drowning* can result from overhumidification, which allows water to collect in tubing and then provides a growth medium for bacteria or suffocates the infant.

➤ *Hypothermia* and *increased oxygen consumption* can result from administering cool oxygen.

➤ *Metabolic* and *respiratory acidosis* may follow inadequate ventilation.

➤ *Pressure ulcers* may develop on the infant's head, face, and around the nose during prolonged oxygen therapy.

➤ A *pulmonary air leak* (pneumothorax, pneumomediastinum, pneumopericardium, interstitial emphysema) may develop spontaneously with respiratory distress or result from forced ventilation.

➤ *Decreased cardiac output* may come from excessive CPAP.

## SPECIAL CONSIDERATIONS

➤ Check ABG levels at least every hour whenever the unstable infant receives high oxygen concentrations and whenever there is a clinical change. If he doesn't respond to oxygen administration, check for congenital anomalies.

➤ Perform neonatal chest auscultation carefully to hear subtle respiratory changes. Also be alert for respiratory distress signs, and be prepared to perform emergency procedures. If required, perform chest physiotherapy and percussion. Follow with suctioning to remove secretions. You will generally discontinue oxygen when the infant's fraction of inspired oxygen ($FIO_2$) reaches room air level and his arterial oxygen stabilizes between 60 and 90 mm Hg. Repeat ABG analysis 20 to 30 minutes after discontinuing oxygen and thereafter following your facility's protocol.

## DOCUMENTATION

➤ Note any respiratory distress that requires oxygen administration, the oxygen concentration given, and the delivery method.

## COMPARING HOME OXYGEN DELIVERY SYSTEMS

If a neonate is discharged on oxygen, the delivery system prescribed may depend on such factors as equipment availability and parental skill levels. Other factors to consider include the liter flow (or oxygen concentration) required and appropriate administration equipment: nasal cannula or catheter, oxyhood, tent, high-flow mask, or nebulizer.

The nasal cannula, which provides a direct flow of oxygen to the nostrils, is the most common oxygen delivery device for home use. It imposes the fewest restrictions on a child attempting to interact with the environment. For instance, attaching extension tubing (up to 50' [15.2 m]) to the cannula allows the child to move freely from room to room. However, the cannula can become dislodged from the nostrils with extensive manipulation. Velcro straps or adhesive dressings can reduce this risk by securing the cannula in the proper position.

Common oxygen sources include the oxygen concentrator, cylinder oxygen, and liquid oxygen. When selecting the appropriate system, the practitioner looks at advantages and disadvantages.

| SYSTEM | ADVANTAGES | DISADVANTAGES |
| --- | --- | --- |
| OXYGEN CONCENTRATOR | | |
| Separates oxygen from ambient air and provides low-flow oxygen | ➤ Cost-effective for the neonate who needs continuous low-flow oxygen | ➤ Can't be used with a high-flow mask or nebulizer<br>➤ Requires electricity<br>➤ Requires an oxygen cylinder as a backup in case of malfunction or power failure<br>➤ Bulky and noisy<br>➤ Emits heat |
| CYLINDER OXYGEN | | |
| Uses oxygen stored as a gas in a cylinder with a valve | ➤ Cost-effective for the neonate who requires high-flow oxygen or intermittent oxygen for up to 12 hours daily<br>➤ Can be used with a high-flow oxygen mask, a nasal cannula, a nasal catheter, or a nebulizer<br>➤ Portable when a small cylinder is used | ➤ Requires a humidification source if the flow must exceed 0.75 L<br>➤ Must be used with caution and kept in a stand or cart; safety cap must be fastened securely |
| LIQUID OXYGEN | | |
| Uses oxygen stored in a liquid state under high pressure in a cylinder with a valve | ➤ Cost-effective for the neonate who needs continuous low- to moderate-flow oxygen<br>➤ Usually can be used with any oxygen delivery method<br>➤ Smaller and more lightweight than other oxygen systems<br>➤ Refillable, portable units available for when the neonate travels | ➤ Humidification source required if flow must exceed 0.75 L<br>➤ May cause burns if oxygen comes into contact with skin during transfer from a stationary to a portable unit<br>➤ Upright position required for cylinder |

➤ Record each change in oxygen concentration and the infant's FIO$_2$ as measured by the oxygen analyzer. Note all checks of oxygen concentration.
➤ Document all ABG values, the times that samples were obtained, the infant's condition during therapy, times suctioned, the amount and consistency of mucus, the type of continuous oxygen monitoring (if any), and any complications.
➤ Note respiratory rate, and describe breath sounds and any signs of additional respiratory distress.
➤ List any patient instructions given to the parents or caregivers and their understanding.

## Phototherapy

### CPT CODE
No specific code has been assigned.

## DESCRIPTION

Phototherapy involves exposing the neonate to light of a specific wavelength that breaks down bilirubin (a pigment of red blood cells [RBCs]) for transport to the GI system and excretion. The range for maximum absorption of bilirubin is 400 to 500 nm and may be delivered by a special halogen light, fluorescent light, or halogen light source directed into a phototherapy blanket (also called a fiber-optic mat). The treatment is commonly given to neonates with hyperbilirubinemia — a symptom of physiologic jaundice, breast-milk jaundice, or hemolytic disease. Phototherapy continues until bilirubin drops to normal levels because unchecked hyperbilirubinemia can lead to kernicterus (deposits of unconjugated bilirubin in the brain cells), permanent brain damage, and even death.

Physiologic jaundice — resulting from the neonate's high RBC count and short RBC life span — may develop in 2 to 3 days after delivery in about 50% of full-term neonates and in 3 to 5 days in about 80% of premature neonates.

Breast-milk jaundice typically develops 3 to 4 days after delivery in about 25% of breast-fed neonates and 4 to 5 days after delivery in less than 5%. Experts think that this hyperbilirubinemia results from reduced calorie and fluid intake (before the mother develops an adequate milk supply) or from constituents in breast milk that reduce bilirubin decomposition. Many practitioners encourage frequent breast-feeding to increase fluid and calorie intake until bilirubin levels reach about 15 mg/dl. After 15 mg/dl, breast-feeding should discontinue for 48 hours while bilirubin levels decrease.

Treatment for hemolytic disease, a much more serious condition, includes phototherapy and exchange transfusions. In pathologic jaundice, which occurs within 24 hours of birth and raises serum bilirubin levels above 13 mg/dl, phototherapy may be used along with appropriate treatment for the underlying cause.

## INDICATIONS

➤ To treat hyperbilirubinemia
➤ To decrease risk of neurotoxicity due to hyperbilirubinemia

## CONTRAINDICATIONS

None known in the presence of hyperbilirubinemia

## EQUIPMENT

Phototherapy unit ◆ photometer ◆ opaque eye mask ◆ thermometer ◆ surgical face mask or small diaper ◆ thermistor (if the phototherapy unit is combined with a temperature-controlled radiant heat warmer) or incubator (if the neonate is small for his gestational age) (optional) ◆ bilimeter ◆ prepackaged eye coverings (optional)

## PREPARATION OF EQUIPMENT

➤ Set up the phototherapy unit about 18″ (46 cm) above the neonate's crib.
➤ Verify placement of the light-bulb shield because this device filters ultraviolet rays and protects the neonate from broken bulbs. If the neonate is in an incubator, place the phototherapy unit at least 3″ (7.6 cm) above the incubator to promote sufficient air flow and prevent overheating. (See *Understanding the phototherapy unit.*)
➤ Turn on the lights. Place a photometer probe in the middle of the crib to measure the energy emitted by the lights. The energy should range between 6 and 8 µw/cm²/nm.

## ESSENTIAL STEPS

➤ Explain the procedure to the parents or caregivers to reduce their anxiety and to ensure cooperation.
➤ Record the neonate's initial bilirubin level and his axillary temperature to establish baseline measurements.
➤ Wash your hands. Place the opaque eye mask over the neonate's closed eyes. Fasten the mask securely enough to stay in place and to prevent the neonate from opening his eyes but loosely enough to ensure circulation and avoid pressure on the eyeballs. This protects the eyes and prevents reflex bradycardia and head molding.
➤ Clean the eyes periodically to remove drainage and check circulation.
➤ Undress the neonate to expose the most skin to the most light. Remember to place a diaper under him and to cover male genitalia with a surgical mask or a small diaper to catch urine and to prevent possible

## UNDERSTANDING THE PHOTOTHERAPY UNIT

Whether you use fluorescent or daylight bulbs, blue lights, or high-intensity quartz lamps in your neonatal phototherapy unit, prepare the neonate in much the same way. Position the unit at a correct distance according to whether the neonate is in a crib, radiant warmer, or incubator (as shown). Take care to expose as much skin surface as possible to as much light as possible because the light decomposes harmful, excess bilirubin in the skin and subcutaneous tissues to a more water-soluble form that is easily excreted from the body.

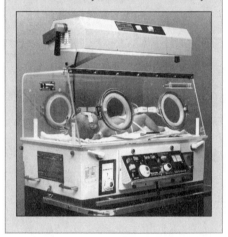

testicular damage from the heat and light waves.
➤ Write orders for the neonate's axillary temperature to be taken every 2 hours to make sure the neonate maintains a normal and stable body temperature.
➤ If the neonate is in a servo-controlled incubator or a radiant warmer, place the thermistor on the neonate's side, and cover it with opaque or reflective tape. This prevents frequent sensor changes and protects the sensor from direct energy.
➤ Check the bilirubin level at least once every 24 hours — more often if levels rise significantly. If you don't use a bilimeter, turn off the phototherapy unit before draw-

ing venous blood for testing because the lights may degrade bilirubin in the blood sample and thereby produce inaccurate test results.

➤ Monitor the neonate closely if the bilirubin level nears 20 mg/dl in full-term neonates, or 15 mg/dl in premature neonates, because these levels may lead to kernicterus. Above this level, transfusion may be required.

➤ Review the neonatal and maternal histories for clues to possible hyperbilirubinemia causes. Also watch for signs of infection and metabolic disorders, and check the neonate's hematocrit for polycythemia. Inspect the neonate for hematoma, bruising, petechiae, and cyanosis. If the phototherapy unit has blue lights, turn them off for the examination because these lights can mask cyanosis.

➤ Prepare parents or caregivers to care for neonate and phototherapy unit in the home.

➤ Phototherapy is typically discontinued when bilirubin levels fall 1.5 to 3 mg/dl below the level at start of therapy, with follow-up testing 6 to 12 hours later.

## PATIENT TEACHING

➤ Explain to the parents or caregivers that phototherapy programs are safe and effective alternatives for treating uncomplicated neonatal jaundice.

➤ Teach parents or caregivers how to perform the procedure, and encourage their compliance.

➤ Explain that testing will continue until results show serum bilirubin at acceptable levels.

➤ Instruct parents or caregivers on how to provide additional warmth, if necessary, by adjusting the warming unit's thermostat.

➤ Instruct parents or caregivers to monitor elimination, note urine and stool amounts and frequency, weigh the neonate twice daily, and watch for signs of dehydration (dry skin, poor turgor, depressed

fontanels) because phototherapy increases fluid loss through stools and evaporation.

➤ Instruct the parents or caregivers to clean the neonate carefully after each bowel movement because the loose green stools that result from phototherapy can excoriate the skin. Advise them not to apply ointment because this can cause burns under phototherapy lights.

➤ Instruct parents or caregivers to feed the neonate at least every 3 to 4 hours and offer water between feedings to ensure adequate hydration and to boost gastric motility. Make sure water intake doesn't replace breast milk or formula as bilirubin is excreted primarily in stool. Take the neonate out of the crib, turn off the phototherapy lights, and unmask his eyes at least every 3 to 4 hours with feedings, if possible, to provide visual stimulation and human contact. Also assess his eyes for inflammation or injury.

➤ Reposition the neonate every 2 hours to expose all body surfaces to the light and to prevent head molding and skin breakdown from pressure.

➤ Provide written instructions at discharge.

## COMPLICATIONS

➤ *Bronze baby syndrome* (an idiopathic darkening of the skin, serum, and urine) may occur and resolves over several weeks without treatment.

➤ *Changes in feeding, activity patterns,* and *hormonal secretions* may follow prolonged therapy. It's important to emphasize that the baby can be removed for feeding and bonding periodically.

➤ *Hypothermia and hyperthymia* may occur because the bulbs add little warmth. Frequent monitoring of skin temperature allows adjustment as needed to compensate.

## SPECIAL CONSIDERATIONS

➤ An option available for bilirubin levels up to 16 mg/dl is a phototherapy blanket. It has a fiber-optic bili-light embedded in the blanket. The blanket is wrapped around the infant so that it touches as much of the infant's skin as possible. The infant can then be dressed, held, and fed without interrupting phototherapy. In addition, the infant doesn't have to wear eye protection. Other advantages are the reduced risk for hyperthermia and dehydration, which may occur with traditional bili-lights.

➤ If the neonate cries excessively during phototherapy, place a blanket roll at each side to give him a feeling of security.

➤ If you have a working diagnosis of breast-feeding jaundice (and suspend breast-feeding temporarily), teach the mother to express milk manually or with a pump. Encourage continued breast-feeding when indicated. Reassure the parents or caregivers by explaining that jaundice is transitory. If possible, arrange for phototherapy treatment in the mother's room to facilitate bonding and to decrease parental anxiety and guilt feelings.

➤ Adding a second spotlight to form a second circle of light or laying the infant on a biliblanket will increase the surface area exposed and thus increase the dose delivered. Again, the irradiance at the level of the infant should be measured and documented. Adding extra, but suboptimal (< 10 µw/cm²/nm), blue, white, or halogen lights from above, below, or the side won't enhance bilirubin level reduction.

➤ Continuous cardiorespiratory monitoring can continue while infant is receiving phototherapy.

## DOCUMENTATION

➤ Document the indications for phototherapy, caregiver instructions given, and any home care arrangements made.

➤ Note the progress of phototherapy, and order assessment every 2 hours with checks to verify that the neonate's eyes remain protected.

➤ Write orders for eye covering changes and eye care.

➤ Monitor records of measured radiant energy — including initially and then every 8 hours, and bilirubin trends.

➤ Note fluid intake and the amount of urine and feces eliminated.

➤ Document any changes in skin appearance and character, in feeding patterns, and in activity level and any changes made to the plan of care.

# Thermoregulation

CPT CODE
No specific code has been assigned.

## DESCRIPTION

A large body surface-to-mass ratio, reduced metabolism per unit area, limited amounts of insulating subcutaneous fat, vasomotor instability, and limited metabolic capacity make all neonates susceptible to hypothermia. To stay warm when he's cold-stressed, the neonate metabolizes brown fat. Unique to neonates, brown fat has energy-producing mitochondria in its cells, which enhance its capacity for heat production.

Brown fat metabolism effectively warms the body but only within a narrow temperature range. Brown fat may be lacking in small-for-gestational-age infants or premature infants. Without careful external thermoregulation, the neonate may become chilled. Hypoxia, acidosis, hypoglycemia, pulmonary vasoconstriction, and even death may result.

Thermoregulation provides a neutral thermal environment that helps the neo-

## UNDERSTANDING THERMOREGULATORS

Thermoregulators preserve neonatal body warmth in various ways. A radiant warmer maintains the neonate's temperature by *radiation*. An incubator maintains the neonate's temperature by *conduction* and *convection*.

### Temperature settings
Radiant warmers and incubators have two operating modes: *nonservo* and *servo*. Temperature controls on nonservo equipment are manually set; a probe on the neonate's skin controls temperature settings on servo models.

### Other features
Most thermoregulators come with alarms. Incubators have the added advantage of providing a stable, enclosed environment, which protects the neonate from evaporative heat loss.

**RADIANT WARMER**

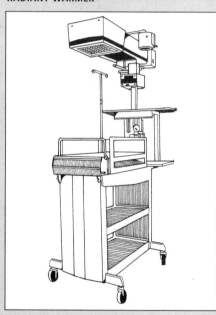

**INCUBATOR**

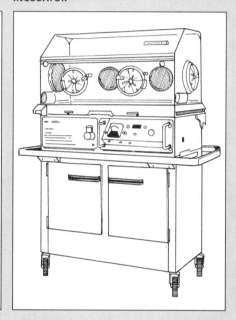

nate maintain a normal core temperature with minimal oxygen consumption and caloric expenditure. Although it varies with the neonate, the average core temperature is 97.7° F (36.5° C).

Two kinds of thermoregulators are common in a hospital nursery: radiant warmers and incubators. The radiant warmer controls environmental temperature while the practitioner gives initial care in the delivery room. Then, when the neonate arrives in the nursery, another radiant warmer may be used until his temperature stabilizes and he can occupy a bassinet. If the temperature doesn't stabilize or if the neonate has a condition that affects thermoregulation, a temperature-controlled incubator will house him. (See *Understanding thermoregulators*.)

## INDICATIONS

➤ To aid a premature or physically stressed infant to maintain a normal core temperature

## CONTRAINDICATIONS

None known

## EQUIPMENT

Radiant warmer or incubator (if necessary) ◆ blankets ◆ washcloths or towels ◆ skin probe ◆ adhesive pad ◆ water-soluble lubricant ◆ thermometer ◆ clothing (including a cap)

## PREPARATION OF EQUIPMENT

➤ Turn on the radiant warmer in the delivery room, and set the desired temperature.
➤ Warm the blankets, washcloths, or towels under a heat source.

## ESSENTIAL STEPS

➤ Explain the procedure to the parents or caregivers and answer any questions they may have.
➤ Continue measures to conserve neonatal body warmth until the patient's discharge.

### In the delivery room

➤ Wash your hands. Place the neonate under the radiant warmer, and dry him with the warm washcloths or towels to prevent heat loss by evaporation.
➤ Pay special attention to drying his scalp and hair. Then, if you take him off the warmer, make sure you cover his head (which makes up about 25% of neonatal body surface) with a ready-made cap to prevent heat loss.
➤ Perform required procedures quickly to reduce the neonate's exposure to cool delivery room air.
➤ Wrap him in the warmed blankets. If his condition permits, give him to his parents or caregivers to promote bonding.

➤ Transport the neonate to the nursery in the warmed blankets. Use a transport incubator when the nursery is far from the delivery room.

### In the nursery

➤ Wash your hands. Remove the blankets and cap, and place the neonate under the radiant warmer.
➤ Use the adhesive pad to attach the temperature control probe to his skin in the upper-right abdominal quadrant. This lets the servo control maintain neonatal skin temperature between 96.8° F and 97.7° F (36° C and 36.5° C). If the neonate will lie prone, put the skin probe on his back to ensure accurate temperature control and avoid false-high readings from the neonate lying on the probe. Don't cover the device with anything because this could interfere with the servo control. Be sure to raise the warmer's side panels to prevent accidents.
➤ Lubricate the thermometer, and take the neonate's rectal temperature on admission to identify a core temperature. Take axillary temperatures thereafter to avoid injuring delicate rectal mucosa. Usually, axillary temperature readings are one degree Fahrenheit lower than the core temperature. Write orders to check axillary temperatures every 15 to 30 minutes until the temperature stabilizes, then every 4 hours to ensure stability.
➤ Write orders to have the neonate sponge-bathed under the warmer only after his temperature stabilizes and his glucose level is normal; leave him under the warmer until his temperature remains stable.
➤ Take appropriate action if the temperature doesn't stabilize. For example, place the neonate under a plastic heat shield or in a warmed incubator — depending on your facility's protocol. Look for objects, such as a phototherapy unit, that may be blocking the heat source. Also check for signs of infection, which can cause hypothermia.

PATIENT-TEACHING AID

# HOW TO GIVE YOUR BABY A BATH

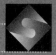

**DEAR PARENT:**

Bath time can be fun — a time to be with your baby, not just to clean up. Remember, your baby won't need a bath every day, but you'll need to wash her face and hands daily. Also wash the genital area every time your baby has a bowel movement or soaks the diaper.

## Getting ready

To avoid rushing and interruptions, set aside a certain amount of uninterrupted time to bathe your baby. Then gather the supplies. You'll need baby soap, shampoo, a bath towel and washcloth, cotton balls, fresh diapers, and clean baby clothes. Baby lotion, petroleum jelly, or powder is optional. If you use powder, don't sprinkle it on the baby; she might inhale it. Apply it from your hand.

Set up the bath area at a comfortable height in a warm, draft-free room.

## Giving a sponge bath

Until the baby's navel (and circumcision, if your baby is a boy) heals, you'll give a sponge bath. First, put a few inches of warm water in a basin.

**1** Keep the baby warm by washing her face and head before removing her clothes. Using only warm water, wash her face and pat it dry. Then moisten a cotton ball in water and clean her eyelids, wiping from the nose toward the ears. Clean the outer part of her ears and nostrils with another moist cotton ball. To avoid possible injury, don't put anything into the inner part of her ears or nostrils.

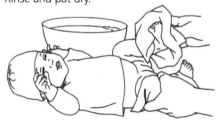

**2** Next, wash your baby's head (about twice a week). Hold her as you would a football (support her head and body with one hand and secure her hips and legs against your side). With your free hand, wet her scalp and apply baby shampoo gently but firmly. Rinse well with a washcloth and rub gently to dry.

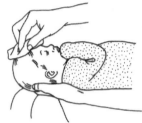

**3** After changing the basin water, remove the baby's clothing. Using your hands, wash her upper and lower body — creases and all — with soap. Care for your baby's navel (and circumcision), following the directions given by your practitioner. Rinse and pat dry. Now turn your baby onto her stomach to wash her back and buttocks. Rinse and pat dry.

**4** Diaper and dress her appropriately for the surroundings. Avoid catching her fingers in sleeves while dressing.

➤ Apply a skin probe to the neonate in an incubator as you would for a neonate in a radiant warmer. Move the incubator away from cold walls or objects.

➤ Perform all required procedures quickly to maintain a neutral thermal environment and to minimize heat loss. Close portholes in the hood immediately after completing any procedure to reduce heat loss. If procedures must be performed outside the incubator, do them under a radiant warmer.

➤ To leave the hospital or to move to a bassinet, a neonate must be weaned from the incubator. Slowly reduce the incubator's temperature to that of the nursery. Check periodically for hypothermia. To ensure temperature stability, never discharge the neonate to home directly from an incubator.

➤ When the normal neonate's temperature stabilizes, dress him, put him in a bassinet, and cover him with a blanket.

## PATIENT TEACHING

➤ Review the reasons for regulating body temperature with the neonate's parents or caregivers. Instruct them to keep him wrapped in a blanket and out of drafts when he isn't in the bassinet, both in the facility and at home. In a warm place, guard against overheating the neonate.

➤ When bathing the neonate, expose only one body part at a time; wash each part thoroughly, and then dry it immediately. (See *How to give your baby a bath.*)

## COMPLICATIONS

➤ *Hypothermia* from ineffective natural or external thermoregulation can inhibit weight gain because the neonate must use caloric energy to maintain his temperature. Hyperthermia can cause increased oxygen consumption and apnea. This is minimized by close monitoring of the neonate and monitoring and adjustment of thermoregulatory units.

## SPECIAL CONSIDERATIONS

➤ Always warm oxygen before administering it to a neonate to avoid initiating heat loss from his head and face.

➤ To prevent conductive heat loss, preheat the radiant warmer bed and linen, warm stethoscopes and other instruments before use, and pad the scale with paper or a preweighed, warmed sheet before weighing the neonate.

➤ To avoid convective heat loss, place the neonate's bed out of direct line with an open window, fan, or an air-conditioning vent.

➤ To control evaporative heat loss, dry the neonate immediately after delivery.

## DOCUMENTATION

➤ Name the heat source, and record its temperature and the neonate's temperature, whenever taken.

➤ Document any complications that result from using thermoregulatory equipment.

➤ List any patient instructions given to the parents or caregivers and their understanding.

# MONITORING

## Apnea monitoring

CPT CODE
No specific code has been assigned.

## USING A HOME APNEA MONITOR

When a neonate will require the use of a home apnea monitor, the parents or caregivers need to be prepared to operate the equipment safely, correctly, and confidently. First, review the neonate's breathing problem with his parents or caregivers. Explain that the monitor will warn them of breathing or heart rate changes.

### Parent and caregiver education
➤ Have the parents or caregivers prepare their home and family for the equipment. A sturdy, flat surface is necessary for the monitor, as well as accessible posting of emergency telephone numbers (practitioner, nurse, equipment supplier, and ambulance).
➤ Teach other responsible family members how to use the monitor safely. Suggest that older siblings, grandparents, babysitters, and other caregivers learn cardiopulmonary resuscitation (CPR).
➤ Instruct the parents or caregivers to notify local service authorities — police, ambulance service, telephone company, and electric company — if their baby uses an apnea monitor

so that alternative power can be supplied if a failure occurs.
➤ Explain to the parents or caregivers how a monitor with electrodes works. Advise them to make sure the respiration indicator goes on each time the neonate breathes. If it doesn't, describe troubleshooting techniques, such as moving the electrodes slightly. Tell them to try this technique several times.
➤ Show the parents or caregivers how to respond to either the apnea or bradycardia alarm. Direct them to check the color of the neonate's oral tissues. If the tissues appear bluish and the neonate isn't breathing, tell them to call loudly and touch him — gently at first, then more urgently as needed. Tell them to stop short of shaking him. If he doesn't respond, urge them to begin CPR.
➤ Also advise the parents or caregivers to keep the operator's manual attached to or beside the monitor and to consult it as needed. Explain that an activated loose-lead alarm, for example, may indicate a dirty electrode, a loose electrode patch, a loose belt, or a disconnected or malfunctioning wire or monitor.

## DESCRIPTION

By signaling when the breathing rate falls dangerously low, apnea monitors can save a neonate who's vulnerable to apnea. Two types of monitors are most commonly used for vulnerable neonates. First is the *thoracic impedance monitor* that uses chest electrodes to detect conduction changes caused by respirations. (The newest models have alarm systems and memories that record cardiorespiratory patterns.) Second is the *apnea mattress,* or *underpad monitor,* that relies on a transducer connected to a pressure-sensitive pad, which detects pressure changes resulting from altered chest movements.

To guard against potentially life-threatening apneic episodes in vulnerable

neonates, monitoring begins in the hospital (or birthing center) and continues at home. (See *Using a home apnea monitor.*)

## INDICATIONS

➤ To monitor infants born prematurely
➤ To monitor infants after a life-threatening medical emergency
➤ To monitor infants with neurologic disorders, neonatal respiratory distress syndrome, bronchopulmonary dysplasia, congenital heart disease with heart failure, a tracheostomy, a personal history of sleep-induced apnea, a family history of sudden infant death syndrome, or acute drug withdrawal

## CONTRAINDICATIONS

None known

## EQUIPMENT

Monitor unit ◆ electrodes ◆ leadwires ◆ electrode belt ◆ electrode gel if needed ◆ pressure transducer pad, if using apnea mattress ◆ stable surface for monitor placement

## ESSENTIAL STEPS

➤ Explain the procedure to the parents or caregivers, as appropriate, and wash your hands.
➤ Place the monitor on a stable surface. Plug the monitor's power cord into a grounded wall outlet. Attach the leadwires to the electrodes, and attach the electrodes to the belt. If appropriate, apply conduction gel to the electrodes. (Or apply gel to the neonate's chest, place the electrodes on top of the gel, and attach the electrodes to the leadwires. Then secure the belt.)
➤ To hold the electrodes securely in position, wrap the belt snugly but not restrictively around the neonate's chest at the point of greatest movement — optimally at the right and left midaxillary line about ¾" (2 cm) below the axilla. Be sure to position the leadwires according to the manufacturer's instructions.
➤ Follow the color code to connect the leadwires to the patient cable. Then connect the cable to the proper jack at the rear of the monitoring unit.
➤ Turn the sensitivity controls to maximum to facilitate tuning when adjusting the system.
➤ Set the alarms according to recommendations so that an apneic period lasting for a specified time activates the signal.
➤ Turn on the monitor. If the monitor has two alarms — one to signal apnea, one to signal bradycardia — both will sound until you adjust the monitor and reset the alarms according to the manufacturer's instructions.
➤ Adjust the sensitivity controls until the indicator lights blink with each breath and heartbeat.
➤ If you use an apnea mattress, assemble the monitor and pressure transducer pad according to the manufacturer's directions.
➤ Plug the monitor into a grounded wall outlet. Then plug the cable of the transducer pad into the monitor.
➤ Touch the pad to make sure it works. Watch for the monitor's respiration light to blink.
➤ Follow the manufacturer's instructions for pad placement.
➤ If you have difficulty obtaining a signal, place a foam rubber pad under the mattress, and sandwich the transducer pad between the foam pad and the mattress.
➤ If you hear the apnea or bradycardia alarm during monitoring, immediately check the neonate's respirations and color, but don't touch or disturb him until you confirm apnea.
➤ If he's still breathing and his color is good, readjust the sensitivity controls or reposition the electrodes, if necessary.
➤ If he isn't breathing, but his color looks normal, wait 10 seconds to see if he starts breathing spontaneously. If he isn't breathing and he appears pale, dusky, or blue, immediately try to stimulate breathing in these ways: Sequentially, place your hand on the neonate's back, rub him gently, or flick his soles gently. If he doesn't begin to breathe at once, start cardiopulmonary resuscitation (CPR). Encourage parents or caregivers to take a CPR course. (See *How to perform CPR on a baby*.)

## PATIENT TEACHING

➤ Teach parents or caregivers that the apnea monitor is a machine that monitors the heartbeat and breathing. It has small
*(Text continues on page 448.)*

PATIENT-TEACHING AID

# How to Perform CPR on a Baby

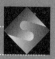

DEAR PARENT:

What would you do if your baby started choking or stopped breathing? Would you panic? Or would you swiftly clear his airway, start cardiopulmonary resuscitation (CPR), and call the ambulance within the first minute?

Use these guidelines to familiarize yourself with CPR technique. They aren't intended as a quick course in CPR. The best training comes from a certified course given by the American Heart Association or the Red Cross.

## Open the airway

**1** Check the baby for obvious injury, then gently shake him to see if he's unconscious. If he is, lay him on his back on a hard surface.

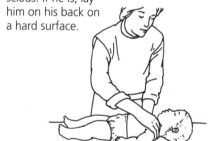

**2** Shout for help. Send someone to dial 911 or call an ambulance. If you are alone, start CPR for 1 minute then dial 911 or call an ambulance. If the baby doesn't appear to have a head or neck injury, use the *head-tilt, chin-lift* maneuver to open his airway: Put your closest hand on his forehead; then, placing the middle and index fingers of your other hand on his chin, tilt back his head and lift his jaw. Don't overextend his neck or press on his throat.

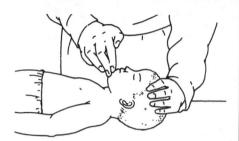

If you suspect a head or neck injury, use the *jaw-thrust* maneuver to open his airway: Get behind the baby's head and put your elbows on the hard surface. Place the middle and index fingers of each hand under his lower jaw, resting your thumbs on the corners of his mouth. Now lift his jaw (his tongue will lift up too). If his tongue was obstructing his airway, this maneuver alone will restore breathing.

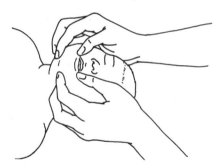

## Check breathing

**1** Once you've opened the airway, put your ear near the baby's mouth and nose. Listen for breath sounds and wait for the feel of air on your cheek. Is his chest rising and falling? If he's breathing, keep his head tilted back to keep his airway open. And watch his breathing carefully.

*(continued)*

## HOW TO PERFORM CPR ON A BABY *(continued)*

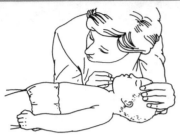

**2** If he still isn't breathing, start CPR: Put your mouth over his mouth and nose, making a tight seal.

Begin ventilation (breathing for him). Blow a puff of air into his mouth. Inhale, blow another puff, inhale. Give only enough breath to make his chest rise; too much can become harmful.

If the first two ventilations don't work, reposition his head and try again. If he still doesn't breathe, he might have an object in his airway (see "Clearing the airway in a conscious baby").

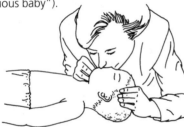

### Check for signs of circulation

**1** Quickly scan the baby for any sign of movement. With your ear next to the baby's mouth, look, listen, and feel for normal breathing or coughing.

**2** If the baby is not breathing normally, coughing, or moving, immediately begin chest compressions. To place your fingers correctly, imagine a line connecting the baby's nipples. Put the index finger of your free hand on the breastbone just below the center of this line, and put your middle and ring fingers next to it.

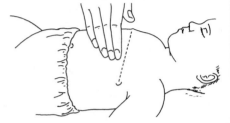

**3** Lift your index finger off the chest. Now press the chest five times, compressing ½ to 1 inch. Release pressure after each compression so the chest returns to normal position, but don't remove your fingers.

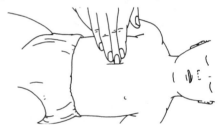

**4** Keep your fingers on the baby's chest, and, using the *head-tilt*, *chin-lift* maneuver, start ventilating him again. Compress five times, then ventilate once — keep repeating for 20 cycles.

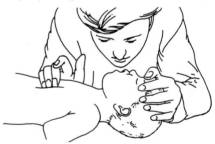

## HOW TO PERFORM CPR ON A BABY *(continued)*

**5** After 20 cycles of compressions and ventilations, recheck for signs of spontaneous breathing or circulation. If there are none, continue CPR by giving one ventilation, then resuming the cycle of five compressions and one ventilation. Recheck every few minutes. If the baby is breathing, watch him closely and keep his airway open by keeping his head tilted back.

### Clearing the airway in a conscious baby

**1** Stand up, put one leg forward, and place the baby face down, straddling your forearm. Hold your arm against your thigh and his head near your knee, and hold his jaw firmly.

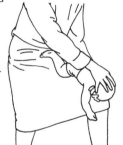

**2** With the heel of your other hand, deliver five sharp blows between his shoulder blades.

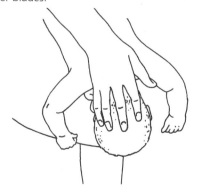

**3** Using both hands, turn the baby over, supporting his back and head. Now, transfer him to your other thigh, keeping his head lower than his body.

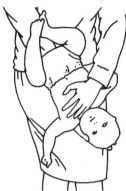

**4** Put two or three fingers just below the nipple line. Press his chest five times, compressing ½ to 1 inch. Release pressure after each compression to allow the chest to return to normal position, but don't remove your fingers. Alternate back blows with chest thrusts until the baby coughs out the object or becomes unconscious. If the baby becomes unresponsive, attempt CPR. Each time the airway is opened, look for the obstructing object and remove it if you see it.

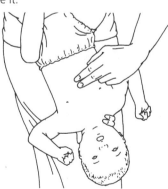

wires, also called leads or electrodes, that attach to small adhesive dots or an electrode belt.

➤ Instruct parents or caregivers not to apply lotions and powders to skin under the adhesive dots or the electrode belt as this will increase the likelihood that the electrodes will fall off and set off the alarm.

➤ Instruct parents or caregivers how to operate the monitor, what actions to take when the alarms sounds, how to troubleshoot problems with the monitor, and how to contact emergency assistance (both emergency medical system and technical assistance). Teach them how to test the alarm system, position the sensor properly, and set the controls properly.

➤ Advise all caregivers to take a course to learn infant CPR.

## COMPLICATIONS

➤ *Apneic episode* resulting from upper airway obstruction may not trigger the alarm if the neonate continues to make respiratory efforts without gas exchange. However, the monitor's bradycardia alarm may be triggered by a decreased heart rate resulting from the vagal stimulation (which accompanies obstruction).

Always compare the clinical picture with the information on the monitor. Initiate CPR as needed.

## SPECIAL CONSIDERATIONS

➤ To ensure accurate operation, don't put the monitor on top of any other electrical device. Make sure it's on a level surface and can't be bumped easily.

➤ Avoid applying lotions, oils, or powders to the neonate's chest because they could cause the electrode belt to slip. Periodically check the alarm by disconnecting the sensor plug. Then listen for the alarm to sound after the preset time delay.

➤ If you're using a thoracic impedance monitor without a bradycardia alarm, you may interpret bradycardia during apnea as shallow breathing. That is because this type of monitor fails to distinguish between respiratory movement and the large cardiac stroke volume associated with bradycardia. In this case, the alarm won't sound until the heart rate drops below the apnea limit.

## DOCUMENTATION

➤ Record the indications for apnea monitoring, caregiver instructions given, and home care arrangements made.

➤ Record all witnessed alarm incidents, actions taken, and outcomes. Include the time and duration of apnea and describe the neonate's color and the stimulation measures implemented.

➤ Document any patient instructions given to the parents or caregivers and their understanding.

## Transcutaneous PO$_2$ monitoring

CPT CODES
94760   *Noninvasive ear or pulse oximetry for oxygen saturation; single*
94761   *Noninvasive ear or pulse oximetry for oxygen saturation; multiple determinations*

## DESCRIPTION

A transcutaneous partial oxygen pressure (TCPO$_2$) monitor measures the amount of oxygen diffusing through skin from capillaries directly beneath the surface. This measurement, which correlates closely with the infant's partial pressure of arterial oxygen, supplements traditional methods (observing skin color and taking periodic arterial blood gas [ABG] measurements) for detecting hypoxemia and hyperoxemia.

The monitor relies on a tiny electrode sensor applied to the skin. This sensor — a metallic, oxygen-sensitive device — warms to between 107.6° F and 115° F (42° C and 46° C). As the electrode's temperature increases (typically, to slightly higher than skin temperature), so does capillary blood flow. The increased vasodilation in cutaneous vessels enhances oxygen diffusion, which the electrode measures. This procedure is widely used in neonatal intensive care units by staff nurses trained to use the monitor.

Because neonatal skin is thin with little subcutaneous fat, TCPO$_2$ monitoring produces accurate findings. Another device for monitoring arterial oxygen levels is the pulse oximeter. (See *Neonatal pulse oximetry*.)

## INDICATIONS

➤ To assess oxygenation or ventilation
➤ To quantitate the response to diagnostic and therapeutic interventions

## CONTRAINDICATIONS

### Relative
➤ Shock or hypoperfusion
➤ Adhesive allergy
➤ Poor skin integrity

## EQUIPMENT

TCPO$_2$ monitor and electrode ◆ cotton balls ◆ soap and water ◆ alcohol sponge ◆ adhesive ring for electrode

## PREPARATION OF EQUIPMENT

➤ Set up the monitor, and calibrate it, if necessary, following the manufacturer's instructions.

### NEONATAL PULSE OXIMETRY

Another noninvasive technique for monitoring oxygenation is pulse oximetry. The sensor of the pulse oximeter, which is attached to the neonate's foot, measures beat-to-beat arterial oxygen saturation. Normally, oxygenation values should drop no lower than 90%.

Arterial blood gases should be ordered every 3 to 4 hours and correlated with the oximetric values for a reliable overview of the neonatal status.

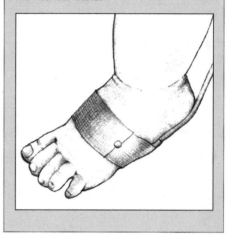

➤ Ensure that the strip chart recorder works properly.

## ESSENTIAL STEPS

➤ Explain the procedure to the parents or caregivers to reduce their anxiety and to ensure cooperation.
➤ Wash your hands, and decide where to place the electrode. Choose a flat site, with good capillary blood flow, few fatty deposits, and no bony prominences. Common sites include the infant's upper chest, abdomen, and inner thigh.
➤ Clean the site first with a cotton ball and soap and water. Then wipe the site

with an alcohol sponge to remove dirt and oils and to ensure good electrode contact.

➤ Dry the skin, attach the adhesive ring to the electrode, and moisten the skin site with a drop of water, according to the manufacturer's instructions, to seal out all air.

➤ Place the electrode on the site, and make sure that the adhesive ring is tight.

➤ Set the alarm switches and the electrode temperature according to the manufacturer's instructions or facility policy.

➤ Expect the monitor reading to stabilize in 10 to 20 minutes. Normal oxygen pressures range from 50 to 80 mm Hg, but normal values also vary with the infant and the equipment. $TCPO_2$ monitors usually have digital readouts and strip chart recorders to show trends.

## PATIENT TEACHING

➤ Inform parents or caregivers that $TCPO_2$ monitoring is a term used for a noninvasive and continuous monitoring device. A probe is placed on the skin; it warms the skin then detects the oxygen level in the underlying arteries.

➤ Advise parents or caregivers that it's normal for values to vary with neonatal movement or crying.

➤ Instruct parents or caregivers in how to keep the infant warm. Conserving heat decreases energy demands on the infant and increases the validity of the monitor.

➤ Inform the parents or caregivers that it will be necessary to take periodic arterial blood samples as they are more accurate than the monitor.

## COMPLICATIONS

➤ *Burns* and *blisters* from the electrode and *skin reactions* to the adhesive ring can develop. Careful removal and site rotation minimizes this risk.

## SPECIAL CONSIDERATIONS

➤ Expect $TCPO_2$ values to vary with neonatal movement and treatment. Also expect them to drop markedly whenever the infant cries vigorously. But be prepared to start resuscitation if a sudden, significant drop in $TCPO_2$ pressure occurs.

➤ $TCPO_2$ monitoring doesn't replace ABG measurements because it doesn't give information about partial pressure of arterial carbon dioxide and pH.

➤ Placing the probe on a poorly perfused area or bony prominence can result in falsely decreased levels on the monitor.

➤ The probe site should be changed every 4 hours.

➤ Shock or hypoperfusion may cause inaccurate results because peripheral blood flow decreases as blood is shunted to the heart, brain, and lungs.

## DOCUMENTATION

➤ Document the indications for monitoring and the level for the high and low alarms to be set at.

➤ Place graphic or printout results on the infant's chart.

➤ Record the range of values observed during monitoring in your notes.

➤ Record any skin disorders related to the electrode such as blisters or skin loss. Document interventions and outcomes.

➤ Document a clinical evaluation, including perfusion, pallor, skin temperature, and probe site appearance.

➤ List any patient instructions given to the parents or caregivers and their understanding.

# SPECIAL PROCEDURES

## Circumcision

**CPT CODE**
*54150  Circumcision, using clamp or other device; newborn*

## DESCRIPTION

Steeped in controversy and history, circumcision — the removal of the penile foreskin — is thought to promote a clean glans and to minimize the risk of phimosis (tightening of the foreskin) in later life. It's also thought to reduce the risk of penile cancer and the risk of cervical cancer in sexual partners, although the American Academy of Pediatrics (AAP) has contended since 1971 that no valid medical reason exists for routine circumcision. Currently, the AAP is continuing its studies on the effects of circumcision.

In Judaism, circumcision is a religious rite (known as a *bris*) performed by a *mohel* on the 8th day after birth, when the neonate officially receives his name. Because most neonates are discharged before this time, the *bris* rarely occurs in the hospital.

One method of circumcision involves removing the foreskin by using a Yellen clamp to stabilize the penis. With this device, a cone that fits over the glans provides a cutting surface and protects the glans penis. Another technique uses a plastic circumcision bell (Plastibell) over the glans and a suture tied tightly around the base of the foreskin. This method prevents bleeding. The resultant ischemia causes the foreskin to slough off within 5 to 8 days. This method is thought to be painless be-

## PENILE ANATOMY

Being aware of penile anatomy can help avoid traumatizing internal structures such as the urethra or resecting too much prepuce.

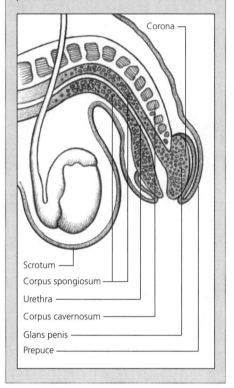

cause it stretches the foreskin, which inhibits sensory conduction.

## INDICATIONS

➤ To satisfy religious requirement
➤ To fulfill parental choice

## CONTRAINDICATIONS

### Absolute
➤ Neonates who are ill or who have bleeding disorders
➤ Ambiguous genitalia

## PERFORMING LOCAL ANESTHESIA

The neonate does experience pain during circumcision. The neural pathways that relay pain, the cortex and subcortex that perceive pain, and the neurotransmitters are all functioning before birth. Research has shown that neonatal circumcision produces increases in heart rate, blood pressure, plasma cortisol levels, crying, wakefulness and irritability, and decreases in the transcutaneous partial pressure of oxygen for up to an hour after the procedure. Local anesthesia reduces or eliminates these changes.

To perform local penile anesthesia, draw up the anesthetic (such as 0.8 ml of 1% lidocaine without epinephrine) into a tuberculin syringe with a 27G needle. Insert the needle halfway along the penile shaft on each side.

Infiltrate the lidocaine in a band or ring around the penis.

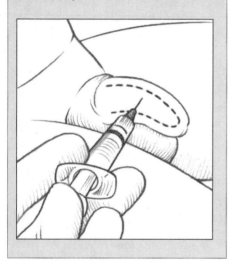

➤ Congenital anomalies of the penis, such as hypospadias or epispadias (because the foreskin may be needed for later reconstructive surgery)

## EQUIPMENT

Circumcision tray (contents vary but usually include circumcision clamps, various sized cones, scalpel, probe, scissors, forceps, sterile basin, sterile towel, and sterile drapes) ◆ povidone-iodine solution ◆ restraining board with arm and leg restraints ◆ sterile gloves ◆ petroleum gauze ◆ sterile 4″ × 4″ gauze pads ◆ sutures, plastic circumcision bell, antimicrobial ointment, and overhead warmer (optional) ◆ tuberculin syringe ◆ 27G needle ◆ local anesthetic such as lidocaine without epinephrine ◆ alcohol swabs

## PREPARATION OF EQUIPMENT

### For circumcision using a Yellen clamp
➤ Assemble the sterile tray and other equipment in the procedure area.
➤ Open the sterile tray and pour povidone-iodine solution into the sterile basin.
➤ Using aseptic technique, place sterile 4″ × 4″ gauze pads and petroleum gauze on the sterile tray.
➤ Arrange the restraining board and direct adequate light on the area.

### For circumcision using a plastic circumcision bell
➤ Although you won't need to assemble a circumcision tray, do assemble sterile gloves, sutures, restraining board, petroleum gauze and, if ordered, antibiotic ointment.
➤ A *mohel* usually brings his own equipment.

## ESSENTIAL STEPS

➤ Explain the procedure to the parents or caregivers, answer any questions they may have, and obtain informed consent.

➤ Withhold feeding for at least 1 hour before the procedure to reduce the possibility of emesis or aspiration, or both.

➤ Wash your hands, and place the neonate on the restraining board, and restrain his arms and legs. Don't leave him unattended.

➤ Comfort the neonate as needed.

➤ Inspect the penis for abnormalities and identify the location of the meatus on the glans. Drape the neonate. (See *Penile anatomy*, page 451.)

➤ If no abnormalities are detected, you may anesthetize the penis. First, clean the insertion site with an alcohol swab. Prepare a tuberculin syringe, 27G needle with lidocaine without epinephrine. Insert the needle around the midpoint of the penile shaft. Infiltrate in a band or ring pattern as you withdraw the needle. (See *Performing local anesthesia*.)

➤ After putting on sterile gloves, clean the penis and scrotum with povidone-iodine, moving from the tip of the glans toward the body, covering an area approximately 3 inches in diameter around the base of the penis, as well as the entire penis.

### Using a Yellen clamp

➤ Apply a Yellen clamp to the penis, loosen the foreskin, insert the cone under it to provide a cutting surface and to protect the penis, and remove the foreskin. (See *Performing a circumcision*, pages 454 and 455.)

➤ Alternatively, a plastic bell may be used. (See *Using a plastic bell*, page 456.)

➤ Cover the wound with sterile petroleum gauze to prevent infection and control bleeding.

➤ Remove the neonate from the restraining board, and check for bleeding.

➤ Show the neonate to his parents or caregivers to reassure them that he's all right.

➤ Write instructions for his care postcircumcision:

– Place the neonate in a side-lying position, rather than prone, to minimize pressure on the excisional area.

– Leave him diaperless for 1 to 2 hours to observe for bleeding and to reduce possible chafing and irritation.

– Once the neonate is rediapered, his diaper should be changed as soon as he voids. If the dressing falls off, clean the wound with warm water to minimize pain from urine on the circumcised area. Don't remove the original dressing until it falls off (usually after the first or second voiding).

– Check for bleeding every 15 minutes for the 1st hour and then every hour for the next 24 hours. If bleeding occurs, apply pressure with sterile gauze pads. You should be notified if bleeding continues.

– Avoid leaving the neonate under the radiant warmer after placing petroleum gauze on the penis because the area might burn.

– Apply diapers loosely to prevent irritation. At each diaper change, apply antimicrobial ointment, petroleum jelly, or petroleum gauze until the wound appears healed.

– Watch for drainage, redness, or swelling. Don't remove the thin, yellow-white exudate that forms over the healing area within 1 to 2 days. This normal incrustation protects the wound until it heals in 3 to 4 days.

– Don't discharge the neonate until he has voided.

## PATIENT TEACHING

➤ Inform the parents or caregivers that the circumcision site may appear yellow in light-skinned neonates and lighter than the surrounding skin in dark-skinned neonates. Tell them that this signifies healing and isn't a cause for concern.

➤ Instruct the parents or caregivers to observe the circumcision site regularly for pus or bloody discharge, which may indicate delayed healing or infection. If these signs occur, the parents or caregivers should notify you.

## PERFORMING A CIRCUMCISION

When performing a circumcision, you may find it helpful to use clock positions as reference points. Place hemostat on very small segments of the prepuce (be sure not to clamp onto the glans) at the 3 o'clock and the 9 o'clock positions, and assert gentle traction. Gently insert a straight hemostat between the prepuce and the glans to the depth of the corona (the rounded proximal border of the glans penis). Open the hemostat, and gently sweep it in both directions in a circumferential motion. Avoid going deeper than the corona or traumatizing the urethra.

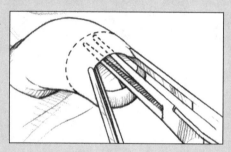

Raise the hemostat away from the glans, forming a tent. Inspect underneath the tented area to ensure that no part of the glans is in the way.

Take the straight hemostat and carefully clamp the dorsal aspect of the prepuce in the vertical line of the penis from one-third to one-half of the total distance to the corona. Wait 1 minute for hemostasis to occur and then remove the straight hemostat.

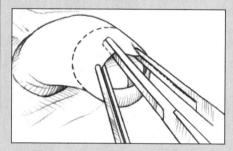

Immediately tent the skin again with straight scissors and cut along the center of the indentation left by the clamped hemostat,

making a dorsal slit. Be careful not to cut past the indentation as this will result in excessive bleeding.

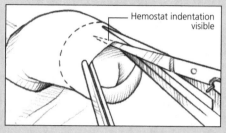

Hemostat indentation visible

Gently retract the prepuce from the glans and lyse any adhesions with 4″ × 4″ gauze or hemostat, taking care to go slightly beyond the incision line to minimize bleeding and provide a cosmetically pleasing result. If the foreskin will not retract, repeat the last two steps, only slightly deeper.

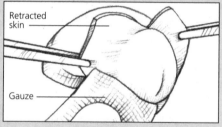

Retracted skin

Gauze

Place the cone over the glans and apply gentle pressure to the distal end or stem of the cone. At the same time, use the attached curved hemostat to ease the prepuce over the cone. The cone should sit between the glans and the prepuce against the corona. Suture the edges of the prepuce to the cone and release the hemostat.

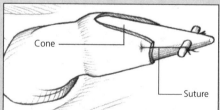

Cone

Suture

Insert the cone and the prepuce into the Yellen clamp, tighten slightly, verify placement (prepuce is even all around and the dorsal slit is fully visible inside the instrument), then tighten firmly. Position the scalpel at an angle slightly higher than horizontal. Press firmly against the cone and glide completely around the cone, being sure to penetrate all skin and mucosal layers. Remove all tissue within the instrument as this may become a source of infection.

Immediately release the penis from the clamp and check for bleeding. Hemostasis may be enhanced by applying pressure, topical epinephrine, silver nitrate, or Gelfoam to the site of the bleeding. If this is ineffective, refer the patient immediately to a urologist.

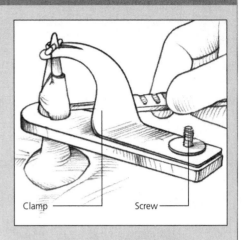

Clamp            Screw

➤ Tell the parents or caregivers that the rim of the device used for circumcision may remain in place after discharge from the hospital. Reassure them that the rim will fall off harmlessly in 3 or 4 days. However, if the rim doesn't fall off after 1 week, tell them to notify you, because a retained rim may lead to infection.

## COMPLICATIONS

➤ *Infection* and *bleeding* may occur after circumcision, and are treated locally. If they don't resolve, further evaluation and work-up is indicated.

➤ *Scarring* or *fibrous bands* may result when the skin of the penile shaft adheres to the glans. The most severe complications are urethral fistulae and edema. Incomplete amputation of the foreskin can follow application of the plastic circumcision bell. These neonates should be referred to a surgeon or pediatrician quickly to increase the likelihood of a good outcome.

## SPECIAL CONSIDERATIONS

➤ Always be sure to show parents or caregivers the circumcision before discharge so they can ask any questions and so you can teach them how to care for the area.
➤ If the neonate's mother has human immunodeficiency virus (HIV) infection, circumcision should be delayed until the neonate's HIV status is known. The neonate whose mother has HIV infection has a higher-than-normal risk of infection.

## DOCUMENTATION

➤ Note the time and date of the circumcision, procedure utilized, condition of the site, how the infant tolerated the procedure, and any parent or caregiver teaching.
➤ Document any excessive bleeding or complications along with actions taken and outcomes.
➤ Note that options along with potential adverse effects and complications were discussed in detail. State that parent(s) or guardian desired circumcision.

## USING A PLASTIC BELL

An alternative method of circumcision utilizes a plastic bell after the dorsal slit is made. Using this method, the distal prepuce will become ischemic, then atrophic, eventually dropping off in 5 to 8 days. The prepuce will drop off with the plastic bell attached, leaving a clean, well-healed excision.

First slide the plastic bell device between the foreskin and the glans penis; verify placement.

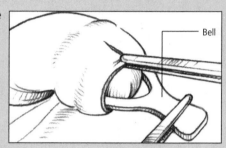

Find the bell indentation (at the coronal edge of the glans), and apply the suture lightly. After reverifying the amount of skin to be removed and that the plastic bell can move freely on the glans penis, tighten the suture for 30 seconds before tying to promote hemostasis.

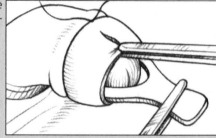

Excise the prepuce ⅛″ distal to the suture. Cut the suture to about ½″.

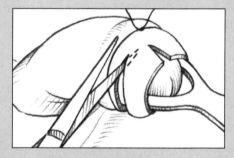

Holding the plastic bell in one hand, gently bend the stem portion with the other hand until it snaps.

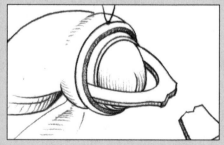

# Suprapubic bladder aspiration

CPT CODE
*51000   Aspiration of bladder by needle*

## DESCRIPTION

The objective of this procedure is to obtain a sterile urine specimen from an infant or young child (up to age 2). Until age 2 the bladder is located in the abdomen, and as the child reaches age 2, the bladder is much lower in the pelvis and thus more difficult to penetrate with this approach.

This procedure is indicated in neonates and young children who present with vague yet worrisome symptomatology where there is concern of urinary tract infection or to rule out sepsis. Infants and young children do not tend to localize infection well and their ability to verbally tell the practitioner how they feel is limited. In addition, this age group does not tend to have a well-developed immune system and thus are at increased risk for urinary tract infections and subsequent bacteremias.

## INDICATIONS

➤ To obtain urine from infants who will not void on command
➤ To collect urine from infants who are severely ill and need definitive diagnosis immediately
➤ To obtain urine from children who have had several urine specimens that equivocally show bacturia

## CONTRAINDICATIONS

### Absolute

➤ Infants with skin infections, especially located at or near the site of the needle insertion point

### Relative

➤ Infants and young children with a history of a bleeding abnormality or an abnormal coagulopathy
➤ Infants or young children with known genitourinary or abdominal tract abnormalities such as ileus, peritonitis, necrotizing enterocolitis, or obstruction

## EQUIPMENT

EMLA cream anesthetic (eutectic mixture of lidocaine 2.5% and prilocaine 2.5% in an emulsion) ◆ 4″ × 4″ transparent dressing (such as Tegaderm) ◆ povidone-iodine solution ◆ 70% rubbing alcohol ◆ four sterile 4″ × 4″ gauze pads ◆ two pairs of sterile gloves ◆ 3-ml sterile syringe ◆ 22G 1″ needle ◆ sterile urine container ◆ restraining board with arm and leg restraints ◆ radiant warmer, if the infant is very young ◆ one or two small sterile towels ◆ sharps container

## PREPARATION OF EQUIPMENT

➤ Assemble all of the equipment in the room. Have the infant under a radiant warmer to decrease loss of heat during the procedure.

## ESSENTIAL STEPS

➤ Explain to the parents or caregivers the steps in the procedure for obtaining a sterile urine specimen. Discuss the need to make a definitive diagnosis so that the child can be treated appropriately and quickly.
➤ Be sure to check the child's record for any history of allergy to iodine products prior to using these products.
➤ Obtain an informed consent explaining the risks, time it takes to do the procedure, and the benefits of doing the procedure. Answer any questions the parents or caregivers may have.

➤ If desired, apply a liberal amount of EMLA cream just above where the needle is to be inserted. Apply the sterile transparent dressing over the creamed area. Allow area to remain untouched for at least 30 minutes. Tell the parents or caregivers that you will perform the procedure when the area is numb in 30 minutes.

➤ Place infant on the restraining board, and restrain his arms and legs, making sure that the straps are secure but not overly tight. The infant should be in the supine, frog-legged position. Make sure that the board is padded to decrease the chance of burns from the heating of the restraining board.

➤ Wash and dry hands thoroughly, and put on two pairs of gloves. The first pair will be used during the percussion and prepping phase of the procedure. Inspect the skin for any irritations or sores. Place the small sterile towel across the legs and perineum of the infant or child to ensure maintenance of the sterile field during the procedure. If the umbilical cord is oozing or moist, another sterile towel should be placed over the abdomen, exposing only the lower abdomen.

➤ Determine that the child has not voided in the last hour. The typical infants' kidneys produce 1 to 2 ml/kg/hour of urine.

➤ To ensure that the infant does not void during the procedure, an assistant can gently apply pressure to the urethra (female) through the rectum or by gentle pressure directly to the male penis.

➤ Locate the symphysis pubis. Now move your gloved hand approximately 1 to 2 cm in midline. You should feel a full bladder.

➤ Moisten one 4″ × 4″ gauze pad with povidone-iodine solution and another one with the 70% alcohol solution. Using a circular motion, wipe with the povidone-iodine solution, from the most medial to approximately 2″ to 4″ on all sides from the site, cleaning the area with a gentle touch. Remember infant skin is often thin and fri-

able. Allow the area to dry for approximately 1 to 2 minutes.

➤ Next take the 4″ × 4″ gauze pad that is moistened with alcohol and repeat the procedure. Allow the skin surface to dry. Remove the first pair of gloves.

➤ Take the 1″ needle and attach it to the 3-ml syringe, and pull back slightly on the plunger. Using your sterile gloved hand, relocate the bladder. (See *Performing suprapubic bladder aspiration*.)

➤ Hold the syringe with the needle perpendicular or slightly caudally to the bladder. Penetrate the skin at the selected site of the bladder, and begin to draw back on the plunger, using gentle, slow pressure.

➤ Stop advancing the needle when the urine begins to flow. This will decrease the possibility of puncturing the posterior bladder wall. In a small infant you may only get 1 to 2 ml of urine as your sample. Insert the urine in the sterile urine container.

➤ If no urine is obtained, remove the needle and wait 30 minutes before repeating the procedure.

➤ After removing the needle, remove the transparent dressing and cover the entry site with a sterile 4″ × 4″ gauze, and apply gentle pressure for 1 to 2 minutes. Discard the syringe and needle in the sharps container.

➤ Remove gloves and wash and dry your hands. Then remove the bindings from the restraining board, diaper the infant, and gently swaddle him in a receiving-type or small blanket.

## PATIENT TEACHING

➤ Reassure the parents or caregivers that the infant should have little pain and no limitation in activity after the procedure. They may hold the infant immediately afterwards.

➤ After the procedure is completed, explain what will be done to care for the in-

## PERFORMING SUPRAPUBIC BLADDER ASPIRATION

To locate the bladder, first find the symphysis pubis. Palpate 1 to 2 cm above the symphysis pubis in midline to detect the bladder. Often there is a transverse crease at the exact location where you will be penetrating the skin. Take the 1" needle and attach it to the 3-ml syringe and pull back slightly on the plunger. Using your sterile gloved hand, relocate the bladder by palpating 1 to 2 cm above the symphysis pubis in midline.

Hold the syringe with the needle perpendicular or slightly caudally to the bladder. Penetrate the skin and begin to draw back on the plunger, using gentle, slow pressure. Stop advancing the needle when the urine begins to flow.

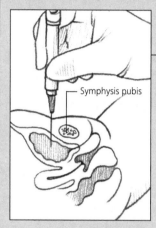

Symphysis pubis

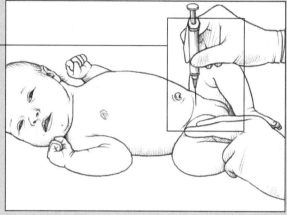

fant and treat him until the results of the culture are obtained (in 24 to 48 hours).

➤ Show the parents or caregivers how to change the diaper and check the bladder area after the procedure. Tell them that they can remove the dressing with the next diaper change.

➤ Instruct parents or caregivers to contact you for any signs of infection, such as fever greater than 100° F or low temperature less than 96° F, extreme irritability, somnolence or lethargy, lack of desire to eat as usual, or bleeding at the site of the puncture.

➤ Tell the parents or caregivers that they may see a slight darkening of the urine (microscopic hematuria), but this should clear within 12 to 24 hours after the procedure.

## COMPLICATIONS

➤ *Transient microscopic hematuria* (resolves without treatment) can develop from the procedure.

➤ *Infection* secondary to needle puncture may be caused by this procedure; this is minimized with good sterile technique.

➤ Rare *perforation of the bowel* may require antibiotics or rare *hematoma or damage to retroperitoneal structures* may develop. Both require consultation with a specialist.

## SPECIAL CONSIDERATIONS

➤ Infants and young children do experience some pain from any needle puncture. The infant may receive liquid acetaminophen or liquid ibuprofen if able to take oral medication.

➤ Developmentally, the infants and young children who would be having the procedure are in the formative stages of trust versus mistrust. Be sure to talk to them and handle them in a kind and loving manner.

## DOCUMENTATION

➤ Document the indication for the procedure as well as the date and time the procedure started.

➤ Record the vital signs of the infant; the preprocedure activities, such as placing on the restraining board under an infant warmer; and the actual draping, skin cleaning, and chemicals used to clean the area.

➤ Record the actual procedure by noting where and how deep the needle was inserted into the abdomen. Be sure to chart how deep the needle was (approximately) when urine was obtained and any signs of bleeding that occurred at the time of the procedure.

➤ Chart the appearance and quantity of urine obtained from the bladder.

➤ Document the appearance of the site and the dressing application when procedure was completed. Note in charting that the infant was covered or dressed and returned to his parents, caregivers, or the nurse (if in-patient).

➤ List any complications such as bleeding at the site or swelling over the area.

➤ Note the time the procedure was terminated.

➤ Document any patient instructions given to the parents or caregivers if child is being seen in the office and sent home afterwards.

# APPENDICES
# SELECTED REFERENCES
# INDEX

# APPENDIX A: RECOMMENDED BARRIERS TO INFECTION

The list below presents the minimum requirements for using gloves, gowns, masks, and eye protection to avoid contacting and spreading pathogens. It assumes that you wash your hands thoroughly in all cases. Refer to your facility's guidelines and use your own judgment when assessing the need for barrier protection in specific situations.

**KEY**

 Gloves

 Gown

 Mask

 Eyewear

## Bleeding or pressure application to control it

 if soiling likely

 if splattering likely

 if splattering likely

## Cardiopulmonary resuscitation

 if splattering likely

 if splattering likely

 if splattering likely

## Central venous line insertion and venisection

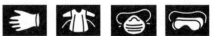

## Central venous pressure measurement

Chest drainage system change

 if splattering likely

 if splattering likely

 if splattering likely

Chest tube insertion or removal

 if soiling likely

 if splattering likely

 if splattering likely

Colonoscopy, flexible sigmoidoscope

Coughing, frequent and forceful by patient (direct contact with secretions)

Dialysis, peritoneal (skin care at catheter site)

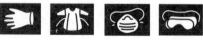

Dressing change for burns

Dressing removal or change for wounds with little or no drainage

Dressing removal or change for wounds with large amounts of drainage

 if soiling likely

Fecal impaction, removal of

Gastric lavage

 if soiling likely

 if splattering likely

Incision and drainage of abscess

 if splattering likely

 if splattering likely

Injection, joint or nerve

Intubation or extubation

if splattering likely

if splattering likely

if splattering likely

Invasive procedures (lumbar puncture, bone marrow aspiration, paracentesis, liver biopsy) outside sterile field

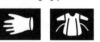

Irrigation, indwelling urinary catheter

Irrigation, vaginal

if soiling likely

Irrigation, wound

if soiling likely

if splattering likely

if splattering likely

I.V. or intra-arterial line insertion, removal, or tubing change at catheter hub

if splattering likely

if splattering likely

if splattering likely

Lesion biopsy or removal

Linen, changing visibly soiled

Nasogastric tube insertion or irrigation

  if soiling likely

  if splattering likely

  if splattering likely

Ostomy care, irrigation, and teaching

  if soiling likely

Pelvic examination and Papanicolaou test

Pressure ulcer care

  if soiling likely

Specimen collection (blood, stool, urine, sputum, wound)

Suctioning, nasotracheal or endo-tracheal

  if soiling likely

  if splattering likely

  if splattering likely

Suctioning, oral or nasal

Tracheostomy suctioning and cannula cleaning

  if soiling likely

  if splattering likely

  if splattering likely

Wound packing

  if soiling likely

# Appendix B: Resources for Professionals, Patients, and Caregivers

## General health care Web sites

➤ www.healthfinder.gov — from the U.S. government; this large searchable database has links to Web sites, support groups, government agencies, and not-for-profit organizations that provide health care information for patients.

➤ www.healthweb.org/ — from a group of librarians and information professionals at academic medical centers in the Midwest United States; offers searchable database of evaluated Web sites for patients and health care professionals.

➤ www.medmatrix.org/reg/login.asp — includes journal articles, abstracts, reviews, conference highlights, and links to other major sources for health care professionals.

➤ www.mwsearch.com — named Medical World Search, this site searches thousands of selected medical sites.

## Organizations

➤ American Academy of Family Physicians — includes "Family Medicine Online," offering handouts and other resources to patients and health care professionals, plus links to other sites: www.aafp.com

➤ Joint Commission on Accreditation of Healthcare Organizations (JCAHO): www.jcaho.org

## Government agencies

➤ Agency for Healthcare Research and Quality (AHRQ)/National Guideline Clearinghouse: www.ahcpr.gov, TDD (888) 586-6340, hearing impaired only

➤ Centers for Disease Control and Prevention — check under "Topics A to Z": www.cdc.gov

➤ Department of Health and Human Services (DHHS): www.dhhs.gov

➤ Food and Drug Administration: www.fda.gov

➤ Health Care Financing Administration (HCFA): www.hcfa.gov

➤ National Center for Complementary and Alternative Medicine: http://nccam.nih.gov/

➤ Specialized Information Services/U.S. Government Resources (online listing of government bureaus with links to their sites): http://sis.nlm.nih.gov/tehwwg.cfm

## Links to Spanish-language sites

➤ Agency for Healthcare Research and Quality (AHRQ): www.ahcpr.gov (click on Información en español)

➤ CANCERCare, Inc.: www.cancercareinc.org (click on Información en español)

➤ CancerNet: http://cancernet.nci.nih.gov/sp_menu.htm

➤ Healthfinder: www.healthfinder.com (click on español)

➤ Immunization Action Coalition, Screening Questionnaire for Adult Immunization: www.immunize.org (click on Spanish)

## Condition-specific sites

### AGING

➤ Administration on Aging: www.aoa.dhhs.gov
➤ Agency on Aging: www.aoa.dhhs.gov
➤ American Society on Aging (ASA): www.asaging.org
➤ National Institute on Aging: www.nih.gov/nia, (800) 222-2225, TTY (800) 222-4225

### AIDS/HIV/STDS

➤ CDC National Prevention Information Network: www.cdcnpin.org
➤ HIV/AIDS Treatment Information Service (ATIS): http://sis.nlm.nih.gov/aids/aidstrea.html or www.hivatis.org: (800) TRIALS-A (874-2572), (800) 448-0440 (Spanish available), TTY (888) 430-3739
➤ JAMA Women's Health Sexually Transmitted Disease Information Center: www.ama-assn.org/special/std/std.htm
➤ National AIDS Hotline (24 hours): (800) 342-AIDS, Spanish (800) 344-SIDA, TTY (800) 243-7889
➤ Office of AIDS Research (OAR): http://sis.nlm.nih.gov/aids/oar.html

### ALLERGIES AND ASTHMA

➤ Allergy and Asthma Disease Management Center: www.aaaai.org/aadmc/
➤ Allergy and Asthma Network — Mothers of Asthmatics, Inc.: www.aanma.org, (800) 878-4403
➤ Allergy, Asthma, and Immunology Online: www.allergy.mcg.edu
➤ American Academy of Allergy, Asthma, and Immunology: www.aaaai.org, (800) 822-2762
➤ Global Initiative for Asthma: www.ginasthma.com
➤ JAMA's Asthma Information Center: www.ama-assn.org/special/asthma
➤ Joint Council of Allergy, Asthma, and Immunology: www.jcaai.org

➤ National Asthma Education and Prevention Program: www.nhlbi.nih.gov/nhlbi/othcomp/opec/naepp/naeppage.htm
➤ National Institute of Allergy and Infectious Diseases: www.niaid.nih.gov

### ALZHEIMER'S DISEASE

➤ Agency for Healthcare Research and Quality (AHRQ) Early Alzheimer's Disease/Clinical Practice Guideline/Patient and Family Guide: www.ahcpr.gov/clinic/alzcons.htm
➤ AHRQ's Recognition and Assessment Guideline: www.ahcpr.gov/clinic/alzover.htm
➤ Alzheimer Europe: www.alzheimer-europe.org/
➤ Alzheimer's Association: www.alz.org, (800) 272-3900
➤ Alzheimer's Disease Education and Referral (ADEAR) Center: www.alzheimers.org, (800) 438-4380
➤ AlzWell Caregiver Page: http://www.alzwell.com/

### ARTHRITIS

➤ American Autoimmune Related Diseases Association, Inc. (AARDA): www.aarda.org/
➤ American College of Rheumatology: www.rheumatology.org
➤ Arthritis Foundation: www.arthritis.org, (800) 283-7800
➤ National Institute of Arthritis and Musculoskeletal and Skin Diseases: www.nih.gov/niams

### ATTENTION DEFICIT HYPERACTIVITY DISORDER

➤ National Attention Deficit Disorder Association (ADDA): www.add.org

### CANCER

➤ American Cancer Society (ACS): www.cancer.org, (800) ACS-2345
➤ CANCERCare, Inc.: www.cancercareinc.org, (800) 813-HOPE

➤ CANCERLit Topic Searches (National Cancer Institute): cnetdb.nci.nih.gov/cancerlit.shtml
➤ CancerNet (National Cancer Institute): http://cancernet.nci.nih.gov
➤ Cancer News on the Net: www.cancernews.com
➤ Cancer Trials — National Cancer Institute: http://cancertrials.nci.nih.gov
➤ National Breast Cancer Awareness Month: www.nbcam.org
➤ National Cancer Institute, International Cancer Information Center: (800) 4-CANCER or (800) 422-6237
➤ National Center for Chronic Disease Prevention and Health Promotion: www.cdc.gov/nccdphp/cancer.htm
➤ National Comprehensive Cancer Network: www.nccn.org
➤ Susan G. Komen Breast Cancer Foundation: (800) 462-9273
➤ Y-Me National Breast Cancer Organization: www.y-me.org, (800) 221-2141; (800) 986-9505 (Español)

### CARDIAC

➤ American Heart Association: www.americanheart.org, (800) 242-8721
➤ Mayo Health Oasis Heart Resource Center: www.mayohealth.org
➤ National Heart, Lung, and Blood Institute: www.nhlbi.nih.gov
➤ National Stroke Association; (800) STROKES

### DIABETES

➤ American Association of Diabetes Educators (AADE): www.aadenet.org, (800) 338-3633
➤ American Diabetes Association: www.diabetes.org
➤ Diabetes self-care equipment for the visually impaired: Palco Labs, Inc. (800) 346-4488, www.palcolabs.com
➤ Joslin Diabetes Center: www.joslin.harvard.edu/wlist.html

➤ National Institute of Diabetes and Digestive and Kidney Diseases: www.niddk.nih.gov

### DISABILITIES

➤ University of Virginia: General Resources About Disabilities, http://curry.edschool.virginia.edu/go/cise/ose/resources/general.html;
Assistive Technology Resources, http://curry.edschool.virginia.edu/go/cise/ose/resources/asst_tech.html

### ELDER ABUSE

➤ National Center for Crime Victims: www.nvc.org
➤ National Center on Elder Abuse (NCEA): www.gwjapan.com/NCEA (case-sensitive Web address)

### GASTROINTESTINAL

➤ American Liver Foundation: (800) GO LIVER (465-4837)
➤ National Institute of Diabetes & Digestive & Kidney Diseases: www.niddk.nih.gov, (301) 654-3810
➤ National Kidney Foundation: www.kidney.org; national office: (800) 622-9010

### MUSCULOSKELETAL

➤ American College of Foot and Ankle Surgeons: (888) 843-3338
➤ Amputee Coalition of America: (888) AMP-KNOW (267-5669)
➤ National Association of Physically Handicapped, Inc.: www.naph.net
➤ National Institutes of Health, Osteoporosis and Related Bone Diseases National Resource Center: (800) 624-BONE
➤ National Osteoporosis Foundation: www.nof.org
➤ www.amputee-support-online.com — provides information, magazines, discussion groups, addresses of support groups, and other items of interest to amputees.

NEUROLOGY

➤ ALS Association, National Office: www.alsa.org; information and referral service, (800) 782-4747; all others (818) 880-9007
➤ ALS Association of Massachusetts: (800) 258-3323
➤ American Brain Tumor Association: www.abta.org, (800) 886-2282
➤ Association of Late-Deafened Adults, Inc., 10310 Main St., #274, Fairfax, VA 22030; TTY (404) 289-1596, fax (404) 284-6862
➤ EAR Foundation/Meniere's Network, American Academy of Otolaryngology, One Prince St., Alexandria, VA 22314; (703) 836-4444
➤ National Association of the Deaf: NADinfo@nad.org
➤ National Federation of the Blind: www.nfb.org; 1800 Johnson Street, Baltimore, MD 21230; (410) 659-9314
➤ National Institute of Neurological Disorders and Stroke (NINDS): www.ninds.nih.gov
➤ National Institute on Deafness and Other Communication Disorders (NIDCD): www.nih.gov/nidcd

PEDIATRICS

➤ CFUSA-Cystic Fibrosis USA: www.cfusa.org
➤ Children with Diabetes: www.childrenwithdiabetes.com
➤ Cystic Fibrosis Foundation: www.cff.org, (800) FIGHT CF, (800) 344-4823
➤ Cystic Fibrosis Mutation Data Base: www.genet.sickkids.on.ca/cftr
➤ Down's Heart Group: www.downs-heart.downsnet.org
➤ Down Syndrome: www.healthlinkusa.com/93ent.htm
➤ Emory University Sickle Cell Information Center (24 hours): www.emory.edu (enter "sickle cell" in the search box), (404) 616-3572

➤ Families of S.M.A. (Spinal Muscular Atrophy): www.fsma.org, (800) 886-1762
➤ Growth Charts for Children with Down Syndrome Web site: www.growthcharts.com
➤ Internet Resources for Special Children (IRSC): www.irsc.org
➤ National Institute of Child Health and Human Development (NICHD): www.nichd.nih.gov
➤ NPAN, the National Pediatric AIDS Network: www.npan.org
➤ Spina Bifida Association of America: www.sbaa.org, (800) 621-3141
➤ United Cerebral Palsy UCPnet: www.ucpnatl@ucpa.org, (800) 872-5827

PSYCHIATRY

➤ American Psychological Association: www.apa.org, (800) 374-3120
➤ National Alliance for the Mentally Ill: www.nami.org, (800) 950-NAMI (6264)
➤ National Depressive and Manic-Depressive Association: www.ndmda.org, (800) 826-3632
➤ National Mental Health Association: www.nmha.org, (800) 969-6642

RESPIRATORY

➤ American Association for Respiratory Care: www.aarc.org
➤ American Heart Association: (800) 242-8721 (smoking cessation information)
➤ American Lung Association: www.lungusa.org, (800) LUNG-USA (local affiliates answer)
➤ National Emphysema Foundation: http://emphysemafoundation.org

SKIN

➤ National Pressure Ulcer Advisory Panel (NPUAP) (information on the PUSH tool and monitoring ulcers): www.npuap.org

➤ Wound Care Information Network — information for patients and professionals, including support groups: www.medicaledu.com

➤ Wound Care Institute, Inc. — newsletter, free products for financial hardships: www.woundcare.org, (305) 919-9192

➤ Wound, Ostomy, and Continence Nurses Society: www.wocn.org, (888) 224-WOCN

## SUBSTANCE ABUSE

➤ Al-Anon and Alateen: www.al-anon. alateen.org, (888) 4AL-ANON (425-2666) (Spanish and French language options)

➤ Alcoholics Anonymous: www.alcoholics-anonymous.org (Spanish and French language options)

➤ Narcotics Anonymous World Services: www.wsoinc.com

➤ National Council on Alcoholism and Drug Dependence: (800) NCA-CALL (622-2255)

➤ National Institute on Alcohol Abuse and Alcoholism: www.niaaa.nih.gov, (301) 443-3860

➤ Office on Smoking and Health Centers for Disease Control and Prevention: www.cdc.gov/tobacco

➤ Substance Abuse and Mental Health Services Administration: www.samhsa.gov

## WOMEN'S HEALTH

➤ American College of Cardiology: www.acc.org

➤ American Heart Association: http://women.americanheart.org

➤ American Medical Women's Association: www.amwa-doc.org

➤ JAMA's Women's Health Information Center: www.ama-assn.org/womh

➤ Johns Hopkins Intelihealth: www. intelihealth.com/specials/htMain.htm (search for "women and heart disease")

➤ Office on Women's Health/U.S. Public Health Service: www.4women.gov/owh

➤ Womens' Heart Initiative (WHI): www.nhlbi.nih.gov/whi

# Appendix C: MEDICAL ENGLISH-SPANISH TRANSLATIONS

## Positioning and preparation

| | |
|---|---|
| Bend over backward. | Dóblese Ud. hacia atrás. |
| Bend over forward. | Dóblese Ud. hacia adelante. |
| Lean backward. | Recuéstese Ud. |
| Lean forward. | Inclínese Ud. hacia adelante. |
| Lie down. | Acuéstese Ud. |
| Lie on your back. | Acuéstese Ud. boca arriba. |
| Lie on your: | Acuéstese Ud.: |
| –side | –de lado. |
| –left side | –del lado izquierdo |
| –right side. | –del lado derecho. |
| Lie on your stomach. | Acuéstese boca abajo. |
| Roll over. | Dé Ud. una vuelta. |
| Sit down. | Siéntese Ud. |
| Sit up. | Enderécese Ud. |
| Stand up. | Párese Ud. |
| Turn to the side. | Voltéese Ud. hacia un lado. |
| Keep your feet together. | Mantenga Ud. los pies juntos. |
| Tighten your muscle. | Tense Ud. el músculo. |
| Turn to the right. | Voltéese Ud. hacia la derecha. |
| Turn to the left. | Voltéese Ud. hacia la izquierda. |
| Lift up your arms. | Levante Ud. los brazos. |
| Make a fist. | Cierre Ud. el puño. |
| Don't move. | No se mueva. |
| When I tell you, hold your breath. | Cuando le diga, contenga Ud. el aliento. |
| Don't breathe (hold your breath). | No respire (contenga el aliento). |
| Breathe. | Respire Ud. |

| | |
|---|---|
| Once more. | Una vez más. |
| Are you pregnant? | ¿Está Ud. embarazada? |
| Don't talk. | No hable Ud. |
| Say "AAHH." | Diga Ud. "AAAA." |
| Whisper. | Murmure Ud. |
| I need to put a tourniquet on your arm. | Tengo que ponerle un torniquete en el brazo. |
| You'll feel pain like a pinprick. | Ud. sentirá un dolor como un alfilerazo. |
| You must drink this liquid before the test. | Ud. tiene que tomarse este líquido antes de la prueba. |
| You must drink this liquid during the test. | Ud. tiene que tomarse este líquido durante la prueba. |
| We must give you an enema before the test. | Tenemos que ponerle una enema (lavativa) antes de la prueba. |
| You must hold the enema in until we're finished with the test. | Ud. tiene que retener la enema (la lavativa) hasta que terminemos con la prueba. |
| You may go to the bathroom when we tell you. | Ud. puede ir al baño cuando le digamos. |
| Is your bladder very full? | ¿Tiene Ud. la vejiga muy llena? |
| You can't empty your bladder until the test is finished. | Ud. no puede vaciar la vejiga hasta que la prueba se termine. |

## Physical examination

| | |
|---|---|
| I'm going to examine your: | Le voy a reconocer: |
| – skin. | – la piel. |
| – hair. | – el cabello. |
| – nails. | – las uñas. |
| – head and neck. | – la cabeza y el cuello. |
| head. | la cabeza. |
| nose. | la nariz. |
| mouth. | la boca. |
| throat. | la garganta. |
| neck. | el cuello. |
| – eyes. | – los ojos. |
| – ears. | – los oídos. |
| – respiratory system. | – el sistema respiratorio. |
| chest. | el pecho. |
| lungs. | los pulmones. |
| – cardiovascular system. | – el sistema cardiovascular. |
| heart. | el corazón. |

| | |
|---|---|
| pulse. | el pulso. |
| –gastrointestinal system. | –el sistema gastrointestinal. |
| abdomen. | el abdomen. |
| rectum. | el recto. |
| –urinary system. | –el sistema urinario. |
| bladder. | la vejiga. |
| kidneys. | los riñones. |
| –reproductive system. | –el sistema reproductivo. |
| breasts. | las mamas or los senos. |
| pelvis. | la pelvis. |
| penis. | el pene. |
| testicles. | los testículos. |
| –nervous system. | –el sistema nervioso. |
| reflexes. | los reflejos. |
| –musculoskeletal system. | –el sistema musculoesquelético. |
| arms. | los brazos. |
| legs. | las piernas. |
| –immune system. | –el sistema inmunológico. |
| –endocrine system. | –el sistema endocrino. |
| I'm going to take your: | Voy a medirle: |
| –vital signs. | –los signos vitales. |
| –blood pressure. | –la presión sanguínea. |
| –pulse. | –el pulso. |
| –temperature. | –la temperatura. |
| I'm going to take a blood sample. | Voy a tomarle a Ud. una muestra de sangre. |
| You need to provide a urine specimen. | Tiene Ud. que darnos un espécimen de orina. |
| I'm going to inspect your _____. | Le voy a examinar _____. |
| I'm going to auscultate (listen to) your _____. | Le voy a auscultar _____. |
| I'm going to palpate your _____. | Le voy a palpar _____. |
| I'm going to percuss your _____. | Le voy a percutir _____. |
| Are you comfortable? | ¿Está Ud. confortable? |
| Does this hurt? | ¿Le duele a Ud. esto? |
| –Where does it hurt? | –¿Dónde le duele a Ud.? |

## Examination with instruments

| | |
|---|---|
| I'm going to use: | Voy a usar: |
| –a measuring tape to measure your: | –una cinta métrica para medirle: |

| | |
|---|---|
| arm. | el brazo. |
| leg. | la pierna. |
| belly. | el vientre. |
| hand. | la mano. |
| head. | la cabeza. |
| chest. | el pecho. |
| – an ophthalmoscope to examine your eyes. | – un oftalmoscopio para examinarle los ojos. |
| – an otoscope to examine your ears. | – un otoscopio para examinarle losoídos. |
| – a penlight to look in your eyes. | – una linterna de bolsillo para examinarle los ojos. |
| – a scale to weigh you. | – una báscula (balanza) para medir su peso. |
| – a sphygmomanometer to take your blood pressure. | – un esfigmomanómetro para medirle la tensión sanguínea arterial. |
| – a stethoscope to listen to your: | – un estetoscopio para escuchar: |
| lungs and breathing. | sus pulmones y su respiración. |
| heart. | su corazón. |
| – a syringe to take a blood sample. | – una jeringa para obtener una muestra de sangre. |
| – a thermometer to take your temperature. | – un termómetro para tomarle la temperatura. |
| – a tongue blade to examine your mouth and throat. | – un depresor de lengua para examinarle la boca y la garganta. |
| – a tuning fork to test your hearing. | – un diapasón para examinarle el oído. |
| – a vaginal speculum to perform a pelvic examination and examine your vagina. | – un espéculo vaginal para hacerle un examen de la pelvis y de la vagina. |
| – a visual acuity chart to test your sight. | – gráfica simplificada para medir su agudeza visual. |

## Testing

### GENERAL TESTS

| | |
|---|---|
| I have ordered: | Yo he pedido que se le haga: |
| – a biopsy. | – una biopsia. |
| – a blood test. | – un análisis de la sangre. |
| – a blood culture. | – un cultivo de la sangre. |
| – a computed tomography scan. | – una tomografía computerizada. |
| – an endoscopy. | – una endoscopia. |
| – a magnetic resonance imaging scan. | – una resonancia magnética. |
| – an ultrasound. | – un ultrasonido. |
| – a urinalysis. | – un urinálisis (or un análisis de orina). |
| – an X-ray. | – una radiografía. |

–allergy tests.     –pruebas de alergia.
–a neck X-ray.     –una radiografía del cuello.
–a nose culture.     –un cultivo de la nariz.
–a skull X-ray.     –una radiografía del cráneo.
–a throat culture.     –un cultivo de la garganta.
–a glaucoma test.     –un examen de glaucoma.
–a vision test.     –un examen de la vista.
–a hearing test.     –un examen de la audición.

### RESPIRATORY TESTS

I have ordered:     Yo he pedido que se le haga:
–an arterial blood gases test.     –gases de la sangre arterial.
–a bronchoscopy.     –una broncoscopia.
–a chest X-ray.     –una radiografía del tórax.
–a lung scan.     –un ultrasonido pulmonar.
–pulmonary function tests.     –una prueba de la función pulmonar.
–a pulse oximetry.     –una oximetría del pulso.

### CARDIOVASCULAR TESTS

I have ordered:     Yo he pedido que se le haga:
–an arteriogram.     –un arteriograma.
–a blood test for:     –un análisis de la sangre para:
    cardiac enzymes.         enzimas cardiacas.
    cholesterol.         colesterol.
    partial thromboplastin time.         tiempo de tromboplastina parcial.
    prothrombin time.         tiempo de protrombina.
    triglycerides.         triglicéridos.
–a cardiac catheterization.     –un cateterismo cardiaco.
–an electrocardiogram.     –un electrocardiograma.
–a Holter monitor.     –monitoreo Holter.
–a stress test.     –un examen de estrés.
–a venogram.     –un venograma.

### GASTROINTESTINAL TESTS

I have ordered:     Yo he pedido que se le haga:
–an abdominal ultrasound.     –un ultrasonido abdominal.
–a barium enema.     –una enema de bario.
–a barium swallow.     –tragar bario.
–a blood test for:     –un análisis de la sangre para:
    amylase.         amilasa.
    liver enzymes.         enzimas del hígado.
–a cholangiogram.     –un colangiograma.

| | |
|---|---|
| – a cholecystogram. | – un colecistograma. |
| – a colonoscopy. | – una colonoscopia. |
| – a gastric analysis. | – un análisis gástrico. |
| – a gastroscopy. | – una gastroscopia. |
| – a liver biopsy. | – una biopsia del hígado. |
| – a sigmoidoscopy. | – una sigmoidoscopia. |
| – a spleen scan. | – una visualización del bazo por ecos de ultrasonidos. |
| – a stool culture. | – un cultivo de la defecación. |
| – an upper GI series. | – una serie gastrointestinal superior. |

RENAL AND UROLOGIC TESTS

I have ordered:
– a blood test for:
   blood urea nitrogen.
   creatinine.
   electrolytes.
– a cystoscopy.
– an excretory urography.
– a renal biopsy.
– a retrograde pyelogram.
– a urine culture.

Yo he pedido que se le haga:
– un análisis de la sangre para:
   nitrógeno y urea sanguínea.
   creatinina.
   electrolitos.
– una cistoscopia.
– una urografía excretora.
– un cultivo renal.
– un pielograma retrógrado.
– un cultivo de la orina.

GENITOURINARY TESTS

I have ordered a:
– breast biopsy.
– breast examination.
– cervical biopsy.
– mammogram.
– Papanicolaou test.
– pelvic examination.
– pregnancy test.
– prostate examination.
– prostatic biopsy.
– rectal examination.
– semen analysis.
– vaginal culture.

Yo he pedido que se le haga:
– una biopsia de la mama.
– un reconocimiento de los senos.
– una biopsia cervical.
– un mamograma.
– una prueba Papanicolaou.
– un reconocimiento pélvico.
– un análisis de embarazo.
– un reconocimiento de la próstata.
– una biopsia de la próstata.
– un reconocimiento del recto.
– un análisis del semen.
– un cultivo vaginal.

NEUROLOGIC TESTS

I have ordered:
– a brain scan.
– a cerebral arteriogram.

Yo he pedido que se le haga:
– un ultrasonido cerebral.
– un arteriograma cerebral.

– a computed tomography scan of the brain.
– an electroencephalogram.
– a lumbar puncture.
– a myelogram.

– una tomografía computerizada del cerebro.
– un electroencefalograma.
– una punción lumbar.
– un mielograma.

MUSKULOSKELETAL TESTS

I have ordered:
– an arthroscopy.
– a bone biopsy.
– an electromyogram.
– a muscle biopsy.
– an X-ray of the:
    ankle.
    arm.
    back.
    elbow.
    foot.
    hand.
    hip.
    knee.
    leg.
    shoulder.
    wrist.

Yo he pedido que se le haga:
– una artroscopia.
– una biopsia del hueso.
– un electromiograma.
– una biopsia del músculo.
– una radiografía de:
    el tobillo.
    el brazo.
    la espalda.
    el codo.
    el pie.
    la mano.
    la cadera.
    la rodilla.
    la pierna.
    el hombro.
    la muñeca.

HEMATOLOGIC BLOOD TESTS

I have ordered a:
– blood test for:
    blood cell count.
    differential blood cell count.
    red blood cell count.
    white blood cell count.
    clotting times.
    hematocrit.
    hemoglobin level.
    hepatitis B.
    human immunodeficiency virus (HIV).
    platelet count.
– bone marrow biopsy.

Yo he pedido que se le haga:
– un análisis de la sangre para:
    recuento sanguíneo.
    recuento diferencial de las células de sangre.
    recuento de los glóbulos rojos de la sangre.
    recuento de los glóbulos blancos de la sangre.
    el tiempo de coagulación.
    hematócrito.
    el nivel de hemoglobina.
    hepatitis tipo B.
    virus de inmunodeficiencia humana (VIH).
    recuento de plaquetas.
– una biopsia de la médula ósea del hueso.

## ENDOCRINE TESTS

| | |
|---|---|
| I have ordered: | Yo he pedido que se le haga: |
| – an analysis of: | – un análisis de: |
|    adrenal function. |    la función adrenal. |
|    ovarian function. |    la función ovárica. |
|    parathyroid function. |    la función paratiroidea. |
|    pancreatic function. |    la función pancreática. |
|    pituitary function |    la función de la pituitaria. |
|    testicular function. |    la función testicular. |
|    thyroid function. |    la función de la tiroides. |
| – a blood test for: | – un análisis de sangre para revisar: |
|    serum calcium level. |    el nivel de calcio. |
|    serum glucose level. |    el nivel de glucosa. |
|    fasting glucose level. |    el nivel de glucosa en abstención. |
|    glucose tolerance. |    la tolerancia a la glucosa. |
|    glycosylated hemoglobin level. |    el nivel de hemoglobina glucosilatada. |
|    2-hour postprandial glucose level. |    el nivel de glucosa dos-horas posprandial. |
|    serum hormone levels. |    niveles hormonales. |
|    serum phosphorus concentration. |    niveles de fósforo. |

## MEDICATION INSTRUCTIONS

| | |
|---|---|
| Don't eat or drink anything after midnight before the test. | No coma ni beba nada después de medianoche antes de la prueba (del examen). |
| Don't eat or drink anything after _____ a.m. | No coma ni beba nada después de las _____ de la mañana. |
| Don't eat or drink anything after _____ p.m. | No coma ni beba nada después de las _____ de la tarde (or la noche). |
| You may take your usual medicine in the morning with a small amount of water. | Ud. puede tomarse todas sus medicinas habituales en la mañana con una cantidad pequeña de agua. |
| You may take all of your usual medicine in the morning with a small amount of water except _____. | Ud. puede tomarse todas sus medicinas habituales en la mañana con una cantidad pequeña de agua con la excepción de ____. |

# SELECTED REFERENCES

## GENERAL

Actis Dato, G.M., et al. "Surgical Management of Flail Chest," *Annals of Thoracic Surgery* 67(6):1826-27, June 1999.

Barker, L.R., et al. *Principles of Ambulatory Medicine*, 5th ed. Baltimore: Lippincott Williams & Wilkins, 1999.

Baum, G.L., et al. *Textbook of Pulmonary Diseases*, 6th ed. Philadelphia: Lippincott Williams & Wilkins, 1998.

Chapeski, A. "Simple Cure for the Ingrown Toenail," *Australian Family Physician* 27(4):299, April 1998.

Cole, C.R., et al. "Heart-rate Recovery Immediately After Exercise as a Predictor of Mortality," *New England Journal of Medicine* 341(18):1351-57, October 1999.

Colyar, M.R., and Ehrhardt, C.R. *Ambulatory Care Procedures for the Nurse Practitioner*. Philadelphia: F.A. Davis Co., 1999.

Ferri, F.F. *Practical Guide to the Care of the Medical Patient*, 4th ed. St. Louis: Mosby–Year Book, Inc., 1998.

Fletcher, G.F., et al. "Current Status of ECG Stress Testing," *Current Problems in Cardiology* 23(7):353-423, July 1998.

Galvin, I. *The Diagnosis of Diffuse Lung Disease*. New York: McGraw-Hill Book Co., 1999.

Greenberg, M.D., and Rosen, C.L. "Evaluation of the Patient with Blunt Chest Trauma: An Evidence Based Approach," *Emergency Medicine Clinics of North America* 17(1):41-62, February 1999.

Heppenstall, B., and Tan, V. "Well-leg Compartment Syndrome," *Lancet* 354(9183):970, September 1999.

Herf, C., et al. "Meningococcal Disease: Recognition, Treatment and Prevention," *Nurse Practitioner* 23(8):30, 33-36, 39-40, August 1998.

Ikard, R.W. "Onychocryptosis,"*Journal of the American College of Surgeons* 187(1): 96-102, July 1998.

Jarvis, C. *Physical Examination and Health Assessment*, 3rd ed. Philadelphia: W.B. Saunders Co., 2000.

Kee, W.D. "Postdural-puncture Headache," *Lancet* 354(9179):680, August 1999.

Larsen, L.C., and Cummings, D.M. "Oral Poisonings: Guidelines for Initial Evaluation and Treatment," *American Family Physician* 57(1):85-92, January 1998.

Lewis, A.M. "Orthopedic and Vascular Emergencies," *Nursing99* 29(12):54-57, December 1999.

Marino, P.L. *The ICU Book*, 2nd ed. Baltimore: Lippincott Williams & Wilkins, 1998.

Mattox, K.L., et al., eds. *Trauma*, 4th ed. New York: McGraw-Hill Book Co., 1999.

Mayberry, J.C., et al. "Surveyed Opinion of American Trauma Surgeons on the Prevention of the Abdominal Compartment Syndrome," *Journal of Trauma* 47(3):509-14, September 1999.

Meek, S., and White, M. "Subungual Haematomas: Is Simple Trephining Enough?" *Journal of Accident and Emergency Medicine* 15(4):269-71, July 1998.

Meyer, N. "Using Physiologic and Pharmacologic Stress Testing in Evaluation of Coronary Artery Disease," *Nurse Practitioner* 24(4):70-72, 75-76, 78, April 1999.

Mollica, M.B. "Chronic Exertional Compartment Syndrome of the Foot: A Case Report," *Journal of the American*

*Podiatric Medical Association* 88(1):21-24, January 1998.

*Mosby's Medical, Nursing, & Allied Health Dictionary,* 5th ed. St. Louis: Mosby–Year Book, Inc., 1998.

Nebelkopf, H. "Abdominal Compartment Syndrome," *AJN* 99(11):53-56, 58, 60, November 1999.

*Nursing Procedures,* 3rd ed. Springhouse, Pa.: Springhouse Corp., 2000.

Pearl, L.B., and Trunkey, D.D. "Compartment Syndrome of the Liver," *Journal of Trauma* 47(4):796-98, October 1999.

Pettersson, E., et al. "Evaluation of a Nurse-Run Asthma School," *International Journal of Nursing Studies* 36(2):145-51, April 1999.

Proehl, J.A. *Emergency Nursing Procedures,* 2nd ed. Philadelphia: W.B. Saunders Co., 1999.

Robinson, D.L., and McKenzie, C.L. *Procedures for Primary Care Providers.* Philadelphia: Lippincott Williams & Wilkins, 1999.

Rosen, P., ed. *Emergency Medicine: Concepts and Clinical Practice,* 4th ed. St. Louis: Mosby–Year Book, Inc., 1998.

Simon, A., et al. "Manual Versus Mechanical Compression for Femoral Artery Hemostasis after Cardiac Catheterization," *American Journal of Critical Care* 7(4):308-13, July 1998.

Swain, R., and Ross, D. "Lower Extremity Compartment Syndrome: When to Suspect Acute or Chronic Pressure Buildup," *Postgraduate Medicine* 105(3):159-62, 165, 168, March 1999.

Tintinalli, J.E., et al., eds. *Emergency Medicine: A Comprehensive Study Guide,* 5th ed. New York: McGraw-Hill Book Co., 2000.

Uphold, C.R., and Graham, M.V. *Clinical Guidelines in Family Practice,* 3rd ed. Gainesville, Fla.: Barmarrae Books, 1998.

Wong, D.L., et al. *Whaley & Wong's Nursing Care of Infants and Children,* 6th ed. St. Louis: Mosby–Year Book, Inc., 1999.

Yamada, T., et al., eds. *Textbook of Gastroenterology,* vol. 1 & 2, 3rd ed. Philadelphia: Lippincott Williams & Wilkins, 1999.

## PEDIATRICS

Melson, K.A., et al. *Maternal-Infant Care Planning,* 3rd ed. Springhouse, Pa.: Springhouse Corp., 1999.

Merenstein, G.B., and Gardner, S.L. *Handbook of Neonatal Intensive Care,* 4th ed. St. Louis: Mosby–Year Book, Inc., 1998.

Pillitteri, A. *Maternal & Child Health Nursing: Care of the Childbearing & Childrearing Family,* 3rd ed. Philadelphia: Lippincott Williams & Wilkins, 1999.

## OBSTETRICS AND GYNECOLOGY

Barker, L.R., et al. *Principles of Ambulatory Medicine,* 5th ed. Philadelphia: Lippincott Williams & Wilkins, 1999.

Harman, J.H. Jr., and Kim, A. "Current Trends in Cervical Ripening and Labor Induction," *American Family Physician* 60(2):477-84, August 1999.

Toubia, N. *Caring for Women with Circumcision: A Technical Manual for Health Care Providers.* New York: Research Action and Information Network for the Bodily Integrity of Women (RAINBO), 1999.

Wald, N.J., et al. "Integrated Screening for Down's Syndrome Based on Tests Performed During the First and Second Trimester," *New England Journal of Medicine* 341:461-67, August 1999.

Wing, D.A., et al. "A Comparison of Orally Administered Misoprostol with Vaginally Administered Misoprostol for Cervical Ripening and Labor Induction," *American Journal of Obstetrics and Gynecology* 180(5):1155-60, May 1999.

Youngkin, E.Q., and Davis, M.S., eds. *Women's Health: A Primary Care Clinical Guide,* 2nd ed. Stamford, Conn.: Appleton & Lange, 1998.

# INDEX

i refers to an illustration; t refers to a table.

i refers to an illustration; t refers to a table.

i refers to an illustration; t refers to a table.

i refers to an illustration; t refers to a table.

i refers to an illustration; t refers to a table.

i refers to an illustration; t refers to a table.

i refers to an illustration; t refers to a table.

i refers to an illustration; t refers to a table.

i refers to an illustration; t refers to a table.

i refers to an illustration; t refers to a table.

i refers to an illustration; t refers to a table.

i refers to an illustration; t refers to a table.

i refers to an illustration; t refers to a table.

i refers to an illustration; t refers to a table.

i refers to an illustration; t refers to a table.

i refers to an illustration; t refers to a table.

i refers to an illustration; t refers to a table.